BSAVA Manual of
Feline Practice
A Foundation Manual

Editors:

Andrea Harvey
BVSc DSAM(Feline) DipECVIM-CA MRCVS

Small Animal Specialist Hospital, 1 Richardson Place,
North Ryde, Sydney, NSW 2113, Australia
and International Society of Feline Medicine
(Australasian Representative)

Séverine Tasker
BSc BVSc(Hons) PhD DSAM DipECVIM-CA
PGCertHE MRCVS

Senior Lecturer in Small Animal Medicine,
School of Veterinary Sciences and The Feline Centre,
Langford Veterinary Services, University of Bristol,
Langford, Bristol BS40 5DU

Published by:

British Small Animal Veterinary Association
Woodrow House, 1 Telford Way,
Waterwells Business Park, Quedgeley,
Gloucester GL2 2AB

A Company Limited by Guarantee in England
Registered Company No. 2837793
Registered as a Charity

Published 2013
Reprinted 2014, 2015, 2017, 2018, 2020, 2022
Copyright © 2022 BSAVA

Illustrations on pages 150, 156, 160, 228, 376 and 473 were drawn by S.J. Elmhurst BA Hons
(www.livingart.org.uk) and are printed with her permission.

A catalogue record for this book is available from the British Library.

ISBN 978-1-905319-39-8

The publishers, editors and contributors cannot take responsibility for information provided on dosages and
methods of application of drugs mentioned or referred to in this publication. Details of this kind must be verified in
each case by individual users from up to date literature published by the manufacturers or suppliers of those
drugs. Veterinary surgeons are reminded that in each case they must follow all appropriate national legislation
and regulations (for example, in the United Kingdom, the prescribing cascade) from time to time in force.

Printed in the UK by Cambrian Printers Ltd, Pontllanfraith NP12 2YA
Printed on ECF paper made from sustainable forests

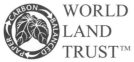

WORLD LAND TRUST™

www.carbonbalancedpaper.com
CBP006075

Carbon Balancing is delivered by World Land Trust, an international conservation
charity, who protects the world's most biologically important and threatened
habitats acre by acre. Their Carbon Balanced Programme offsets emissions
through the purchase and preservation of high conservation value forests.

17395PUBS22

Other titles in the BSAVA Manuals series

For further information on these and all BSAVA publications, please visit our website:
www.bsava.com

Contents

SECTION 3: Management of common disorders

Quick reference guides

Contributors

Natalie Barnard BVetMed CertVD DipECVD MRCVS
Langford Veterinary Services, University of Bristol, Langford, Bristol BS40 5DU

Esther Barrett MA VetMB DVDI DipECVDI MRCVS
Wales and West Imaging, Jubilee Villas, Tutshill, Chepstow, Gwent NP16 7DE

Vanessa Barrs BVSc(Hons) MVetClinStud MACVSc(Small Animal) FANZCVSc(Feline) GradCertEd(Higher Ed)
Valentine Charlton Cat Centre (B10), Faculty of Veterinary Science, The University of Sydney, NSW 2006, Australia

Julia A. Beatty BSc(Hons) BVetMed PhD FANZCVSc(Feline) GradCertEd(Higher Ed) MRCVS
Valentine Charlton Cat Centre (B10), Faculty of Veterinary Science, The University of Sydney, NSW 2006, Australia

Sarah M.A. Caney BVSc PhD DSAM(Feline) MRCVS
Vet Professionals Limited, Midlothian Innovation Centre, Roslin, Midlothian EH25 9RE

Martha Cannon BA VetMB DSAM(Feline) MRCVS
The Oxford Cat Clinic, 78A Westway, Botley, Oxford OX2 9JU

Marge Chandler DVM MS MANZCVSc DipACVN DipACVIM DipECVIM-CA MRCVS
University of Edinburgh, Hospital for Small Animals, Easter Bush Veterinary Centre, Roslin, Midlothian EH25 9RG

Luca Ferasin DVM PhD CertVC PGCert(HE) DipECVIM-CA (Cardiology) GPCert(B&PS) MRCVS
Specialist Veterinary Cardiology Consultancy, 148 Swievelands Road, Biggin Hill, Westerham, Kent TN16 3QX

Myra Forster-van Hijfte DVM CertSAM CertVR DipECVIM-CA MRCVS
North Downs Specialist Referrals, The Friesian Buildings 3 & 4, The Brewerstreet Dairy Business Park, Brewer Street, Bletchingley, Surrey RH1 4QP

Darren Foster BSc BVMS PhD FACVSc
Small Animal Specialist Hospital, 1 Richardson Place, North Ryde, Sydney, NSW 2113, Australia

Laurent S. Garosi DVM DipECVN MRCVS
Davies Veterinary Specialists, Manor Farm Business Park, Higham Gobion, Hertfordshire SG5 3HR

Mark Goodfellow MA VetMB CertVR DSAM DipECVIM-CA MRCVS
Davies Veterinary Specialists, Manor Farm Business Park, Higham Gobion, Hertfordshire SG5 3HR

Danièlle A. Gunn-Moore BSc BVM&S PhD FHEA MACVSc MRCVS
University of Edinburgh, Hospital for Small Animals, Easter Bush Veterinary Centre, Roslin, Midlothian EH25 9RG

Vicky Halls RVN DipCouns MBACP Member of the Association of Pet Behaviour Counsellors
PO Box 269, Faversham ME13 3AZ

Andrea Harvey BVSc DSAM(Feline) DipECVIM-CA MRCVS
Small Animal Specialist Hospital, 1 Richardson Place, North Ryde, Sydney, NSW 2113, Australia
and International Society of Feline Medicine (Australasian Representative)

Angie Hibbert BVSc CertSAM DipECVIM-CA MRCVS
The Feline Centre, Langford Veterinary Services, University of Bristol, Langford, Bristol BS40 5DU

Geraldine B. Hunt BVSc MVetClinStud PhD FACVSc
Department of Veterinary Surgical and Radiological Sciences, University of California, Davis, CA 95616-8745, USA

Albert E. Jergens DVM PhD DipACVIM
Department of Veterinary Clinical Sciences, College of Veterinary Medicine, Iowa State University, Ames, IA 50010, USA

Rachel M. Korman BVSc GPCertFelP MANZCVSc
Veterinary Specialist Services, Underwood, Queensland 4119, Australia

Sorrel J. Langley-Hobbs MA BVetMed DSAS(O) DipECVS MRCVS
Department of Veterinary Medicine, University of Cambridge, Madingley Road, Cambridge CB3 0ES

Michael R. Lappin DVM PhD DipACVIM
Department of Clinical Sciences, Colorado State University, 300 West Drake Road, Fort Collins, CO 80523, USA

Dan Lewis MA VetMB CertVA DipACVECC MRCVS
Petmedics, Priestley Road, Worsley, Manchester M28 2LY

Susan Little DVM DipABVP(Feline)
Bytown Cat Hospital, Ottawa, Ontario, Canada

Jill E. Maddison BVSc DipVetClinStud PhD FACVSc MRCVS
The Royal Veterinary College, Hawkshead Lane, North Mymms, Hertfordshire AL9 7TA

Richard Malik DVSc DipVetAn MVetClinStud PhD FACVSc FASM
Centre for Veterinary Education, The University of Sydney, Level 2, Veterinary Science Conference Centre B22,
The University of Sydney, NSW 2006, Australia
and Double Bay Veterinary Clinic, 125 Manning Road Woollahra, Sydney, NSW 2025, Australia

Lisa Milella BVSc DipEVDC MRCVS
The Veterinary Dental Surgery, 53 Parvis Rd, Byfleet, Surrey KT14 7AA

Natasha Mitchell MVB DVOphthal MRCVS
Eye Vet, Crescent Veterinary Clinic, Dooradoyle Road, Limerick, Ireland

Jo Murrell BVSc(Hons) PhD DipECVAA MRCVS
School of Veterinary Sciences and Langford Veterinary Services, University of Bristol, Langford, Bristol BS40 5DU

Nicki Reed BVM&S Cert VR DSAM(Feline) DipECVIM-CA MRCVS
University of Edinburgh, Hospital for Small Animals, Easter Bush Veterinary Centre, Roslin, Midlothian EH25 9RG

Suzanne Rudd DipAVN Med RVN
The Feline Centre, Langford Veterinary Services, University of Bristol, Langford, Bristol BS40 5DU

Margie Scherk DVM DipABVP(Feline)
catsINK, Vancouver, BC, Canada

Kerry E. Simpson BVM&S Cert VC FACVSc PhD MRCVS
The Feline Expert, London

Séverine Tasker BSc BVSc(Hons) PhD DSAM DipECVIM-CA PGCertHE MRCVS
School of Veterinary Sciences and The Feline Centre, Langford Veterinary Services, University of Bristol,
Langford, Bristol BS40 5DU

Samantha Taylor BVetMed(Hons) CertSAM DipECVIM-CA MRCVS
International Cat Care, Taeselbury, High Street, Tisbury, Wiltshire SP3 6LD

Kathleen Tennant BVetMed CertSAM CertVC FRCPath MRCVS
Langford Veterinary Services, University of Bristol, Langford, Bristol BS40 5DU

David Yates BVSc MRCVS
Hospital Director, RSPCA Greater Manchester Animal Hospital, 411 Eccles New Road, Salford M5 5NN

Foreword

It is a great privilege to be able to introduce this first *BSAVA Manual of Feline Practice*. The need for such a manual is self-evident – cats replaced dogs as the most commonly kept companion animal many years ago, and their popularity continues to expand. In the face of this there has never been a more important time for clinicians to understand cats, their diseases and their management.

In developing this Manual, the authors and editors have done a truly wonderful job. It is often said that if you need a job doing, you should ask a busy person. Well that is very applicable here – Séverine Tasker and Andrea Harvey are two of the leading international feline clinicians and clinical researchers, yet despite their already heavy workload they have found the time to assemble a team of excellent authors from around the world, and have produced a truly outstanding volume. Those who have written or edited books, or have contributed as authors, know only too well that this sort of thing is a labour of love, and I cannot begin to imagine the number of hours of work that have gone into producing this Manual. However, because the editors and assembled panel of authors are grounded in clinical work, this is an immensely useful and practical book. Beautifully illustrated, and full of quick reference tips and guides, this Manual is set to become one of the most well used books in any clinical library.

I am delighted and honoured to commend this book to you – I have the utmost personal and professional respect for the editors and they, together with the other authors, have assembled a Manual that will prove to be an invaluable clinical aid for all who are fortunate enough to own a copy. By keeping this book close by, and using it on a regular basis, I have no doubt that any practitioner will benefit enormously from the information and practical advice it contains and, perhaps even more importantly, the health and wellbeing of many cats with whom we share our lives will be improved.

Andrew Sparkes BVetMed PhD DipECVIM MRCVS
Veterinary Director, International Cat Care and
International Society of Feline Medicine

Preface

A good feline practitioner is not just someone who has good knowledge of feline medicine and surgery, but is someone who takes a holistic and empathetic approach to the care of cats, considering their unique needs at every step of their management.

The aim of this new foundation level *BSAVA Manual of Feline Practice* is to provide an easily accessible source of practical and clear advice regarding the approach and management of a wide variety of common feline problems encountered in first opinion practice. Our aim is for the Manual to be used within the consulting room/ward/theatre as a step-by-step guide, rather than being an exhaustive reference text. It is designed to be an essential tool for any veterinary surgeon that sees feline cases, whether they are a new graduate, a practitioner with a special interest in cats, or a mixed practice vet just seeing the occasional cat, and also for veterinary students undertaking clinical training. The Manual gives enough information to allow any vet to deal very competently with common feline problems, giving guidance on where to go for further information if required. Where appropriate, guidelines are also given as to the best steps when financial limitations exist, and when referral should be considered. In veterinary practice there is never just one way to perform a technique or manage a condition, but giving too many different options can be confusing to the busy practitioner with a case in front of them. In this Manual we have striven to produce one clear set of instructions for different techniques or treatments, according to author preferences, in order to make the Manual straightforward to use.

The Manual starts with a section on effective feline practice, which provides an overview of issues that enable every feline case to be dealt with in an optimal and minimally stressful manner for both the cat and the client. Gold-standard preventive healthcare guidelines focusing on a life-stage approach are included, together with a practical user-friendly discussion of therapeutics including antibiotic use, analgesia and anaesthesia. A problem-oriented section then follows, in which easy-to-follow step-by-step guides to investigating and/or managing common problems are presented; emergency problems are described separately to provide quick and easy access. The final section of the book is systems-based, containing more detailed information on the management of common disorders encountered in feline practice.

A unique feature of all sections of the Manual are the Quick Reference Guides; these present practical techniques or treatments in an easy-to-follow step-by-step format, with clear colour photographs illustrating each step whenever possible. These 'QRGs' are sufficiently detailed to enable a practitioner to perform a technique or treatment effectively and with confidence, even if performing it for the first time. They cover a wide range of topics, including: emergency thoracic radiography, neurological examination, tooth extraction, enucleation, prepubertal neutering of kittens, pinnectomy, skin cytology, thoracocentesis, liver biopsy, treatment of hypocalcaemia, and inserting a chest drain.

A large number of international authors have been involved in the Manual, all carefully chosen for their knowledge and practical expertise in different areas of feline practice. As Editors, we have worked hard to bring their contributions together into a book that is relevant, practical, clear and a must-have for any veterinary surgeon seeing feline cases. We have tried to get the balance right between what is, and isn't, included in the book, as well as pitching the level of detail appropriately for different subjects, but we would very much welcome feedback on this at **publications@bsava.com** so that future editions can evolve to further fulfil the needs of the readers.

We are truly grateful to everyone who has helped make this new Manual possible. The excellent contributions of the authors, and their patience in responding to our often numerous queries, especially in relation to making the content as practically useful as possible, are much appreciated. The BSAVA Publications team is also thanked for its patience and enthusiasm for the project, as is Tracy Dewey of the Photography Unit of the University of Bristol Veterinary School, for provision of many of the excellent photographs used in the Manual. These combined efforts have enabled our vision to be realised. Finally we wish to thank our family, friends and colleagues, who have shown incredible support over the three years of this project; in particular our partners, Steve Tasker and Richard Malik, and Séverine's children, Amélie and Loïc.

We sincerely hope that you find the Manual useful, and most importantly, that your feline patients will benefit from it.

Andrea Harvey
Séverine Tasker

January 2013

The cat-friendly practice

Margie Scherk

Introduction

In order to work cooperatively with cats, in which the fight or flight response is triggered so easily, we need to engender empathy, based on an understanding of their nature and innate behaviours, i.e. to see things from a cat's perspective.

We are taught a lot about how to perform techniques, how to make a diagnosis and what therapies are appropriate, but often this objectifies the patient. Our own experiences as a patient in the human healthcare system hopefully include caring and competent professionals but may also include feeling less than cherished as unique individuals. Do we feel *cared* for or merely 'processed' in a professional and polite manner? Is the person interacting with you truly empathetic, or only sympathetic? Are WE processing our patients, checking them off in our minds or on the day sheet as we 'complete' the procedure or office call?

And what about the environment? In human hospitals, are gowns and paper-covered examination beds designed for our comfort or for the healthcare team? Similarly, in veterinary clinics, are stainless steel cages and tables designed for the comfort of our patients or for ease of disinfection, height and durability?

Understanding feline behaviour

Working with feline patients, whose social structure is very different from those of humans and dogs, provides interesting challenges to the veterinary practitioner. Cats are able to function completely efficiently as solitary creatures but they *do* have complex and changing social interactions, which are much more intricate than that of a herd or pack species.

What makes a cat a cat?

The first step in developing a cat-friendly environment is to be able to imagine, from the patient's perspective, what it might be experiencing within the environment, as this will guide its response (Figure 1.1). To do this, one needs to understand some very basic but critical differences between other species (including humans) and domestic cats:

- Cats are **predatory as well as preyed upon**. They are predators of small birds, rodents, rabbits, insects, earthworms, small reptiles, etc., but are also potential prey to any bird larger than a pigeon. This is important to recognize because, when frightened, cats respond defensively in order to try to escape and/or protect themselves. These physical cues are often misinterpreted as being indicative of aggression when in fact they reflect fear.

- Being **obligate carnivores** has affected everything about cats – from their dentition and lack of salivary amylase, to the size of their stomach, the speed of GI transit, their hunting behaviour, solitary feeding and even their social structure. They are anatomically and physiologically adapted to eating 10–20 small meals throughout the day and night. Under stressful situations, cats will refuse a novel food; under other circumstances, the same cat may be very adventuresome and choose a new diet over their familiar food.

- Cats are **solitary, not social hunters**. The drive to hunt is independent from the need to eat. Hence, ready availability of food does not stop them killing birds or mice; it merely makes them gain weight. On average, a cat needs 10–15 attempts before it can achieve a successful kill; thus the drive to eye, stalk, pounce and kill is permanently turned on, or else a cat in the wild would starve.

- Cats are very **scent-sensitive**. When they rub against humans, it is to maintain an affiliative colony odour; this may be incorrectly interpreted as a request for food! Smells need to be reassuring within their territory and cats spend a lot of time re-marking, via different methods, to assure the security of their home territory.

- Cats have **casual encounters**. Cats (in general) interact with us frequently and at a low intensity or casually.

- Relying on their **'fight or flight' or adrenaline (epinephrine) response**, cats will attempt to escape situations viewed as dangerous. If they have the opportunity, rather than fight, they will flee or hide. Fear promotes survival by causing the individual to avoid danger. From the perspective of a cat, humans in a veterinary setting are

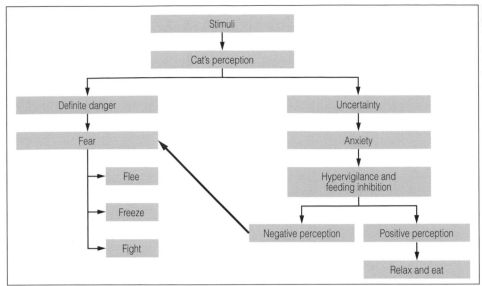

1.1

The progression of emotional states and responses that a cat may experience when frightened/stressed. (Adapted from Gourkow, 2004)

threatening and what they do is dangerous. Accordingly, one of the great challenges to veterinary personnel on a daily basis is the frightened and defensive cat. It is essential to remember at all times not to become frightened oneself and that this small creature feels threatened. Because cats are small and live independently, they can not afford to get hurt; they therefore try to avoid physical confrontation at all costs and attempt to intimidate, using sounds and posture as much as possible. To work with cats in a way that makes them feel secure and willing to cooperate, it is necessary to try to imagine what it is like to be a cat. How can our interactions and the physical space we work in be adjusted to reduce the strangeness and threat that cats appear to experience in the veterinary clinic?

Recognizing feline body language and communication

Given the chance, cats choose to avoid conflict by avoiding proximity. They try to maintain distance from any other animals (including humans) that are not in their social group through olfactory cues (marking with urine and scent gland secretions). Should a potentially unfriendly animal or person come within sight, cats use an elaborate repertoire of body and tail postures, facial expressions and vocalizations to attempt to convince that individual to GO AWAY. Only if those signals are not respected, and the cat can neither flee nor hide, will it fight in order to defend itself and the resources within its territory. Cats will use a combination of the following modes of communication in any situation. Learning to look for these, interpret them and react appropriately will improve the clinic experience.

Tactile cues

Tactile communication such as rubbing, grooming, or kneading indicates affiliative friendly relationships. Through rubbing, the transfer of scent maintains the 'family' or colony. Grooming of another cat is generally restricted to its head and neck; it may precede a playful attack, be conciliatory, or be part of hygiene. Kneading and treading occurs in kittens, as a regressive behaviour in adults, or as a component of sexual interaction.

The neck bite/scruffing is a signal that is used in three contexts: transporting a young kitten; part of sexual mounting; and as a means to dominate another cat in a fight.

PRACTICAL TIP

The use of scruffing by veterinary staff resembles the attempt of another cat to dominate in a fight and does not belong in a conciliatory, respectful cooperative setting.

Olfactory cues

The role of smell and scent is an aspect of feline communication that is difficult for humans to appreciate. Cats are very scent-sensitive. It has been estimated that the size of the olfactory epithelium in cats can be up to 20 cm^2 whereas humans have only 2–4 cm^2 of olfactory epithelium. Scent signals may be left by several methods: urine spraying, cheek marking of an object or individual, scratching to leave scent from glands below pads, and midden (leaving a deposit of faeces uncovered in a strategic place). Olfactory cues are frequently used by cats and have the advantage over visual cues of persisting over time, thus allowing for remote communication without direct interaction and its potential for conflict. Olfactory cues also have the ability to be utilized in circumstances of poor visibility (e.g. night time, heavy vegetation). The disadvantage of olfactory communication is that the sender has no control over a message once it has been deposited; it can not be altered or removed, and no adjustments can be made in response to the recipient's reaction. Urine marking in the home is an attempt to signal to the other cats that 'I was here' and to establish a routine so that the cats can keep a distance by time-sharing the same space without needing to come into conflict. However, every time a person cleans up the urine, they defeat this attempt at communication!

Due to humans' poor olfactory sense, veterinary staff cannot appreciate some of the messages a feline patient may be experiencing or providing and are unable to fathom the overwhelming olfactory messages that the clinic experience must represent to the cat.

Visual cues: body language

Body language (including tail position) and facial expression are extremely effective at maintaining or increasing distance between hostile individuals. This requires an unobstructed view, adequate ambient light and, unlike olfactory cues, that the two individuals are in the same space together. Body posture conveys the overall picture of relaxation or fear but facial expression (eyes, ears, whiskers, mouth, visibility of teeth) provides the finer details *and* changes more rapidly. Thus, in a clinic setting, for the veterinary team to understand the mental/emotional state of an individual patient, to avoid provoking them and getting hurt, it is extremely important to watch and interpret facial changes, including some that may be very subtle to the untrained eye.

Posture: As a species that would generally lead a solitary existence in the wild, survival depends on speed, stealth, self-reliance and outsmarting others. The latter means that cats may 'say one thing but mean another'. When they appear to be aggressive, it is generally a means to hide their fear; 'stoicism' hides vulnerability, and these subtle changes in behaviour can mask significant illness. For example:

- A body posture that suggests confidence and physical prowess often actually represents a frightened cat, trying to keep a threat at a distance to avoid the necessity for physical confrontation. The arched back 'Halloween cat' typifies this façade of confidence and increased size (Figure 1.2, bottom right).
- The attempt to make oneself smaller, on the other hand, to minimize threat and evade attention, is portrayed by a crouch and withdrawal stance (Figure 1.2, bottom left). Note that the weight remains on all four paws so that flight/chase is quickly possible. A cat who is feeling less fearful does not need to be on his/her feet.
- The posture of the cat in Figure 1.2, top right

illustrates a confident but threatening state of mind. It is uncommon to see this 'stalker' in the clinic setting; this cat will not hesitate to attack and lacks fear.
- The cat shown in Figure 1.2, top left indicates a relaxed and confident cat that will respond with curiosity or be neutral in interactions.

Rolling: Rolling has several presentations. The social roll is an invitation to interact; the cat lies on its side. An extremely fearful threatened cat will roll to expose its abdomen, with all four feet ready for self-defence and showing all of its weapons (nails and teeth). Such a cat will often be screaming, and may urinate or defecate.

Tail position: Tail position allows observation of communication from further away. Tail up, happy Js (i.e. hooked-shaped tails) and a tail quiver are all greeting behaviours. A tail tucked to one side is part of becoming less visible, as in a crouch and withdrawal stance. A bottlebrush, pilo-erected tail is part of threat/bluff behaviour.

Facial expressions: Facial expressions can change more rapidly than body posture and can be more subtle; they should, therefore, be observed closely. Cats have extremely mobile ears.

- When the ears are facing forward, a cat is listening and is generally relaxed or alert but not emotionally aroused (Figure 1.3, top left).
- Turned laterally/flat 'aeroplane ears' indicate that the cat is more fearful/threatened (Figure 1.3, centre left).
- When the ears are held back and tight to the head, the cat is feeling very threatened/frightened. As shown in Figure 1.3, bottom left this cat will have a partially open or fully open mouth and be hissing, spitting, yowling or screaming. This cat will protect itself using teeth and claws, if the perceived threat level is not reduced.

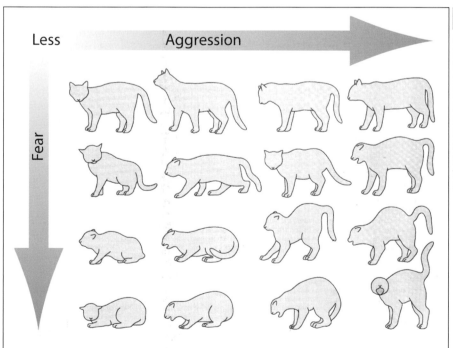

1.2 Body posture. An increase in emotional arousal from contented to aggressive is shown from left to right; a state of fearfulness increases from the top to the bottom. (Reproduced from Little S (2012) *The Cat: Clinical Medicine and Management* with the permission of Elsevier. Adapted from Bowen J and Heath S (2005) *An Overview of Feline Social Behaviour and Communication* (Saunders); which was adapted in turn from Leyhausen P (1979) *Cat Behaviour* (Garland).)

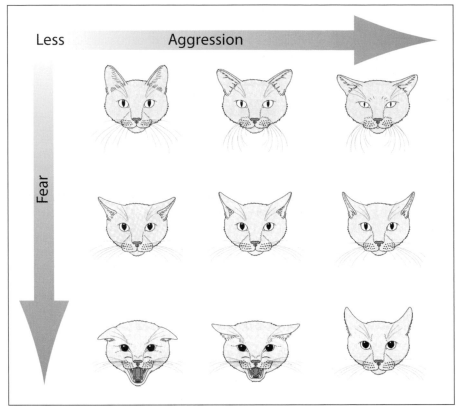

1.3 Facial expressions. The relaxed cat's face is shown in the top left-hand corner. When frightened and feeling the need to defend itself, the expressions change as depicted from left to right; when fearful but less aggressive, they change as shown from top to bottom of the diagrams. (Reproduced from Little S (2012) *The Cat: Clinical Medicine and Management* with the permission of Elsevier. Adapted from Bowen J and Heath S (2005) *An Overview of Feline Social Behaviour and Communication* (Saunders); which was adapted in turn from Leyhausen P (1979) *Cat Behaviour* (Garland).)

■ Ears turned back but erect indicates the most reactive and aggressive state (Figure 1.3, top right). In this case, the mouth will be closed and the cat will be emitting a low growl with or without swallowing. This is the cat that may suddenly attack.

Vocalization
This form of communication requires the presence of the recipient and can change rapidly. As with other forms of signalling, cats have a well developed repertoire to convey a need or wish for increasing distance between individuals. These include: growl, yowl, snarl, hiss, spit, gurgle, long miaow, wah-wah and pain shriek. The sounds made for socialization are: trill/chirrup, purr, puffing, prusten, chatter, miaow and sexual calling. The cat who is open-mouthed screaming is highly emotionally aroused but likely to be less aggressive than the cat who is emitting a closed-mouthed growl or partially closed-mouthed wah-wah.

Social structure
Cats are not completely solitary, asocial creatures but they are emotionally capable of surviving alone and do not require social contact. In the wild, the number of feral cats living together is dependent on the availability of resources: food, water, privacy and safety, latrine (toileting area) and sexual partners. This results in reduced competition and a social structure that does not require sharing or taking turns, so there is no need for a linear hierarchical structure. Stress is minimal unless there is a threat from a stranger for one of the resources. Thus, communication and aggression have largely developed to keep distance between individuals and to prevent contact with outsiders. The natural grouping, should there be enough resources, is a colony of related female cats with their young,

which they will jointly defend and nurse. Males are relegated to the periphery and vie for the prime breeding spot; only one tom usually lives with the group.

The challenges of housing cats together
Forcing cats to live together in a human household generally results in stress, as they have to share their home territory and resources with cats that they are not related to. The picture of many cats eating together is not a reflection of community but rather reflects the core need to eat; aggressive behaviours are suppressed in order to obtain food. The consequences of the chronic stress of being forced to share their territory with other cats outside their social group may be manifested as over-grooming, urine spraying (to try to define time- and space-sharing), overeating, or other behavioural disorders. Lack of enough safe water stations may result in dehydration. If a cat does not have hiding places and perches that are sufficiently hidden or apart from the other cats, then it is perpetually vulnerable and unable to have some control over its environment; this results in a state of stress. Individuals predisposed to stress-aggravated conditions (such as idiopathic cystitis, inflammatory bowel disease, allergy) may experience disease flare-ups.

Environmental adaptations in the home

The goal is to provide an environment that, from the cat's perspective, is safe and secure and has adequate resources that do not require facing the risk of ambush. This will utilize three-dimensional space. Hiding places and perches can be readily created by placing towels or bedding on top of cabinet surfaces, refrigerators or bathroom counters. One must be cognizant of the (perceived) potential for ambush and therefore cupboards or corner perches without a second exit, or litter boxes with hoods, are to be avoided. A consistently safe environment consists not only of food, water and shelter, but also predictable routines, sounds and scents. A cat, like any other individual, needs to feel safe and in control of its own circumstances. More information on environmental enrichment can be found at: http://indoorpet.osu.edu/cats/.

It should be remembered that opportunities to express hunting behaviour are also a basic need for a cat. If a cat does not have the opportunity to hunt, then toys that meet appropriate criteria are small (prey-sized), make high-pitched squeaks or cheeps and/or move in a rapid, unpredictable fashion. Also, allowing cats to hunt for their food (bowl) or using a feeding toy (e.g. feeding ball, puzzle feeder; Figure 1.4) are mentally stimulating.

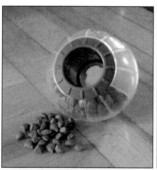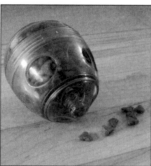

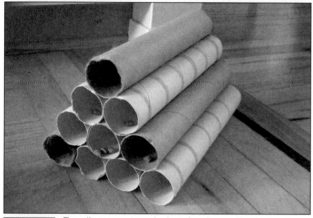

1.4 Feeding toys can help stimulate cats through hunting behaviour. Many types are commercially available, or they can be homemade.

Reducing the threat of the clinic experience from the cat's perspective

Recognizing, reading and understanding feline body language is critically important in reducing a patient's fear when in the clinic. It also allows veterinary staff to respond to the cat in a respectful manner. **Staff should avoid using signals that are perceived as hostile (e.g. scruffing, making shushing or hissing sounds, directly staring at a cat).**

In order to begin to appreciate what the clinic experience is like for a cat, it is useful to try to imagine what it might be like to be a cat, and to think about everything around us from a cat's perspective.

Imagine:

- Walking on four feet
- Jumping five or more times your height
- Perceiving the world in overlapping clouds of smell
- Having much better vision in dim lighting
- Grooming yourself with your tongue
- Locating sound by rotating your ears
- Having poor close-up vision and using your whiskers to locate things
- Having a tail!

Reducing the stress of travelling to the vet
Going to the clinic appears to be a frightening experience for many cats, and begins at home. Imagine the scenario from the cat's perspective:

'The carrier comes out, your owner is nervous, they chase you around and try to push you into the carrier. You resist, but are unable to run away, and resort to self-defence, scratching your owner. Having done this you feel anxious. Human sweat, stress, maybe blood and other smells make you feel so apprehensive that you soil yourself! Eventually you are in the carrier. Everyone is exhausted. Then you are moved into a 'car' that moves without you moving. You become a bit nauseous; certainly you are scared. You cry out repeatedly. You vomit. Then the 'car' stops and you get carried on a noisy and unfamiliar street and into a place with overwhelming smells and sounds, and a room full of predators! You are aroused and anxious… look out!'

This stress can be reduced or, in the case of a new cat, prevented by teaching/habituating the cat to associate positive experiences with the carrier and the car (and even the clinic).

- Leaving the carrier out, so that the cat sees it routinely and enters it for food treats or other rewards, can dampen the initial tension and fight or flight response. Multi-use items such as the Hide Perch & Go box can be assembled into a carrier (Figure 1.5).
- A carrier should open from the top for ease of removing the cat or examining it within the base of the box (Figure 1.6). Having a side opening for the cat to walk through willingly, in addition to the opening at the top, is ideal.
- The carrier should be secured within the car with a seatbelt; the front passenger seat is not suitable for a carrier due to possible airbag expansion.
- Carriers should be covered with a towel or blanket when being carried to and from the car and within the veterinary clinic.
- Taking the cat on short car rides that are unassociated with the clinic also helps recondition the negative associations with the clinic.
- Finally, taking the cat to the clinic to be fussed over or only to get a treat will help teach the cat that the clinic isn't necessarily a horrible place.
- All of these positive associations can be assisted by a reward.

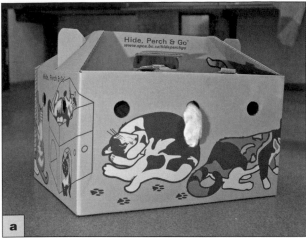

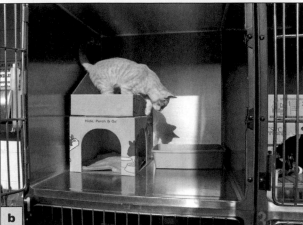

1.5 The Hide Perch & Go box is produced by the British Columbia Society for the Prevention of Cruelty to Animals. These carriers may be used for perching and hiding at home and then **(a)** reassembled into a carrier retaining the cat's own scent and the familiarity of a pleasant sleeping place from their home. **(b)** In the clinic setting, the carrier can revert into a place to perch or hide in the cage. While coated with a plastic coating made from recycled water bottles, these carriers do not hold up to significant soiling or moisture from urine or water. (© Craig Naherniak, BC SPCA)

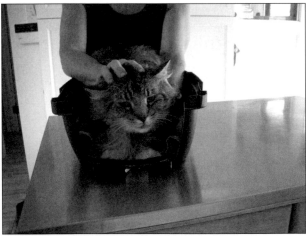

1.6 Familiarity with the base of the carrier can provide a sense of security that generally reduces the cat's need to defend itself. The walls of the carrier base and the bedding allow the cat to partially hide. For veterinary examination, this will reduce the need for manual restraint. By removing the top of the carrier, there is no need to displace the cat and occasion the unpleasant sensation of being moved.

Recognizing fearful cats: the continuum of fearful states

There is a progression between emotional states, whether positive or negative. In the clinic setting, four negative states can be recognized: anxiety, fear, frustration and depression. By recognizing the state a cat is in, veterinary staff can act to reduce its level of fear, etc, as well as making appropriate changes in the cage or other environments to help the cat to relax. Figures 1.2 and 1.3 show the body and face postures associated with these states, as well as with relaxation when the person changes their approach technique; further information is available in the AAFP and ISFM feline-friendly handling guidelines (Rodan *et al.*, 2011; www.isfm.net).

Anxiety

> *Imagine that it is night time. You are alone at home, in bed and are falling asleep when you hear an unfamiliar and unexpected sound in your home. Your adrenaline levels rise, your heart rate increases and your hearing becomes acute. You dare not move and you watch every shadow. Your imagination is racing. You are anticipating danger.*

When cats lose control over their environment, are surrounded by unfamiliar smells or novel objects, are handled by strangers, have procedures performed on them, hear loud sounds and experience sudden movements, they experience anxiety. Their eyes may either be wide open or squeezed shut (feigning sleep); their ears and body may be flattened, whiskers are retracted, and their tail is tucked close to the body. Their heart and breathing rates are increased. They stay at the back of the cage, in their litter box or under their towel, trying to make themselves small or invisible.

Fear

> *Imagine that it is night time. You are alone at home, in bed and are falling asleep when a stranger walks into your room! He is holding something that might be a weapon. Your heart is racing and your mind is spinning through possible ways to get away or defend yourself if you can't escape. You may shout or scream. You are terrified!*

Cats in a clinic setting are regularly handled by strangers, and experience discomfort and pain from the procedures performed (e.g. handling, restraint, catheterization, injections, cystocentesis, giving oral medication). The fearful cat will flatten its ears back against its head, and its eyes will be fully open to assess the danger. The cat may hiss or scream. The tail is tight into the body but the cat's whiskers are reaching forward and out to assess distance. The cat's heart and breathing rates are increased. It may quiver/shake, salivate and may urinate or defecate. The cat is attempting to defend/protect itself initially by warning the 'attacker' away (hiss, spit, quick strikes with claws out). When/if the approach is continued without changing the signals, the cat may expose all of its weapons: 18 nails and 30 teeth.

Frustration and depression

> *Imagine being in a prison cell, you have none of the things you are used to having around you and you don't have the ability to correct this situation. The bed you have to sleep on is uncomfortable, the place is noisy, it smells bad, the food isn't to your liking, you can't call your friends, there is nothing to do. Your routines are disrupted so that meal times and family don't show up when you expect them to. Regardless of your actions, no one seems to understand you and your wishes are not being granted.*

A frustrated cat may shred paper, chew the bars of the cage, be unpredictable (friendly and then aggressive or not interactive), and may vocalize a lot. It may pace or attempt to escape at every opportunity. Turning everything upside down may be an attempt for a frightened cat to hide or could be an expression of frustration. An individual who is less outgoing will show frustration by over-grooming, pawing at a corner of the kennel, overeating, or chewing/sucking non-edible items. Incessant kneading may also be a stereotypic expression of frustration.

This is a very unrewarding and frustrating state. Unrelieved, it may result in depression. Depression may manifest itself as being withdrawn and listless, sitting with the head hanging, not grooming, anorexia, and/or showing little or no interest in things going on outside the cage.

The physical environment: feline-friendly modifications
Looking back to the clinic environment:

- What can be done to reduce the stress and threat level of the physical and social environment?
- What things or events assault the five senses of a cat?
- How can we make positive changes to these?

Figure 1.7 summarizes some of the main threats to cats in the clinic environment, and makes some suggestions of how those threats may be reduced. This is not an exhaustive list, but rather is a starting point. Veterinary surgeons need to evaluate their own individual clinics, from the cat's perspective, to identify further potential threats, and to find practical solutions that will work in their individual situations.

Feline facial pheromone F3 (e.g. Feliway) can be very helpful. Diffusers releasing pheromones can be plugged into every room: the waiting room, consultation rooms, treatment area and hospital ward. Diffusers need to be replaced on a monthly basis, so this should be added to the monthly duty list. Additionally, it is beneficial to spray pheromone F3 into a patient's cage or carrier 30 minutes before placing the cat into it. Hands and clothing can also be sprayed before going to examine a distressed cat, but it is important to leave enough time after application for the carrier agent in the spray to evaporate before examining or handling the cat.

Waiting areas
It is *very* important to keep cats away from other cats, and away from dogs, as much as possible. **Avoiding direct visual contact with other animals is essential.** Avoiding cats hearing other animals is ideal, but this is often more difficult to achieve. Wherever possible, a separate quiet seating area should be provided that is only for clients with cats (Figure 1.8). If this is not possible, cat carriers should remain covered (with, for example, a towel or blanket) and be held or placed away from curious noses or fingers. Relaxing music, an aquarium, or a running water fountain can contribute to a calm atmosphere. The more the client relaxes, the more the cat will relax.

Consultation rooms
Having at least one dedicated cat consultation room is beneficial, so that a suitable cat-friendly environment can be maintained with appropriate equipment and without the smells of dogs. Room design should provide enough space that the cat can explore the room safely without getting caught under or behind immobile furniture; the cat may choose to stay inside the carrier however. The examination can be performed on the clinician's lap, on the client's lap, on the floor, on a bench or on a warm, non-slippery table.

Sense	Threat	Possible methods to reduce threat
Smell	Dogs, other cats, fear pheromones, chemicals, alcohol, disinfectants, deodorizers, blood, urine, anal gland secretions, pus, etc.	Keep away from dogs and other cats where possible. Use feline pheromone F3 infusers in the waiting area, consultation room, treatment area and cat ward, making sure they are replaced monthly. When rubbing alcohol is used, wipe off excess; using medial saphenous vein reduces the proximity of the alcohol to the cat's face
Hearing	Barking, frightened cats, clippers, running water, cage doors closing, phones, computer printers, spray bottles, strange voices, any unfamiliar sounds	Examine cats away from other animals. Keep away from barking dogs and other busy noisy areas of the clinic. Sound-proof whenever possible. Avoid clipping fur unless necessary and use quiet clippers. If for venepuncture/catheterization, consider using the medial saphenous vein so the noise and sensation are away from the cat's face. Cover the pins on the cage doors with intravenous tubing to reduce the metallic closing noise. Spray cleaning cloths or paper towels away from the cat, bringing the cloth to the surface rather than the spray bottle for wiping surfaces
Sight	Strange people wearing lab coats and uniforms (scrubs), dogs, unfamiliar cats, equipment approaching the cat's face, reflections on tables, cage walls, bright lights, etc.	If feasible, wear 'civilian' clothing. Reduce reflections by covering part of the cage door with a towel. Allow the cat to hide (bed, box) wherever possible and keep it out of direct sight of dogs and other cats. Minimize the number of people in sight of the cat at all times. Avoid shining bright lights at cats (apart from ocular exam)
Taste	Unfamiliar foods when frightened, bitter	Avoid changing diet while in clinic unless medically required
Touch	Cold, slippery, wet	Provide warm soft surfaces to cover the floor of the cage and the examination/treatment table

1.7 Recognizing threats to cats, and how they can be reduced in the clinic.

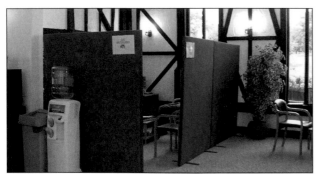

1.8 It is desirable for cats to wait in a completely separate waiting area or room where possible, out of sight, sound and smell of dogs. This is often not achievable in a mixed practice but most practices are able to find a way of at least providing some separation between dogs and cats, such as partitioning off an area of the waiting room. (Courtesy of Andrea Harvey and Davies Veterinary Specialists)

The optimal location will be the one the cat feels most comfortable in. If the cat chooses to remain in the bottom of the carrier (see Figure 1.6), the surface it is placed upon must be stable. To remove or minimize olfactory cues, disinfectants or mild soaps should be used that themselves have minimal scent, and veterinary staff should avoid wearing perfumes and aftershaves to avoid contributing to sensory overload.

The position of lights during any restraint of a cat for a procedure should be considered. For example, if raising the cat's head to take a jugular blood sample, it is important to avoid forcing the cat to look into a bright light on the ceiling.

Hospital wards

It is important to ensure that direct visual contact with other animals, including other cats, is avoided at all times, be it while in the hospital cage, on an examination table, or being carried around the clinic. Banks of cages should not be opposite each other or angled around a corner, and examination tables should not be placed in front of ward cages.

Lighting: The lighting within the ward should be carefully considered. If lights are mounted on a track and are moveable, they should be directed away from the cages so that they are not shining on to the cats. This will also help to reduce reflections on the walls of the cage. In addition, when a person approaches a cat in a cage, they may block out the light, and this will create a bigger change in light if the lights within the ward are very bright. People should approach the cage in such a way as to avoid casting too much of a shadow over the cat.

Caging: The larger the cage, kennel or bedroom the better; even a cage measuring 60 cm x 60 cm x 60 cm does not allow for a large enough litter tray that cats will feel comfortable using. It is very important to have a place for a cat to hide and to be able to perch/observe when they want to, yet be far enough away from their latrine. Food and water bowls also need to be placed away from the litter tray and not under the nose of a patient who is feeling nauseous. Vertical height can be used to separate perching from litter areas, while taking an individual's agility into consideration. Thus a 'kitty condo' (Figure 1.9) offers many advantages.

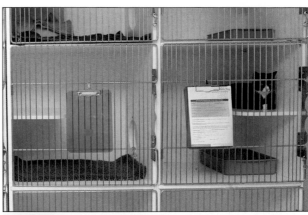

1.9 The pens of this 'kitty condo' have two sections side by side; the partitions have openings for the cat to move through. Shelves are present to allow perching, and the space allows separation of the litter tray and food bowl. (Courtesy of Anne Fawcett)

Laminate material is preferable for cat cages, as stainless steel cages are not only cold but also reflective and noisy. However, if using stainless steel cages, a towel hung over part of the cage door can reduce reflection from the walls. An easy first step to decreasing the noise created by opening and closing stainless steel cage doors is to put rubber stoppers on the front of the cage, or wrap a small piece of bandage or intravenous tubing around the latch pins. A warm non-slip surface, such as a towel, blanket or other type of bedding, should cover the floor of the cage (Figure 1.10).

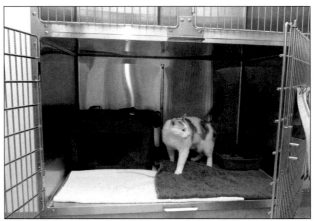

1.10 A good cat cage environment. The cage is big enough to allow good separation of litter tray and food/water. (A food/water bowl is not present in this image but would ideally be placed diagonally opposite the litter tray.) The floor of the cage is fully covered with a warm comfortable bed, and the cat's own basket is within the cage, providing a familiar place to hide and a raised surface to perch on. (Courtesy of Anne Fawcett)

Ideally, the bed should be slightly raised off the floor. Any material that is soft and insulates against cold is suitable. It should be textured and dry rather than smooth, so that the cat can knead it. It should hold scent from the cat's pads. Towels and fleece fabric are ideal. While cat beds are lovely at home, because of their size they may be impractical to put through the laundry every day. A simple towel under the cat, with a second towel (rolled lengthwise) wrapped as a tube (like a doughnut) around the cat, works just as well (Figure 1.11).

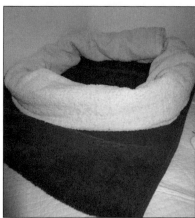

1.11

A simple and effective cat bed has been made using a flat towel for the base and a second towel rolled up lengthwise and wrapped in a circle to form the sides. (Courtesy of The Feline Centre, Langford Veterinary Services, University of Bristol)

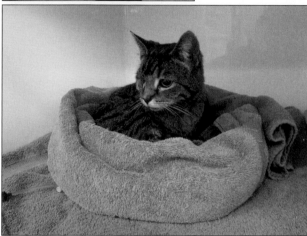

- An item to hide in
- An item to perch on
- An item to rub on for scent marking, and preferably an item from home that already has their own and other familiar scents on
- If the cat is well enough, toys to stimulate hunting (e.g. those for batting, pouncing, throwing up in the air)
- Scratching opportunities (e.g. carpet or corrugated cardboard near the litter box) if cats are hospitalized for any length of time.

Having a soft thick rope or a toy tied to the cage door will increase the chance that a person will interact with the cat when they walk by the cage.

Treatment/procedures area

The same concepts apply as described for other areas:

- The treatment table should have a non-slip warm surface
- Towels and blankets work well both to cover the table and to provide a chance for the cat to hide
- Cats should be positioned so that they do not see other animals
- Noises should be kept to a minimum and energy should be calm rather than 'busy'
- Examination lights should be positioned so they do not shine directly into a cat's face
- Personnel should avoid direct eye contact with the cat.

Equipment

In line with the preceding discussion, equipment in the cat-friendly practice should generally be small, discrete, streamlined and quiet. Listed below are things that are required or useful to have.

- **Food and water bowls:** metal or sturdy glass, low and wide.
- **Large towels of various thicknesses.** Towels are useful for providing warmth and to eliminate slippery surfaces and reflections. They are comforting and can be used to bundle a frightened patient gently to provide comforting restraint for examination and procedures. A towel rolled lengthwise and shaped into a circle on top of another towel acts as a cosy bed (Figure 1.11), and allows the cat to partially hide, while being less bulky for the laundry. Towels also help to buffer noise.
- **Scales:** accurate paediatric or cat-specific.
- **Clippers:** silent and light and, ideally, cordless.
- **Thermometer:** digital with a flexible tip. Thermometer covers are a good idea for cleanliness as well as the client's awareness that the practice is cautious about hygiene.
- **Stethoscopes:** should have a small enough diaphragm to enable auscultation (see QRG 1.5) of different regions of the chest in a small patient (e.g. paediatric). An acrylic stethoscope head (Figure 1.12) can be very helpful for hearing subtle lung sounds through fur and even bandages.
- **Otoscope tips:** small, paediatric otoscope tips can be used with the appropriate otoscope head.

Food and water bowls should be low and wide so that whiskers do not touch the edges. Metal or sturdy glass bowls are preferable to plastic for cleaning purposes, and plastic can give the water a tainted taste. Alternatively, for food, disposable paper plates make a good feeding surface. Unless there is a medical reason otherwise, cats should be offered the food that they are familiar with receiving at home. Calculation of energy requirements for hospitalized cats is discussed in QRG 1.1. Food and water bowls may be raised and attached securely to the cage door to keep them away from the litter tray.

Litter trays must be kept meticulously clean, and a type of litter used to suit the cat's preference. The client could be asked to bring some litter from home to enhance familiarity. If a cat is not using the litter tray, it may be helpful to place the cat in a quiet room with a full-sized litter tray, as it may feel too vulnerable or awkward using the small tray in the cage.

The cat's sense of vulnerability while in the hospital cage can be significantly reduced by providing it with a place to hide and/or perch. The cat's own carrier (without the door/gate), a sturdy cardboard or plastic box that is turned on its side, or a specialist container (see Figure 1.5) will give the cat the option of hiding inside or sitting on top. Various types of bed are also available that can provide the cat with a place to hide, e.g. an igloo-type bed. Even hanging a towel over part of the cage door will give the cat the chance to hide and feel less threatened.

The cat should be enabled to exert some control over the amount of exposure to activities taking place in front of its cage and given an opportunity to engage in a wider range of behaviours, by providing:

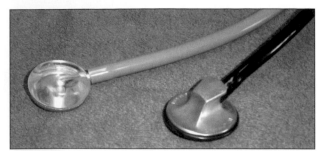

1.12 The acrylic stethoscope head (left) provides better acoustics for subtle lung sounds compared to a standard stethoscope head.

- **Blood pressure monitor:** Doppler system is ideal, with appropriate cuffs and headphones (see QRG 5.18.1). In an anaesthetized patient, Doppler or oscillometric methods are reliable. In conscious cats, however, not all oscillometric devices correlate with values obtained telemetrically in patients weighing <11 kg, and Doppler, or PetMap or Memoprint (both high-definition oscillometry) methodology should be used.
- **Hypodermic needles size 25 G through 16 G.** Size 16 G are useful for marrow aspiration and intraosseous needle placement. 18–20 G are useful for subcutaneous fluid administration. For blood collection, use 22–25 G (lengths: 5/8, 1 inch); 1½ inch 22 G or 23 G needles are used for cystocentesis.
- **Intravenous catheters:** 22 G is the most commonly used size.
- **Butterfly needles:** can be good for collecting small volumes of blood and are also useful for administering intravenous drugs when a catheter is not desired.
- **Red rubber or white silicone** (softer but more expensive) **feeding tubes.** Sizes 14–16 Fr are used for oesophageal feeding tubes; sizes 3–5 Fr may be used for naso-oesophageal feeding or as an indwelling urethral catheter if a shorter, polyurethane catheter is not available. Size 5 is also suitable for transoral airway lavage sampling. Size 14 is useful for colonic lavage and for administering enemas.
- **Padded collars** for stabilizing an oesophagostomy tube in place (Figure 1.13).
- **Multiple-use injection port ('prn') adaptor** (Figure 1.14): preferable to a three-way stopcock or clamp to close the end of a feeding tube (either gastric or oesophageal) as is less bulky. Also useful on intravenous catheters.
- **Paediatric (0.5 ml) blood collection tubes** (EDTA and serum separator tubes): are very helpful for smaller volumes of blood (e.g. difficult collection, a very small cat, or when numerous samples are taken over sequential days). Using standard tubes for small blood volumes will create undesirable errors and artefacts.
- **Haematocrit tubes and clay:** with the appropriate centrifuge for assessing PCV, total solids (TS), % buffy coat and serum colour. A **refractometer** is needed for TS. This simple set-up is more accurate than using an in-house chemistry analyser. PCV and TS should ideally be assessed at least once a day for patients on fluid therapy in order to be able to determine fluid adjustments.

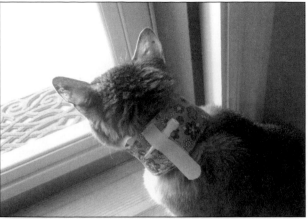

1.13 A padded collar, such as this Kitty Kollar, can be used to hold an oesophagostomy tube in place. A circular protective pad is slipped over the tube between the skin and the collar. The tube is then passed through a buttonhole opening, capped off with a prn adaptor (see Figure 1.14) and then fixed in place under a Velcro tab. These collars are soft and can be laundered readily. They come in a variety of fabric patterns and may be better accepted by cats than routine bandaging.

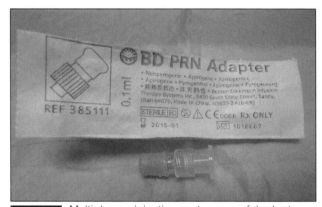

1.14 Multiple-use injection ports are useful adaptors for intravenous catheters or feeding tubes. (Courtesy of Loïc Legendre)

- **Blood typing methods:** e.g. cards or other kits (see QRG 20.1).
- **Glucometer:** Alpha-trak has been validated for cats. Other hand-held glucometers may be used but should be validated against the reference laboratory's hexokinase blood glucose evaluations.
- **Aerosol inhaler adaptor:** e.g. Aerokat (see QRG 10.1).
- **Nail covers:** e.g. SoftPaws, to protect the skin from self-induced trauma.
- **Fluid pumps:** small and able to be hung on the cage door rather than take up space in the kennel or be a frightening object on a pole outside the cage.
- **Syringe pump:** or burettes, for the administration of blood or other products that will be given over a short time period. This allows products to be piggy-backed to the existing intravenous set-up without disrupting it.
- **Useful in-house testing systems:** e.g. InPouch Feline TF growth culture media are specific for *Tritrichomonas foetus* identification and ideal for in-clinic use if this is quicker and more cost-effective than sending a sample externally for PCR, in-house FeLV and FIV tests.

- **Pheromone diffusers and sprays.** Plug in a diffuser in the waiting room, every consultation room, the treatment area and the hospital ward. Spray the carrier and cage 30 minutes before putting a patient into it. Spray your hands and clothing before going in to examine a distressed cat but be sure to do this with enough time for the carrier agent in the spray to evaporate.

General approach and handling

The goal is to handle the patient respectfully and provide an appeasing environment. This is achieved by reducing threats, thereby lowering the cat's need to react defensively. **Scruffing is an unnecessary act of dominance that does not promote a good, harmonious relationship with the patient.**

The handler's body language

The key to handling feline patients successfully is always to think about how you will be perceived from the cat's perspective, and to be careful not to mimic the behaviour of a predator or an aggressive cat.

- Consider your own body language and tone of voice very carefully, and pay close attention to how they may be perceived by the cat.
- Be ready to modify your behaviour/body language/ voice if they appear to be threatening to the cat.
- Always move slowly and use a calm tone.
- Do not show fear or anxiety outwardly.

The aggressive cat makes itself large and has an upright stiff-legged stance (see Figure 1.2); so it helps to approach cats with the opposite body language, i.e. making yourself small (e.g. sitting down, crouching or sitting on the floor) with a relaxed stance. The aggressive cat or predator will stare threateningly directly into the eyes of the frightened cat. Therefore, to be less threatening, cats should be examined from behind and, other than for the ophthalmic evaluation, direct facial staring should be avoided.

The aggressive cat growls and uses low tones. Staff need to take care not to say 'shush' or 'pssst' to a cat to try to calm it, as this is the equivalent of a hiss. Instead, use light, upper-register tones, perhaps chirruping as cats do when they are relaxed with conspecifics. Likewise, short repetitive sounds should be avoided as these may resemble spitting rhythms. Purrs, trills, and chirrups are all social welcoming sounds.

Getting a cat out of a carrier or hospital cage

It is important to follow the principles above, so that the cat feels less threatened before any physical contact is made. Some information can be obtained before removing the cat from the carrier, such as weighing within the carrier, observing the cat's demeanour, and counting the respiratory rate. With a top-opening carrier, or one where the lid can be removed, it may be possible to examine the cat within the carrier, without removing it at all (see Figure 1.6).

Never tip or shake a cat out of a carrier. If the cat must be removed:

- Allow the cat an opportunity to get out of the carrier of its own accord.

- If the cat is within a bed in the carrier, it may be easier to lift the cat out of the carrier within the bed, so that it still feels safe and secure, it can partially hide, and direct physical contact is avoided.
- Disassemble the carrier (Figure 1.15) and either remove the cat, or examine it in the base of the carrier.
- Remember that when you reach into the carrier you will block off light and may appear as a looming frightening predator. Try to approach the opening from the side so that some light still enters.
- Do not block off every chance of escape; if the possibility to have some control over the environment and situation exists, the cat will be much more cooperative.

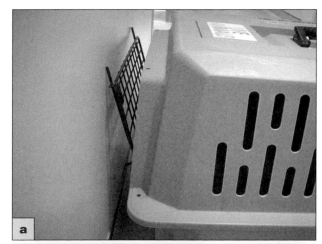

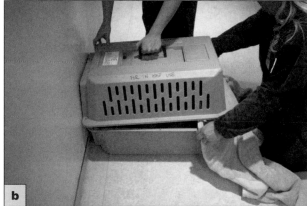

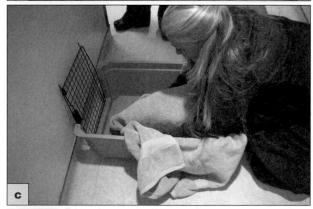

1.15 Removing an anxious cat from a carrier. **(a)** Place the carrier close to a wall with the door facing the wall and unscrew the bolts. **(b)** Ask an assistant to lift up the carrier lid/top towards the wall, so that the gate falls towards the wall and away from the cat. **(c)** Quietly place a towel over the cat and lift it out. Alternatively, the cat may be examined within the base of the carrier.

When removing a cat from a hospital cage:

- Where possible turn the cat around by swivelling its bed, so that the cat is facing away from you, and will therefore feel less threatened
- Removing the cat within its bed or box will reduce physical contact and make it feel safer and more secure while being moved
- Ensure that, as you remove the cat from the cage, you do not force it to face other cats in nearby cages.

General handling

Because cats rely on flight and fight for survival, and are not reliant on others, when it comes to restraint, LESS IS MORE. Cats inherently resist intimate handling and restraint. By confining them, we take away their sense of control and cause them to react. It is very easy to condition negative emotional responses; bags, masks and gloves all carry the scents of previous similarly terrified patients plus other sundry smells (anal gland secretion, pus, blood, halitosis, etc.) Use of a towel is usually all that is needed to 'burrito' a cat for protection of the handler (Figure 1.16). Remember, a cat would rather flee – or hide – than attack.

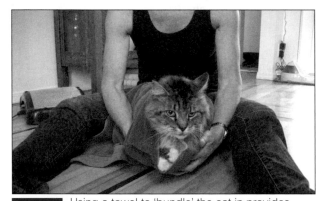

1.16 Using a towel to 'bundle' the cat in provides secure, yet minimal and comfortable, restraint.

When cats feel secure and safe, even through just being able to hide their faces in the handler's elbow or a towel, they will allow most procedures to be performed. A comprehensive examination, blood pressure evaluation, body temperature measurement and blood and urine collection can all be done without even moving the cat out of its bed, or bottom half of the carrier, in most cases. It is important to try to keep all four paws to the floor (table or lap) and avoid changing the cat's position as much as possible.

Allowing the cat to maintain a sense of control over the experience greatly reduces distress and its feeling of needing to defend itself. If a patient struggles, rather than hold it more tightly or ask another person to help with restraint, it can help to allow the cat more freedom:

- Rather than insisting on a cat being completely in lateral recumbency for a procedure, many will struggle less and appear to be more comfortable when their front end is allowed to be in a more natural position. The abdomen and hindlimbs can be easily accessed in this posture for various procedures (e.g. cystocentesis, abdominocentesis, medial saphenous venepuncture (Figure 1.17) and lateral saphenous venepuncture (Figure 1.18).

- Avoid restraining the cat's forelimbs over the edge of a table for jugular venepuncture; for an already frightened individual, additional lack of support under paws is frightening. Allowing the patient to have all four feet on a stable surface (floor, table) so that he/she feels able to flee, should it be necessary, helps to reduce anxiety (Figure 1.19)
- Try to move at the cat's pace, watch its responses and adjust accordingly.
- Reward desired behaviour with a treat or a stroke/rub.

Further guidance on handling for some common procedures can be found in QRG 1.2.

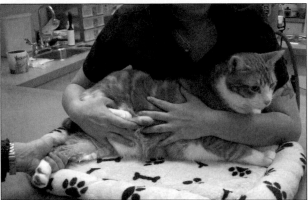

1.17 Positioning for access to the medial saphenous vein for venepuncture or intravenous catheterization.

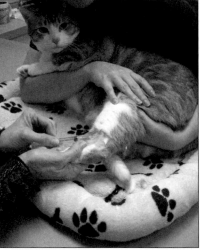

1.18 Positioning for access to the lateral saphenous vein for venepuncture or intravenous catheterization.

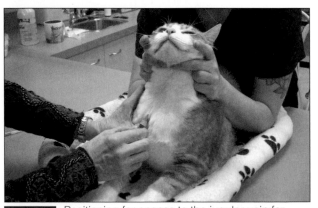

1.19 Positioning for access to the jugular vein for venepuncture, without stretching the cats' forelimbs over the edge of the table.

Taking the history

Cats mask illness and pain extremely well and the signs are often subtle. Listening carefully to clients is extremely important as they may detect small changes intuitively that represent real problems. By asking open questions, one elicits a more detailed history than using closed questions. For example: 'Have you noticed any changes in the contents of the litter box?' evokes a yes/no answer; whereas asking 'What does his stool look like? Is it hard pellets, moist logs, cow-pie or coloured water? When did you first notice this?' elicits much more detailed information.

1. **Find out what the client's main concern is.** If the visit is of a preventive nature, ask if the client has noticed anything since the last visit that concerns them, even if it has resolved. Encourage the client to elaborate. Once the specific concern has been discussed, unless the patient requires immediate problem-directed medical attention, a series of general questions may be asked.
2. **General questions should encompass:**
   a. Appetite (amount as well as frequency and pattern of eating):
      – Is there any change in how the food is being eaten (dropping food, chewing on one side of the mouth, etc.)?
      – What is being fed currently (brands, dry, moist, raw, scraps, treats)?
      – If the diet has been changed, it is helpful to find out why it has been changed.
      – When is food available (free choice, two meals a day, etc.)?
      – Is there any other cat, dog, child who might be perceived as a competitor for the food?
      – Does the cat have access to any other food?
      – Does the cat hunt?
   b. Amount being drunk (water, milk):
      – Where is the water dish?
      – In a multicat home, how many and where are the dishes placed?
   c. Bowel movements (consistency, frequency, colour):
      – Be sure to find out if there are multiple cats and if a litter tray is used or not.
      – Also be sure that the person you are interviewing is the person responsible for cleaning the litter tray
   d. Amount and frequency of urination:
      – As for (c)
   e. Changes in activity level:
      – Kittens should be very active and playful whereas a young adult will be less so.
      – Have they noticed any changes in how the cat moves, jumps (up or down) or climbs (up or down)?
   f. Changes in grooming:
      – A decrease may reflect illness, pain, dehydration
      – An increase may reflect anxiety, pain
   g. Changes in interactions with people or other animals.

An example of a history form is given on page 16.

Examination

It is important first to watch the cat from a distance to see how it is moving and how it is interacting with the environment and the owner. Temperature, pulse, respiration rate and blood pressure may be ascertained immediately, or postponed until after the examination has been completed if the patient is anxious.

Every cat should undergo a nutritional assessment, including **bodyweight** and **body condition score** (Figure 1.20). As ill or injured cats preferentially lose lean body tissue (protein), a **muscle condition score** may also be useful (Figure 1.21). By 12–15 months of age, a cat should reach its adult weight. By noting slight changes in weight, either increases or decreases, one can follow trends and hopefully avert significant problems such as lipidosis or obesity, and detect malabsorption of nutrients or catabolism of cancer at an earlier stage.

One simple technique for detecting subtle changes in weight is measuring bodyweight at every visit and calculating the percentage change:

$$\% \text{ change} = \frac{\text{previous weight} - \text{current weight}}{\text{previous weight}} \times 100$$

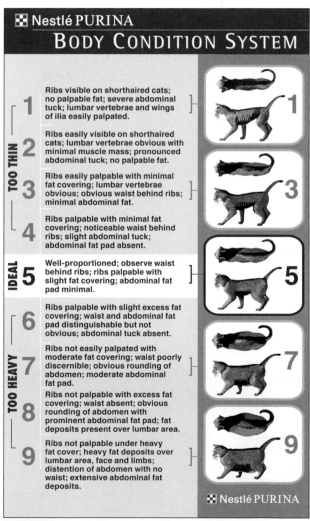

1.20 9-point body condition scale for cats. (© Nestlé Purina PetCare and reproduced with their permission)

3 Normal muscle mass
Muscles are easily palpated over the tempo-ral bones, ribs, lumbar vertebrae, and pelvis bones. No bony prominences are visible when the patient is viewed from a distance.

2 Moderate muscle wasting
Upon palpation, a thin layer of muscle covering the temporal bones, ribs, lumbar vertebrae, and pelvic bones is present. Bony prominences are slightly visible from a distance.

1 Marked/severe muscle wasting
No muscle covering the temporal bones, ribs, lumbar vertebrae, and pelvic bones is present upon palpation. Bony prominences are highly visible from a distance.

Overcoat syndrome
Clinically, body condition score (BCS) and MCS are not directly related because of the over-coat syndrome. This syndrome occurs when an animal has less muscle and more fat, mak-ing an MCS of 1 or 2 look relatively normal. Suspect the overcoat syndrome when the his-tory and physical examination findings do not match. Palpation is required for a diagnosis of overcoat syndrome. Although some areas of the body may feel relatively normal (as shown at right), marked wasting is felt over bony prominences.

skin
fat
muscle
bone

Overcoat

1.21   Determining muscle condition score. (Reproduced with permission from Buffington *et al.*, 2004.)

Handling

Again, it is important to allow the cat to maintain a sense of control, and to use appropriate non-threatening body language, minimal restraint (see QRG 1.2), and react appropriately to changes in the cat's body language if it begins to feel distressed.

This author chooses to sit on the floor with her patients in the nest made by her legs and facing away from her (Figure 1.22) or in the base of their carrier (see Figure 1.6). Another approach is to examine the cat on the client's lap or, if a table must be used, keeping the cat in its carrier so that it has some familiar smells surrounding it.

PRACTICAL TIPS

- Regardless of positioning, remember to face the cat away from you so that you are less like an aggressive cat staring at them
- The best place to examine a cat is the place he/she wants to be

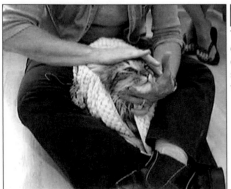

1.22

The author examining a cat while seated on the floor.

Physical examination

As with any other species, performing the physical examination in a standardized manner ensures that nothing will be overlooked. Using an examination sticker (Figure 1.23) or sheet (see example on page 17) helps by making sure everything is recorded. When a cat is frightened, the order of the examination may need to change to reduce stress. If the patient shows signs of pain during examination (see Chapter 3), it is necessary to re-evaluate the site to which the discomfort appeared to be related in order to verify whether pain is present.

Physical Exam

1) Attitude/Appearance	2) Oral Cavity/Teeth	3) Mucous Membranes	4) Integumentory
☐N ☐A ☐NE	☐N ☐A ☐NE	☐N ☐A ☐NE	☐N ☐A ☐NE
		Colour _____	
BCS _____ /9	Breath odour _____	CRT _____ SEC	Skin tent: Present ☐
		Moisture _____	Absent ☐
5) Eyes	6) Ears	7) Cardiovascular	8) Respiratory
☐N ☐A ☐NE	☐N ☐A ☐NE	☐N ☐A ☐NE	☐N ☐A ☐NE
9) Gastrointestinal	10) Musculoskeletal	11) Lymph Nodes	12) Urogenital
☐N ☐A ☐NE	☐N ☐A ☐NE	☐N ☐A ☐NE	☐N ☐A ☐NE
13) Nervous System	14) Pain ☐Y	Cuff	
☐N ☐A ☐NE	_____/10 ☐N	BP _____ Size _____ Limb _____	

T _____ PR _____ HR _____ RR _____ Wt _____ % wt Δ _____

Fed ☐ AM ☐ PM ☐ Free choice

Diet _____

☐ Indoors ☐ Outdoors ☐ Contact with others _____	N = Normal
	A = Abnormal
	NE = Not Examined

1.23   Using an adhesive examination sticker in the medical record ensures that nothing is overlooked during an examination. It becomes part of the record, as opposed to a longer sheet that may fall out.

1. Start the physical examination at the head, but do so from behind the cat. Evaluate the overall appearance and symmetry.
2. Look at the eyes and eyelids; using the ophthalmoscope, look at the fundus, lens, iris and anterior chamber (see QRG 1.3).
3. Check for discharge at, and symmetry of, the nostrils.
4. Stroke the nose, cheeks and forehead to feel for lumps and excoriations.
5. Lift each lip to look at the teeth. Check mucous membrane colour and moisture, and capillary refill time.
6. Open the mouth to look at the position and state of the tongue, gums and oropharynx; place a finger between the mandibular rami elevating the tongue to look underneath it. Smell the breath. (See QRG 1.4).
7. Palpate the submandibular lymph nodes and salivary glands and feel along the jaw for lumps.
8. Palpate the neck region, including along the trachea deep to the thoracic inlet for asymmetry or enlargements that might reflect thyroid gland changes. This may be done in cats of all ages but must be included in the examination of any mature cat over 7–8 years of age.
9. Using an otoscope, examine the ear canals of the cat, looking also for any obvious debris around the ear. If there are ear mites and you let the otoscope's light warm the ear canal for a while the mites will start to move.

10. Auscultate the thorax. The cat provides some unique anatomical characteristics that should be considered (see QRG 1.5).
11. Palpate the abdomen, imagining what each structure should feel like and where it should lie. Start by feeling the right and left kidneys; the right one should be located more cranially than the left.
12. With your fingers behind the ribcage, feel for the liver margins; they should have crisp rather than rounded margins and be almost tucked under the ribcage.
13. Slide your hand underneath the ventral abdomen, reaching your fingers dorsally. Gently pressing them together and pulling downwards, you should feel the loops of intestine slip through your fingers. Normal bowel loops slide easily and are thin, approximately 1 mm in thickness. The descending colon lies parallel to and just below the lumbar spine.
14. Assess the consistency of the contents of both small and large intestines. Note any generalized or regional thickening of bowel walls.
15. With your hand in the same position, identify the bladder in the caudal ventral abdomen.
16. Check whether any abdominal lymph nodes are obvious. Assess regional lymph nodes (groin, popliteal, axillary). Normally they are very small and rather flat.
17. Palpate each limb for swelling or pain.
18. Look at the perineal region: check the anal gland openings, vagina or prepuce, and rectal area.
19. Lastly, assess skin elasticity over the scapular area. Leave this to last because it may be misinterpreted as an attempt to control or subjugate if the cat is fearful. Pick up a tent of skin and twist it 180 degrees; release it promptly. In a young or adult well hydrated cat, the skin should 'snap' back quickly into its original place. Any delay is indicative of dehydration; the longer the delay, the greater degree of dehydration is present. In neonates and in elderly cats this test is not as useful and stool consistency may be a more reliable assessment of hydration.

A full neurological examination can be performed if indicated (see QRG 1.6). Practical tips for blood sampling are given in QRG 1.7.

Normal clinical parameters
Normal values on clinical examination are listed in Figure 1.24.

References, further reading and resources

Buffington CA, Holloway C and Abood K (2004) *Manual of Veterinary Dietetics.* Saunders, St. Louis.
Carney H, Little S, Brownlee-Tomasso D *et al.* (2012) AAFP and ISFM feline-friendly nursing care guidelines. *Journal of Feline Medicine and Surgery* **14**, 337–349 [also available at www.catvets.com and www.isfm.net]
Garosi LS (2005) Neurological examination. In: *BSAVA Manual of Canine and Feline Neurology, 3rd edn,* ed. S Platt and N Olby, pp. 1–23. BSAVA Publications, Gloucester
Garosi LS (2009) Neurological examination of the cat: how to get started. *Journal of Feline Medicine and Surgery* **11**, 340–348
Gourkow N (2004) *The Emotional Life of Cats: A Manual for Improving the Psychological Well-being of Shelter Cats.* BCSPCA, Vancouver
Leyhausen P (1979) *Cat Behaviour.* Garland STMP Press, New York
Mould JRB (2002) Ophthalmic examination. In: *BSAVA Manual of Canine and Feline Ophthalmology, 2nd edn,* ed. S Petersen-Jones and S Crispin, pp. 1–12. BSAVA Publications, Gloucester
Rochlitz I (2009) Basic requirements for good behavioural health and welfare in cats. In: *BSAVA Manual of Canine and Feline Behavioural Medicine,* ed. D Horwitz and D Mills, pp. 35–48. BSAVA Publications, Gloucester [a selection of client handouts is available to members at www.bsava.com]
Rodan I, Sundahl E, Carney H *et al.* (2011) AAFP and ISFM feline-friendly handling guidelines. *Journal of Feline Medicine and Surgery* **13**, 364–375 (also available at www.catvets.com and www.isfm.net)

Useful websites

American Association of Feline Practitioners (www.catvets.com) – contains information about the Cat Friendly Practice scheme, amongst a wealth of other further information on feline topics, including free downloads of the AAFP/ISFM feline friendly handling and nursing care guidelines
CATalyst Council (www.catalystcouncil.org) – contains helpful videos on different aspects of cat handling
Feline Advisory Bureau (www.fabcats.org) – contains useful information, particularly for owners, breeders and boarding catteries
International Society of Feline Medicine (www.isfm.net) – contains information about the Cat Friendly Clinic accreditation scheme, amongst a wealth of other further information on all feline topics, including free downloads of the AAFP/ISFM feline friendly handling and handling and nursing care guidelines

Parameter	Reference values
Body temperature	38.0–39.2°C
Heart rate	120–180 beats/min in clinic; may be lower at home. Pulse rate should be the same as heart rate
Respiration rate	24–36 breaths/min in clinic; at home 16–30 breaths/min
Body condition score (BCS)	4/9 to 5/9
Capillary refill time (CRT)	<2 seconds
Systolic blood pressure (BP)	120–150 mmHg is normal; agitation may or may not cause this to be increased (see Chapter 5.18)
Skin tenting	In young and adult cats, there should be no delay in skin elasticity. Kittens and elderly cats often have a delay in skin elasticity

1.24 Normal findings on clinical examination of an adult cat.

Clinical history

WellCat *for life*

Date: .... Case number: .... Cat's name: ....

Owner's name: .... Clinician: ....

BACKGROUND

Age: .... Sex: .... Breed: .... Time in owner's possession: ....

Acquired from: ☐ Breeder ☐ Rescue centre ☐ Other: ....

Other cats: ☐ No ☐ Yes How many? .... Any problems? ....

HABITAT

Environment: ☐ Indoor ☐ Indoor/Outdoor ☐ Limited outdoors ☐ In at night ☐ Outdoor only

Litter tray: ☐ No ☐ Yes Type of litter used: ....

Cat fighting: ☐ No ☐ Yes ....

Hunting: ☐ No ☐ Yes ....

Access to toxins: ☐ No ☐ Yes ....

NUTRITION

Last fed: .... am/pm

Diet: ☐ Dry cat food ☐ Wet cat food ☐ Both ☐ Other ....

Food type/brand normally fed: ....

Favourite foods or dislikes: ....

ROUTINE PREVENTIVE HEALTHCARE

Vaccinations: ☐ FHV/FCV/FPV ☐ FeLV

Last vaccination given: ☐ ≤15 months ☐ <36 months ☐ >36 months ☐ Never ☐ Unknown

Worming (which product and when): ....

Flea treatment (which product and when): ....

Retrovirus status: ☐ FeLV+ ☐ FeLV– ☐ FIV+ ☐ FIV– When: ....

PREVIOUS PROBLEMS

....

....

....

CURRENT PROBLEMS

....

....

....

CURRENT STATUS

Attitude/demeanour: ....

Appetite: .... Thirst: ....

Urination: .... Defecation: ....

Any vomiting? ....

Respiratory signs (coughing, breathing difficulty, sneezing, nasal discharge): ....

Mobility: ....

Behaviour: ....

An example of a clinical history sheet. (© Feline Advisory Bureau/ISFM)

Physical examination

WellCat *for life*

Date: .... Case number: .... Cat's name: ....

Owner's name: .... Clinician: ....

Temperature: .... Pulse rate: .... Respiratory rate: ....

1 BODYWEIGHT
Current (kg): .... Previous (and date): .... % change: ....

2 BODY CONDITION SCORE
☐ 1 Very thin ☐ 2 Underweight ☐ 3 Ideal weight ☐ 4 Overweight ☐ 5 Obese

3 ATTITUDE
☐ Bright and alert ☐ Quiet but alert ☐ Lethargic ☐ Dull ☐ Hyperactive

☐ Other: ....

4 FACE
☐ Normal ☐ Head tilt ☐ Abnormal (eg, wounds, swelling, asymmetry) ....

5 EYES
☐ Fully open, bright, clear of discharge, swelling and redness

☐ Pupils normal size, symmetrical, normal pupillary light reflex

Conjunctiva and sclera: ☐ Normal ☐ Pale ☐ Hyperaemic ☐ Icteric

Abnormalities (cornea, iris, lens): ....

Retinal exam required? ☐ No ☐ Yes Findings: ....

6 EARS
☐ Normal ☐ Abnormal (smell, discharge, wax, mites): ....

Otoscope examination required? ☐ No ☐ Yes: ....

7 NOSE
☐ Normal ☐ Abnormal (swelling, asymmetry, discharge – one or both nostrils, purulent/

serous/haemorrhagic): ....

8 HYDRATION
Skin tenting: ☐ Normal ☐ Abnormal

Mucous membranes: ☐ Normal ☐ Dry/tacky % Dehydrated: ....

9 MOUTH
Dentition: ☐ Deciduous ☐ Adult Abnormal eruption? ☐ Yes ☐ No

Tartar: ☐ Mild ☐ Moderate ☐ Severe

Gingivitis: ☐ Mild ☐ Moderate ☐ Severe

Stomatitis: ☐ Mild ☐ Moderate ☐ Severe

Tongue: ☐ Normal ☐ Abnormal (ulcers, masses, foreign bodies wrapped around)

Palate: ☐ Normal ☐ Abnormal (ulcers, masses, foreign bodies)

Pharynx and tonsils: ☐ Normal ☐ Abnormal (inflammation, foreign bodies, masses)

10 MUCOUS MEMBRANES
☐ Pink ☐ Pale ☐ Icteric ☐ Congested

Capillary refill time: ☐ Normal ☐ Abnormal: ....

11 SUPERFICIAL LYMPH NODES
Submandibular: ☐ Not palpable ☐ Palpable ☐ Enlarged

Prescapular: ☐ Not palpable ☐ Palpable ☐ Enlarged

Popliteal: ☐ Not palpable ☐ Palpable ☐ Enlarged

12 NECK
Palpable goitre: ☐ No ☐ Yes ⇒ ☐ Unilateral ☐ Bilateral

Size and position: ....

13 RESPIRATORY TRACT
Respiratory rate and effort, noise: ☐ Normal ☐ Abnormal ....

Anterior rib spring: ☐ Normal ☐ Reduced

Percussion: ☐ Normal ☐ Dullness ☐ Increased resonance

Auscultation: ☐ Normal ☐ Abnormal (wheezes, crackles, increased lung sounds)

14 CARDIOVASCULAR SYSTEM
Heart rate: ....

Heart apex beat: ☐ Normal ☐ Abnormal (displaced? any thrill?)

Rate/rhythm: ☐ Bradycardia ☐ Tachycardia ☐ Gallop ☐ Dysrhythmia

Murmur: ☐ No ☐ Yes ⇒ grade: ..../VI Systolic/diastolic

Point of maximum intensity? L/R, base/apex

Pulse: ☐ Normal ☐ Weak ☐ Bounding ☐ Deficits

Difference between L and R pulses? ☐ Yes ☐ No

15 ABDOMEN
Compression: ☐ Normal ☐ Abnormal (mass, pain)

Liver: ☐ Normal ☐ Abnormal (enlarged, mass, firm/soft, irregular, pain)

Kidneys: ☐ Normal ☐ Abnormal (inc/dec size, irregular, unequal size, firm, pain)

Intestines: ☐ Normal ☐ Abnormal (abnormal contents, mass, pain)

Bladder: ☐ Normal ☐ Abnormal (loss of tone, very firm, distended, thickened, painful)

☐ Other findings (eg, masses, pain): ....

16 COAT AND SKIN (mark abnormalities on diagrams)
☐ Coat normal

☐ Abnormal (hair loss, flea dirt, dandruff): ....

☐ Skin normal

☐ Abnormal (nodules, swellings, lumps): ....

ventral   dorsal

17 MUSCULOSKELETAL SYSTEM
☐ No concerns

☐ Other (weakness, stiffness, lameness): ....

Further assessment required? ☐ No ☐ Yes: ....

18 CENTRAL AND PERIPHERAL NERVOUS SYSTEMS
☐ No concerns ☐ Other: ....

Further assessment required? ☐ No ☐ Yes: ....

SUMMARY (problems, differentials, treatment and monitoring)

ADDITIONAL FINDINGS

An example of a physical examination sheet. (© Feline Advisory Bureau/ISFM)

QRG 1.1 Calculation of energy requirements for ill cats

by Marge Chandler

Calculation of an ill hospitalized cat's energy requirements begins with estimation of the **resting energy requirement** (RER), which estimates the cat's calorie (kcal) requirements at rest in a thermoneutral environment. Energy requirements are expressed as kilocalories (kcal) of metabolizable energy (ME) or joules (J) of ME (where 1 J = 4.18 kcal).

For any cat:
$$RER_{(kcal/day)} = bodyweight^{0.75}_{(kg)} \times 70$$

For cats >2 kg, the following estimation can be used:
$$RER_{(kcal/day)} = (30 \times bodyweight_{(kg)}) + 70$$

For both calculations, the actual current bodyweight is used, not the patient's ideal bodyweight.

Previously, the RER was multiplied by a factor of 1.2 to 2.0 to obtain an **illness energy requirement** (**IER**) to provide the extra calories thought to be necessary for the hypermetabolism of illness or injury. However, energy requirements in hospitalized dogs and people are actually very similar to RER levels, and it is assumed that this is also the case for hospitalized cats, with certain exceptions. Human patients whose energy needs are known to be 1.2–2.0 times RER include those with head trauma and severe burns. Cats with hyperthyroidism are also likely to have elevated energy requirements, although this has not been studied.

In a patient that has not been eating for several days, neither enteral nor parenteral supplementation should be started immediately at full RER:

1. On Day 1 provide about 1/3 of the RER, divided into several small meals or tube-fed boluses.
2. If this is well tolerated, 2/3 of the RER is fed on the Day 2.
3. The full RER is given from Day 3.

For cats that are **overweight**, a weight loss programme should not be initiated until the cat is otherwise healthy. Animals that are ill or injured catabolize protein as an energy source, and this may be especially true for cats as even when healthy they use more protein for energy than do dogs or people. A fat ill or injured cat that is losing weight will also lose more protein, which compromises the immune system, the cardiovascular system, and the ability to heal.

QRG 1.2 Handling techniques for simple procedures

by Suzanne Rudd

It is vital for the clinician to be aware that the most successful handling and restraint for procedures relies not just on the way the cat is handled or restrained for the particular procedure, but on having taken prior measures to ensure that the cat is as relaxed as possible prior to beginning handling for the procedure, as discussed in this chapter. The importance of this cannot be emphasized enough and it will make a significant difference to handling cats for procedures.

Furthermore, it is essential that the environment in which the cat is being handled and having procedures performed, is kept as quiet as possible, with no other animals and minimal personnel nearby. Sudden noises and movements should be avoided, and nervous cats provided with the opportunity to partially hide whenever possible. If these basic guidelines are adhered to, the majority of cats will allow simple procedures to be performed with very minimal restraint.

The most minimal restraint possible should always be attempted first. The heavier the restraint used, the more likely the cat will resist. If a cat needs slightly firmer restraint, first consider the positioning on the table. Cats can be held more securely at the edge and end of a table than in the middle of it. The cat should be allowed to sit calmly on a non-slip surface or, preferably, a blanket.

Blood sampling

Blood sampling can often be performed with very minimal restraint; sometimes the most wriggly cats will allow blood sampling without their legs even being held. However, the safety of the handler(s) and sampler is vital, and every cat should be judged on an individual basis. Many cats will require more restraint, but still with minimal force so that they can feel in control, safe and secure. Holding a cat's legs for blood sampling can still be done in a way that the cat feels safe and secure, simply by placing an index finger between the forelimbs so that they are not squeezed together and allowing the cat to have all four feet on the table. Many cats do not like being lifted and so ensuring all four feet are on solid ground will increase the cat's feeling of security enormously. Blood sampling technique (see QRG 1.7) is also important in maintaining the cat in a relaxed demeanour.

Note: If the handler is right-handed it is generally easier to hold the cat to their right side; if left-handed, restraint will be easier holding the cat to the left side of the body. The following guidelines are written for right-sided restraint and should be reversed for holding the cat to the handler's left side.

Jugular vein

Standard positioning

- Having followed the general guidelines for ensuring that the cat is as relaxed as possible, very minimal restraint should be tried first.

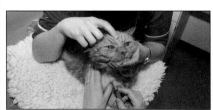

The handler has positioned herself so that the cat is in front of them, with their body leaning over the cat's body and their forearm tucking the cat's hindquarters in towards them. The cat is facing away from the handler. This makes the cat feel secure and prevents it from walking backwards, without any restraint as such. Leaving the cat's limbs unrestrained may be possible in some cats. Often gentle stroking on the top of the head or bridge of the nose can also help to keep cats relaxed during blood sampling. ▶

QRG 1.2 *continued*

- Some cats will prefer to sit within a bed with sides or a sack-type bed, so that the bed itself is providing the restraint rather than the handler. This is particularly worth trying in cats that are hospitalized and already using such a bed, as it allows them to be lifted out of the cage within the bed and not have to be removed from the bed before, during or after the procedure.
- Some nervous cats will be much more relaxed if they are allowed to hide their head underneath a blanket held by the handler.
- If slightly more control of the limbs is required and the cat reacts adversely to having its limbs held, gentle restraint within a blanket or towel may be achievable.

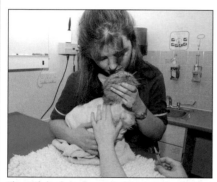

The cat's body is covered with a towel and the cat held gently so that its limbs are still relatively unrestrained, rather than being firmly wrapped in the towel.

- Or slightly more restraint may be required.

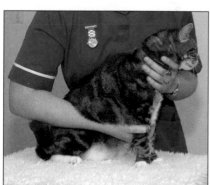

The handler places their right arm around the hindquarters of the cat and uses their right hand to slowly take hold of its forelimbs. The forelimbs are approached from the caudal aspect of the limbs, with the thumb wrapping around the right forelimb, index finger between the limbs, and second finger wrapping around the left forelimb. The forelimbs are held midway along the radius and ulna, as too close towards the paws will irritate the cat. The cat's feet should be allowed to rest on the table, as this will give the cat a greater feeling of security than placing its feet over the table edge. The handler's left hand is used to hold the cat's head by placing the index, middle and ring fingers under the cat's mandible and the thumb behind the cat's skull.

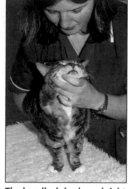

The handler's body and right shoulder are rotated slightly over the top of the cat's body, whilst using the right elbow to tuck in the cat's hindquarters towards the handler's body. This should be close and in line with the cat's back, but no pressure should be put on the back. The cat's head is elevated slightly to allow access for the blood sampler. When the blood sample is about to be taken, the middle and ring fingers may need to be lifted slightly to allow the blood sampler better visualization of the vein. It may also be necessary to increase the grip around the mandible with the index finger, to ensure better control of the head.

- For further control the handler may wish to bring their head further towards the top of the cat's head; however, **this should only be done with extreme caution** and if the handler is confident that they know how the cat is going to respond.

Upside down technique

This technique is useful for cats that jump during needle insertion, and/or when applying local anaesthetic cream to the venepuncture site has failed to help blood sampling. It is also useful in kittens and brachycephalic breeds, where holding the head in the correct position can be more challenging.

Bedding material or a blanket must always be placed on the table for this technique, to provide comfort for the cat's spine.

As with the standard technique, the cat should be restrained at the end of the table rather than in the middle to allow for better control. The cat is allowed to sit on the blanket, and the handler's right arm used to wrap around its hindquarters, holding the forelimbs with the right hand**.** The cat is brought into the handler's body for extra control.

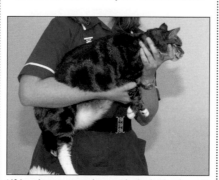

Lifting the cat up and towards the body; the cat should rest on the forearm.

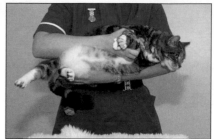

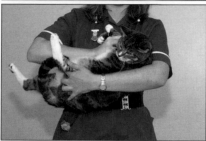

The cat is turned over slowly and smoothly, letting go of its head so that the cat then moves on to the handler's left forearm. They should still be holding the cat's forelimbs with the right hand.

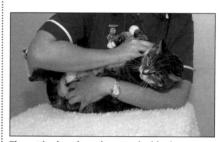

The cat is placed gently on to the blanket, wrapping the right arm around its hindquarters whilst still holding the forelimbs with the right hand.

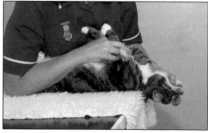

The left arm is slid out from the back of the cat's head, and the head taken hold of again by placing the thumb across the mandible and the fingers around the top of the cat's head. The blood sampler may prefer the handler to continue to hold the cat's head whilst they raise the vein and take the sample.

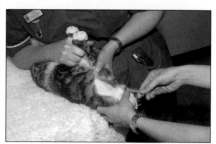

Alternatively, the blood sampler may wish to take hold of the cat's head themselves, allowing the handler to raise the jugular vein with their left hand.   ▶

QRG 1.2 *continued*

Dyspnoeic cats

Minimal but effective restraint is used, ensuring that the cat's mouth is not held closed and thereby giving it the opportunity to breathe through its mouth. The handler is positioned slightly further back to the rear of the cat and their right arm placed around the cat's body and forelimbs (see above).

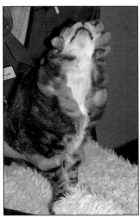

The handler takes hold of the cat's head from above the skull with the left hand. The thumb and index finger can grip around the cat's zygomatic arches and then tilt the head slightly upwards. This restraining technique will not feel as controlled as the others described, but it will allow the cat to breathe effectively, making it less stressful for it and thereby facilitating blood sampling by increasing the likelihood of staying still.

Cephalic vein catheterization

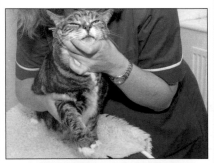

The handler wraps their right arm around the cat's hindquarters and extends the cat's right forelimb by placing fingers behind the cat's elbow and the thumb over the dorsal aspect of the cat's radius. The left hand should hold the cat's head by holding its mandible with the index finger and placing the thumb behind the head. Ideally the cat's left forelimb should be placed on the table unrestrained.

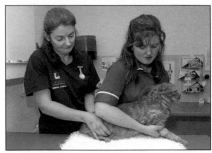

If there is risk of injury due to not restraining the left forelimb, this can be held by the little finger on the right hand, hooking the left forelimb underneath the right forelimb.

Blood pressure measurement

Techniques for measuring blood pressure are described in QRG 5.18.1.

Forelimb

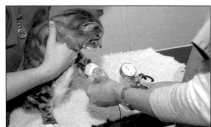

The cat can be held as for cephalic catheterization (above), but more relaxed restraint can be used and the cat's forelimb does not need to be extended as far forward. Some cats prefer their forelimb to be left down on the table and unrestrained; this method should be tried if they react to their forelimb being held off the table. The cat's head also does not need to be restrained; the cat can be prevented from moving forward by gently supporting its chest.

Some cats that are relaxed within a bed with sides or the bottom half of a cat carrier will allow blood pressure measurement *in situ* without any additional restraint. It is preferable to try this first, as sometimes these cats will become more resistant if any restraint is attempted.

Tail

Some cats tolerate blood pressure measurement better using the tail, whilst other cats may dislike their tail being handled. For cats that tolerate it well, this method can allow blood pressure assessment with very little restraint.

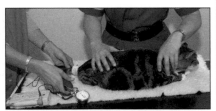

The handler's hands can be placed gently over the cat's shoulders and hindquarters to prevent sudden jumping or movement, though even less restraint may be needed in very relaxed cats. Placing the cat on a comfortable bed always encourages it to settle more than when placed on a bare table.

Lateral recumbency

When restraining a cat in lateral recumbency it is advisable to have two people for the restraint: one for the front half of the cat, and the other for the back half. Soft bedding or a blanket should be used for the cat to lie on for comfort.

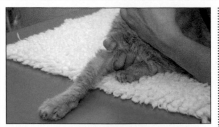

The cat should be turned with the cat standing across the body of handler 1, who should take hold of the forelimbs with one hand and place their other hand under the cat's chin for support and safety. Handler 2 should take hold of the hindlimbs.

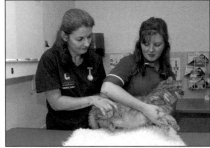

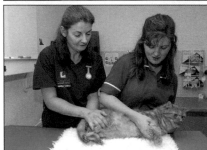

The cat is gently turned over into lateral recumbency. If tolerated, handler 1 can adjust the restraint of the legs by holding them separately and allowing the cat to rest its head on their arm. Both handlers should always hold the cat's legs midway along the limbs, as cats are often very sensitive to having their paws touched.

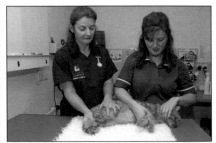

If the cat is less cooperative or there is a risk of injury to the handler, the forelimbs can be held in one hand whilst the other hand is gently placed across the cat's neck and fingers under the mandible. ▶

QRG 1.2 *continued*

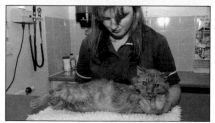

When less restraint is required, cats will often be more relaxed if they are able to have some free head movement, as this allows them to feel more in control and therefore more relaxed. It is possible to restrain a relaxed cat effectively with a single handler. However, it is preferable to have two handlers to allow gentle restraint whilst also being able to provide comfort by gently stroking the top of the cat's head and bridge of the nose; stroking in this way will often even result in cats going to sleep during ultrasonography.

Medial saphenous vein catheterization

Restraint for this procedure should be approached using the same technique as for restraining in lateral recumbency (see above).

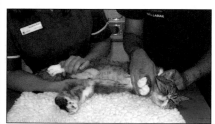

Handler 1 can hold the forelimbs in one hand leaving the other hand to restrain the head as necessary. Handler 2 should hold the hindlimbs separately, ensuring that the uppermost hindlimb is either flexed or extended slightly caudally to allow good visualization of the medial aspect of the lower hindlimb. To extend the leg and raise the medial saphenous vein, handler 2 must hold the lower hindlimb above the stifle and take a careful but firm grip around the femur. An alternative is for a single handler to allow the cranial part of the cat to remain in sternal recumbency (see Figure 1.17), whilst the person placing the catheter extends and holds the hindlimb.

Thoracocentesis

Restraint for thoracocentesis should be done with extreme care so as not to cause excessive stress to the cat, especially as dyspnoea may be present. Thoracocentesis technique is described in QRG 4.2.4.

The cat should be provided with something comfortable to sit on, such as soft bedding or a blanket. The cat is encouraged to lie down in sternal recumbency by gently sliding the forelimbs forward or using other tactics such as stroking the cat down its back to encourage it to settle in that position. Using excessive force to get the cat to lie down will usually only result in resistance and increased stress. Note that sedation may be required for this procedure if the cat becomes distressed (see Chapter 3).

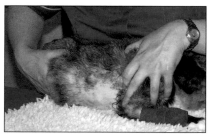

The cat should be lying across the handler's body so that they can use their body to support the cat and aid restraint. One hand should be placed across the shoulders of the cat whilst using the fingers to gently slide and keep the forelimb forward. The other hand should be used to support the hindlimbs and to keep the cat close to the handler's body. It may be useful for the handler to lean over the cat slightly for further restraint so that it does not jump as the needle is inserted.

Procedures performed in a standing position

As noted above, most cats will be more relaxed if their paws can remain on the table, and therefore some cats will tolerate procedures better if allowed to stand using minimal restraint, rather than being restrained in lateral recumbency. Suitability will be dependent on the procedure being performed and the cat's individual preference.

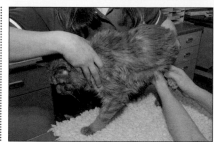

Performing cystocentesis (see QRG 4.11.4). The handler uses her hands across the shoulders and around the hindquarters to keep the cat's body close to her. Very little pressure is put on the cat but having the handler's hands in this position does help to prevent the cat from jumping as the needle enters the abdominal cavity. If needed, the handler's left hand can also be used to hold the cat's left hindlimb caudally if access to the bladder is not easy.

WARNING

Whilst minimal restraint is advised, it should be ensured that the procedure can be performed safely while the needle is in the abdominal cavity.

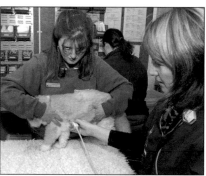

Performing cursory thoracic ultrasonography on a cat with respiratory difficulties, looking for signs such as the presence of pleural fluid. Here the handler uses her hands across the cat's shoulders and around its hindquarters to gently keep the cat's body close to her. Very little pressure is put on the cat, so that stress and further respiratory compromise are avoided.

QRG 1.3 Examining the eye
by Natasha Mitchell

Eye examination is best carried out using a systematic step-by-step approach, in a quiet examination room that can be darkened when required. The patient should be minimally restrained. It is preferable to avoid sedation as it causes the third eyelids to protrude, hindering examination, and also alters test results. Cats that resist may be wrapped, burrito-style, in a towel. **Both eyes should be examined, even when only one appears to be abnormal.** More details on ophthalmic examination can be found in the *BSAVA Guide to Procedures in Small Animal Practice* and the *BSAVA Manual of Canine and Feline Ophthalmology*.

Equipment

- Focal light source – penlight torch or Finhoff transilluminator
- Magnification – direct ophthalmoscope; otoscope; loupe
- Condensing lens 20 to 30 diopter
- Non-toothed forceps for examining behind the third eyelid

QRG 1.3 *continued*

- Tonometer (e.g. Schiøtz, Tonopen)
- Mydriatic (dilates pupils) – tropicamide 0.5% (single-use vials available)
- Fluorescein dye strips
- Topical local anaesthetic – proxymetacaine 0.5% single-use vials
- Schirmer tear test paper strips
- Swabs for bacterial culture and virus isolation
- Lacrimal cannulae (sterile disposable plastic or metal)

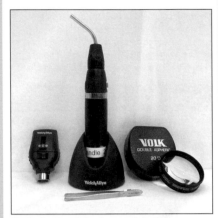

Clockwise from left: direct ophthalmoscope; Finhoff transilluminator; condensing lens; forceps.

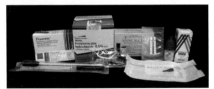

Disposables for ophthalmic examination.

Examination with the room lights on

While taking a thorough history the cat is allowed to acclimatize to the consulting room. Facial and eye symmetry is noted at this time, along with blepharospasm and ocular discharge.

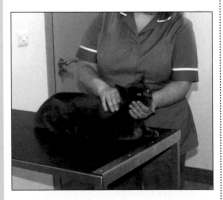

Close inspection of the eye and adnexa (periocular structures) is then carried out, using a focal light source. It is best to proceed from external to internal. The eyelids, conjunctiva, lacrimal punctae, cornea, anterior chamber, iris, pupil and lens are examined.

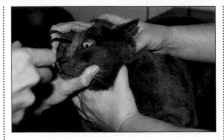

Neuro-ophthalmic examination

The neurological examination (see QRG 1.6) includes the following:

- **Menace response** – covering one eye at a time and taking care not to create wind currents. This tests: retina, optic nerve (cranial nerve (CN) II, sensory), contralateral optic tract and contralateral forebrain, ipsilateral cerebellum and facial nerve (CN VII, motor) to close eyelids. Absent in kittens <10–12 weeks.

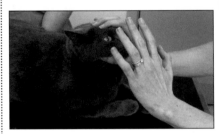

- **Pupillary light reflex (PLR)** – carried out while examining with the focal light source. This tests: retina, optic nerve (CN II, sensory) and parasympathetic section of oculomotor nerve (CN III, motor). Normally both pupils constrict equally and rapidly; the PLR in the eye being illuminated is the *direct* pupillary response, whilst that in the other pupil is the *consensual* response. The PLR is a subcortical reflex and may be normal in a cortically blind cat.
- **Palpebral reflex** – elicited by touching the medial canthus with a finger. Tests: maxillary division of trigeminal nerve (CN V, sensory) and its connection to the facial nerve (CN VII, motor) to cause a blink
- Like the PLR, the **dazzle reflex** is a subcortical reflex; it is a bilateral, partial blink in response to a bright light. The anatomical pathway is poorly understood but it requires functional retina, optic and facial nerves. It is a useful substitute for the menace response if there is an opacity in the visual axis (e.g. cataract).
- **Tracking response** is useful for assessing whether vision is absent or present. Cotton wool balls are dropped from a height beside the patient. A cat with normal vision will usually watch the ball fall; as this is noiseless it cannot be misinterpreted as use of the other senses. Cats can choose to ignore any stimulus however.

Examination with the room lights off (minimizes reflections)

Distant direct ophthalmoscopy

This involves observing the tapetal reflection from both eyes from an arm's distance away.

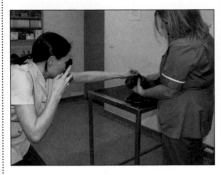

It is a very useful technique for quickly picking up abnormalities such as:

- Anisocoria (difference in pupil size)
- Absence of tapetal reflection (something in the way, e.g. cataract)
- Nuclear sclerosis/cataract: nuclear sclerosis does not obstruct the bright tapetal reflection, whereas a cataract causes a black shadow
- Focal opacities, e.g. corneal pigmentation
- Aphakic crescent; with lens luxation, a moon-shaped crescent of tapetal hyper-reflectivity can be seen.

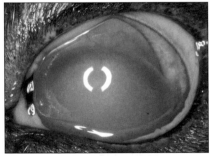

A large round white lens occupies the majority of the anterior chamber, due to a cataractous anterior lens luxation. A bright green crescent of tapetal reflection is present within the visible pupil above the ventrally positioned luxated lens; this aphakic crescent is pathognomonic for lens luxation.

Examination of anterior segment with magnification

Using the direct ophthalmoscope set at 12–20 diopters, or an otoscope or magnifying loupes, a more careful examination of the anterior segment is carried out. Attention is paid to finer details, such as distichia or ectopic cilia on the eyelids, opacities on the cornea, turbidity in the anterior chamber, etc. ▶

QRG 1.3 *continued*

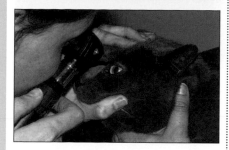

Examination of the fundus

Dilating the pupils with one drop of 0.5% tropicamide makes fundus examination much easier; it takes 20 minutes to take effect and has a duration of action of 4–12 hours.

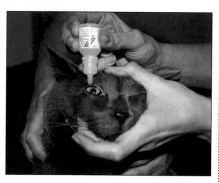

- Using **close direct ophthalmoscopy**, a magnified, upright image is obtained. The direct ophthalmoscope is used on the zero diopter setting and held as close to the observer's eye as possible. The light intensity should be reduced with the rheostat to minimize discomfort to the cat, and thereby improve cooperation. The observer needs to be as close to the cat's eye as possible to get a good image, ideally just 1–3 cm away. The optic nerve, retinal blood vessels and any fundus lesions can be seen in great detail, although the limited field of view makes examination difficult.

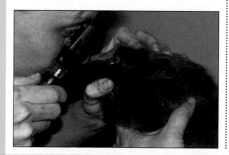

- Using a focal light source and condensing lens, **indirect ophthalmoscopy** allows for a much wider field of view so that the fundus is easier to examine. The technique needs to be practised; the image obtained is virtual and inverted but is easy to interpret. The handler gently holds the eyelids open and directs the gaze of the cat towards the observer. The observer positions themselves an arm's length from the eye and holds the light source next to their eye. The tapetal reflection is first obtained from the eye, and then the condensing lens is dropped into the plane of view (convex side towards the observer) approximately 2–4 cm in front of the cat's eye. The fundus image should fill the lens.

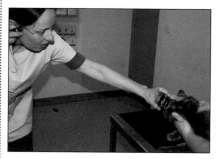

Additional diagnostic tests

Schirmer tear test

STT results are quite variable in cats, but a value of <10 mm wetting per minute is considered abnormal in the presence of ocular surface disease, such as ocular discharge, conjunctival hyperaemia or corneal opacities.

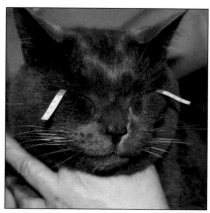

Fluorescein dye

Fluorescein is used to highlight corneal ulcers. It will not stain intact corneal epithelium or Descemet's membrane. Stain uptake indicates corneal stromal staining due to corneal ulceration. Since Descemet's membane does not take up the stain, a lack of uptake within an ulcer indicates descemetocele formation, an ocular emergency (see Chapter 8). Observing stain uptake is greatly enhanced by examining with a blue light. The dye should appear at the nares in 5–10 minutes. This confirms the patency of the nasolacrimal duct, and is termed a positive Jones test. The absence of fluorescein dye at the nares is not diagnostic for blockage of the nasolacrimal duct, as it may drain into the pharynx.

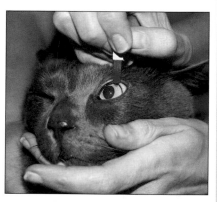

Tonometry

Measurement of intraocular pressure (IOP) is very useful for the diagnosis of glaucoma (raised IOP, usually >25 mmHg), uveitis (lowered IOP, usually <10 mmHg) and for monitoring response to treatment.

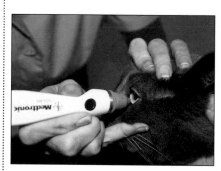

QRG 1.4 Examining the mouth in a conscious cat

by Lisa Milella

The aim of the conscious oral examination is to obtain a tentative diagnosis and help formulate a treatment plan. The cat is examined on a table with a non-slip surface. It is important to have good lighting when examining the mouth. Oral examination of a conscious animal is limited to visual inspection and some digital palpation. Gentle technique is essential, as some cats may have dental pain or discomfort. If the cat has painful areas in the mouth, examination may be difficult. The owner must be made aware that the mouth can only be fully examined, and the true extent of oral disease evaluated, with the cat under a general anaesthetic (see QRG 7.1).

1 Approach the cat from the side or from behind. Gently make contact with the cat and stroke its head prior to examining the mouth.

2 Examine the cat's head externally, assessing for any asymmetry. In cases of a tooth root abscess, for example, the area of the nose below the eye may be swollen; or in cases of an oral tumour, a swelling may be obvious on one side.

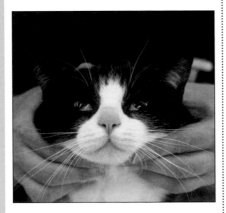

3 Gently palpate the facial muscles, facial bones and salivary glands.

4 Palpate the lymph nodes: the mandibular and retropharyngeal nodes at the angle of the jaw, as well as the cervical chain extending down the neck to the prescapular lymph node. The retropharyngeal lymph nodes may only be palpable if enlarged. An enlarged lymph node may indicate infection or inflammation.

5 Gently hold the jaws closed and retract the lips. Do **not** pull on the fur to retract the lips.

6 Lift the lips and examine the buccal surfaces of the teeth and oral mucosa.

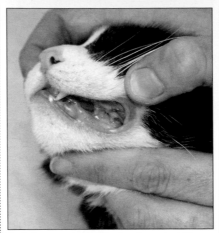

Technique used to lift the lips; here gingivitis with calculus accumulation is present.

7 Examine the occlusion. Is this normal for the breed or are there any signs of any soft tissue trauma due to malocclusion?
Check:

- The incisor relationship – the lower incisors should occlude palatal to the uppers. Occasionally brachycephalic breeds, such as Persians, have a reverse scissor bite, where the lower incisors occlude labial to the upper incisors
- The canine interlock – the lower canine should occlude in the diastema between the upper canine and third incisor

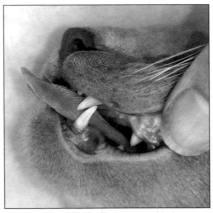

Canine malocclusion: the upper canine is too rostral; the lower canine is therefore occluding more lateral and distal than its normal position, resulting in the cusp catching the upper lip and causing ulceration.

- Premolar alignment – the teeth should interdigitate and the distal occlusion should be such that the mandibular premolars and molars occlude on the palatal surface of the maxillary premolars
- The position of individual teeth.

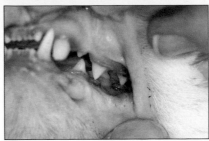

Soft tissue trauma to the gingival tissue of the mandible has resulted from a premolar malocclusion (common in British Shorthairs); the cusps of the maxillary premolars have caused ulceration of the mucosa. Note also the fractured upper left canine tooth.

8 Check the mucous membranes for inflammation and ulceration. Check for any swelling of the buccal mucous membranes, gingival tissues or oral mucosa. Is the gingival margin inflamed, swollen or receded?

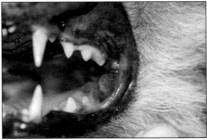

Swelling of the buccal mucosa resulting from contact of the maxillary fourth premolar on a non-healing extraction site.

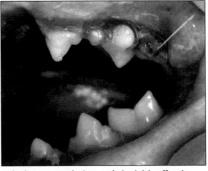

Calculus accumulation and gingivitis affecting the maxillary premolars.

9 Check for missing teeth or extra teeth. Check the crown for defects such as fractures or resorptive lesions (see Chapter 7). Check to see whether any of the teeth are mobile by digital manipulation. Check the calculus coverage on individual teeth *versus* the whole mouth.

10 Approach the cat from the side. Place one hand over the muzzle, with the forefinger and thumb placed ▶

QRG 1.4 *continued*

just behind the upper canine teeth. Press the lips gently into the oral cavity while tilting the head slightly upwards.

11 Place a finger from your other hand on the lower incisors and exert gentle pressure to open the mouth. Do **not** use the fur under the mandible to try to pull the jaw down.

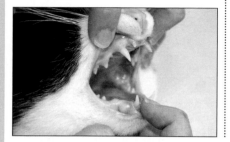

12 Examine the mucous membranes of the hard palate.

13 Examine the oropharynx (soft palate, palatoglossal arch, tonsillary crypts, tonsils and fauces) .

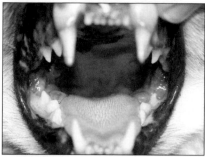

Inflamed lateral glossopalatine folds and caudal mucosa. Pus accumulation can be seen between the mandibular molars and buccal mucosa.

14 The lingual and palatal surfaces of the teeth can be briefly evaluated.

15 Gently place pressure externally between the mandibles to lift up the tongue and examine it.

QRG 1.5 Thoracic examination and auscultation
by Kerry Simpson

Equipment

The ideal stethoscope for auscultation of the cat has a small head, i.e. infant or paediatric stethoscope; although electronic stethoscopes can produce a comparable sound.

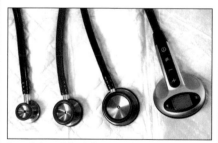

From left to right: infant, paediatric, Master Classic II, 3M electronic stethoscope.

Patient preparation

- Quiet room with minimal people present.
- The cat should be allowed to sit in a comfortable position, on a non-slip surface.

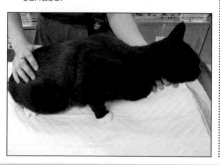

Technique

1 Palpate the thoracic wall for any traumatic injuries, masses or conformational abnormalities. Note the location and strength of the apex beat.

2 Assess chest compliance by gently compressing the cranial thorax between your fingers and thumb lateral-to-lateral. Some clinicians prefer to use both hands with fingers together. The thorax should be relatively 'springy', particularly in younger cats. A non-compliant thorax is expected in a very old cat, but can also indicate soft tissue masses (e.g. anterior mediastinal lymphoma) or fluid within the cranial thoracic cavity.

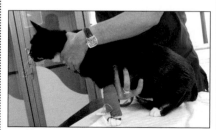

3 Auscultate the heart. The heart lies in a very sternal position in the cat, with the majority of murmurs being noted in the parasternal region; auscultation should include careful evaluation of this area. Therefore auscultation of both left and right parasternal regions, starting cranial to the forelimbs and gently moving the stethoscope caudally, can improve murmur detection. With

traditional stethoscopes, the diaphragm is the most useful side, auscultating the majority of sounds, whilst the bell is preferable for auscultation of low-frequency sounds.

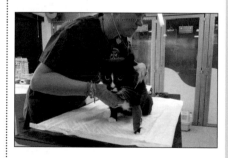

4 If gentle restraint is necessary, auscultating the heart whilst lifting the cat can alter the cat's focus for long enough to allow a thorough cardiac examination. Purring can sometimes occlude heart sounds. There are many tricks to stop purring; the author prefers to turn on a tap, lift the cat and, whilst listening to the heart, gently approach the tap still holding the cat. ▶

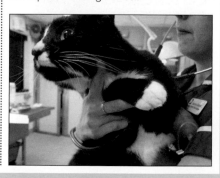

QRG 1.5 *continued*

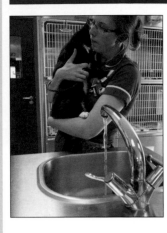

5 Note the cardiac rhythm. Normal and abnormal heart sounds are illustrated below.

6 Assess for pulse deficits by palpation of the femoral pulse (both left and right, sequentially) at the same time as auscultating the heart. Additionally, assess the timing and quality of a peripheral pulse (e.g. metatarsal).

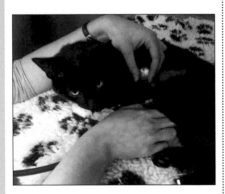

7 Inspect the jugular vein for signs of distension or pulsation. These may indicate increased right atrial pressure (distended and pulsatile) or pleural effusion (distended but not pulsatile).

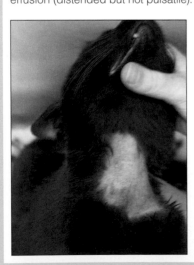

8 Auscultate the lungs using a grid approach (see Chapter 4.2) to assess the lung fields. Note the location of any adventitious lung sounds.

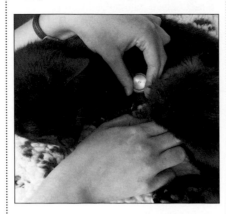

9 Percuss the thorax by placing the fingers of one hand flat on the cat's chest and tapping the middle finger with two fingers of the opposite hand, whilst running the finger in contact with the thoracic wall down the ribcage. The thorax should be resonant over the lung fields. Increased resonance can occur with air trapping (pneumothorax or asthma). Decreased resonance can occur with fluid or soft tissue masses within the thoracic cavity.

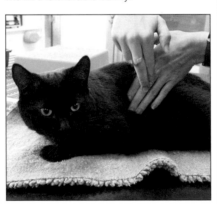

Normal heart sounds

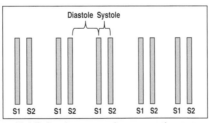

S1 ('lub'): first heart sound: occurs at the start of systole; associated with closure of the atrioventricular (mitral and tricuspid) valves.

S2 ('dub'): second heart sound: occurs at the end of systole; corresponds to closure of semilunar (aortic and pulmonic) valves but is due to vibrations produced by opening of the AV valves, early muscular relaxation and acceleration of blood in the great vessels.

Abnormal heart sounds

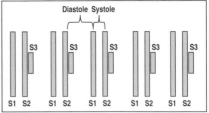

S3 ('dub'): third, but abnormal, heart sound: heard as a gallop sound immediately following S2 (dub), i.e. lub (S1)-pause-dub (S2) dub (S3). Sound is caused by early diastolic filling and cannot be heard in normal cats. An audible S3 implies poor compliance (as in restrictive cardiomopathy), mitral regurgitation or an accelerated filling velocity (as seen with high atrial pressures).

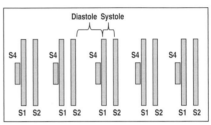

S4 ('le'): fourth, but abnormal, heart sound: produced by atrial systole. It is heard if the atrium contracts against a distended or non-compliant ventricle (as in volume overload). Therefore, it is audible as a gallop sound occurring immediately before the first heart sound (i.e. lelub-pause-dub). In addition, cats may present with combination gallops, in which both S3 and S4 can be heard.

Murmurs

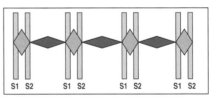

The majority of murmurs auscultated in cats are systolic ('lub-shush-dub'); they may be dynamic (present only at higher heart rates) or static. Generally the 'shape' of the murmur cannot be described, as the cat's heart rate is too high.

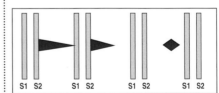

Diastolic and continuous murmurs are rare and typically represent severe and/or congenital disease. The most common cause of an early diastolic murmur is aortic regurgitation. Continuous murmurs are typically associated with congenital diseases such as patent ductus arteriosus.

QRG 1.6 Performing a neurological examination
by Laurent Garosi

A veterinary surgeon with limited experience may not be able to interpret neurological findings accurately, but being able to perform the neurological examination and record the findings is important as it then allows them to seek advice from a specialist and/or further information from other sources.

The aims of the neurological examination are:

- To assess whether the clinical signs observed refer to a nervous system lesion
- To determine the location of a lesion within the nervous system
- To aid consideration of what type of disease processes could explain the neurological signs
- To assess the severity of the neurological signs.

Hands-off examination

The cat should be permitted to walk freely on the floor of a quiet consulting room, to adapt to this new environment. This allows hands-off assessment of mentation, posture and gait, which can all give vital clues that may be missed if the cat is placed straight on the examination table.

State of consciousness, awareness and behaviour

Disturbances of state of consciousness are classified in order of increasing severity as:

- Depression
- Lethargy
- Obtundation
- Stupor (semicoma)
- Coma.

Common changes in the level of awareness and behaviour include:

- Disorientation
- Aggression
- Vocalizing
- Circling
- Compulsive walking
- Head pressing.

The owner is usually the best judge of subtle changes in the patient's behaviour in its normal environment and should be questioned about that. Home video recordings of any abnormal behaviour can also be very useful (see also Chapter 5.24).

Posture and body position at rest

Abnormal postures should be evaluated, e.g.:

- Head tilt – associated with vestibular disorders (see Chapter 5.16)
- Head turn – associated with ipsilateral forebrain lesions
- Ventroflexion of the neck – associated with neuromuscular disorders (e.g. hypokalaemic polymyopathy, myasthenia gravis), thiamine deficiency, or severe cervical spinal cord grey matter lesion
- Spinal curvature – kyphosis or lordosis.

Attention should also be given to:

- The position of joints
- Limb stance
- Tail posture
- Presence of voluntary tail movement.

Gait evaluation

The aim is to determine whether the cat is:

- Ataxic (uncoordinated)
- Paretic (weak)
- Lame.

Ataxia is defined as an uncoordinated gait and can arise from a peripheral nerve or spinal cord lesion (general proprioceptive ataxia), a vestibular lesion (vestibular ataxia) or a cerebellar lesion (cerebellar ataxia) (see Chapter 5.6).

Two qualities of **paresis** can be distinguished: upper motor neuron (UMN) and lower motor neuron (LMN) paresis.

- UMN paresis causes a delay in the onset of protraction, which is the swing phase of the gait. It is frequently associated with ataxia.
- LMN paresis reflects degrees of difficulty in supporting weight, and varies from a short stride to complete inability to support weight causing collapse of the limb whenever weight is placed on it. LMN paresis does not cause ataxia. Care must be taken, as many cats can have an apparent plantigrade stance (crouched posture) in a perceived hostile environment such as a consultation room.

Lameness may be caused by neuromuscular disease or by an orthopaedic disorder (see Chapter 5.23). The limb(s) involved should be noted.

Hands-on examination

Postural reactions

The aim is to detect subtle deficits that were not obvious on gait evaluation. This is best evaluated by hopping response, wheelbarrowing, extensor postural thrust and tactile placing, as paw position testing (or 'knuckling' response) can be very difficult to assess in cats.

- Hopping response: The normal cat responds to hopping by quickly replacing the limb under its body as it is moved laterally. The hopping movement should be smooth and fairly rapid, and not irregular or excessive. The thoracic limbs should be carefully compared. The pelvic limbs should then be tested.

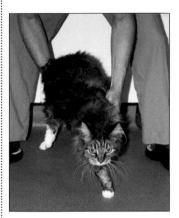

- Wheelbarrowing: This is performed with the neck extended and the pelvic limbs elevated, moving the cat forwards.

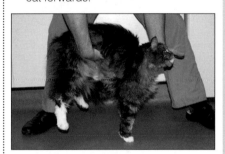

- Extensor postural thrust: The cat is lowered to the floor, hindlimbs first, whilst holding up the forequarters. The hindlimbs should extend as they contact the floor and take a step backwards
- Tactile placing: When the carpal (forelimb) or metatarsal (hindlimb) area makes contact with the edge of a table, the cat should immediately place its foot on to the table surface.

Together with gait evaluation, postural reaction testing helps to show how many limbs are involved and therefore to narrow down the lesion localization:

- If all four limbs show abnormalities on gait evaluation and/or postural reaction testing, the lesion is likely to be cranial to T3 spinal cord segments (brainstem, C1–C5 or C6–T2 segments) or generalized polyneuropathy, junctionopathy or polymyopathy.
- If only pelvic limbs are involved on gait evaluation and/or postural reaction testing, then the lesion is ▶

QRG 1.6 *continued*

likely to be located in the T3–L3 spinal cord segments, L4–S1 segments or peripheral nerve roots/ nerve of the pelvic limbs.

Spinal reflexes, muscle tone and size

Spinal reflex evaluation helps to narrow down the lesion localization further by testing the integrity of the cervicothoracic intumescence (C6–T2 segments) and lumbosacral intumescence (L4–S3 segments), as well as respective segmental sensory and motor nerves that form the peripheral nerve, and the muscles innervated.

- Lesions at the level of these intumescences, or affecting the peripheral nervous system, result in LMN signs in the muscles innervated, i.e. loss of segmental spinal reflexes (e.g. withdrawal, patellar) as well as reduced muscle tone and size.
- Lesions cranial to the intumescences (UMN dysfunction) will result in normal to increased segmental spinal reflexes (due to release of the inhibitory modulatory effect of the UMN on the LMN).

The withdrawal reflex and the patellar reflex are the most reliable spinal reflexes to test in cats. Others (e.g. triceps, biceps, extensor carpal radialis, gastrocnemius) are more difficult to test and to interpret. Spinal reflex testing is best performed with the cat in dorsal recumbency between the thighs of the examiner.

Withdrawal reflex:

- A noxious stimulus is applied by pinching the nail bed or digit with the fingers or haemostats. This stimulus causes a reflex contraction of the flexor muscles and withdrawal of the tested limb.
- If this withdrawal reflex is absent, individual toes can be tested to detect whether specific nerve deficits are present.
- Reduced or absent withdrawal reflexes are consistent with an LMN (i.e. neuromuscular) disorder.

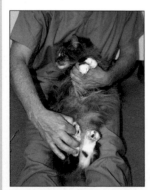

The withdrawal reflex is best performed with the cat in dorsal recumbency between the thighs of the examiner.

Patellar reflex:

- The patellar ligament is hit. This should cause a reflex contraction of the quadriceps muscle and extension of the stifle joint.
- Evaluation of extensor tone on the pelvic limb can be used as a control in cats with ambiguous patellar reflex, as it involves the same neuroanatomical components (femoral nerve and quadriceps muscle).
- Reduced or absent patellar reflex is consistent with an LMN (i.e. neuromuscular) disorder.

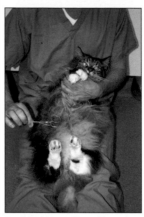

Testing the patellar reflex using the handles of artery forceps to tap the patellar ligament. As with the withdrawal reflex, it is best performed with the cat in dorsal recumbency between the thighs of the examiner. This position allows the stifle to be slightly flexed, and the two sides to be compared.

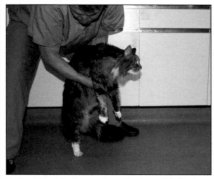

Evaluation of extensor tone in the pelvic limb. The ability to support weight on the tested limb is determined while the contralateral limb is lifted off the ground.

Nociception testing

Nociception is tested by pinching the digits on the cat's paw with the fingers. A behavioural response, such as turning the head or attempting to bite, indicates conscious pain perception. If no response is elicited using fingers, the test should be repeated with haemostats to ensure that the response is absent. *Note that withdrawal of the limb is only the flexor reflex and should not be taken as evidence of pain sensation.* Although it only defines the degree of dysfunction and not the degree of structural damage, nociceptive testing has significant prognostic value in cases of spinal cord or peripheral nerve lesions.

Cranial nerve (CN) evaluation

Menace response (see also QRG 1.3)

This tests the ipsilateral retina, ipsilateral optic nerve (CN II), optic chiasm, contralateral optic tract, contralateral forebrain, ipsilateral cerebellum and ipsilateral facial nerve (CN VII). The expected response is a closure of the eyelid. The response is absent in kittens <10–12 weeks.

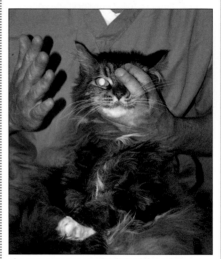

The menace response is elicited by making a threatening gesture towards the eye of the cat with one hand while blindfolding the contralateral eye.

Visual placing response

The visual placing response of the forelimbs requires intact visual and motor pathways and can be useful in assessing visual function in a cat where the menace response is ambiguous. It is tested by carrying a cat towards a tabletop. On approaching the surface the cat will reach out to support itself on the table before its paw touches the table.

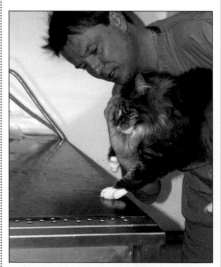

Each eye can be tested separately by covering the eye contralateral to the one being tested. This response requires intact visual pathways, mentation and postural control of the thoracic limbs.
▶

QRG 1.6 *continued*

Evaluation of pupil size and symmetry

Pupillary size and equality should be assessed in ambient light as well as in darkness. Normal pupils should be symmetrically shaped and equal to each other in size. This is a test of the parasympathetic (mediates constriction of pupil) and sympathetic (mediates dilation of pupil) supply to the eye.

In cats with pupils of unequal size (anisocoria) or shape (dyscoria), primary or secondary anatomical or mechanical abnormalities (e.g. iris atrophy, uveitis, glaucoma) must be ruled out before consideration is given to a neurological dysfunction. Which pupil is abnormal can be determined by checking the pupillary light reflex (PLR; see QRG 1.3) and determining whether the asymmetry in pupil size increases in bright light (larger pupil is the abnormal one) or in complete darkness (dark adaptation test; smaller pupil is the abnormal one).

Trigeminal nerve (CN V)

The trigeminal nerve (CN V) provides sensory innervation of the face (cutaneous elements as well as the cornea, mucosa of the nasal septum and mucosa of the oral cavity) and motor innervation of the masticatory muscles (temporalis, masseter, medial and lateral pterygoid, and rostral part of the digastric muscles).

- **Motor function** of CN V is assessed by evaluating the size and symmetry of the masticatory muscles and testing the resistance of the jaw to opening the mouth.
- **Sensory function** of CN V (sensation of the face) can be individually tested by the corneal reflex (ophthalmic branch; retraction of globe and eyelid closure when cornea is gently touched with moistened cotton bud), the palpebral reflex (ophthalmic or maxillary branch when touching the medial or lateral canthus of the eye, respectively), the response to nasal stimulation (ophthalmic branch) (see below), and by pinching the skin of the face with haemostat forceps and observing an ipsilateral blink or facial twitch.

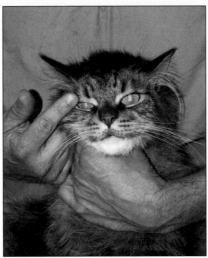

The palpebral reflex is elicited by touching the medial canthus of the eye and observing a reflex closure of the eyelids. The afferent arm of the reflex is mediated by the trigeminal nerve (CN V sensory) while the efferent arm is mediated by the facial nerve (CN VII motor).

- Nasal stimulation: the inside of one of the two nostrils is stimulated using a pair of forceps or a pen while the cat's eyes are masked to prevent any visual input. The expected response is a withdrawal movement of the head and neck. This tests the sensory component of CN V as well as the brainstem and contralateral forebrain.

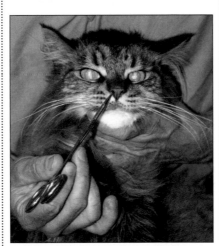

Response to stimulation of the nasal mucosa; the cat's eyes should be masked, as described above.

Facial nerve (CN VII)

- The facial nerve (CN VII) provides motor innervation to the muscles of facial expression. Its function is assessed by observing the face for movement and symmetry of the ears, eyelids, lips and nostrils.
- The facial nerve also provides the motor response (efferent part) of the following tests:
  - Palpebral reflex (CN V afferent)
  - Corneal reflex (CN V afferent)
  - Menace response (CN II afferent)
  - Pinching of the face (CN V afferent).
- The Schirmer tear test (STT) can evaluate the parasympathetic supply of the lacrimal gland associated with CN VII (see QRG 1.3).

Oculovestibular reflex and pathological nystagmus

Oculocephalic reflex testing is best performed by holding the cat at arm's length and rotating its head from side to side. This tests: vestibular receptors in the inner ear; the vestibulocochlear nerve (CN VIII); medial longitudinal fasciculus in the brainstem; and cranial nerves involved in movement of the globe (CN III, IV and VI). Physiological nystagmus (oculovestibular reflex) is normal. It consists of a slow phase, where the eyes move away from the direction of head rotation, and a fast phase, where they move back in the direction of head rotation. Loss of physiological nystagmus indicates a lesion in one of these areas.

In the absence of any head movement, nystagmus should never be present in a normal animal. Pathological nystagmus can be: spontaneous (observed when the head is in a normal position at rest); and/or positional (observed when the head is held in different positions, such as to either side, dorsally or ventrally, or by placing the animal upside down on its back).

Nystagmus is usually classified on the basis of the direction of the fast movement (occurring away from the side of the lesion). It may be horizontal, vertical or rotatory. Central vestibular disease may cause any of these, while peripheral vestibular disease can only cause horizontal or rotatory nystagmus.

QRG 1.7 Blood sampling: practical tips
by Martha Cannon

Handling and patient positioning

The principles of cat-friendly handling outlined in this chapter should be applied. QRG 1.2 provides further advice on restraint of cats for blood sampling.

Blood samples are most commonly collected from the jugular or cephalic vein.

- The jugular vein is usually preferred, as it is large enough to allow a sample to be withdrawn rapidly without requiring excessive negative pressure. This minimizes the incidence of haemolysis and blood clots within the sample. ▶

QUICK REFERENCE GUIDES

QRG 1.7 *continued*

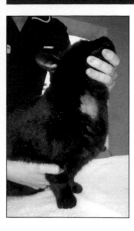

- Some cats resent being restrained with their neck extended; these cats may be more tolerant of restraint for collection from the cephalic vein.

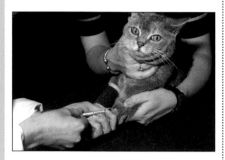

- Wrapping the cat in a large towel will help to control all the limbs when collecting a jugular sample; or, for cephalic vein sampling, the target limb can be excluded from the towel.

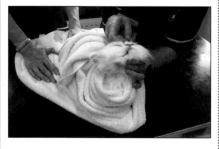

- Fear-aggressive cats, or cats that are especially wriggly, can be restrained for jugular sampling by placing them on their side or on their back, controlling the limbs with the hands and body, or wrapping the cat in a towel. The person holding the cat then raises the vein, while the person taking the blood restrains the head, extends the neck, and inserts the needle into the vein in a craniocaudal direction.

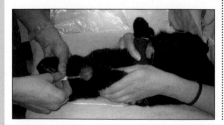

- A similar method also works well for small kittens.

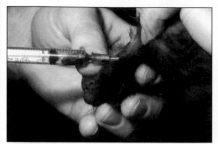

(Courtesy of The Feline Centre, Langford Veterinary Services, University of Bristol)

Preparing the site

- A generous area of skin is clipped over the target vein, enough to allow identification of the vein, and the direction in which it runs.
  - Many cats are frightened by the noise of the clippers. Battery-operated models often make less noise and some are specifically designed to be quiet; these are less robust than standard models but are adequate for clipping small amounts of fur from over the vein in conscious cats.
  - Switch the clippers on at a distance from the cat while talking to it, to mask the initial noise.
  - If the cat is fear aggressive or particularly nervous, consider using the cephalic vein rather than the jugular vein so the region can be clipped with curved scissors.
- Applying a local anaesthetic cream or spray to the skin may help to reduce resistance from the cat:
  - Intubeaze local anaesthetic spray will take effect within a few minutes
  - Local anaesthetic creams (e.g. EMLA) should be liberally applied to shaved skin, covered with an occlusive dressing and left for 15–20 minutes to take effect.
- Prepare the site with a cotton wool swab soaked in spirit.

Raising the vein

For a jugular sample the blood sampler raises the vein with one hand by applying *gentle* pressure to the jugular groove, at around the level of the thoracic inlet. Firm pressure is not required, and will be resented by the cat.

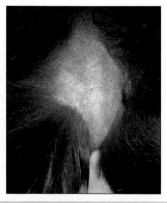

For a cephalic sample the person holding the cat raises the vein by wrapping a thumb around the forelimb just distal to the elbow, and then gently rotating the wrist to encourage the vein on to the cranial aspect of the forelimb. For fear aggressive or agitated cats using a tourniquet will allow the handler to concentrate on holding the limb still.

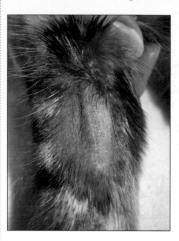

Collecting the sample

Use a 23 or 25 G hypodermic needle attached to an appropriately sized empty syringe. 2.5 ml of blood is adequate for most diagnostic panels and a small syringe is easier to manipulate than a larger one.

1 Introduce the needle, bevel upwards, into the vein, following the line of the vein. In cats the vein is very near the surface. To avoid passing the needle right through the vein press the needle gently against the skin over the vein to indent it slightly.

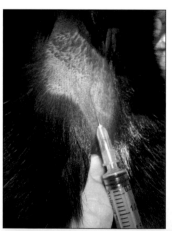

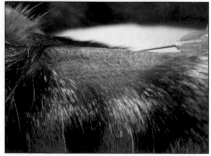

▶

QRG 1.7 *continued*

2 Advance the needle through the skin and into the vein, keeping it almost parallel to the surface.

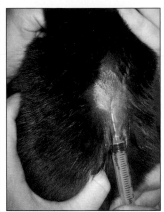

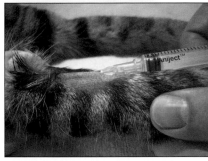

3 Apply gentle negative pressure to the syringe and watch for blood in the hub of the needle.

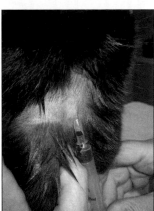

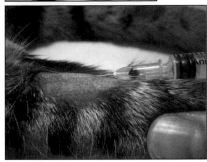

4 If no blood is present in the hub, try gently redirecting the needle to enter the vein, but avoid large sweeping movements. If necessary withdraw the needle and start again with a fresh needle. Fine-gauge needles soon become blunt if they are used to penetrate the skin more than once.

5 Use very gentle negative pressure (e.g. approx 0.3 ml of vacuum) to draw blood from the cephalic vein, as it is more collapsible than the jugular vein. The cephalic vein will empty as you withdraw blood, so as the vein flattens out release the negative pressure to allow it to refill and then apply gentle negative pressure again.

All images © Martha Cannon unless stated otherwise

Preventive healthcare: a life-stage approach

2

Susan Little

Feline life stages

The current approach to feline wellness care includes a focus on six specific life stages to assess risk factors and specific age-related healthcare needs. These life stages, with relevant health problems and issues for discussion with owners, can be summarized as:

- Kitten (birth to 6 months):
  - Congenital and inherited defects (see Chapter 15)
  - Lifestyle choices
  - Identification
  - Nutrition
  - Neutering
  - Primary vaccination programme
- Junior (7 months to 2 years):
  - Prevention of infectious diseases
  - Illnesses associated with outdoor access (e.g. bite wounds, trauma)
  - First vaccination booster
  - Obesity prevention; adjust nutrition plan after neutering
  - Start collection of minimum database results
- Prime (3 to 6 years):
  - Ensure owners understand need for continuing wellness examinations, even for apparently healthy indoor cats
  - Common medical problems include obesity, oral disease, lower urinary tract disease, gastrointestinal disease, cardiac disease
  - Regular monitoring of minimum database
- Mature (7 to 10 years):
  - Common medical problems include obesity, diabetes mellitus, chronic kidney disease, hypertension, hyperthyroidism (Figure 2.1), cancer, oral disease
  - Awareness of subtle signs of illness for early detection and intervention (see Figure 2.3)
  - Consider wellness examinations every 6 months or as needed, according to health status
- Senior (11 to 14 years):
  - Signs of ageing *versus* signs of disease; e.g. dulling senses of vision and hearing are due to ageing but weight loss is more likely a sign of disease

  - Additional common medical problems include cognitive dysfunction, arthritis
  - Concurrent diseases are common
  - Monitor for and diagnose causes of weight loss
  - Frequent wellness examinations (at least every 6 months)
- Geriatric (15 years and older):
  - Importance of weight maintenance
  - Ensure quality of life
  - Palliative care, end-of-life decisions (see QRG 2.5)
  - Frequent wellness examinations – at least every 6 months but more frequently if dictated by health status.

Specific healthcare recommendations by life stage are summarized in Figure 2.2. However, it is important to remember that individual cats and body systems

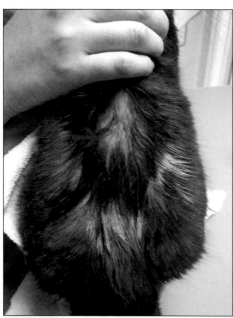

2.1 This 10-year-old cat has a visibly enlarged thyroid gland. Not all cats with hyperthyroidism have such obvious gland enlargements; palpation of the thyroid gland should be a routine part of the examination for all cats from about the age of 7 years to facilitate early disease detection.

Life stage	General	Behaviour, environment [a]	Medical, surgical	Elimination	Nutrition, weight management [b,c,d]	Oral health [e]	Parasite control	Vaccination [f,g]
Kitten: Birth to 6 months	Congenital and genetic diseases; breed predispositions to disease. Claw care and grooming	Lifestyle choices; discuss 'resources' and toys. Teach simple commands. Acclimate to car and pet carrier	Discuss sterilization, age to perform surgery	Litter box set-up, cleaning. Discuss normal elimination	Discuss growth requirements, healthy weight management. Introduce to variety of foods, flavours	Acclimate to handling mouth. Educate about dental care; start tooth brushing	Deworm every 2 wk from 3–9 wk of age, then monthly until 6 months. Faecal exam at least twice in first year of life	Administer core vaccines, other vaccines according to risk factors. Vaccinate for rabies in accordance with local laws
Junior: 7 months to 2 years	Collect a thorough medical history. Monitor for common health problems such as asthma, intestinal disease, diabetes mellitus	Discuss social interactions with other pets, people; regular handling of mouth, ears, feet	Discuss benefits of minimum database for monitoring health	Confirm litter box appropriate for growing cat Identify & correct litter box problems	Monitor for weight increase. Adjust caloric intake after sterilization. Feed to moderate body condition	Monitor, discuss ongoing needs	Faecal exam at least once per year. Ongoing parasite control based on lifestyle, risk factors	Ongoing reassessment of vaccine needs according to lifestyle. Continue core vaccines, others as indicated
Prime/adult: 3 to 6 years	Collect a thorough medical history. Monitor for common health problems such as asthma, intestinal disease, diabetes mellitus	Review environmental enrichment. Discuss ways to keep active	Monitor for subtle changes. Discuss mobility	Identify & correct litter box problems	Feed to moderate body condition. Monitor for weight gain			
Mature: 7 to 10 years	Increase frequency of examinations. Educate owner on changes associated with ageing and common diseases in the age group	Discuss access to litter box, bed, food, water	Discuss mobility. Monitor for signs of illness	Ensure easy access to litter box with changes in mobility				
Senior: 11 to 14 years		Discuss changing environmental needs. Educate about changes in behaviour & illness	Regular review of medications, diet, supplements	Adjust litter box size, height, location, cleaning, etc., as required to meet changing needs	Monitor for weight loss. Adjust diet and feeding management as needed	Monitor for oral tumours, other sources of oral pain		
Geriatric: 15 years +		Discuss access to litter box, bed, food, water. Signs of cognitive dysfunction. Discuss quality of life						

2.2 Important focal points for feline wellness examinations by life stage. (Adapted from Vogt *et al.*, 2010.) Sources: [a] Overall *et al.* (2005); [b] WSAVA Nutritional Assessment Guidelines Task Force (2011); [c] Baldwin *et al.* (2010); [d] Freeman *et al.* (2011); [e] Holmstrom *et al.* (2005); [f] Day *et al.* (2010); [g] Richards *et al.* (2006).

age at different rates, so that a cat may develop a condition not typically associated with its life stage. In addition to life-stage considerations, lifestyle is also important when assessing risk factors and healthcare needs. The clinician should learn to question owners carefully about each cat's environment, access to outdoors and contact with other cats. Recently, the link between stressors (e.g. change in routine, change in cat population, visitors to the home) and signs of illness in cats (e.g. anorexia, vomiting, diarrhoea, house soiling) has been established definitely (Stella *et al.*, 2011).

In addition to the life-stage-specific recommendations, certain topics are important enough to review with the owner at every wellness examination. These include:

- Subtle signs of sickness in cats (Figure 2.3)
- The importance of preventive healthcare and health monitoring for early disease detection and intervention
- Identification (e.g. microchip, collar and tag)
- Pet insurance
- Preparation for pet care/evacuation during natural disasters (e.g. severe weather, earthquake, fire)
- Environmental enrichment
- Medications (both prescribed and non-prescription), supplements, nutraceuticals, botanicals, homeopathic remedies, etc.
- Litter box/tray management
- Feeding management and weight control
- Benefits of oral healthcare
- Zoonotic diseases.

- Inappropriate elimination behaviour
- Changes in social interactions with other cats or their owners
- Changes in activity
- Changes in sleeping patterns
- Changes in food or water consumption
- Unexplained weight loss or weight gain
- Changes in grooming habits
- Signs of stress, e.g. hiding away, unexplained aggression
- Changes in vocalization
- Bad breath

2.3 Subtle signs of sickness in cats. (Adapted from *Subtle Signs of Sickness*, www.healthycatsforlife.com)

The American Association of Feline Practitioners (AAFP) and the American Animal Hospital Association (AAHA) have published an excellent resource to guide veterinary surgeons in providing appropriate life-stage care for cats (Vogt et al., 2010). Information on life-stage care is also included in the International Society for Feline Medicine's 'WellCat *for Life*' programme (www.isfm.net).

General preventive healthcare recommendations

Frequency of examination
While the optimal frequency of health examinations for cats is unknown, it is generally accepted that healthy adult cats should be examined at least once per year. Owners should be educated to understand that changes in health status may occur rapidly and that cats may not show signs of illness until a problem is advanced. The AAFP, AAHA and ISFM recommend 6-monthly examinations for cats 7 years of age and older. Cats with prior or ongoing health problems may need more frequent examination, based on the disease and their health status.

Minimum database monitoring
The goal of monitoring a minimum database (MDB) in apparently healthy cats is early disease detection and intervention (Figure 2.4). MDB testing can also be used to detect problems before procedures requiring sedation or anaesthesia. Although no specific recommendations exist for frequency of MDB monitoring,

	Kitten/ Junior (2 years or less)	Adult (3–6 years)	Mature (7–10 years)	Senior/ Geriatric (11 years or older)
Complete blood cell count, differential				
Serum chemistries, electrolytes				
Complete urinalysis				
Total T4				
Blood pressure				
FeLV/FIV testing				
Faecal flotation				

2.4 Recommendations by life stage for tests to be carried out for a minimum database. Green = recommended; yellow = optional; red = not recommended. (Adapted from Vogt *et al.*, 2010.)

annual testing allows the clinician to establish a baseline for the individual patient and to monitor trends over time. However, routine testing also increases the chance of finding test results that are outside the laboratory's normal reference range but clinically insignificant; interpretation therefore requires clinical judgement, taking into account the context of the individual patient. The old adage 'treat the patient, not the test result' remains highly relevant in this age of abundant laboratory data.

Retrovirus testing
Feline leukaemia virus (FeLV) and feline immunodeficiency virus (FIV) are among the most common causes of infection in cats (see Chapter 19), although prevalence in the general cat population varies by geographical location and risk factors. Guidelines for prevention and management of retroviral infection have been published in Europe and North America. In general, the retroviral status of all cats should be known. For example, all newly acquired cats and kittens should be tested, as well as sick cats (including those with bite wounds and oral inflammatory disease). Cats and kittens should be tested before vaccination against FeLV or FIV. This is for several reasons, for example: if a cat is positive for FeLV, there is no point in vaccinating against FeLV (same for FIV); if an undiagnosed infected cat is vaccinated, once it is diagnosed it may appear that the vaccine failed to prevent infection when in reality the cat was already infected at the time of vaccination. It is also appropriate to test cats at ongoing risk of infection for FeLV and FIV (if not FIV-vaccinated) annually for early disease detection.

Genetic testing
Testing for genetic diseases, disease predispositions, or certain traits (e.g. response to drug therapy, blood type) is likely to become a more important part of feline medicine as the feline genome is explored. About 250 genetic diseases are known in the cat, many with close parallels to human diseases. At the time of writing, more than a dozen genetic tests are available for the cat, but only a few are important to the clinician. Currently, genetic testing is largely based on risk assessment by breed and can be used:

- To help breeders eliminate or reduce the prevalence of disease
- To identify cats with possible problems before purchase or adoption
- To provide information to enable an individual monitoring plan for early detection and intervention.

Most laboratories allow for submission of DNA samples collected by cheek (buccal) swabs (Figure 2.5). Examples of genetic testing that might be important for some newly acquired cats and kittens include hypertrophic cardiomyopathy (Maine Coon, Ragdoll), polycystic kidney disease (Persians and related breeds), progressive retinal atrophy (Abyssinian, Somali, Siamese and related breeds), blood type (British Shorthair, Cornish and Devon Rex, Birman and other breeds) and pyruvate kinase deficiency (Abyssinian, Somali, Singapura, Bengal). Test results should become part of the cat's medical record.

Examples of resources for feline genetic testing
- Langford Veterinary Services
  http://www.catgenetics.co.uk
- University of Pennsylvania, Section of Medical Genetics
  http://research.vet.upenn.edu/penngen
- University of California Veterinary Genetics Lab
  http://www.vgl.ucdavis.edu
- VetoGene, University of Milan
  http://www.vetogene.com
- Genlab Niini
  Tirri Niini, Dr.med.vet; Helsinki, Finland

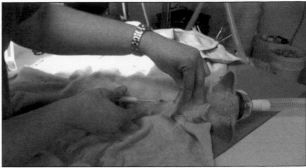

2.6 Both permanent and visible identification should be provided for all cats. This kitten is receiving a microchip at the time of spay surgery. Even indoor cats should be identified in case of escape or loss.

Indoor *versus* outdoor lifestyle

Debates over whether cats should be kept totally indoors reflect geographical, cultural and personal differences. Access to the outdoors provides a more stimulating environment, but also carries risks of trauma and infectious diseases. In addition, predation of wildlife by cats is often unacceptable, especially in areas where endangered species live. An indoor-only lifestyle removes these issues, but brings risks of compromised welfare (e.g. behaviour problems) and illness (e.g. obesity, idiopathic cystitis) due to a stressful or sterile environment. A compromise may be supervised (e.g. walking on a leash; Figure 2.7) or controlled (e.g. cat-safe enclosure) outdoor access.

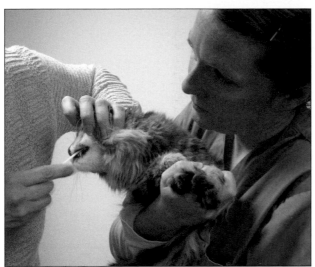

2.5 DNA tests for genetic diseases and various traits are becoming more commonly available. This cat is having a DNA sample collected using a cytology brush to harvest cheek cells; ordinary cotton tip applicators (cotton buds) work just as well. This Maine Coon cat is being tested for hypertrophic cardiomyopathy risk.

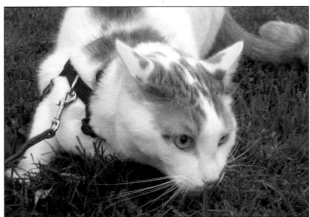

2.7 Safe access to the outdoors can increase mental stimulation and provide a source of environmental enrichment. This cat has been trained to walk on a leash. *Cats should never be left outdoors unattended while on a leash.* (Courtesy Heather MacDonald.)

Identification

The benefits of both permanent (e.g. microchip; Figure 2.6) and visible (e.g. collar and tag) identification should be discussed with pet owners, even those whose cats are considered to be indoor-only. In North America, only about 2% of lost cats are returned to owners; a major contributor to this low return rate is lack of identification. The International Standards Organization (ISO) microchip standards have been adopted by several regions (e.g. Canada, Europe, Asia, Australia). Cats travelling to countries that have adopted ISO standards should be implanted with the appropriate microchip.

The microchip identification number should be part of a cat's medical record. The microchip should be scanned at each wellness examination to verify its position and that it is functioning. Newly adopted cats and kittens should be scanned to determine whether a microchip has previously been implanted. Recommendations for the use of microchip scanners include:

- Remove collars and tags before scanning
- Perform scanning away from computers, metal tables, fluorescent lights
- Pass the scanner over the cat in different directions and multiple times.

Environmental enrichment

When cats must live totally indoors, environmental enrichment is critically important for welfare and health maintenance. Indoor cats need places to climb, scratch, sleep and hide (Figure 2.8).

Many cats do not like to compete for resources (food, water, hiding and sleeping places). In a multi-cat environment, there must be enough space to provide individual food and water stations, as well as multiple opportunities to hide, sleep, perch, and play with stimulating toys (Figure 2.9). More information on environmental enrichment is available from the Ohio State University College of Veterinary Medicine's *Indoor Pet Initiative* website (http://indoorpet.osu.edu); see also Further reading.

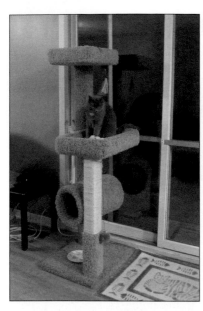

2.8

Cats that live totally indoors need places to sleep, climb, perch and hide. Ideal 'cat trees' are tall and sturdy, and provide multiple levels for one cat at a time to perch. Situating a 'cat tree' in front of a window provides opportunities for bird watching.

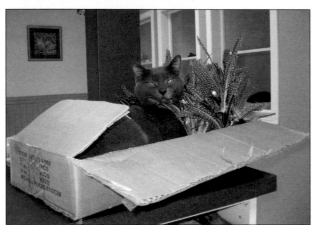

2.9 One component of environmental enrichment for indoor cats is providing stimulating toys and play opportunities. Many cats like toys that mimic birds. Other opportunities to play and explore can be very simple, such as a cardboard box.

Vaccination

Vaccination reduces feline morbidity and mortality, and also serves to protect humans against zoonotic disease (e.g. rabies). Guidelines for vaccination of cats have been published by three international panels since 2006, and two summary documents have been produced (Figure 2.10). In most countries, however, a minority of cats are protected and ongoing efforts must be made to vaccinate more animals.

Vaccination is a medical procedure and is not without risks. Adverse events may be: local or systemic; mild to severe or fatal; peracute, acute, subacute or chronic. However, most adverse events associated with vaccination are mild and temporary (e.g. lethargy with or without fever) and occur in <1% of vaccinated cats. However, although serious and life-threatening adverse events (e.g. hypersensitivity reactions, injection-site sarcomas) are rare, informed owner consent for vaccination is important.

Data on duration of immunity are not available for all vaccines. When available, such data have influenced the abandonment of annual revaccination intervals and have encouraged the licensing of products with longer revaccination intervals in some countries. The predictive value of antibody titres to

American Association of Feline Practitioners
■ Richards JR, Elston TH, Ford RB *et al.* (2006) The 2006 American Association of Feline Practitioners Feline Vaccine Advisory Panel report. *Journal of the American Veterinary Medical Association* **229**, 1405–1441

European Advisory Board on Cat Diseases: *Journal of Feline Medicine and Surgery* vol. 11, 2009
ABCD guidelines on prevention and management of: ■ *Bordetella bronchiseptica* infection in cats (Egberink H, Addie D, Belak S *et al.*) pp. 610–614   ■ *Chlamydophila felis* infection (Gruffydd-Jones T, Addie D, Belak S *et al.*) pp. 605–609   ■ Feline calicivirus infection (Radford AD, Addie D, Belak S *et al.*) pp. 556–564   ■ Feline herpesvirus infection (Thiry E, Addie D, Belak S *et al.*) pp. 547–555   ■ Feline immunodeficiency (Hosie MJ, Addie D, Belak S *et al.*) pp. 575–584   ■ Feline infectious peritonitis (Addie D, Belák S, Boucraut-Baralon C *et al.*) pp. 594–604   ■ Feline leukaemia (Lutz H, Addie D, Belak S *et al.*) pp. 565–574   ■ Feline panleucopenia (Truyen U, Addie D, Belak S *et al.*) pp. 538–546   ■ Feline rabies (Frymus T, Addie D, Belak S *et al.*) pp. 585–593

World Small Animal Veterinary Association
■ Day MJ, Horzinek MC and Schultz RD (2010) WSAVA guidelines for the vaccination of dogs and cats. *Journal of Small Animal Practice* **51**, 338–356

2.10 Published vaccination guidelines.

determine the need for revaccination is unclear and may not be equal for each pathogen.

Consensus has been agreed upon by the three international panels on certain points:

■ Vaccines should not be given needlessly
■ An annual health examination should be conducted, even if vaccination is not being performed
■ Owners should be educated in order to give informed consent
■ Adverse events associated with vaccination should be reported to the product manufacturer and to regulatory authorities
■ Vaccines are categorized as **core** (where vaccination of all cats is justified) and **non-core** (where vaccination is justified based on risk assessment) (Figure 2.11)

Core: recommended for all cats
■ Feline calicivirus   ■ Feline herpesvirus   ■ Feline panleucopenia virus   ■ Rabies depending on geographical area, local laws and/or travel requirements

Non-core: recommended for cats at risk
■ *Bordetella bronchiseptica*   ■ *Chlamydophila felis*   ■ Feline immunodeficiency virus   ■ Feline leukaemia virus

Not generally recommended
■ Feline infectious peritonitis

2.11 Vaccine categories.

- Revaccination can be extended beyond annual intervals where supportive data exist; although choices should also be based on individual risk factors rather than attempting to formulate protocols suitable for every cat in every situation.

Vaccines

Commercially available vaccines may be infectious or non-infectious:

- **Infectious vaccines:**
  - Modified-live, e.g. some vaccines for feline calicivirus (FCV), feline herpesvirus (FHV), feline panleucopenia virus (FPV)
    - Contain avirulent or attenuated organisms
    - Administered by injection or intranasally
    - Usually do not contain adjuvant
  - Live virus-vectored recombinant, e.g. recombinant canarypox-vectored FeLV vaccine
    - Contain non-pathogenic virus vectors
    - Administered by injection
    - Usually do not contain adjuvant
- **Non-infectious vaccines**
  - Killed whole organisms, e.g. some vaccines for FCV, FHV, FPV
    - Do not contain live organisms, cannot cause disease
    - May be less effective at inducing immune responses at mucosal surfaces (respiratory, gastrointestinal tracts) than infectious vaccines
    - Slower onset of immunity than infectious vaccines
    - Administered by injection
    - Usually contain adjuvant
  - Subunit, e.g. some FeLV vaccines
    - Contain inactivated recombinant organisms or purified antigens
    - Administered by injection
    - Often contain adjuvant.

Vaccines should always be stored and prepared with strict adherence to the manufacturer's guidelines; other preparation guidelines include:

- Administer with single-use syringes and needles of the appropriate size
- Completely dissolve reconstituted vaccines before drawing into the syringe
- Reconstituted vaccines should be used within 30 minutes of preparation
- Spilled vaccine should be cleaned from the cat's fur with alcohol and from contaminated surfaces with an appropriate disinfectant.

Administration

Routes: Available routes of administration include:

- **Injection:**
  - Subcutaneous or intramuscular, depending on manufacturer's recommendations
  - The subcutaneous route has been recommended to avoid delay in detecting injection-site reactions, should they occur
- **Intranasal:**
  - For some respiratory pathogens
  - Induces local and systemic immunity
  - Not available in all countries

WARNING

A vaccine must be administered by the route stipulated by the manufacturer. A modified-live vaccine for FHV that is designed to be given subcutaneously can cause disease if some of the product is licked from the hair coat and ingested.

Sites: Adjuvants are chemicals that are included in vaccines to enhance the immune response. Adjuvanted vaccines have been associated with local inflammatory reactions at injection sites, although the degree of inflammation varies among products. The role of inflammation in the development of injection-site sarcomas (see Chapter 21) is controversial and may only occur in certain predisposed individuals. In general, clinicians are advised to use the least inflammatory products available and to avoid multiple vaccinations at a single site. Administering injectable vaccines at specific body sites has been recommended in order to monitor site reactions and facilitate management of sarcomas if they develop:

- Right forelimb – lateral, below elbow, as distal as possible: FPV, FHV, FCV (with or without *Chlamydophila felis*)
- Right hindlimb – lateral, below stifle, as distal as possible: rabies
- Left hindlimb – lateral, below stifle, as distal as possible: FeLV, FIV (with or without any other antigen except rabies).

Record-keeping: Details of vaccination should be recorded in the medical record:

- Name of product, manufacturer
- Serial/lot number
- Expiration date
- Date administered
- Vaccine type
- Administration site and route.

If a swelling develops at an injection site, owners should be instructed to notify the clinician. Biopsy of the mass is warranted (incisional, wedge, multiple cores) if any of the following criteria are met (3-2-1 rule; see also Chapter 21):

- Mass is present 3 months after vaccination
- Mass is >2 cm in diameter
- Mass is increasing in size after 1 month.

Protocols

Generic guidelines for primary vaccination of kittens (unless directed otherwise by the manufacturer) are as follows.

- Most kittens receive initial vaccinations at 8–9 weeks of age, but vaccination may begin as early as 6 weeks when warranted (e.g. shelters, orphan kittens, endemic disease environments).
- Primary core vaccines should be administered at 3–4-week intervals until 16 weeks of age.
- If 6 weeks or longer have elapsed since the previous dose, at least two further doses of vaccine should be administered, 3–4 weeks apart.
- After the primary series, the next vaccination is one year later.

For primary core vaccination of cats or kittens over 16 weeks of age, two doses of vaccine are administered on average, at an interval of 3–4 weeks (unless directed otherwise by the manufacturer), with the next vaccination one year later.

A summary of feline vaccination recommendations from the AAFP, WSAVA and European Advisory Board on Cat Diseases (ABCD) panels is shown in Figure 2.12. Although the optimal interval between the initial and subsequent doses on primary vaccination is unknown, current recommendations are to administer vaccines at a minimum interval of 2 weeks and a maximum interval of 4 weeks. Any brand of vaccine may be used for revaccination.

Special considerations

- **Kittens:** Maternally derived immunity may interfere with vaccination; it typically wanes by 9–12 weeks of age, although this may happen earlier (<6 weeks) or later (up to 16 weeks). The latter results in the recommendation to give a final vaccine to kittens at 16 weeks of age for FPV, FCV and FHV (Figure 2.12).
- **Surgery and anaesthesia:** Vaccination can be performed at the same time as surgical sterilization if necessary, as response to vaccination will not be affected.
- **Senior and geriatric cats**: It is not known whether older cats respond to vaccination in the same manner as younger cats; however, current recommendations are that healthy older cats and those with stable chronic diseases receive vaccines according to the same guidelines as for younger cats.
- **Pregnant and lactating queens:** Most vaccines have not been evaluated for safety or efficacy in

this group, so routine vaccination of these cats should be avoided. However, in some circumstances, vaccination may outweigh risks; if pregnant queens must be vaccinated, killed virus vaccines are recommended.
- **Cats with pre-existing illness:** Cats with acute illness, debilitation or high fevers should not be vaccinated, but vaccination of a cat with chronic stable illness may be justified. In shelters, vaccination in the face of mild to moderate illness may be indicated for infection control.
- **Vaccination of cats infected with FeLV or FIV:** Although ability to respond to vaccination may be impaired compared with uninfected cats, otherwise healthy retrovirus-infected cats should be vaccinated with core vaccines as for uninfected cats, and with non-core vaccines only when justified; many experts recommend use of only non-infectious products (e.g. killed vaccines) in these patients.
- **Cats receiving corticosteroids:** Studies evaluating safety and efficacy of vaccination in these patients are lacking, so concurrent use of corticosteroids at the time of vaccination should be avoided. However, this is not always practical for cats on long-term therapy and in these cases vaccination is often performed.
- **Cats with prior adverse effects:** Revaccination should only be performed after serious consideration of the risks and benefits. A different product, type or route of administration is recommended; only one vaccine should be administered at a time and a 3-week interval should be allowed before another vaccine is administered if required. Patients may be monitored in the clinic for 4–6 hours. Patients may be treated with an antihistamine (e.g.

Vaccine	Initial series: kittens (<16 weeks)	Initial series: adults (or kittens >16 weeks)	Boosters
Core vaccines			
FPV	First dose at 8 wk (or as early as 6 wk); then q3–4wk until 16 wk old	Two doses, 3–4 wk apart	1 year after last kitten vaccine; then no more often than q3yr
FHV + FCV	First dose at 8 wk (or as early as 6 wk); then q3–4 wk until 16 wk old	Two doses, 3–4 wk apart	1 year after last kitten vaccine; then no more often than q3yr unless high risk perceived (e.g. entry into boarding cattery; multi-cat household)
Rabies	Start as early as 12 wk; then 1 year later	Two doses, 1 year apart	Annually, or q3yr, depending on local laws and product licensing
Non-core vaccines			
FeLV	Start as early as 8 wk; then 3–4 wk later	Two doses, 3–4 wk apart	1 year after last kitten vaccine; then annually for cats at ongoing risk (ABCD recommends booster vaccines q2–3yr after 3–4 years of age)
FIV	Start as early as 8 w; then q2–3wk for two additional doses (three doses required in total)	Three doses, 2–3 wk apart	1 year after last kitten vaccine; then annually for cats at ongoing risk
Chlamydophila felis	Start as early as 8–9 wk; then 3–4 wk later	Two doses, 3–4 wk apart	Annual for cats at ongoing risk
Bordetella bronchiseptica	Single dose as early as 4 wk	Single dose	Annual for cats at ongoing risk
FIP [a]	First dose at 16 wk; then 3–4 wk later	Two doses, 3–4 wk apart	Annual booster recommended by vaccine manufacturer

2.12 Summary of feline vaccination recommendations from the AAFP, WSAVA and ABCD vaccine guideline groups. (Data from Rodan I and Sparkes A, 2012.) [a] Please note this vaccine is not generally recommended as there is insufficient evidence of clinically relevant protection.

diphenhydramine 2 mg/kg i.m.) and corticosteroid (e.g. dexamethasone 5 mg/cat i.m.) 20 minutes before vaccination.
■ **Cats entering a boarding facility** (Figure 2.13): Since this is a higher risk situation, it may be prudent to ensure that the last vaccination against FHV and FCV occurred within the previous 12 months. If required, a booster vaccination may be given 2–4 weeks prior to entering the facility.

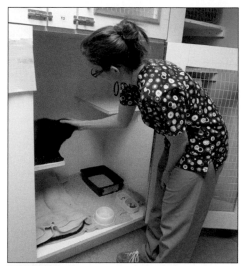

2.13 Cats may be boarded at a boarding cattery or at other boarding facilities, such as veterinary hospitals, for various reasons. These represent higher risk situations for infectious diseases than the home environment, so that core vaccinations should be up to date before entering the facility.

Surgical sterilization

Prepubertal neutering
Puberty occurs between 4 and 21 months of age in female cats and between 8 and 10 months in males; there are significant benefits to surgical sterilization before the onset of puberty. Early neutering refers to sterilization carried out between 6 and 16 weeks of age, and is now commonly practised as veterinary surgeons gain experience with paediatric anaesthesia and surgery (see QRGs 2.2–2.4). Many international veterinary organizations support early neutering.
The benefits of prepubertal neutering include:

■ Effective population control
■ Pre-adoption or pre-sale surgery to avoid owner non-compliance
■ Easier surgeries (less bleeding, improved visualization of organs, shorter surgery times) and shorter recovery times
■ Lower postoperative complication rates
■ Avoidance of stress and costs of spaying females in oestrus, while pregnant, or with pyometra
■ Reduction in risk of mammary adenocarcinoma by 91% when females are spayed before 6 months of age (Overley *et al.*, 2005).

Several long-term studies have confirmed that early neutering is not associated with increased risk of disease, including lower urinary tract disease and behaviour problems. An excellent summary of the issues involved can be found in a policy statement from The Cat Group (www.fabcats.org/cat_group).

Suggested ages for neutering in various situations include:

■ **Pedigree kitten from breeder:**
  • Rarely re-homed before 14 weeks
  • Allow 2–3 weeks to adapt to new home, so neutering may occur around 16 weeks
  • Some breeders neuter kittens before re-homing them
■ **Non-pedigree kitten from private home:**
  • Often re-homed at about 8 weeks
  • Should receive primary vaccination series before neutering
  • Schedule surgery following last vaccination – at about 16 weeks
■ **Kitten from rescue organization:**
  • Often re-homed at about 8 weeks
  • Schedule surgery following last vaccination – at about 16 weeks
  • May be neutered before re-homing
■ **Feral kitten:**
  • If caught before 7 weeks of age, may be re-homed and treated as for rescue kittens
  • If part of trap/neuter/release programme, neuter and vaccinate as early as 6–7 weeks
  • Identification such as ear-tipping is recommended.

Parasite control
Control of parasites is important not only for the health of the cat but also to prevent zoonotic disease. Unfortunately, owner awareness of these issues is often low. The clinician should become familiar with the most important feline endo- and ectoparasites in their practice area, as there are considerable geographical differences in prevalence.
The Companion Animal Parasite Council (CAPC; www.capcvet.org) and the European Scientific Counsel for Companion Animal Parasites (ESCCAP; www.esccap.org) publish guidelines on the diagnosis and prevention of parasitic infections of dogs and cats.

■ Both recommend starting prophylactic roundworm and hookworm treatment at 3 weeks of age, repeating every 2 weeks until 9 weeks of age.
■ Year-round broad-spectrum parasite control, typically with a monthly product, should be instituted for cats at risk of infection.
■ In heartworm endemic areas, monthly products that have efficacy against heartworm and roundworm (as well as fleas) are recommended. In low-risk situations, treatment a minimum of 4 times per year is recommended. In areas where heartworm is absent, such as the UK, prophylaxis is unnecessary.
■ Regular faecal examinations (2–4 times in the first year of life, 1 or 2 times per year in adults) should also be performed. Faecal flotation/centrifugation techniques (e.g. using zinc sulphate or modified Sheather's sugar solution) are considered the most reliable screening tests for endoparasites.

Ectoparasites
The most common ectoparasites are discussed in Figure 2.14; flea control products are discussed further in Figure 2.17.

Group	Common species	Common clinical signs	Diagnosis	Treatment and control	Comments
Ear mites	*Otodectes cynotis*	Coffee ground discharge, pruritus	Direct examination, cerumen (wax) smear	Clean ear canal to allow topical medications to penetrate. Otic steroid for pruritus. Concurrent use of otic miticide and whole body flea control. Treat affected and in-contact cats for at least 4 wks	Kittens at highest risk
Fur mites and lice	Most common mites: *Dermanyssus gallinae*, *Lynxacarus radovsky*, chiggers (*Eutrombicula*, *Walchia americana*), and *Cheyletiella* spp. Only one species of louse: *Felicola subrostratus*	Pruritus, skin eruptions, crusting and scaling, alopecia	Visual inspection of hairs, skin scrapings, flea combings, hair trichograms, acetate tape preparations, faecal examinations, response to treatment	Bathe to remove debris, excess scales, egg cases and nits from hair coat. Whole body topical treatments: lime sulphur rinses, fipronil spray, pyrethrin sprays. OR systemic treatments: ivermectin (0.2–0.4 mg/kg orally q24h for 4 wk); milbemycin (0.5–2 mg/kg orally q24h for 4 wk); selamectin q2wk for 3 treatments	
Fleas	*Ctenocephalides felis* (>90%)	Alopecia, scaling, papular eruptions ± crusting, areas of self-trauma, or asymptomatic (see Chapter 6)	Clinical signs, flea combing (fleas, flea eggs, flea excreta)	Nitenpyram (1 mg/kg orally q24–48h) for up to 4 weeks until fleas no longer seen, plus monthly spot-on treatments; or just monthly spot-on treatments; or sprays. Environmental treatment. Young kittens: Products are authorized for early use in some countries: fipronil spray (from 2 days of age) – apply spray to a cloth or cotton wool and wipe the kitten, avoiding the eyes and mucous membranes; lufenuron (from 6 wk); nitenpyram (from 4 wk, at least 0.9 kg); selamectin (from 6 wk); in areas where no authorized products are available for very young kittens, consider use of a water-based pyrethrin spray authorized for cats (apply to towel and wrap kitten's body, excluding the head, in the towel) and aggressive flea combing (See also Figure 2.17 and Chapter 6)	Often found year-round, even in cold climates, even on indoor cats. Young, old and severely debilitated cats are most at risk. Can cause severe flea bite anaemia in kittens. Associated with tapeworm infestation, bartonellosis
Ticks	Various, depending on geographical location	Small nodular reactions at site of attachment, otitis, or asymptomatic	Physical examination (Figure 2.15)	Manual removal: grasp as close to the skin as possible with fine forceps or tick remover; extract using slow, steady pressure. *Do not* crush, twist or jerk out of the skin as may result in exposure to pathogens within tick or cause its head to detach and stay in skin, which may cause infection or granuloma formation. Topical fipronil	Often not noticed by owners. May transmit infectious agents (e.g. *Cytauxzoon felis*, *Ehrlichia* spp.)
Demodex mites	*Demodex cati*: not considered contagious; may be associated with current disease (e.g. diabetes mellitus, hyperadrenocorticism, retrovirus infection, toxoplasmosis, immune-mediated disease, neoplasia). *Demodex gatoi*: highly contagious, lives in superficial stratum corneum	Lesions may be localized to otitis or generalized. Alopecia, scaling and crusting, erythema, pruritus	Skin scrapings (Figure 2.16); ear swab cytology, hair trichogram	Topical: twice-weekly lime sulphur rinses, alone or with systemic treatment. Systemic: ivermectin (200 µg/kg orally q24h) for 4–8 wk; milbemycin (0.5 mg/kg orally q24h) for 4–8 wk. Treat all in-contact cats. *Isolate cats with D. gatoi*	

2.14   Common ectoparasites of cats.

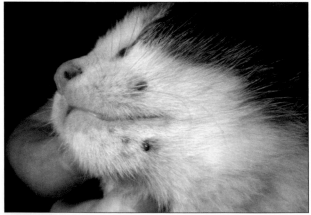

2.15   Ticks are most commonly found on the head and neck.

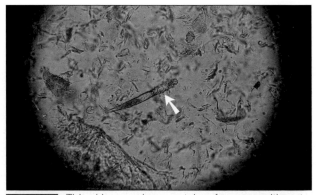

2.16   This skin scraping was taken from a pruritic cat infected with FIV. Numerous long slender mites (such as the one arrowed in this field) were found and identified as *Demodex cati*.

Drug	Application	Effective against	Comments
Imidacloprid	Spot-on	Fleas	Not absorbed systemically
Imidacloprid with moxidectin	Spot-on	Fleas, heartworm, ear mites, hookworms, roundworms	
Fipronil	Spray, spot-on	Fleas, ticks	Safe in breeding, pregnant, lactating cats
Selamectin	Spot-on	Fleas, heartworm, ear mites, hookworms, roundworms	Safe in breeding, pregnant, lactating cats
Nitenpyram	Oral	Adult fleas	Safe in breeding, pregnant, lactating cats. Can be used with imidacloprid, fipronil, lufenuron, pyrethrins
Metaflumizone	Spot-on	Fleas	
Dinotefuran (with pyriproxifen)	Spot-on	Fleas	

2.17 Summary of commonly used flea control products in cats. Products should always be administered in accordance with licensing and manufacturer's recommendations.

Endoparasites

The most common endoparasites and their treatments are discussed in Figures 2.18 to 2.21.

Parasite	Common clinical signs	Diagnosis	Transmission and control	Comments
Giardia	Acute or chronic small or large bowel diarrhoea; profuse diarrhoea with mucus; or asymptomatic	Faecal wet mount (trophozoites, cysts), faecal flotation (cysts), faecal antigen testing, polymerase chain reaction (PCR)	Ingesting cyst-contaminated faeces, grooming an infected cat, contaminated fomites. Control includes cleaning contaminated environmental surfaces and bathing animals to prevent re-infection	Infection more common in young cats and cats in densely populated multi-cat environments. Some genotypes have zoonotic potential
Cystoisospora (formerly *Isospora*)	Diarrhoea ± vomiting, weight loss, poor growth	Faecal flotation (oocysts)	Ingestion of oocysts. Environmental control important (low population density, cleaning and disinfection, reduce faecal contamination)	Kittens and sick young adults most likely to show clinical signs
Tritrichomonas foetus	Plasmacytic–lymphocytic and neutrophilic colitis; chronic foul-smelling large bowel diarrhoea with increased frequency of defecation, mucus, blood, flatulence; irritated anal mucosa; faecal incontinence	Warm fresh faeces required for faecal wet mount; colon flush to identify trophozoites and for culture; PCR	Ingestion of trophozoites from faeces. No cyst form. Control in multi-cat environments difficult due to re-infection; strict isolation and treatment of infected cats required	Most common in young pedigree cats and in multi-cat environments. Clinical signs most common in kittens and young adults
Toxoplasma gondii	Prenatal infection: hepatomegaly, ascites, dyspnoea, fever. Postnatal infection: inflammatory ocular disease, dyspnoea, fever, ascites, stiff gait, hyperaesthesia, neurological deficits. Most cats have no clinical signs	Oocysts difficult to find on faecal exam as are shed for short time after infection; 4-fold rise in IgG over 2–3-wk period or high IgM titre suggests infection; PCR on tissue, blood, aqueous humour, CSF samples	Ingestion of infected tissues or oocysts, transplacental. Feed only canned or dried commercial diets or well-cooked table food; avoid raw or undercooked meats. Do not allow cats to hunt. Control rodent populations	Cat is definitive host. Risk of infection increased in immunosuppressed cats, e.g. with retroviral infection or receiving immunosuppressive drug therapy. Severe disease seen in transplacentally infected kittens. *Zoonotic*

2.18 Common protozoal parasites of cats.

Drug	Dosage	Route	Susceptible parasites
Azithromycin	10 mg/kg q24h for 10 days minimum	Oral	*Cryptosporidium*
Febantel	56.5 mg/kg q24h for 5 days	Oral	*Giardia*
Fenbendazole	50 mg/kg q24h for 5 days	Oral	*Giardia*
Metronidazole	25 mg/kg q12h for 7 days	Oral	*Giardia*
Nitazoxanide	25 mg/kg q12h for 5–28 days	Oral	*Giardia, Cryptosporidium*
Paromomycin	125–165 mg/kg q12h for 5 days	Oral	*Giardia, Cryptosporidium*
Ponazuril	20–50 mg/kg q24h for 1–2 days	Oral	*Cystoisospora*
Ronidazole	30 mg/kg q24h for 14 days	Oral	*Tritrichomonas foetus*
Sulfadimethoxine	50 mg/kg once; then 25 mg/kg q24h for 14–21 days	Oral	*Cystoisospora*
Trimethoprim/sulphonamide	30 mg/kg q12h for 14 days	Oral	*Cystoisospora*

2.19 Antiprotozoal drugs and doses. Products should always be administered in accordance with licensing and manufacturer's recommendations. (Adapted from Javinsky, 2012)

Group	Common species	Common clinical signs	Diagnosis	Transmission and control	Comments
Roundworms	*Toxocara cati, Toxascaris leonina*	Often asymptomatic	Faecal flotation (eggs)	Infective larvae, paratenic hosts (accidental hosts, e.g. humans, rodents, etc), transmammary. Eggs highly resistant in the environment. Routine prophylaxis recommended even if faecal examination negative	Infection very common; kittens and young adults at highest risk. *Important zoonosis (visceral and ocular larva migrans)*
Tapeworms	*Dipylidium caninum*		Observation of mature worms in faeces, proglottids on perineum	Fleas as intermediate hosts. Flea control important for prevention	
	Taenia taeniaeformis		Observation of proglottids on perineum, faecal flotation (eggs)	Intermediate hosts (rodents, lagomorphs)	
Lungworms	*Aelurostrongylus abstrusus*	Often asymptomatic; heavy infections may result in coughing, dyspnoea, anorexia, weight loss	Observation of first-stage larvae in faeces using Baermann technique	Snails and slugs are intermediate hosts; cats more likely to be infected by eating transport hosts (e.g. birds, rodents). Control is by prevention of hunting. Most effective treatments may be moxidectin or emodepside (e.g. in combination products)	Infection most common in cats that hunt and can be found worldwide
Hookworms	*Ancylostoma, Uncinaria*	Weight loss, poor growth, diarrhoea, melaena, anaemia (especially in kittens with high worm burdens)	Faecal flotation (eggs)	Cutaneous penetration of larvae, ingesting larvae, ingesting an infected paratenic host (e.g. rodents). No transplacental or transmammary transmission	*Zoonotic*
Heartworm	*Dirofilaria immitis*	Vomiting, anorexia, weight loss, lethargy, cough and dyspnoea (heartworm-associated respiratory disease), sudden death or anaphylaxis when adult worms die. Many infections asymptomatic	May be difficult; often requires combinations of tests. Heartworm antigen and antibody testing (should be performed together), echocardiography, radiography	Intermediate host (mosquito). Routine prophylaxis recommended in endemic areas. Adulticide therapy not recommended	Cats more resistant to infection than dogs but still susceptible. Infection typically with very few worms (1–3). Pulmonary response predominates. Infection worldwide (but not UK); endemic in some countries (e.g. most of USA). Indoor cats may be infected

2.20   Common helminth parasites of cats.

Drug	Dosage	Route	Susceptible parasites
Emodepside with praziquantel	3 mg/kg once	Topical	Roundworms, heartworm, tapeworms
Epsiprantel	2.75 mg/kg once	Oral	Tapeworms
Febantel with praziquantel and pyrantel	15 mg/kg once	Oral	Roundworms, heartworm, tapeworms
Fenbendazole	50 mg/kg q24h for 3–5 days	Oral	Roundworms, heartworm, *Taenia* spp., lungworm
Flubendazole	22 mg/kg q24h for 2–3 days	Oral	Roundworms, heartworm, tapeworms
Piperazine	110 mg/kg; repeat in 3 weeks	Oral	Roundworms
Praziquantel	5 mg/kg once	Oral or s.c.	Tapeworms
Pyrantel pamoate	5–20 mg/kg; repeat in 3 weeks	Oral	Roundworms, heartworm
Pyrantel with praziquantel	1 tablet/4 kg once	Oral	Roundworms, heartworm, tapeworms
Selamectin	6 mg/kg once	Topical	Roundworms, heartworm

2.21   Spectrum of activity and doses of selected anthelmintics. Products should always be administered in accordance with licensing and manufacturer's recommendations. (Adapted from Javinsky, 2012)

Nutrition and weight management

Cats are obligate carnivores that normally consume small, frequent meals. The natural diet (primarily rodents) is relatively high in protein and fat and low in carbohydrates. Cats have a higher protein requirement than dogs and require certain animal-derived nutrients in their diet (e.g. the amino acid taurine). Energy and nutrient requirements depend on factors such as age, activity, and reproductive status. Home-prepared diets can be formulated but should be evaluated by a nutritionist to ensure that they are complete and balanced. Feeding raw foods is discouraged to prevent disease transmission. Kittens are strongly influenced in food preferences by those of the queen and also by the type of diet fed at weaning. Exposing kittens to a variety of foods (including wet and dry foods) is important to increase the chance that a new diet will be accepted later in life should a diet change be required. Although knowledge of feline nutrition is still evolving, many types of specialized diets are available for cats at different life stages or with various diseases. Nutritional status is now called the 'fifth vital sign' and both AAHA and WSAVA have recently published nutritional assessment guidelines that should be consulted.

General recommendations

Recommendations for feeding management include:

- Mimic normal feeding behaviour by providing food in foraging devices (e.g. food balls (Figure 2.22) or puzzle feeders) or providing food in multiple novel locations
- Feed multiple small meals to older kittens and adults, rather than feeding *ad libitum*
- Locate food and water away from litter boxes
- Ensure each cat in a multi-cat home has its own food and water station
- Provide large water bowls.

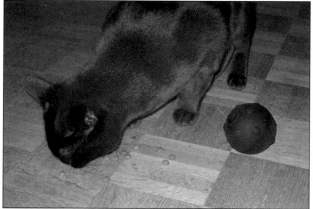

2.22 Food balls or food puzzles can be used to encourage natural foraging behaviours and expenditure of energy in pursuit of food. Many types are available, and owners may need to experiment to find one that their cat will interact with.

Changing diets

If a cat must be moved on to a new diet, the transition should be performed slowly, especially where cats have become fixated on one type or flavour of food. Further recommendations include the following.

- It is easiest to change to a new food that is similar in texture and shape to the old food.
- Avoid changing a cat's diet when it is stressed by pain, illness or while hospitalized or boarding. Wait until the cat's condition is improved, it is eating normally, and it is at home to effect the transition to a new diet.
- Educating owners about realistic expectations can help improve compliance, as it may take several weeks for some cats to accept a new food. The cat's bodyweight should be monitored during diet transitions. The old diet should be reintroduced for a few weeks if weight loss of >10% occurs.
- Meal feeding may make the transition to a new diet easier than *ad libitum* feeding, as the cat is more likely to be hungry at meal times. The transition to meal feeding can be made by leaving food out for 1 hour two or three times per day. It is often easiest to start this during the time of day when the owner is normally away from home and cannot be tempted to feed the cat off schedule.

- The new food should be offered along with the old food, rather than abruptly discontinuing the old food. Ideally, both foods should be in the same type of familiar bowl. The new food may have to be offered for several days to a week, or longer, before the cat will try it. Once the cat starts consuming the new food, the amount of the old food offered should be reduced by a small amount each day, with the aim of moving totally to the new diet over a 1–2-week period.
- Another method of introducing a new diet involves mixing the old and new foods together. For the first few days the cat is offered a mix of 75% current food and 25% new food. Then the ratio is changed to 50:50 for the next few days. By the end of the first week, it may be possible to offer 25% old diet and 75% new diet. The amount of the new food is increased thereafter, until the cat is consuming 100% of the intended diet.
- Cats must be exposed to both the smell and the taste of a new food to overcome neophobia. If the new diet is a canned food, it may be helpful to smear a small amount on a front paw to encourage the cat to lick and taste the food.
- Enhancing the smell and flavour of the new food can be accomplished by warming it slightly, or by adding small quantities (approximately 1 tablespoon) of tuna or clam juice, or low-salt chicken broth.

Weight management

More than a third of cats in most countries are either overweight or obese. Obesity (Figure 2.23) is associated with increased disease risks (e.g. diabetes mellitus) and treating obesity once it develops is difficult. Therefore, attention should be focused on prevention through owner education about the nutritional needs of cats and normal feeding behaviours. In particular, owners should be counselled that eating is not a social event for cats as it is for people, and feeding should not be used to replace other types of interactions between owner and cat.

Neutering is an important contributing factor, due to hormonal changes and decreased caloric requirements (by over 25%). Therefore, adjustment of diet type and feeding practices in the post-neutering period are critical for prevention of weight gain. Important factors include:

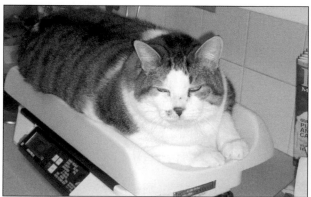

2.23 An alarming number of pet cats are overweight or obese. Prevention of obesity starts early in life, around the time of surgical sterilization. Cats should be weighed and body condition scored (see Figure 1.20) at every opportunity.

- Careful calculation of daily caloric requirements (see QRG 2.1); the amounts indicated on food packaging are too generous
- Careful measurement of daily food allotments (weighing dry diets may be more accurate than using a measuring cup)
- Feeding multiple small meals instead of *ad libitum* feeding
- Changing from a growth diet to an adult maintenance diet at the appropriate time
- Regular monitoring of bodyweight and body condition score or body mass index.

Litter box/tray management

Litter preferences probably reflect the desert habitat of the domestic cat's ancestor, the African wild cat, as litters with characteristics similar to sand are still preferred by cats today. The reason cats will use a litter box at all is probably related to their preference for burying their waste. Many types of cat litter are now available, including clumping, biodegradable (e.g. wood pellets, recycled newspaper) and silica gel litters. A few studies have evaluated cat preferences for litter material, and concluded that clumping type litters are preferred by most cats. In a multi-cat household, cats may have different litter preferences, so that more than one type of litter may be required.

Citrus appears to be an offensive odour to cats, so citrus-scented litters are best avoided. Odour control additives may be important; research has indicated that cats prefer litters with activated carbon. Other common recommendations for litter boxes include the following.

- Cleanliness is important: each box should be scooped out at least once daily. Clay litters should be completely changed and the box washed weekly, clumping litters every other week. Strongly scented cleaners (e.g. bleach, pine cleaners) should be avoided; hot water alone or with a mild detergent is recommended.
- The minimum number of litter boxes in a home is commonly recommended as the number of cats plus 1. One large litter box is not the same as having two smaller ones! Even in a single cat home, there should be a minimum of two litter boxes, as some cats prefer to urinate and defecate in separate areas. Litter boxes should be in multiple sites rather than concentrated in one location, especially in multi-cat homes.
- Litter boxes should not be too small (Figure 2.24). A common recommendation is that the box should be 1.5 times the body length of the cat; although no data exist to substantiate this, many behaviourists recommend large boxes. Many commercial litter boxes are too small, especially for large-breed cats or overweight cats; plastic storage boxes with low sides are useful for these cats.
- Covered boxes are controversial; they are not acceptable to all cats as they may trap odours and may lead to decreased scooping and cleaning ('out of sight, out of mind'). In addition, in a multi-cat home, a covered box may be an opportunity for ambush and attack by another cat, though this can be avoided by cutting a second opening in the cover.

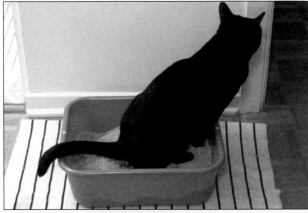

2.24 This cat litter box, a converted plastic dishwashing bowl, is smaller than the recommended size of 1.5 times the length of the cat. Commercially available litter boxes are also often too small.

- Boxes should be placed in easily accessible locations but also areas that are quiet and not near noisy appliances; boxes should not be placed immediately next to food and water. Lighting should be considered; if the location of the box is totally dark (especially at night), a night lamp should be added.
- Owners should not disturb a cat when it is in the box, and children and other animals should also be prevented from interfering with the litter box. Cats should not be caught while in the box in order to perform unpleasant tasks, such as administer medication, trim claws, or be put in a cat carrier.
- Modification of the box may be required in special circumstances, such as with arthritic senior cats. A box with lower sides or construction of a ramp can be very helpful. Young kittens also may require boxes with lower sides until they are older.

Behavioural needs by life stage

- **Kittens (birth to 6 months):**
  - Strong play needs must be met; toys allow kittens to practise normal predatory behaviours
  - Inter-cat social play peaks at about 12 weeks of age, after which object-oriented play becomes more important
  - Play should be directed toward toys and not owners' hands or feet
  - The primary socialization period is from about 3 to 9 weeks of age
    - Kittens should have positive experiences with people during this period
    - Kittens should be exposed to a variety of stimuli and normal situations, such as:
      - Handling to trim nails or examine the mouth
      - Children, other cats, other pets (Figure 2.25)
      - Cat carriers and car trips
    - Positive behaviours should be rewarded and punishment avoided.
- **Junior (7 months to 2 years):**
  - Continue acclimation of the cat to handling for nail trims, oral examinations, grooming, etc.
  - Inter-cat aggression may develop, starting at about 2 years of age, and lead to inappropriate

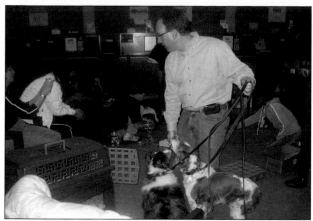

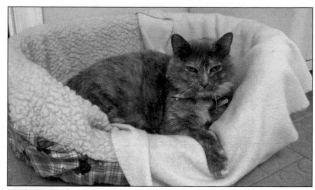

2.26 Senior and geriatric cats often have mobility problems. Resources such as favourite beds or sleeping spots should be made accessible and should be well padded for comfort.

2.25 The primary socialization period for kittens is between 3 and 9 weeks of age. In this 'kitten kindergarten' class, young kittens are being taught to accept handling, are acclimating to cat carriers and car rides, and are being socialized to other people, other cats and to dogs. (Courtesy of Steve Dale)

elimination, urine spraying, and fighting (see Chapter 18)
- Owners must be educated to provide adequate space and resources in multi-cat homes
- Synthetic feline pheromone diffusers placed in each room where the cat spends time may also be helpful.

■ **Adult/prime (3 to 6 years) and Mature (7 to 10 years):**
- A decline in play activity may occur
  - Owners should be encouraged to provide stimulating environments and regular play sessions (2 or 3 sessions of 15 minutes each daily)
  - A decline in roaming, fighting and predatory behaviour may occur in cats with access to the outdoors
  - A decline in sexual activity and fertility may occur in intact cats.

■ **Senior (11 to 14 years):**
- Behaviour changes (e.g. inappropriate vocalization, change in litter box habits) may be indicative of medical problems
- Owners should be educated that behavioural changes may not be due to 'old age'
- Arthritis and other painful conditions are common and may lead to decreased mobility, inappropriate elimination, and decreased interactions with other pets and people
  - Ramps can be used to facilitate access to favourite high places
  - Litter boxes can be moved to one floor of the home
  - Litter boxes should be large with a low lip for easy access.

■ **Geriatric (15 years and older):**
- Attention must be paid to ensure litter box, food, water, and sleeping places are easily accessed (Figure 2.26)
- Owners should be educated about signs of cognitive dysfunction such as increased vocalizing (see Chapter 18), attention-seeking or reclusiveness, and altered sleep patterns. Owners should assist with grooming as needed

(i.e. regular brushing, wiping with a damp cloth)
- Owners should be assisted in assessing quality of life and end-of-life planning (see QRG 2.5).

References and further reading

Baldwin K, Bartges J, Buffington T *et al.* (2010) AAHA nutritional assessment guidelines for dogs and cats. *Journal of the American Animal Hospital Association* **46**, 285–296

Curtis T (2007) Environmental enrichment for cats. *Compendium on Continuing Education for the Practicing Veterinarian* **29**, 104–106

Day MJ, Horzinek MC and Schultz RD (2010) WSAVA guidelines for the vaccination of dogs and cats. *Journal of Small Animal Practice* **51**, 338–356

Ellis SLH (2009) Environmental enrichment: Practical strategies for improving feline welfare. *Journal of Feline Medicine and Surgery* **11**, 901–912

Epstein M, Kuehn NF, Landsberg G *et al.* (2005) AAHA senior care guidelines for dogs and cats. *Journal of the American Animal Hospital Association* **41**, 81–91

Freeman L, Becvarova I, Cave N *et al.* (2011) Nutritional assessment guidelines. *Journal of Small Animal Practice* **52**, 385–396

Herron ME and Buffington CA (2010) Environmental enrichment for indoor cats. *Compendium on Continuing Education for the Practicing Veterinarian* **32**, E1–E5

Holmstrom SE, Bellows J, Colmery B *et al.* (2005) AAHA dental care guidelines for dogs and cats. *Journal of the American Animal Hospital Association* **41**, 277–283

Javinsky E (2012) Gastrointestinal parasites. In: *The Cat: Clinical Medicine and Management,* ed. S Little, pp. 496–512. Elsevier Saunders, St. Louis

Levy J, Crawford C, Hartmann K *et al.* (2008) American Association of Feline Practitioners' feline retrovirus management guidelines. *Journal of Feline Medicine and Surgery* **10**, 300–316

Little S, Bienzle D, Carioto L *et al.* (2011) Feline leukemia virus and feline immunodeficiency virus in Canada: recommendations for testing and management. *Canadian Veterinary Journal* **52**, 849–855

Overall K, Rodan I, Beaver B *et al.* (2005) Feline behavior guidelines from the American Association of Feline Practitioners. *Journal of the American Veterinary Medical Association* **227**, 70–84

Overley B, Shofer FS, Goldschmidt MH, Sherer D and Sorenmo KU (2005) Association between ovariohysterectomy and feline mammary carcinoma. *Journal of Veterinary Internal Medicine* **19**, 560–563

Pittari J, Rodan I, Beekman G *et al.* (2009) American Association of Feline Practitioners Senior Care Guidelines. *Journal of Feline Medicine and Surgery* **11**, 763–778

Richards JR, Elston TH, Ford RB *et al.* (2006) The 2006 American Association of Feline Practitioners Feline Vaccine Advisory Panel report. *Journal of the American Veterinary Medical Association* **229**, 1405–1441

Rodan I and Sparkes A (2012) Preventive health care for cats. In: *The Cat: Clinical Medicine and Management,* ed. S Little, pp. 151–180. Elsevier Saunders, St. Louis

Seksel K (2009) Preventive behavioural medicine for cats. In: *BSAVA Manual of Canine and Feline Behavioural Medicine, 2nd edn,* ed. DF Horwitz and DS Mills, pp. 75–82. BSAVA Publications, Gloucester

Stella JL, Lord LK and Buffington CAT (2011) . Sickness behaviors in response to unusual external events in healthy cats and cats with feline interstitial cystitis. *Journal of the American Veterinary Medical Association* **238**, 67–73

Vogt AH, Rodan I, Brown M *et al.* (2010) AAFP-AAHA: Feline life stage guidelines. *Journal of Feline Medicine and Surgery* **12**, 43–54

WSAVA Nutritional Assessment Guidelines Task Force (2011) WSAVA Nutritional Assessment Guidelines. *Journal of Feline Medicine and Surgery* **13**, 516–525

QRG 2.1 Calculation of energy requirements for life stages and weight management
by Marge Chandler

Calculation of daily energy requirements begins with calculating the **resting energy requirement (RER),** which estimates the cat's calorie requirements at rest in a thermoneutral environment. Energy requirements are expressed as kilocalories of metabolizable energy (kcal ME) or joules (J) of ME (where 1 J = 4.18 kcal).

$$RER_{(kcal/day)} = bodyweight^{0.75}_{(kg)} \times 70$$

Or, for cats >2 kg:

$$RER_{(kcal/day)} = (30 \times bodyweight_{(kg)}) + 70$$

For both calculations, the actual current bodyweight is used, not the patient's ideal bodyweight.

The RER is then multiplied by a factor related to the cat's life stage, to account for growth, pregnancy, lactation, or adult maintenance.

The caloric content of cat foods may be found by contacting the manufacturer; producers of premium foods usually provide full nutritional information to veterinary practices. If an owner wishes to feed a homemade diet it should be formulated and balanced by a veterinary nutritionist.

Adult MER

The maintenance energy requirement (MER) for adult cats can be calculated as follows:

- For minimally active indoor cats: MER = 1.0 to 1.2 x RER
- For active neutered cats: MER = 1.2 to 1.4 x RER
- For active sexually intact cats: MER = 1.4 to 1.6 x RER

Several other formulae are available for estimating feline adult MER but many veterinary nutritionists use the formulae given above to calculate MER for an adult cat that is not a breeding queen.

The most important part of estimating caloric requirements is the awareness of the **individual variation of MER** among cats; it can be 40% above or below the calculated value, and thus regular assessment of body condition score (see Figure 1.20) and bodyweight is vital to ensure that MER calculations are appropriate. Thus, ranges for calculation of MER have been provided above; a decision on which figure to start with can be reached based on clinical judgement of the cat's activity and body condition. After neutering, most cats require fewer calories due to the metabolic changes induced; prevention of obesity is a major aim in feeding the appropriate MER to cats.

Pregnancy

Pregnant queens require 25–50% more energy than the MER. Unlike dogs or humans, queens gain weight throughout pregnancy compared to primarily in later gestation.

- A queen's requirements are met by initially providing 1.6 x RER and gradually increasing to 2 x RER over pregnancy.

Free-choice feeding of a high-quality, high-energy food (4–5 kcal/g dry matter of diet) is recommended to meet their increased energy needs.

Lactation

Lactation is the most energy-demanding period for a queen.

- Energy requirements increase when the kittens are born and reach a peak around 6 weeks after parturition. At this peak, queens may require 2–6 x RER, depending on the number of kittens and the amount of milk they are consuming. It is often best to feed queens *ad libitum*, as they will usually then consume appropriate energy requirements.

Feeding during lactation should take into account both the needs of the queen and the intake of the kittens, which will have begun eating solid food at around 3 weeks of age. Kittens are usually fully weaned at around 8 weeks, after which the queen can be transitioned back to MER, unless she needs to regain body condition in which case additional food can be given.

Growth

The energy requirement of kittens and junior cats depends upon their age, with the kcal requirement per kg of bodyweight decreasing with increasing age.

Age	kcal requirement per kg of bodyweight	Examples
6–20 weeks	250	1.4 kg; 350 kcal/day
4–6.5 months	130	2.3 kg; 300 kcal/day
6.5–8.5 months	100	2.7 kg; 270 kcal/day
8.5–11 months	80	3.2 kg; 256 kcal/day

As for adults, kittens should be fed to an appropriate bodyweight and not allowed to become too fat. Monitoring body condition scores and weight is important.

Overweight cats

Weight loss programmes for obese cats may be based on their current 'fat weight' or on their ideal weight. Using the current weight may be easier than estimating the ideal weight.

1. A starting point is to use the calculation of 90% of the MER for the cat's current weight.
2. After 2 weeks, reweigh the cat to see whether it has lost 0.5–1% of initial bodyweight per week.
3. If not, decrease the caloric intake to 80% of MER for current weight.
4. After 2 weeks, reweigh the cat to see whether it has lost 0.5–1% of initial bodyweight per week.
5. If not, decrease the caloric intake to 70% of MER for current weight.
6. After 2 weeks, reweigh the cat to see whether it has lost 0.5–1% of initial bodyweight per week.
7. If not, decrease the caloric intake to 60% of MER for current weight.

The amount fed should not be below 60% of MER for the current weight. Hepatic lipidosis is a serious risk if weight loss is too rapid.

The feed should be a calorie-restricted diet designed for weight loss, as decreasing the amount of the cat's usual diet may not provide enough protein, minerals or vitamins. Other considerations to increase energy expenditure by increasing activity should also be considered.

Thin cats

This situation is usually best solved by getting owners gradually to increase the amount fed to the cat, usually by adding lunch or a late evening meal, depending on the current feeding regime. However, many thin cats are already being fed to satiety, so consideration should be given to feeding an energy-dense diet.

References, further reading and resources

German A (2010) Obesity and weight management. In: *BSAVA Manual of Rehabilitation, Supportive and Palliative Care: Case Studies in Patient Management*, ed. S Lindley and P Watson, pp. 60–77. BSAVA Publications, Gloucester

Hand MS, Thatcher CD, Remillard RL, Roudebush P and Novotny BJ (2010) *Small Animal Clinical Nutrition, 5th edn*. Mark Morris Institute, Topeka, KS

Harvey A and Taylor S (2012) *Caring for an Overweight Cat*. Available at catprofessional.com

National Research Council (2006) Energy. In: *Nutrient Requirements of Dogs and Cats*, pp. 28–48. The National Academies Press, Washington DC

For information on formulating homemade diets, see https://secure.balanceit.com/index.php

QRG 2.2 Prepubertal neutering of kittens
by David Yates

Both male and female cats have traditionally been neutered at 6 months of age, but there is a strong case for neutering earlier. Veterinary surgeons working with feral cats may neuter kittens as early as 8 weeks of age, but 'early neutering' is generally considered to be at around 4 months of age (rather than the traditional 6 months).

Prepubertal neutering allows effective population control, prevents females from 'calling', reduces hunting, straying and fighting behaviours (the latter can be associated with cat bite abscesses, transmission of infections such as FIV) and reduces the risk of diseases associated with entire females, such as pyometra and pregnancy problems. Complicating factors to surgery, such as pregnancy, are eliminated; and postoperative morbidity is reduced compared to conventional neutering. Early neutering also provides an ideal opportunity to carry out other procedures such as microchipping.

Prepubertal surgery is simple. Early neutering essentially uses similar methodology to the neutering of older cats, although certain considerations are important, such as conserving heat and landmarks for surgery (see below and QRGs 2.3 and 2.4).

Prepubertal neutering is an elective surgical procedure. Kittens should be healthy prior to surgery. For owned animals, vaccination is recommended prior to hospitalization but this may not be possible in a shelter environment.

To minimize stress during hospitalization, keep littermates together.

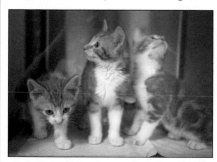

It is safe to withhold food for up to 3 hours before anaesthesia; this reduces the risk of hypoglycaemia and does not result in other problems. Water should be available until premedication.

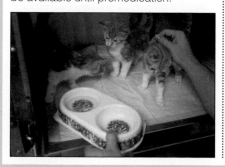

The high surface area to volume ratio (compared to adult cats) may increase the likelihood of hypothermia. Heated cages are invaluable. Ensure kittens are warmed prior to premedication to minimize heat loss. Reflective foil sheets and a heated operating table (37°C) are effective measures for heat preservation. Other heating mechanisms are available.

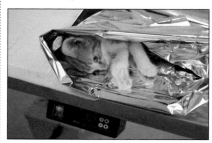

Full details of premedication and anaesthesia protocols for early neutering are given in Chapter 3.

- Keep surgical and preparation time to a minimum.
- Dosing anaesthetic agents using body surface area may be more reliable than on a bodyweight basis.
- Ensure that all equipment needed is ready prior to injecting anaesthetic agents.
- The use of injectable intramuscular anaesthetic combinations including ketamine may necessitate corneal protection; an ocular lubricating agent can be applied to the eyes.

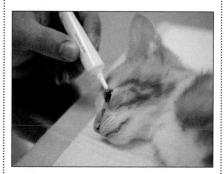

Non-cuffed endotracheal tubes (from 2 mm internal diameter) are recommended for kittens. The author does not use a laryngoscope in such small patients. Provide oxygen via the endotracheal tube from an appropriate breathing system (see Chapter 3).

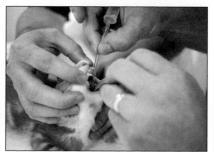

Littermates are recovered as a group. Particular attention must be given to avoiding problems due to dissimilar recovery rates. For example, the nursing team should be vigilant against kittens lying on each other prior to full recovery.

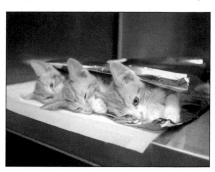

Kittens should be offered food when they are able to stand. This is likely to be about an hour after induction of anaesthesia. Prompt feeding mitigates against the risks of hypothermia and hypoglycaemia. Anaesthetic combinations that include midazolam may improve postoperative food intake.

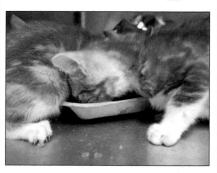

Kittens should be returned promptly to their owners; this reduces both stress and the risk of infectious disease.

QRG 2.3 Prepubertal neutering of males: castration

by David Yates

1 Screen kittens for cryptorchidism before anaesthesia, by palpation for both testes. After gentle palpation in the inguinal region, the prepubertal testis, being both small and mobile, is moved into the scrotal position.

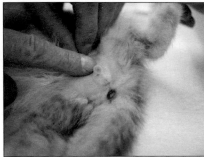

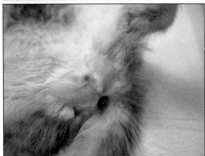

This kitten had a single scrotal testis on palpation.

If this is not possible, or no testes can be found, cryptorchidism is diagnosed, and surgery will need to be postponed. The developed testis will be found more readily at sexual maturity (~6 months).

2 Under general anaesthesia (see Chapter 3), a vertical incision is made on each side of the scrotum to facilitate exposure of the testis.

3 In a **closed castration** the tunic beneath the skin is kept intact.

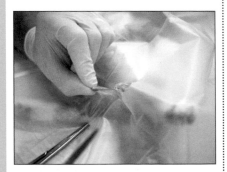

■ One method of closed castration involves the formation of a knot in the vaginal tunic, containing the vas deferens and blood vessel, around mosquito forceps; the closed forceps

are twisted around the vaginal tunic and the forceps are then opened slightly to grasp the vaginal tunic close to the testis. The forceps are then clamped shut, the testis is removed by cutting along the forceps with a scalpel, and the vaginal tunic is then pushed off over the end of the forceps to make a secure knot in the vaginal tunic. The forceps are then removed.

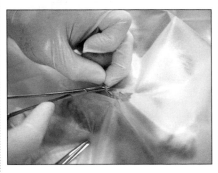

■ Alternatively, an absorbable suture material (e.g. 1.5 metric (4/0 USP) polyglecaprone 25) can be used to ligate the vas deferens and blood vessel within the vaginal tunic before the testis is removed by cutting with scissors.

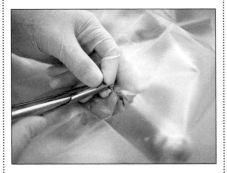

If an **open castration** technique is used, the tunic is incised with a scalpel.

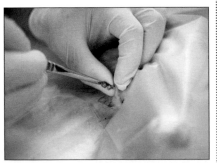

■ The fibrous attachment of the tunic to the testis is broken down using forceps.

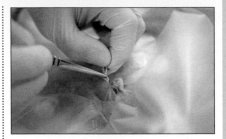

■ The blood vessel is separated from the vas deferens by breaking down the loose connective tissue between them; the testis remains attached to the blood vessel.

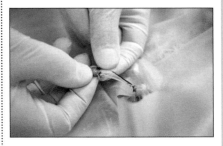

■ Five or six square knots are made using the vas deferens and blood vessel; this ensures adequate haemostasis. Care must be taken to avoid excess traction and cord or vessel damage. The vas deferens and blood vessel are then cut a few millimetres distal to the knots.

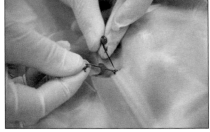

4 The scrotum is gently raised to return the tunic within it. The skin edges are lightly compressed with a sterile swab to check for haemorrhage, and to ensure no tissue protrusion. The small scrotal incisions heal rapidly without the need for sutures.

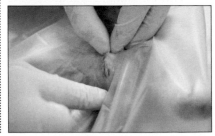

QRG 2.4 Prepubertal neutering of females: ovariohysterectomy

by David Yates

1 Under general anaesthesia and before surgery the bladder should be gently expressed to: improve visualization of the abdominal cavity; reduce the likelihood of urination (and patient cooling) on recovery; and improve postoperative comfort. This is particularly important if α2-agonists (medetomidine, dexmedetomidine) are used as they have a diuretic effect (see Chapter 3).

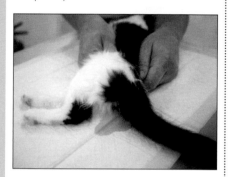

2 The kitten is placed in dorsal recumbency (or a left flank approach can be used). The landmarks for the skin incision (and therefore clipping) include the umbilicus (left cross) and bony pubic brim (right cross). The location of the 10–15 mm incision is determined by the age of the patient (the younger patient has a more caudal incision):

- Kittens <12 weeks: the incision is centred two-thirds of the distance from the umbilicus to the pubic brim (centre of incision shown as black dot on photo)
- Kittens >12 weeks: the centre of the incision is halfway between the umbilicus and the pubic brim (not illustrated).

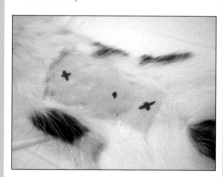

Patient cooling is minimized by:

- Reduced area of clipping
- Minimal wetting
- Avoiding alcohol-based products; instead chlorhexidine gluconate 4% w/v (Hibiscrub) is applied to the clipped skin using cotton wool moistened in warm water.

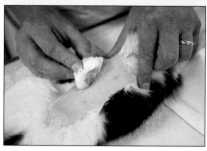

3 The linea alba is carefully incised using a reversed scalpel blade to avoid any internal damage. In some spays on very young kittens, an appreciable amount of clear abdominal fluid (SG <1.020) may be present. This may be removed with a sterile swab.

4 The uterine body is located between the urinary bladder and descending colon.

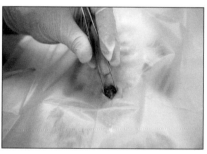

5 The left uterine horn is then identified and gently elevated from the abdomen.

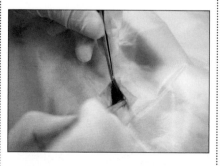

6 The left ovary is then elevated and the ovarian pedicle clamped.

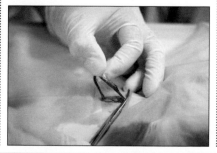

- Note the following features of prepubertal neutering in females:
  - The relatively large ovary
  - The excellent exposure
  - Minimal fat.

7 Three clamps are placed on to the ovarian pedicle, and a single clamp on the proper ligament (between the ovary and uterine horn).

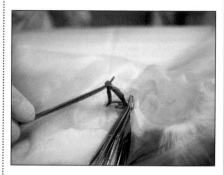

8 An absorbable ligature (e.g. 1.5 metric (4/0 USP) poliglecaprone 25) is placed around the bottom clamp and tightened into the crush as the bottom clamp is removed. A scalpel is used to cut above the two remaining clamps beneath the ovary. The top clamp is removed and the crushed tissue grasped with forceps. The final clamp is then removed and the ligature returned to the abdomen, checking haemostasis is adequate.

9 The clamps attached to the proper ligament (background of photo) are retracted caudally to display the broad and round ligament. Two additional clamps (foreground) may be placed to allow separation of the relatively avascular broad and round ligaments from the uterine horn.

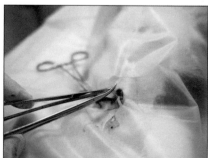

10 The forceps holding the proper ligament are retracted caudally to expose the remaining (right) uterine horn. The uterine horn is then traced cranially to reveal the remaining ovary. The process of ovarian ligation, as described above, is repeated.

▶

QRG 2.4 *continued*

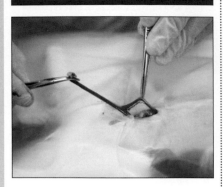

11 The uterine body is exposed using caudal traction on the forceps attached to both the proper ligaments. Midline exposure of the uterine body is superior to the flank approach.

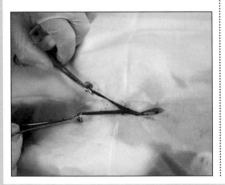

12 The vagina is ligated using 1.5 metric (4/0 USP/PhEur) poliglecaprone 25. A second ligature may then follow into the crush, using a 3-clamp method described above (not shown).

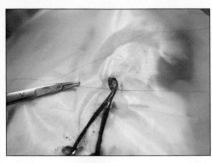

13 The vaginal stump is checked for bleeding by holding it with forceps, before returning it to the abdomen if no bleeding occurs. Repeat ligation is required if bleeding is apparent.

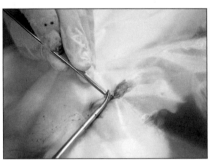

14
- The muscle is closed with absorbable suture material (e.g. 2 metric (3/0 USP/PhEur) polydioxanone) using a continuous pattern.
- The subcutaneous tissue is apposed using interrupted absorbable sutures (e.g. 1.5 metric (4/0 USP/PhEur) poliglecaprone 25). Occasional 'bites' of the muscle sheath when suturing this layer can help reduce tissue 'dead space'.

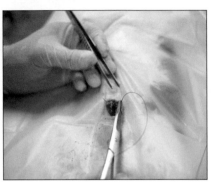

- Subcuticular sutures (or tissue glue) reduce the likelihood of patient interference with the wound.

QRG 2.5 Compassionate euthanasia
by Martha Cannon

A euthanasia consultation is a highly emotional experience for owners and can also be stressful for the veterinary staff involved.

It is essential to handle things as smoothly and professionally as possible to minimize the owner's distress but it is also important to acknowledge that distress, to sympathize, and to reassure the owner that they are doing the right thing and that their emotions are entirely natural.

Be prepared

- All members of staff should be aware of the circumstances so that from the time of their arrival in the practice the owner is handled gently and sympathetically.
- Try to schedule euthanasia consultations for a quiet time of day when the waiting room will not be busy. Allow adequate time and, as far as is possible, make sure that you will not be under time pressure yourself. Euthanasia

consultations should be significantly longer than normal appointments.
- Attend to the client promptly at the appointed time; if you are running late, make sure the client is informed.

Prepare the owner

- Explain to the owner what will happen and ensure that they know what to expect:
  - The speed of action of the injection
  - Their cat's eyes will stay open
  - Their cat is likely to void urine once it is unconscious
  - There may be muscle twitches and respiratory spasms but the cat will be deeply unconscious through them.
- Discuss the options for disposing of the body.
- Some owners may prefer to pay in advance so that they can leave immediately afterwards.

Euthanasia in the practice

- Ensure that there is a private place to discuss the need for euthanasia – and to carry it out.
- Always offer the owner the option to stay with the cat, or to leave the cat with the veterinary surgeon and staff. Ensure that they do not feel under pressure in either direction, and that they feel free to do what feels right for them.

Euthanasia in the home

Many owners will prefer to arrange a home visit for euthanasia. This is less stressful for the cat and the owners but may be more stressful for the veterinary staff involved. Be prepared to take control politely and calmly, even though you are a guest in the owner's home. The owner's choice of situation may not be ideal: ▶

QRG 2.5 *continued*

- Ensure that the cat can be adequately and safely restrained
- Make sure that you have enough light to see what you are doing
- If necessary move the cat to a more appropriate site
- If any of the above is not possible, consider sedating the cat before attempting to administer the pentobarbital.

Administering the injection

In most cases administering pentobarbital into the cephalic vein is straightforward. However, when emotions are running high, and especially if the cat is agitated or severely debilitated, finding a vein can be challenging. Practice and good technique will help, but even the most experienced vet will sometimes struggle.

- If the cat is an inpatient pre-place an intravenous catheter and ensure that it is patent.
- Try to have your best cat nurse on hand to assist you.
- Use a 21 G or 23 G needle to draw up the pentobarbital. Then discard that needle and replace it with a new 23 G or 25 G needle:
  - A small sharp needle will be better tolerated – small needles are rapidly blunted even by a single passage through the rubber stopper of the bottle
  - Pentobarbital stings – an uncontaminated needle will be better tolerated as it passes through the skin.

- Make sure you have adequate light and have clipped off enough fur to see the vein clearly.
- Use a local anaesthetic spray (e.g. Intubeaze) or cream (e.g. EMLA) on the skin and allow adequate time for it to take effect
- Sedate fractious or wriggly cats:
  - 0.4 mg/kg butorphanol i.m. has minimal sedative effect but can make wriggly cats more tolerant of handling and restraint
  - For more fractious cats, an intramuscular combination of butorphanol (0.4 mg/kg) and ketamine (5 mg/kg) will usually provide adequate sedation to allow intravenous access. Addition of a very small volume of medetomidine (e.g. 0.05 ml per cat) will provide even more sedation, but may induce vomiting so is best avoided unless the cat is very fractious. Higher doses of medetomidine should not be used as they will reduce peripheral perfusion, making intravenous injection more difficult.
- For cats with poor peripheral circulation, sedation with intramuscular butorphanol and ketamine (as described above) followed by intrarenal injection of pentobarbital can achieve very peaceful and rapid euthanasia. This route may also be preferred if euthanasia is being carried out single-handed.

After the event

- Spend a little time with the owners, allowing them to reminisce about their cat, try to evoke some happy memories from a time when the cat was well.

- Make **absolutely** sure that the heart beat is absent and that all respiratory spasms have ceased before pronouncing the cat dead and/or releasing the body to the owners.
- Handle the body gently at all times and with the same care that you would use if the cat were still alive.
- Allow the owners some time alone with the body before they leave the building.
- If the owners are taking the body home to bury, or were absent for the euthanasia but are coming to see their cat before disposal, wrap the body in a towel or blanket and arrange it in a comfortable sleeping position before the limbs start to stiffen. Arrange the folds of the blanket so that the head can easily be uncovered, in case the owners or other family members wish to say a final goodbye.
- If the owners are taking the body home to bury, make sure that a suitable box is available in which to place the wrapped body. Often the cat's carrying basket is most appropriate, but remember that if the carrier has a small front-opening door it may be difficult for the owner to get the body out with dignity, especially if it has started to stiffen. Cardboard 'coffins' are available to purchase, but a suitable sized cardboard box or cardboard pet-carrier will usually suffice and will not offend most owners.
- Check that the waiting room is relatively clear, or if possible offer distressed clients the opportunity to leave via a side or back door.
- Always ring the owners, or write to them, to express your condolences after the event.

Practical therapeutics

Jill E. Maddison and Jo Murrell

Introduction

Although cats and dogs are physiologically similar in many respects, and dosing regimens recommended for dogs can frequently be extrapolated to cats, there are some important differences in drug disposition between the two species that can have a profound influence on dosing recommendations. The majority of differences relate to pharmacokinetic differences in drug metabolism, but differences in haemoglobin structure, receptors and behaviour may also be relevant.

Cats tend to be deficient in some glucuronyl transferases that are important for glucuronidation. As a result, drugs that are excreted as glucuronide conjugates in other species (e.g. aspirin, benzoic acid, paracetamol (acetaminophen), morphine and hexachlorophene) may have a prolonged half-life in cats, increasing the risk of toxicity due to drug accumulation. This is not a problem for all drugs that are glucuronidated, as cats are only deficient in certain families of glucuronyl transferases. A drug normally metabolized by glucuronidation may have a wide safety margin, or the drug may be metabolized by a different route in cats (although this can result in toxicity for some drugs, e.g. paracetamol). Sulphation and acetylation, for example, are more developed in cats than in dogs.

Differences between dogs and cats with respect to drug receptor distribution and affinity have been described, with morphine representing the archetypal example. In addition to a slower rate of biotransformation due to the deficiency of glucuronidation in the cat, differences observed in the pharmacodynamic effects of morphine in the cat compared to the dog include CNS stimulation (compared to CNS depression in the dog), much less sensitivity to centrally mediated emesis, and pupillary dilation (compared to miosis in the dog).

The grooming behaviour of cats increases the likelihood that topically applied medications will be ingested. Advantage can be taken of this behaviour by applying medications intended for ingestion (e.g. anthelmintic or antibiotic paste preparations) to accessible parts of the cat's body. However, cats are at greater risk of exposure to deliberately or adventitiously applied topical toxicants such as disinfectants (particularly phenolics that are principally candidates for glucuronidation) or pesticides. Indeed, concentrated preparations of permethrin applied topically to cats can be lethal when ingested.

Figure 3.1 shows drugs not recommended for use in cats and Figure 3.2 shows drugs that are therapeutically useful in cats but may have different dosing/toxicity/activity profiles than in dogs.

It is the responsibility of the veterinary surgeon to comply with all national and local legislation.

Within the UK, medicines should be prescribed in accordance with the Prescribing Cascade:

When no authorized veterinary medicinal product exists for a condition in a particular species, and in order to avoid unacceptable suffering, veterinary surgeons exercising their clinical judgement may prescribe for one or a small number of animals under their care other suitable medications in accordance with the following sequence:

1. A veterinary medicine authorized for use in another species, or for a different use in the same species ('off-label' use).
2. A medicine authorized in the UK for human use or a veterinary medicine from another country with an import certificate from the Veterinary Medicines Directorate (VMD).
3. A medicine to be made up at the time on a one-off basis by a veterinary surgeon or a properly authorized person.

Medication compliance

Cats are notorious for being difficult to medicate – even by professionals. In addition, there are some general problems with compliance that are likely to apply as much to cats as to dogs:

- For a short course of antibacterial tablets given to dogs, 80% of clients will give at least 80% of the drug but 20% will give less, sometimes substantially so

Drug	Adverse effects
Apomorphine	Significant CNS depression
Azathioprine	Bone marrow suppression
Benzocaine (local anaesthetic found in some human topical preparations)	Methaemoglobinaemia. Laryngeal oedema
Cisplatin	Fatal, acute pulmonary oedema
Hexachlorophene (found in surgical scrubs, enemas)	Vomiting. Depression. Ataxia. Paralysis
Paracetamol	Methaemoglobinaemia. Heinz body anaemia
Permethrin	Seizures. Hyperaesthesia. Tremor and muscle fasciculation
Potassium bromide	Lower airway disease of sufficient severity to require euthanasia in some cats
Primidone	High incidence of toxicity: hepatotoxicity; profound sedation. (Efficacy as anticonvulsant questionable)
Propylthiouracil	Lethargy. Weakness. Anorexia. Bleeding diathesis

3.1   Drugs not recommended for use in cats and their adverse effects.

Drug	Differences from dogs/Comments
Aminoglycosides	Cats more sensitive to nephrotoxic and ototoxic effects
Amphotericin	Cats more sensitive to adverse effects including anaphylaxis
Aspirin	Adverse effects: hyperpnoea; hypersensitivity; hyperthermia. Increase the dosing interval, and use lower end of dose range (e.g. 10 mg/kg q72h)
Carprofen	Chronic use not safe due to long half-life. Single use only
Chloramphenicol	Much lower dose than for dogs: 50 mg per cat q12h *versus* 50 mg/kg q12h in dogs
Clindamycin	Oesophagitis and oesophageal stricture may occur after oral administration. Give a small amount of food or water bolus after solid oral medications, or combine capsule contents with a small amount of food
Diazepam	Idiosyncratic hepatotoxicity with oral administration
Digoxin	Cats more sensitive to toxicity. Reduce dose and frequency: 30 µg per cat orally q48h for cats <3 kg; 30 µg per cat orally q24h for cats 3–6 kg; and 30 µg per cat orally q12–24h for cats >6 kg
Doxorubicin	Kidney injury may occur. Histological and echocardiographic evidence of myocardial damage may occur with cumulative doses from 170 mg/m^2, although clinical cardiac disease does not usually occur. Use lower dose (25 mg/m^2) to reduce risk of kidney injury
Doxycycline	Oesophagitis and oesophageal strictures may occur with some preparations from incomplete swallowing of tablets. Follow tablet administration with a small amount of water or food, or administer with butter to ensure tablets are completely swallowed into the stomach
Enrofloxacin	Acute blindness has been reported with (usually but not always) high-dose use; daily and total doses and duration of treatment highly variable but toxicity does appear to be dose-related, and doses should not exceed 5 mg/kg q24h. Risk may be higher in cats with urinary tract infections and concurrent kidney disease. Take care dosing geriatric cats or those with hepatic or renal impairment. The use of other fluoroquinolones is generally preferred in cats
Furosemide	More susceptible to dehydration and electrolyte disturbances, particularly hypokalaemia. Use lower end of dose range (1–2 mg/kg in most cases) when possible, or ensure appropriate potassium supplementation
Griseofulvin	Bone marrow dyscrasia risk increased in FIV-positive cats. Non-reversible ataxia has also been reported
Hydroxycarbamide	Paronychia has been reported in cats but this does not preclude its use
Ketoconazole	Anorexia and gastrointestinal side effects more common
Lidocaine	Cats more commonly develop seizures with systemically administered lidocaine and so this must be used cautiously; administer slowly and monitor effects closely
Megestrol	Adverse effects: mammary hypertrophy and neoplasia; cystic endometritis and pyometra; diabetes mellitus
Metronidazole	Adverse effects: disorientation; ataxia; seizures; blindness
Naloxone	Reversal of opioids with this is unpredictable
Opioids: morphine derivatives (excluding pethidine, butorphanol, buprenorphine)	Inconsistent sedation. Increased risk of excitation. Morphine and methadone are therapeutically useful but may need a lower dose than in dogs
Organophosphate insecticides	Acute toxicity: hypersalivation, vomiting, diarrhoea, muscle tremors. Chronic or delayed toxicity: paresis or paralysis which may or may not be reversible. Use with care, ensure product rinsed off coat
Tetracyclines (oxytetracycline in particular, but not doxycycline)	Adverse effects: hepatic lipidosis; increased ALT activity; ptyalism; anorexia; pyrexia
Thiacetarsamide (used for heartworm)	Adverse effects: drug fever; respiratory distress; fulminant pulmonary oedema

3.2   Drugs that are therapeutically useful in cats but may have different dosing/toxicity/activity profiles than in dogs.

- Compliance with chronic medication regimens has not been measured in veterinary patients but extrapolating from human studies it is likely to be substantially worse
- It has been well established that veterinary surgeons are unable to predict which clients will be compliant; their ability to predict compliant behaviour is no better than chance. It is therefore wise to treat all clients as potentially non-compliant and put in place strategies to enhance compliance
- There are no data on owner compliance with medication given to cats but it would probably not be inappropriate to assume that the compliance level will be if anything worse.

Improving compliance

Based on what is known from veterinary studies and what can be extrapolated from human studies, the following would appear to be reasonable strategies for improving client compliance with the medication prescribed for their cat.

- Ensure that clients have been shown how to administer the medication, and consider dispensing the formulation that best suits the needs of both cat and owner. Cats are much less likely than dogs to take medication hidden in food, though medication specifically developed to give with food is often well tolerated. Pastes and liquids are often easier to administer than tablets, though individuals vary. If the cat has not been medicated before, owners will not know which administration method or route is easiest. Make sure owners are aware there are other choices available and encourage them to contact you about trying another formulation if problems are encountered.
- Studies in the veterinary literature suggest that compliance is lower if clients do not understand the disease being treated and the reason for medication. Where feasible, involve clients in treatment decisions and explain why the medication is being dispensed, the expected outcomes, and the potential consequences of poor compliance.
- Choose treatment regimens that suit the client's lifestyle.
- Ensure that instructions are clear; support verbal instructions with written instructions. Remember that the pill label may not allow sufficient space for adequate directions or may be very difficult to read, especially for elderly clients or those with impaired vision.
- Where possible, avoid medication that has to be administered more than twice daily.
- In one study, pet owners who felt their veterinary surgeon spent a sufficient time on the consultation had a higher compliance level than those who did not. Consultation times in busy practices are by necessity relatively short. To enhance the client's feeling of engagement and being cared for, involve veterinary nurses in enhancing client communication, demonstrating medication administration techniques, educating clients about treatment regimens, and following up on

treatment outcomes. Clients may be more likely to admit to a nurse or technician that they are having difficulties medicating their cat, than to the veterinary surgeon.

Some hints on giving oral medicines to cats are given in QRG 3.1.

Antibacterials

The goal of antibacterial therapy in any species is **to help the body eliminate infectious organisms without toxicity to the host**. It is important to recognize that the **natural defence mechanisms of a patient are of primary importance** in preventing and/or controlling infection. The difficulty of controlling infections in immunocompromised patients emphasizes that antibacterial therapy is most effective when it supplements endogenous defence mechanisms rather than acts as the sole means of infection control. Natural defences include the mucociliary escalator in the respiratory tract, the flushing effect of urination and gut normal flora.

Veterinary surgeons have a responsibility to use antibacterials prudently and rationally, to reduce the risk of emergence of bacterial resistance.

Antibacterial agents do not cause bacteria to become resistant but their use preferentially selects resistant populations of bacteria. Some genes that code for resistance have been identified in bacterial cultures established before antibacterial agents were used. Antibacterial drug resistance can emerge in various ways, the most clinically important being R (resistance) plasmids. R plasmids are cytoplasmic genetic elements that can transfer drug resistance to previously susceptible bacteria. This can occur between species and genera and may involve genes that impart resistance to different classes of antibacterial agents.

Factors influencing drug selection

Antibacterials should not be prescribed for every clinical problem. Neither should they be prescribed *in lieu* of a diagnosis, unless there is reasonable evidence for suspecting a bacterial infection, e.g. clinical signs such as pyrexia, heat, redness and swelling and/or clinical pathological changes such as neutrophilia. However, all of these may occur in non-bacterial disease or in non-infectious diseases such as neoplasia and immune-mediated conditions.

If antibacterial therapy is deemed appropriate, although **culture and susceptibility testing** should ideally be performed before initiating antibacterial therapy, this is often not practical. Thus, more often than not, the clinician needs to **prescribe empirically**. The antibacterial choice should be based on the **most likely organisms to be pathogens at the site of infection,** taking into account **pharmacokinetic and pharmacodynamic factors** discussed below. However, if **therapy fails or immediately recurs once therapy has ceased, culture and susceptibility testing is strongly recommended**.

The clinician should also ensure that the client understands dosing instructions and is able to administer the medication.

This is particularly relevant to cats, who are notoriously difficult to medicate (see QRG 3.1). As a result, often a compromise needs to be made between the ideal antibacterial choice based on susceptibility considerations and the pragmatic consideration of what formulation is most appropriate to ensure good owner compliance.

Key questions

Before using or prescribing antibacterials the following should always be considered:

- Is bacterial infection confirmed or probable?
- Would bacterial infection cause critical illness if it occurred?
- Would the infection progress without treatment?
- Is the patient's condition life-threatening?
- If a bacterial infection seems unlikely, can it be entirely ruled out at the moment?
- Can you predict the type of bacteria and their antimicrobial susceptibility?
- Are there any pharmacokinetic considerations, e.g. tissue penetration?
- Are there any pharmacodynamic considerations at the site of infection that may impair drug action?
- Are there any potential side effects of concern? (see Figures 3.1 and 3.2)
- Are culture and susceptibility testing or cytology indicated?
- Is the client able to administer the drug appropriately?

Methods of bacterial suppression/killing

Antibacterial agents are often described as bacteriostatic or bactericidal:

- **Bacteriostatic drugs** temporarily inhibit the growth of an organism but the effect is reversible once the drug is removed. Hence they work in a **time-dependent** manner (see below). They include tetracyclines, chloramphenicol, non-potentiated sulphonamides, macrolides (e.g. erythromycin, tylosin, azithromycin, clarithromycin) and lincosamides (e.g. lincomycin, clindamycin).
- **Bactericidal drugs** cause the death of the organism. They are preferred in infections that cannot be controlled or eradicated by host mechanisms, because of the nature or site of the infection (e.g. bacterial endocarditis) or because of reduced immunocompetence of the host (e.g. patient receiving immunosuppressive therapy). They include aminoglycosides, cephalosporins, fluoroquinolones, metronidazole, penicillins and potentiated sulphonamides.

However, this classification only really applies under strict laboratory conditions, is inconsistent against all bacteria, and becomes more arbitrary in clinical cases. It is more important to consider the **method** of bacterial killing **(time-dependent *versus* concentration-dependent)** as this can have an impact on drug selection and administration.

- **Time-dependent drugs** (e.g. penicillins, cephalosporins and potentiated sulphonamides) are slowly bactericidal. For the drugs to be clinically effective, the drug concentration at the site of the infection should be **maintained above the minimal inhibitory concentration (MIC) throughout the dosing interval**. Plasma levels should be above MIC for as long as possible (ideally at least 80% of each 24-hour period) to reduce the risk of resistance emerging. As a result, adherence to correct dose timing is important, and clients should be instructed to administer drugs every 24, 12 or 8 hours (as appropriate) rather than once, twice or three times a day.. For these drugs there is little or no advantage (regarding proportion of pathogens killed or duration of post-antibacterial effect) in achieving a peak plasma concentration (C_{max}) to MIC ratio of >2–4:1. Bacteria need to be multiplying for drugs to be effective and these drugs should not therefore be given in combination with bacteriostatic drugs.
- For **concentration-dependent drugs** (e.g. aminoglycosides, fluoroquinolones, metronidazole) the peak concentration achieved (and/or the area under the plasma concentration *versus* time curve) predicts antibacterial success. The higher the C_{max}, the greater the proportion of target bacteria killed and the longer the effect. The C_{max} to MIC ratio should be >8:1. All of these factors have been considered when pharmaceutical companies determine appropriate drug doses. Bacteria do not need to be multiplying to be susceptible to these drugs and so these drugs can be given in combination with bacteriostatic drugs.

Minimal inhibitory concentration

The MIC is the lowest concentration of the drug that will inhibit bacterial growth. Pharmaceutical companies usually use MIC_{90} (concentration that inhibits 90% of isolates of bacterial species of interest) to determine the therapeutic dose. MIC determination is not routinely performed in clinical veterinary laboratories (qualitative culture and susceptibility testing based on disc diffusion are more common), but it may be requested when there are concerns about drug resistance and/or to aid in selection of the most effective antibacterial.

Predicting the bacteria present

Predicting the type of infection involves consideration primarily of the **presumed site of infection**. It may be possible to predict the most common bacterial species that infect a site (e.g. *Escherichia coli* for urinary tract infections, *Staphylococcus* spp. for skin infections). In other cases it can be possible to predict the most common group of bacteria (e.g. obligate and facultative anaerobes in pyothorax and abscesses; Gram-negative plus anaerobes for infections arising from contamination of gastrointestinal contents or originating in gut flora, such as neutrophilic cholangitis). In some cases, however, it is not possible to predict the likely bacteria, or one wishes to cover as many bacterial groups as possible while awaiting culture and susceptibility data. Figure 3.3 gives an overview of common bacterial causes of clinical infections in cats, together with suggested antibacterials to be used.

Diagnosis	Common organisms (less common in parentheses)	Preferred drugs (alternatives in parentheses)
Skin and soft tissue infections		
Pyoderma, pustular dermatitis	*Streptococcus, Pasteurella, Staphylococcus*	Amoxicillin/clavulanate Cephalosporin (Lincosamide) (Doxycycline)
Skin and subcutis mycobacterial infections*	e.g. *Mycobacterium smegmatis, M. fortuitum*	Doxycycline + fluoroquinolones + clarithromycin (3–6 months combination therapy required)
Bite wounds, traumatic and contaminated wounds	Anaerobes, *Pasteurella, Actinomyces*	Clindamycin Amoxicillin 1st generation cephalosporin or cefovicin (Penicillin G) (Doxycycline) (Pradofloxacin)
Anal sac inflammation, abscessation	*Escherichia, Enterococcus, (Clostridium, Proteus)*	Amoxicillin/clavulanate 1st generation cephalosporin or cefovicin Chloramphenicol Trimethoprim/Sulphonamide
Conjunctivitis	FHV, FCV, *Chlamydophila, Mycoplasma*, secondary bacteria	Doxycycline or chloramphenicol (topical and/or systemic)
Respiratory tract		
Upper respiratory tract infections	*Bordetella*, viruses, secondary bacteria (*Mycoplasma*)	Doxycycline Trimethoprim/Sulphonamide (Chloramphenicol)
Bacterial pneumonia*	Obligate anaerobes, *Steptococcus, Pasteurella multocida*, coliforms, (*Actinomyces, Mycoplasma*)	Amoxicillin/clavulanate (if i.v. formulation unavailable, use ticarcillin/clavulanate) Fluoroquinolone + clindamycin Pradofloxacin
Pyothorax*	Obligate anaerobes, *Steptococcus, Pasteurella multocida*, (*Actinomyces, Mycoplasma*)	Amoxicillin/clavulanate (if i.v. formulation unavailable, use ticarcillin/clavulanate), Fluoroquinolone + clindamycin Pradofloxacin
Oral cavity and gastrointestinal tract		
Peridontitis, gingivitis, ulcerative stomatitis	Anaerobes, mixed aerobes	Amoxicillin Metronidazole or metronidazole/spiramycin combination Clindamycin (Doxycycline)
Cholecystitis, cholangitis	Coliforms, anaerobes	Amoxicillin/clavulanate Fluoroquinolones plus metronidazole or clindamycin
Urinary tract		
Lower urinary tract infection, pyelonephritis*[a]	*Escherichia, Proteus, Staphylococcus, Streptococcus, Klebsiella, Pseudomonas, Enterobacter*	Amoxicillin Amoxicillin/clavulanate Trimethoprim/Sulphonamide Cephalosporin (Fluoroquinolone)
Reproductive system		
Mastitis*	*Escherichia, Staphylococcus, Streptococcus*	Trimethoprim/Sulphonamide Fluoroquinolone + clindamycin
Bone		
Osteomyelitis*	*Staphylococcus* (possibly with *Streptococcus, Escherichia, Proteus, Pseudomonas*, anaerobes)	Amoxicillin/clavulanate Lincosamide Cloxacillin/flucloxacillin Fluoroquinolone Cephalosporin
Systemic		
Septicaemia*, bacterial endocarditis*	Various aerobes or anaerobes	Fluoroquinolone plus clindamycin or metronidazole Gentamicin plus cephalosporin or cloxacillin/flucloxacillin
Toxoplasmosis	*Toxoplasma gondii*	Clindamycin Sulphonamide + pyrimethamine
Feline infectious anaemia	*Mycoplasma haemofelis*	Doxycycline Marbofloxacin Pradofloxacin
Bartonellosis	*Bartonella*	Doxycycline (Fluoroquinolones or azithromycin if no response)

3.3 Suggested antibacterial drug selection for feline infections. 'Anaerobes' here signifies bacterial species that are obligate anaerobes; while 'aerobes' denotes aerobic and facultatively anaerobic bacteria. Culture and susceptibility testing should be performed, if possible, prior to initiating therapy for those conditions marked by * and in all other conditions if initial empirical antimicrobial therapy is unsuccessful. [a] Signs of lower urinary tract disease in cats younger than 10 years are rarely due to bacterial infection (less than 5% of cases). Therefore routine use of antibacterials in these cases is not appropriate.

Antibacterial spectrum: Since the bacterial species involved in an infection is often not known when treatment is started, it is frequently useful to consider the spectrum of antimicrobial action related to broad categories of bacteria. Bacteria can be classified based on their staining properties (Gram-negative, Gram-positive, or other) and on the environment in which they grow (aerobic, anaerobic, facultative anaerobic). Combining these can give a useful classification which helps select the most appropriate antimicrobial drug when culture and susceptibility information is not available:

- Gram-positive aerobic bacteria (and facultative anaerobes)
- Gram-negative aerobic bacteria (and facultative anaerobes)
- Obligate anaerobes; both Gram-negative and Gram-positive
- Penicillinase-producing *Staphylococcus* spp.
- Atypical bacterial species (non-Gram-definable):
  - *Rickettsia* spp.
  - *Mycoplasma* spp.
  - *Chlamydophila* spp.
  - *Bartonella* spp.
  - *Mycobacterium* spp.

There are some predictable differences between the susceptibility of Gram-negative and Gram-positive aerobic bacteria but there are no predictable differences between Gram-negative and Gram-positive obligate anaerobic bacteria. In addition, due to its ability to produce penicillinase, *Staphylococcus* can have a very different susceptibility compared with other Gram-positive aerobic bacteria. Figure 3.4 summarizes the antibacterials that have no clinically useful effect and those that have excellent or very good activity, against the different groups of bacteria.

Distribution to the site of infection (pharmacokinetic phase)

To be effective an antibacterial agent must be distributed to the site of infection in adequate concentration and come into intimate contact with the infecting organism.

- For most, but not all, tissues, antibacterial drug diffusion is **perfusion-limited**, i.e. provided the tissue has an adequate blood supply, antibacterial concentrations achieved in serum or plasma are equal to the drug concentration in the extracellular (interstitial) space, unless the drug is highly protein-bound
- Effective antibacterial concentrations may not be achieved in poorly vascularized tissues, e.g. extremities during shock, sequestered bone fragments and endocardial valves

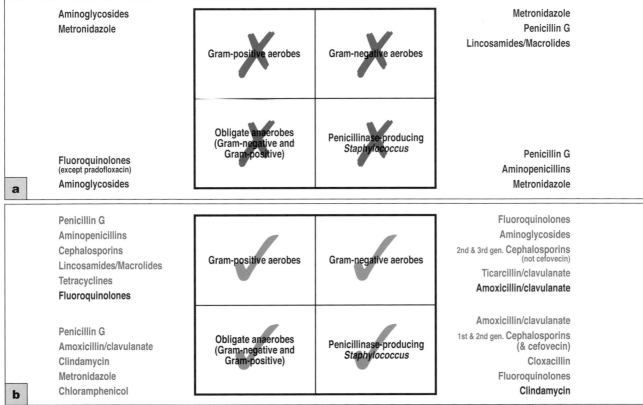

3.4 Antibacterial activity. **(a)** Drug classes with NO clinical useful antibacterial action against most if not all bacterial species in different quadrants. **(b)** Drug classes with EXCELLENT (green) or very good (blue) antibacterial action against many bacterial species in different quadrants. Drugs not designated as red, green or blue for a particular quadrant do have some activity in that quadrant but there are a reasonable proportion of bacterial species that will be resistant to that agent. This does not mean that such drugs are not clinically useful but they may not be the best choice if the therapeutic aim is to maximize antibacterial activity against bacteria in a quadrant because of the nature of the infection or the clinical status of the patient. Examples of such drugs are: 1st generation cephalosporins, cefovicin and amoxicillin (without clavulanic acid) against Gram-negative aerobes and obligate anaerobes; lincosamides (other than clindamycin) against anaerobes; trimethoprim/sulphonamides in all quadrants; and tetracyclines in all quadrants except Gram-positive aerobes (tetracyclines have excellent activity against 'atypical bacteria').

- Drug diffusion to the central nervous system, eye, epithelial lining of the lung (bronchial secretions), prostate and mammary gland, is **permeability-limited**, i.e. the epithelial cell barrier (in which the junctions between cells are tight, particularly in secretory tissues) provides a barrier to drug diffusion and only those drugs that are lipid soluble (and can diffuse through the cell barrier) can effectively penetrate these barriers.

Figure 3.5 provides information on the ability of drugs to penetrate 'difficult' body barriers.

Glucocorticoids

Corticosteroid hormones are produced by the adrenal cortex and classified as glucocorticoids or mineralocorticoids. Glucocorticoid drugs play a central role in the management of allergic skin disease, feline asthma and immune-mediated dermatoses, as well as other immune-mediated diseases affecting the gastrointestinal tract, blood, joints, kidney and other tissues. They are often essential for the successful management of the patient, yet have the potential to cause serious and occasionally life-threatening side effects. In general, **cats are less susceptible to adverse affects than dogs,** despite requiring relatively higher doses to achieve equivalent therapeutic effects.

Glucocorticoids affect carbohydrate, lipid and protein metabolism, and the haemolymphatic system, and also influence water and electrolyte balance to varying degrees. They have potent anti-inflammatory and immunosuppressive effects which are central to their therapeutic actions. The reader is directed to more complete reference sources on the topic: Boothe and Mealey (2001); Day (2008). Synthetic glucocorticoids have been manufactured to increase their anti-inflammatory potency and to reduce mineralocorticoid (sodium and therefore water retention) effects. This has obvious therapeutic advantages but major disadvantages if they are used inappropriately, due to the potential for serious side effects. The more potent the glucocorticoid, the greater its potential for adverse effects. The relative potency of the various glucocorticoids is shown in Figure 3.6.

Polar (hydrophilic) drugs of low lipophilicity		Drugs of moderate to high lipophilicity			Highly lipophilic molecules with low ionization
Acids	*Bases*	*Weak acids*	*Weak bases*	*Amphoteric*	
Penicillins Cephalosporins Beta-lactamase inhibitors	Polymixins Aminoglycosides ■ gentamicin ■ spectinomycin ■ tobramycin ■ streptomycin ■ amikacin	Sulphonamides	Trimethoprim Lincosamides ■ lincomycin ■ clindamycin Macrolides ■ erythromycin ■ tylosin ■ spiramycin ■ tilmicosin	Tetracyclines ■ tetracycline ■ chlortetracycline ■ oxytetracycline	Chloramphenicol Fluoroquinolones ■ enrofloxacin ■ norfloxacin ■ ciprofloxacin Lipophilic tetracyclines ■ minocycline ■ doxycycline Metronidazole Rifampin
These drugs: ■ **Do not readily penetrate 'natural body barriers'** so that effective concentrations in transcellular fluids (CSF, milk, prostatic fluid, bronchial secretions and ocular fluid) will not always be achieved. ■ Adequate concentrations may be achieved in joints, and in pleural and peritoneal fluids. ■ Acidic antibacterials may diffuse into prostate in small concentrations but easily diffuse back into the plasma, rendering these drugs ineffective against clinical prostate infections. ■ Penetration may be assisted by acute inflammation.		**These drugs:** ■ Cross cellular membranes more readily than polar (hydrophilic) drugs so enter transcellular fluids (CSF, milk, prostatic fluid, bronchial secretions and ocular fluid) to a greater extent. ■ Antibacterials that are weak bases will be ion-trapped (concentrated) in fluids that are more acidic than plasma – prostatic fluid, milk, intracellular fluid if lipophilic enough to penetrate (e.g. erythromycin) ■ Penetration into CSF and ocular fluids affected by plasma protein binding as well as lipophilicity; sulphonamides and trimethoprim penetrate effectively, whereas macrolides, lincosamides and tetracyclines do not, the latter probably due to efflux pumps. ■ Tetracyclines do not achieve high concentrations in prostate after systemic administration.			**These drugs:** ■ Cross cellular barriers very readily, meaning that they can reach most tissues and organs. ■ Penetrate into 'difficult' transcellular fluids such as CSF, milk, prostatic fluid, bronchial secretions and ocular fluid. ■ However, chloramphenicol and tetracyclines do not achieve high concentrations in prostate. ■ All penetrate into CSF except tetracyclines and rifampin, which do not, probably due to efflux pumps. ■ All penetrate into intracellular fluids and therefore can be effective against intracellular bacteria including *Bartonella, Brucella, Chlamydophila, Mycobacterium, Rickettsia* and *Staphylococcus* (facultative)

3.5 Physicochemical properties of antimicrobial drugs and effects on tissue distribution.

	Mineralocorticoid potency (per mg)	Glucocorticoid potency (per mg)	Anti-inflammatory equivalent dose (mg) [a]
Cortisone	0.8	0.8	25.0
Hydrocortisone	1.0	1.0	20.0
Prednisolone	0.25	4.0	5.0
Methylprednisolone	Minimal	5.0	4.0
Triamcinolone	0	5.0	4.0
Dexamethasone	Minimal	30.0	0.75
Betamethasone	Negligible	35.0	0.6
Fludrocortisone	100	15	Not relevant

3.6 Relative glucocorticoid (anti-inflammatory) and mineralocorticoid potency of common natural and synthetic corticosteroids administered systemically. [a] The dose of each drug required to achieve the same anti-inflammatory effect (e.g. 20 mg of hydrocortisone is required to achieve the same anti-inflammatory effect as 5 mg of prednisolone).

The duration of action of the synthetic glucocorticoids can be increased by modification of the steroid molecule (Figure 3.7) or by forming a complex with esters of varying degrees of solubility to prolong release after intramuscular or subcutaneous injection (Figure 3.8). The prolongation of effect also means prolongation of suppression of the hypothalamic–pituitary–adrenal axis; there are no clinical advantages that outweigh this problem unless the use of shorter-acting agents is impossible (e.g. fractious animal, animal with a painful mouth, lack of owner compliance). It should also be noted that the **duration of adrenal suppression is greater than the duration of anti-inflammatory effect from depot treatment**.

The mechanism of action of glucocorticoids is similar in dogs and cats. However, cats require different dosing regimens due to differences in anti-inflammatory potency. The cat is considered more 'steroid-resistant' (to the immunosuppressive rather than the adrenosuppressive effects of glucocorticoids) than the dog, which may reflect reduced expression of glucocorticoid-binding receptors in the tissues (skin and liver) of the cat.

Precautions and adverse effects

Glucocorticoids should be avoided or, if use is essential, used with care in:

- **Infections:** Glucocorticoids impair the body's ability to fight infections by inhibiting inflammation and cell-mediated immunity
- **Immature animals:** The effect of glucocorticoids on growth are complex. Administration to immature animals reduces growth by inhibiting linear skeletal growth via catabolic effects on connective tissue and muscle, as well as inhibition of insulin-like growth factor (IGF-1)
- **Patients undergoing bone healing:** Glucocorticoids impair bone healing by inhibiting osteoblast proliferation and synthesis of bone matrix. In addition they stimulate osteoclast activity and antagonize the effects of Vitamin D3
- **Diabetes mellitus:** Glucocorticoids reduce the uptake and utilization of glucose by tissues and may decrease the expression of the insulin receptor in these target cells
- **Pregnancy:** Glucocorticoids can cause abortion, and congenital cleft palates, in dogs – and may do so in cats
- **Corneal ulceration:** Glucocorticoids delay healing by slowing the process of re-epithelialization. They may increase the risk of corneal perforation by enhancing the activity of collagenase produced by leucocytes and by some bacteria such as *Pseudomonas.*

Potential adverse effects include the following:

- Polyuria with polydipsia may occur in cats, but is less common than in dogs.
- Polyphagia and weight gain
- Promotion of gluconeogenesis which can cause hyperglycaemia and diabetes mellitus; this effect is much more common in cats than dogs.
- Gastrointestinal ulceration (especially in the presence of other conditions that increase risk of ulceration e.g. an anaemic cat or a hypotensive cat with possible compromise of gut perfusion, or concurrent NSAID use)
- Suppressed immunological processing of antigens resulting in increased susceptibility to infection or impaired recovery from infection e.g. animals being treated with glucocorticoids have a higher incidence of bacterial infections; in one study 75% of dogs being treated with glucocorticoids for allergic skin disease had clinical or subclinical urinary tract infections.
- Recurrence of latent viral infections in cats who are carriers e.g. herpes virus
- Thin skin, alopecia (long-term use)
- Calcinosis cutis (long-term use)
- Bruising due to reduced collagen synthesis and increased capillary fragility (not commonly observed in cats)
- Hepatomegaly (this is less of a problem in cats than in dogs)
- Septic arthritis (from intra-articular injection).

Duration class [a]	Glucocorticoids and their durations
Short-acting (<12 hours)	Cortisone (8–12 h) Hydrocortisone (8–12 h)
Intermediate-acting (12–48 hours)	Prednisone [b] (12–36 h) Prednisolone (12–36 h) Methylprednisolone (12–36 h) Triamcinolone (24–48 h)
Long-acting (>36 hours)	Dexamethasone (48–72 h) Betamethasone (36–54 h)

3.7 Relative metabolic duration of effects for common glucocorticoids. [a] Duration if drug in a soluble formulation is given orally or parenterally (see Figure 3.8). [b] Prednisone is metabolized in the liver to prednisolone and theoretically should be avoided in liver disease.

Very soluble – released for minutes – intravenous, intramuscular or subcutaneous administration

- Succinate or phosphate:
  - Prednisolone sodium succinate (e.g. *Solu-delta-cortef*)
  - Hydrocortisone sodium succinate (e.g. *Solu-cortef*)
  - Dexamethasone sodium phosphate (e.g. *Dexadreson, Colvasone*)
  - Betamethasone (e.g. *Betsolan soluble*)

Moderately insoluble – released for days to weeks – intramuscular or subcutaneous administration

- Acetate:
  - Prednisolone acetate
  - Methylprednisolone acetate (e.g. *Solu-Medrone*)
- Phenylproprionate
  - Dexamethasone phenylproprionate (e.g. *Dexafort*)
- Isonicotinate
  - Dexamethasone isonicotinate (e.g. *Voren Suspension)*

Poorly soluble – released for 6–8 weeks – intramuscular administration

- Acetonide:
  - Triamcinolone acetonide (e.g. *Vetalog*)

3.8 Glucocorticosteroid esters, solubility (in water) and duration of steroid release. The duration of action of each formulation will be determined by the duration of action of the steroid molecule (see Figure 3.7) OR by the duration of steroid release (shown here) – whichever is the longer. For example: dexamethasone sodium phosphate will have a duration of action of 48–72 hours (depending on dose and individual metabolism) as this is the duration of action of dexamethasone after immediate release from the phosphate ester; whereas methyprednisolone acetate will have a duration of action of 4–6 weeks, as this is the time over which the drug is released from the acetate ester, even though the steroid itself has a duration of action of only 12–36 hours.

Guidelines for use

Dose

Use an **appropriate dose** and the **shortest-acting effective agent** for the effect intended.

> Cats are relatively steroid-resistant and require higher doses than dogs. Doses can usually be doubled compared to dogs, but the **lower end of the dose range should be used whenever possible**; doses at the top end of the dosing range for anti-inflammatory and immunosuppressive effects are not commonly required.

Prednisolone dose ranges in cats to induce remission of clinical signs:

- Anti-inflammatory   1–2 mg/kg/day
- 'Immunosuppressive'   2–4 mg/kg/day
- Cytotoxic   4 mg/kg/day

It is not *clinically* important whether the drug is given once or twice daily, but to improve owner compliance in medicating cats once-daily dosing is preferred. There is no good evidence that splitting the dose reduces side effects, especially at anti-inflammatory doses when it may actually reduce efficacy. However, on the rare occasions that the dose being used is at the top of the 'immunosuppressive' dose range, it is usual to split the dose to give twice-daily dosing.

Dose protocol

It is important to remember that to induce remission of clinical signs or manage their recurrence requires institution of daily therapy at an appropriate anti-inflammatory or immunosuppressive dose to control clinical signs, tapered to reach the **minimum daily dose** that will control signs, followed by alternate-day therapy to manage the disease.

It is also important to recognize that individuals vary greatly in their response to the therapeutic and adverse effects of glucocorticoids and there may be qualitative differences between the effects of different glucocorticoids in the same patient.

Tapering off

Daily therapy for longer than 1–2 weeks, even with short-acting agents such as prednisolone, will suppress the adrenal axis; recovery of this will take longer than 1 week after stopping treatment. Therefore, when treating inflammatory or immune-mediated disease, once the clinical signs are in remission the dose must be tapered off gradually using alternate-day therapy.

There are various regimens proposed for tapering the dose of prednisolone but it should be noted that doses >1 mg/kg/day saturate the cat's ability to fully metabolize the last dose before the next dose is given, and so a true 'adrenal rest' day is not achieved until the dose is below this level. As noted above, the adrenosuppressive effects of long-acting injectable glucocorticoids last longer than the anti-inflammatory effects. Therefore, the adrenal function of patients treated with injectable glucocorticoids is suppressed throughout treatment. This is one reason it is preferable to use oral medication that can be suitably tapered, if at all possible, though this can be difficult to achieve with some feisty felines.

If the patient is receiving >1 mg/kg/day of prednisolone, abrupt cessation of therapy can result in iatrogenic hypoadrenocorticism (Addisonian crisis) as a result of the failure of normal endogenous cortisol production secondary to ACTH suppression by administered glucocorticoids. If glucocorticoid therapy does need to be stopped, e.g. if the patient develops an infection or an additional risk factor results in gastric ulceration, then the dose needs to be tapered before treatment is stopped completely (Figure 3.9). There are no studies to the author's knowledge that have established the optimal way to do this. Since ill cats have higher cortisol levels than healthy cats, likely due to a physiological benefit, reducing the prednisolone dose to around 0.5 mg/kg/day for about a week then 0.5 mg/kg every other day for 1–2 weeks should be reasonably safe. Doses at this level are not immunosuppressive and therefore should not seriously compromise treatment of an infection. If clinically serious ulceration has developed, supportive treatment for this will also be required using ulcer-healing drugs. In these cases faster reduction in the glucocorticoid dose to 0.5 mg/kg every other day immediately may be warranted and safe, especially if the patient is receiving intravenous fluids as part of the symptomatic management of the gastrointestinal signs. Clearly, the glucocorticoid effect of long-acting injectable treatment cannot be stopped or reversed.

For a 4 kg cat needing *immunosuppressive treatment* with 2 mg/kg/day of oral prednisolone:

Induction dose (taking into account dose range and tablet size): 10 mg/day (2 x 5 mg tablets) for 2–4 weeks depending on clinical response (equates to 2.5 mg/kg prednisolone per day; a longer period at this dose may be required). Currently there is no evidence that either once- or twice-daily medication is more effective.

Tapering dose: started once clinical signs are in remission or reasonably controlled for at least a couple of weeks. Tapering is usually done more quickly (e.g. 50% of dose every 1–2 weeks) for cats on anti-inflammatory doses of prednisolone compared to immunosuppressive doses (e.g. 25% every 2–4 weeks), as faster tapering with the latter may be associated with relapse of the immunosuppressive disease.

Example method to reduce dose by 25% every 2–4 weeks:
Reduce to 7.5 mg/day (1½ x 5 mg tablets) for 2–4 weeks, then 5 mg/day for 2–4 weeks, then 5 mg every other day for 2–4 weeks, then 2.5 mg every other day for as long as needed.

Example method to reduce dose by 50% every 2–4 weeks:
10 mg every other day for 2–4 weeks, then 5 mg every other day for 2–4 weeks, then 2.5 mg every other day for as long as needed.

3.9 Tapering of glucocorticoid treatment. Please note that clinician preference varies and that the rate of decrease will be dictated by the clinical response of the cat. Also the tapering doses will be influenced by the size of the cat and the convenience of tablet size. It is not an exact science and clinical judgement and common sense is important. Examples are shown for guidance only.

Gastroprotectants

The concurrent use of gastroprotective drugs in patients treated with glucocorticoids has become common practice but there is little evidence to support it. Glucocorticoid-induced ulceration is rare and almost always associated with additional risk factors which, in most cases, should have precluded glucocorticoid use (e.g. concurrent NSAID administration or use of glucocorticoids in hypotensive patients). There have not to the author's knowledge been relevant studies in cats, but in dogs there is no evidence from at least nine studies of efficacy in preventing steroid-induced ulceration of any anti-ulcerogenic drug including sucralfate, H_2 antagonists (e.g. cimetidine), omeprazole and misoprostol.

Effective feline analgesia

Recognition and alleviation of pain is very important in feline practice. Surveys in small animal practice indicate that analgesic drugs are administered to cats less frequently than to dogs. This is attributed to concerns about side effects of analgesics in cats as well as to difficulties in recognizing and quantifying pain.

Acute pain

Acute pain is generally associated with tissue damage that resolves with tissue healing. Surgery is the most common cause but it can also be caused by acute medical conditions (e.g. pancreatitis) or trauma. The **principle of acute pain management** is to **prevent/limit central and peripheral sensitization;** these are changes in sensory processing in the central and peripheral nervous systems that occur with tissue injury and activation of nociceptive pathways. Sensitization causes a heightened sensitivity to pain, such that effective pain management becomes more difficult to achieve in the individual patient. Sensitization is characterized by:

- **Hyperalgesia:** Increased pain from stimuli that normally provoke pain, both at the site of tissue injury (primary hyperalgesia caused by peripheral sensitization) and in the surrounding uninjured tissue (secondary hyperalgesia caused by central sensitization; manifests as increased sensitivity to gentle palpation around a wound or site of tissue trauma)
- **Allodynia:** Pain due to a stimulus that does not normally provoke pain e.g. touch due to light stroking in a cat
- **Spontaneous pain:** Ongoing pain at the site of tissue damage and surrounding area.

Once established, sensitization can be difficult to reverse, making effective pain management challenging; multi-modal analgesia and pre-emptive analgesia can be used to help provide effective pain relief.

Multi-modal analgesia is the principle of using different classes of analgesic drugs in combination (e.g. an NSAID combined with an opioid). The rationale behind this is that pain pathways involve multiple neurotransmitters and receptors. Administration of one class of analgesic drug alone, which is only able to modulate one aspect of the pain pathway, is therefore unlikely to provide effective pain relief. Different classes of analgesic drugs generally have different side effects; drug combinations are not usually associated with an increased risk of adverse effects as combining different classes of drugs usually allows a lower dose of each individual agent to be used.

Pre-emptive analgesia is the administration of analgesic drugs before the onset of pain (i.e. before activation and modulation of nociceptive pathways).

Experimentally, if noxious input to the central nervous system (CNS) following tissue injury is blocked (e.g. by a local nerve block), central sensitization can be prevented. However, in a clinical context it is usually impossible to prevent all afferent noxious input to the CNS following tissue damage, and in animals with trauma or medical disease the animal is in pain at the time of presentation. However, the principle of pre-emptive analgesia is still favoured.

Recognizing and assessing acute pain
Cats rarely demonstrate obvious signs of acute pain so recognizing pain can be challenging. Furthermore, signs of pain can be similar to signs of stress and anxiety (see Chapter 1), and this needs to be addressed to enable optimal assessment. Knowing the cat's behaviour in the clinic environment prior to the onset of pain (e.g. preoperatively) is vital for allowing a more accurate interpretation of the cat's behaviour when assessing for pain (e.g. postoperatively).

Pain assessment can be achieved by:

- Observing the cat from a distance to see its interaction with the environment, its position and posture in the cage and its facial expression (Figure 3.10a)
- Interacting and talking to the cat and carefully assessing its response to stroking
- If appropriate, application of *gentle* pressure around any (suspected) site of tissue injury (Figure 3.10b).

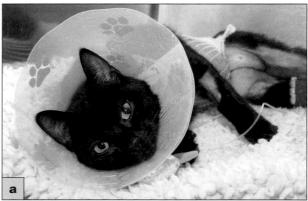

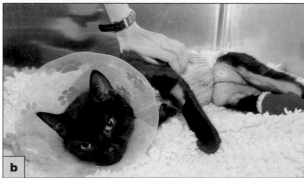

3.10 **(a)** This cat appears to be interested in its surroundings and is relaxed, suggesting that analgesia is adequate after an exploratory laparotomy 5 days earlier. The eyes are fully open and the ears are in a relaxed position, a facial expression that may be indicative of patient comfort. **(b)** It is important to assess the response of the cat to application of gentle pressure around the site of surgery or tissue injury. Note that the cat's facial expression remains relaxed during palpation and the body position appears relaxed and without obvious discomfort.

This approach to pain assessment allows both the emotional aspect of pain (e.g. is the cat depressed, frightened or anxious) and the intensity/location of pain to be evaluated. Gentle palpation around a wound site is a cardinal test of effective analgesia and should not be neglected if at all possible. Cats can appear comfortable from a distance yet show marked sensitivity to wound palpation.

Changes in behaviour and activity that are indicative of pain include the following:

- Hiding in the cage or taking up a position at the back of the cage
- Absence of normal behaviours (e.g. the cat is immobile)
- Aggression or fear
- Hunched, unrelaxed posture
- Failure to groom, indicated by poor coat condition
- Absence of interaction with people
- Failure to eat or drink
- Guarding of an injured body part
- Altered facial expression.

In cats there is preliminary evidence to suggest that flattened ears and a squinting eye position (Figure 3.11) are indicative of pain and that relaxation of facial expression occurs following administration of effective analgesia. Changes in facial expression may reflect both the emotional and sensory aspects of pain, making them a useful indicator.

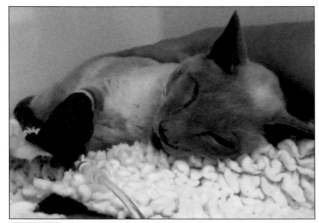

3.11 A cat following repair of a fractured jaw. The cat had received an NSAID preoperatively, a mandibular nerve block with bupivacaine, and intravenous buprenorphine (20 µg/kg) at the end of surgery. On examination the cat was dull and unresponsive to interaction and had closed slanting eyes and very flattened ears. These facial characteristics are thought to indicate pain in cats. Additional analgesia with 0.3 mg/kg methadone (slow i.v. over 1–2 minutes) was given, and the cat then appeared more comfortable.

Quantifying pain: It is helpful to incorporate pain scoring systems into daily clinical practice to quantify pain in individual animals and monitor changes in pain over time. No 'gold standard' pain scoring system is available for cats, so it is important to adopt a technique that is practical for clinical use and is reasonably robust when used by multiple individuals. One example of a pain scoring system for cats is the Colorado State University Feline Acute Pain Scale (Figure 3.12); this is relatively easy to use and takes account of both the intensity and emotional aspects of pain.

Management of acute pain

The classes of analgesic drugs most frequently used in the management of acute pain in cats are:

- Opioids
- NSAIDs
- Alpha-2 adrenoreceptor agonists (α-2 agonists)
- Ketamine
- Local anaesthetic agents, e.g. lidocaine, bupivacaine.

Opioids: Opioids form the backbone of acute analgesia regimens in animals. Although there are many myths associated with opioid administration in cats, they can (and should) be used very safely and effectively. Opioids are classified according to: the opioid receptor to which they bind; their action at the receptor (agonist, partial agonist, antagonist) and duration of action. Opioids that bind to the µ receptor are more efficacious analgesics than those that bind to the κ receptor, and full agonists are more efficacious than partial agonists. The duration of action determines the suitability of different drugs for use in different situations (e.g. fentanyl is a very short-acting opioid that is not suitable for premedication or postoperative analgesia unless given intravenously by continuous rate infusion (CRI)). The pharmacological characteristics of commonly used opioid analgesic drugs in cats are shown in Figure 3.13. Strict regulations exist regarding the purchase, storage and record-keeping of administration of opioids to animals (see *BSAVA Guide to the Use of Medicines* at www.bsava.com).

Selection: Given the myriad of agents available it can be confusing to decide which opioids to store at the practice and when to administer them. Decision-making should be governed by which opioids are authorized for use in animals (including dogs if not cats; see Figure 3.13), analgesic efficacy, and duration of action.

The practice should have **one full µ agonist with a medium duration of action** (e.g. methadone, authorized for dogs but very effective in cats) for management of moderate to severe pain, and **buprenorphine, a partial agonist,** authorized for cats, that is efficacious for the management of moderate pain and has a relatively **long duration of action**. If carrying out invasive surgeries likely to cause severe pain it is also useful to stock fentanyl, which can be given intraoperatively and postoperatively by CRI. Pethidine is authorized for cats, providing comparable analgesia to methadone but only for a very short duration (1–1.5 hours), requiring frequent re-dosing and limiting its usefulness in clinical practice. Morphine is an efficacious analgesic but is not authorized in animals. Butorphanol, a κ agonist, is less efficacious than µ agonists, but can be useful for the management of mild pain or to provide good sedation, in combination with acepromazine or α-2 agonists. The sedative effects of butorphanol are generally considered to be greater than those of buprenorphine.

Factors that determine which opioid to give to individual patients include:

- **Severity of pain**: Use a full µ agonist for moderate (e.g. methadone) to severe (e.g. methadone or fentanyl) pain. For mild to moderate pain, or in cats

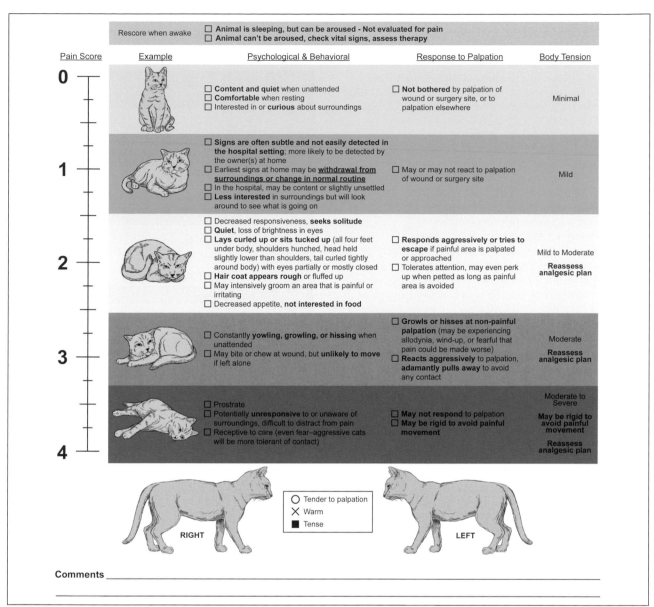

3.12 An example of a pain scoring system for cats. The Colorado State University Feline Acute Pain Scale can be downloaded from the International Veterinary Academy of Pain Management website (www. ivapm.org). The scale should not be used as a definitive pain score, but it is useful to aid decision-making about the severity of acute pain in cats and the requirement for analgesic administration. In general: the assessment begins with quiet observation of the patient in the cage at a distance; this is followed by an assessment of the response of the patient to interaction, including the reaction to gentle palpation of a wound or painful area. Advantages of the scale include: ease of use, with minimal interpretation required; the provision of specific descriptors for individual behaviours decreases interobserver variability. A disadvantage of this scale is the lack of validation by clinical studies comparing it to other scales. (© 2006 PW Hellyer, SR Uhrig, NG Robinson)

Drug	Opioid receptor	Effect	Duration of action	Clinical uses	Marketing authorization in the UK
Buprenorphine	μ	Partial agonist	Long: 6 hours	Premedication and postoperative analgesia	**Authorized for use in cats** and dogs
Methadone	μ	Agonist	Medium: 4–5 hours	Premedication, intra- and postoperative analgesia	Authorized for use in dogs
Morphine	μ	Agonist	Medium: 4–5 hours	Premedication, intra- and postoperative analgesia	Not authorized for use in animals
Pethidine	μ	Agonist	Short: 1–1.5 hours	Premedication and postoperative analgesia	**Authorized for use in cats** and dogs
Fentanyl	μ	Agonist	Short: 10 minutes	Intraoperative and postoperative analgesia	Authorized for use in dogs
Butorphanol	κ	Agonist	Short: 1–1.5 hours	Short duration of perioperative analgesia	**Authorized for use in cats** and dogs
Naloxone	μ	Antagonist	Short: 20–30 minutes	Reversal of opioid overdose	Not authorized for use in cats and dogs

3.13 Pharmacological characteristics of commonly used opioids in cats.

receiving multimodal analgesia, buprenorphine is a good first line opioid analgesic

- **Administration of other analgesic drugs**: Using an opioid in combination with other analgesic drugs (particularly NSAIDs) usually allows the dose of opioid to be reduced or may allow a partial μ agonist (e.g. buprenorphine) to be used instead of a full μ agonist (e.g. methadone) for more severe pain
- **Required duration of action**: For animals that are being discharged and unable to receive further doses of opioid, it is useful to administer a long-acting opioid such as buprenorphine
- **Available routes of administration**: Good evidence suggests that the efficacy of buprenorphine is reduced when given subcutaneously compared to intramuscularly or intravenously. Buprenorphine is also efficacious when given via the oral transmucosal route; when oral transmucosal dosing is preceded by a dose given intravenously or intramuscularly, it is likely to be more effective than reliance on subcutaneous buprenorphine alone. The oral transmucosal route avoids the need for repeated intramuscular injections (see later).

Practical considerations: Opioids are generally unsuitable for oral administration due to first pass metabolism by the liver. Repeated intramuscular administration is painful and should be avoided if possible.

Placement of an intravenous catheter solely for the purpose of drug administration should be considered, to reduce pain associated with frequent administration; *but* pethidine cannot be administered intravenously due to associated histamine release. All other opioids should be given slowly (over 2 minutes) intravenously to cats.

Buprenorphine can be given via the oral transmucosal route, which is non-invasive and well tolerated by cats; here the buprenorphine is given into the cheek pouch or under the tongue to prevent the cat swallowing the drug directly, allowing absorption across the buccal mucous membranes (Figure 3.14). The preservative-free preparation (Vetergesic, Alstoe Animal Health) should be used, as the multi-dose formulation contains a preservative that has an unpleasant taste.

Fentanyl can be given transdermally, but there is evidence to suggest that systemic absorption can be very variable between individuals, and transdermal fentanyl should not be relied upon as a sole means of analgesia.

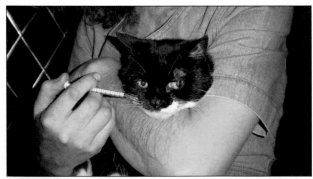

3.14 Oral transmucosal administration of buprenorphine. (Courtesy of Polly Taylor)

Recommended doses of opioids in cats appropriate for different routes of administration are shown in Figure 3.15.

Route	Dose	Frequency of administration
Methadone		
i.v.	0.2–0.4 mg/kg	Repeat dosing every 4–6 hours
i.m.	0.2–0.5 mg/kg	
Morphine		
i.v.	0.2–0.4 mg/kg	Repeat dosing every 4–6 hours
i.m.	0.2–0.5 mg/kg	
Buprenorphine		
i.v.	20 μg/kg	Repeat dosing every 6–8 hours
i.m.	20–30 μg/kg	
Oral transmucosal	20–30 μg/kg	
Pethidine		
i.m.	5 μg/kg	Repeat dosing every 60–90 minutes
Fentanyl		
i.v.	5 μg/kg	Repeat dosing every 15–20 minutes
Transdermal	4–8 μg/kg/h	Apply patch and leave *in situ* for 72 hours. Can replace with a new patch at a different site
Butorphanol		
i.v.	0.2–0.4 mg/kg	Repeat dosing every 60–90 minutes
i.m.	0.4 mg/kg	

3.15 Recommended doses and routes of administration of opioids in cats.

Continuous rate infusion: Administering analgesics by CRI allows the continuous provision of analgesia, avoiding the peaks and troughs in plasma concentration that occur following intermittent bolus administration of analgesics. The following points should be considered.

- Always use controlled administration apparatus (e.g. a syringe driver). Label the drug preparation with the date, patient name, drug, dilution (dilute drugs for CRI in 0.9% NaCl in order to allow low doses of potent drugs to be given accurately by a syringe driver), dose (mg/kg/h) and dose rate (ml/h) (Figure 3.16a).
- Most drugs require a loading dose (given over 1–2 minutes) immediately before starting the CRI to rapidly achieve and maintain a therapeutic plasma concentration of the drug (see Figure 3.18).
- Administer different drugs via different individual infusion apparatus (Figure 3.16b; this allows the dose rates of drugs to be adjusted, started and stopped independently).
- Always place an intravenous catheter prior to starting a CRI (Figure 3.17).
- Check the intravenous catheter at least every 4 hours to confirm that the drug is being delivered correctly intravenously.
- Check the cat frequently for signs of pain (see above) to confirm that the dose rate and drug are providing an appropriate level of analgesia.

- Be aware that there are very few data to support dosing recommendations for analgesic drugs given by CRI in cats (Figure 3.18), particularly when more than one drug is used in combination.

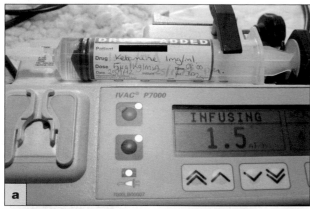

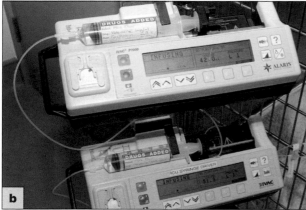

3.16 **(a)** Label syringes with the patient ID, drug name, infusion rate and concentration. This facilitates checking that the correct infusion rate has been set and reduces the likelihood of drug infusion errors (e.g. incorrect drug, dose or patient). **(b)** When delivering more than one drug by CRI, administer them using different syringes and controlled infusion apparatus. This allows the dose rate of each drug to be adjusted independently and also prevents any risk of interactions between drugs caused by mixing in the same syringe or drip bag.

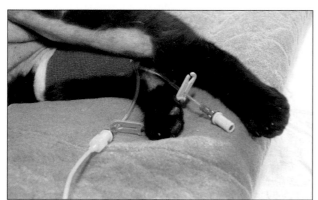

3.17 When delivering more than one type of solution to a cat continuously (e.g. Hartmann's solution and an analgesic drug) it is useful to use an intravenous extension line connected directly to the intravenous catheter, with two ports for drug administration. This allows both solutions to be administered directly, close to the intravenous catheter, preventing mixing of drugs in the fluid line. The ports are colour-coded to allow easy identification of the two lines and use a needleless injection system. This cat is receiving only fluids via one port on the extension set; the other port is for analgesic administration.

Loading dose given immediately before starting CRI	CRI and dilution instructions
Morphine	
0.2–0.4 mg/kg i.v.	Dilute 10 mg/ml morphine to a 1 mg/ml solution with NaCl 0.9%. CRI: 0.1–0.2 mg/kg/h. Accumulation likely after infusions >12 h; reduce dose rate with prolonged administration. Try to switch to intermittent bolus doses of opioids, e.g. methadone, after 24 h infusion
Fentanyl	
5 µg/kg i.v.	Dilute 50 µg/ml fentanyl to a 25 µg/ml solution with NaCl 0.9%. CRI: 2–4 µg/kg/h. Accumulation likely after infusions >12 h; reduce dose rate with prolonged administration. Try to switch to intermittent bolus doses of opioids, e.g. methadone, after 24 h infusion
Dexmedetomidine [a]	
1–2 µg/kg i.v.	Dilute 500 µg/ml dexmedetomidine to a 5 µg/ml solution with NaCl 0.9%. CRI: 1–2 µg/kg/h. Accumulation likely after infusions >12 h; reduce dose rate with prolonged administration
Ketamine [a]	
0.25–0.5 mg/kg i.v.	Dilute 100 mg/ml ketamine to a 2 mg/ml solution with NaCl 0.9%. CRI: 10 µg/kg/min intraoperatively during anaesthesia; reduce to 2–5 µg/kg/min in awake cats. At dose rates <10 µg/kg/min, CNS behavioural effects, such as sedation or 'spacey' behaviour, are unlikely. Accumulation likely after infusions >12 h; reduce dose rate with prolonged administration

3.18 Recommended infusion rates for administration of drugs by continuous rate infusion. All these drugs can be combined for CRI, although choose EITHER morphine OR fentanyl as the opioid. It is recommended to use ketamine and/or dexmedetomidine as an *adjunct* to an opioid CRI, or with opioid bolus dosing, rather than using ketamine or dexmedetomidine alone before the instigation of concurrent opioid therapy. Use the lower end of the suggested range of CRI doses when using more than one drug in combination. Ketamine should be used in preference to dexmedetomidine as an adjunctive agent in cats with cardiovascular disease or systemic disease likely to result in cardiovascular derangements, although it is prudent to avoid ketamine in cats with hypertrophic cardiomyopathy. Ketamine can also be used preferentially when chronic/altered pain states are suspected, as it may reverse or reduce central sensitization. Dexmedetomidine is very helpful to provide analgesia in cats that are very anxious due to the concurrent sedation. [a] This dose recommendation is not supported by robust scientific studies in cats but the author has used it effectively.

Non-steroidal anti-inflammatory drugs: NSAIDs are an essential component of acute analgesia regimens in cats and can be used very effectively in combination with opioids and other adjunctive analgesic agents such as α-2 agonists.

WARNING

Side effects resulting from inappropriate administration of NSAIDs to individual patients can be life-threatening, and the likelihood of adverse effects should be considered in all patients. If the risk is significant, **do not** administer an NSAID; derive analgesia from other classes of analgesic drugs, particularly opioids, which have a much greater therapeutic index with a very low risk of significant adverse effects.

Side effects include:

- **Gastrointestinal ulceration:** Clinical signs include inappetence/anorexia, vomiting (± haematemesis), diarrhoea and lethargy. Probably increased likelihood if cat has a history of gastrointestinal disease or ulceration.
- **Renal ischaemia:** Acute renal dysfunction typically occurs within 7 days of NSAID administration. Increased likelihood of clinically detrimental effects if pre-existing kidney disease is present. Associated with administration of NSAIDs to dehydrated, or hypotensive cats. Ideally measure blood pressure to document hypotension (Doppler systolic arterial blood pressure <90 mmHg), although hypotension may be suspected based on clinical situation (e.g. hypotension common in sepsis, pancreatitis, hypovolaemia, cardiac disease with poor cardiac outputs, or during anaesthesia).
- **Hyperkalaemia:** Potassium retention can occur through the renal effects of NSAIDs; ideally monitor plasma potassium concentration (e.g. after 1–2 days, after 7 days, then every 1–2 months) if NSAIDs are given concurrently with potassium.
- **Hypertension:** Water and sodium retention occur following NSAID therapy; ideally monitor blood pressure regularly (e.g. after 1–2 days, after 7 days, then monthly) in cats with concurrent cardiac disease or pre-existing hypertension (treat hypertension before starting NSAID if possible).
- **Hepatopathy:** Liver dysfunction is a rare idiosyncratic reaction associated with NSAID administration to some cats.
- **CNS effects:** Lethargy and dullness sometimes reported after starting NSAID therapy but usually decreases over time.
- **Altered blood clotting function:** Disturbances in blood clotting are unlikely following acute administration of NSAIDs, but chronic administration of non-cyclo-oxygenase (COX)-2-specific NSAIDs (e.g. meloxicam) is associated with more prolonged blood clotting in dogs, and this is likely to be similar in cats. However, these changes are unlikely to be clinically significant in healthy animals. COX-2-specific drugs (see Figure 3.19) may cause an increased but unquantified risk of thrombosis in cats (due to selective inhibition of prostacyclin production without concurrent inhibition of thromboxane A_2).

Using NSAIDs safely and effectively: The ISFM and AAFP consensus guidelines on long-term use of NSAIDs in cats (Sparkes *et al.,* 2010) provide excellent recommendations, including a justification for optimizing the safe and effective use of NSAIDs in cats of different ages and health status. The following summarizes the key points from these guidelines.

- Never exceed the recommended (authorized) dose of an NSAID.
- Do not administer more than one NSAID at any one time. Allow a wash-out period of 5–7 days between stopping one NSAID drug and starting a different NSAID.
- Never administer NSAIDs concurrently with corticosteroids.

- Do not administer NSAIDs to cats with vomiting or diarrhoea, a history of gastrointestinal ulceration or concurrent gastrointestinal disease that may result in ulceration.
- Do not administer NSAIDs to cats with acute renal dysfunction. Use NSAIDs cautiously in older cats and those with known chronic kidney disease. Be aware that NSAIDs are **not** necessarily contraindicated in cats with *chronic* kidney disease; detailed guidelines on how to use them wisely in this population of cats are given in Sparkes *et al.* (2010). Use the lowest effective dose and monitor renal function carefully, as well as ensuring adequate water intake at all times.
- Do not administer to cats that are hypotensive (Doppler systolic arterial blood pressure <90 mmHg) or in clinical situations in which hypotension is suspected (e.g. sepsis, pancreatitis, cardiac disease), until normal blood pressure (and fluid balance) are restored. Use NSAIDs cautiously before or during anaesthesia, and avoid administration to cats that are at high risk of developing hypotension during anaesthesia until fully recovered and normotensive.
- Use NSAIDs cautiously in animals with liver dysfunction due to the risk of drug accumulation with repeated dosing.
- Do not administer to cats with prolonged blood clotting and avoid COX-2 specific drugs in cats with shortened blood clotting.
- Educate owners about the risks and benefits of NSAID administration; inform them about when to stop NSAIDs (e.g. signs of any of the above side effects) and contact their veterinary surgeon for further advice. An information sheet for owners about using NSAIDs safely in cats is provided in the ISFM and AAFP guidelines.

Selection: The NSAIDs currently authorized in the UK for use in cats are shown in Figure 3.19; they differ in their selectivity for the enzyme COX-2, in authorized duration and timing of administration, and in tissue selectivity.

There has been a drive to develop NSAIDs that are selective for the COX-2 enzyme, with limited inhibition of COX-1. It was believed that this strategy would lead to NSAIDs that would be effective analgesics but without side effects. It is now known that the prostaglandins produced by the different isoforms of the COX enzyme cannot be classified simply as inflammatory or constitutive and it is of particular relevance that COX-2-derived prostaglandins are essential for normal renal homeostasis. Therefore **no currently available NSAID is devoid of side effects**.

There are currently no robust scientific data detailing the relative risk of side effects associated with different NSAID drugs or the benefits of increased COX-2 selectivity. It is generally accepted that a degree of COX-2 selectivity is advantageous in terms of reduced side effects (e.g. choose a COX-2-*specific* or a COX-2-*preferential* NSAID over a non-selective NSAID), and it is possible (but unproven) that COX-2-specific drugs might be associated with reduced GI effects compared to COX-2 preferential NSAIDs. Clinical data describing NSAID safety in the cat is probably more relevant than use of COX-2 selectivity ratios alone to estimate relative safety of different NSAIDs.

Drug	COX-2 selectivity	Authorized for perioperative administration?	Authorized duration of administration	Clinical use
Meloxicam	COX-2 preferential	✓	Short- and long-term administration to cats. Injectable preparation authorized to be followed by oral preparation (suspension) for 4 days	Specific cat preparation available for oral and injectable dosing. Give oral preparation with food. Oral suspension is honey-flavoured to increase palatability
Robenacoxib	COX-2 specific (coxib)	✓	Tablets authorized for 6 days of administration. Injectable preparation not authorized to be followed by tablets	For perioperative use it is recommended to administer the injectable preparation approximately 30 minutes before surgery
Carprofen	COX-2 preferential	✓	Injectable preparation authorized for single dose administration only	
Ketoprofen	Non-selective for COX-1 and COX-2	✗	Injectable and tablet preparations. Injection may be given for 3 consecutive days or injection may be followed by 4 days' treatment with tablets	Do not use in the perioperative period

3.19 Pharmacological and clinical properties of NSAIDs authorized in the UK for administration to cats.

Tissue selectivity refers to the property whereby the NSAID rapidly leaves the circulation following systemic administration and concentrates in the site of inflammation (tissue damage). Target side-effect organs (kidney, gastrointestinal tract, liver) are exposed to the NSAID for a shorter period of time, reducing the likelihood of side effects. All NSAIDs show a degree of tissue selectivity for sites of inflammation, and hence most NSAIDs have a longer duration of action than suggested by their plasma levels. Robenacoxib combines the properties of a short plasma half-life and preferential uptake at sites of inflammation, which minimizes the total time that side effect organs are exposed, although the clinical benefit of this is currently unknown.

As well as pharmacological considerations, other important factors are the formulation and ease of dosing. For example:

- Metacam (Meloxicam, 0.5 mg/ml, Boehringer Ingelheim) is a liquid preparation that is specifically formulated at a concentration to facilitate easy and accurate dosing in cats. Most cats find it very palatable due to the honey flavouring, but it can also be given with food to facilitate administration
- Robenacoxib 6 mg tablets for cats contain yeast flavouring and are also very palatable; many cats will eat them as if they were treats. This is important because robenacoxib is ideally given 45 minutes before or after feeding in order to promote absorption from the gastrointestinal tract.

Perioperative administration: NSAIDs authorized for perioperative administration may be given before the start of surgery (usually around the time of induction of anaesthesia) or at the end of surgery (once the animal is fully recovered from anaesthesia). The advantages of giving an NSAID before surgery (particularly for elective procedures) are that it provides the opportunity for pre-emptive analgesia, which might limit the development of central and peripheral sensitization, and that it contributes to intraoperative analgesia and a multimodal anaesthesia technique. However, should the cat become hypotensive during anaesthesia and surgery, NSAIDs increase the risk of renal dysfunction following anaesthesia due to blockade of protective prostaglandin production in the kidney. Whether or not to administer NSAIDs before surgery is a cost–benefit question that should be assessed for all patients. In healthy cats undergoing routine elective procedures it is acceptable to give an NSAID before the start of surgery (note timing for robenacoxib in Figure 3.19). If there is concern about the potential for hypotension during the perioperative period, NSAID administration should be delayed until the cat is normotensive and fully recovered from anaesthesia.

Alpha-2 adrenoceptor agonists: α-2 agonists are potent sedative and analgesic agents and can be used as adjunctive analgesic agents in healthy cats. They should not be used alone as first line analgesics but rather used in combination with other classes of analgesic. The duration of analgesia following a single dose of dexmedetomidine or medetomidine is short (e.g. dexmedetomidine 10 μg/kg i.m. provides approximately 45 minutes of analgesia); thus, in order to use them effectively they should be given by CRI (see Figure 3.18) using apparatus such as a syringe driver. α-2 agonist-mediated analgesia is synergistic with opioid-mediated analgesia; it is therefore advisable to use α-2 agonists in combination with opioids, given either intermittently or by CRI, though they will cause concurrent sedation (see later). α-2 agonists should only be used in systemically well cats.

Ketamine: Ketamine given in subanaesthetic doses provides analgesia in laboratory animal pain models, but there are very limited data to support dose recommendations for ketamine or analgesic efficacy in cats. Ketamine should be considered an adjunctive rather than a first-line analgesic and is best used in combination with opioids, either by intermittent dosing of 0.25–0.5 mg/kg i.v. or via CRI (see Figure 3.18).

Local anaesthesia: Local anaesthetic techniques (Figure 3.20) provide a very useful adjunct to systemic analgesia in cats, but are most useful during the immediate perioperative period because of practical difficulties associated with re-dosing. Lidocaine and bupivacaine are the agents most widely used in veterinary practice for local nerve blockade. Lidocaine has a quick onset (5–10 minutes) but short duration of action (90–120 minutes). Bupivacaine has a slower onset (20–30 minutes) but a longer duration of action

Technique	Clinical indications	Recommended dose and volume (for a 5 kg cat)
Topical application of lidocaine (acts within 1–2 minutes)	Prior to endotracheal intubation of all cats	1 mg/kg lidocaine (0.1–0.2 ml of 1% solution divided between both sides of larynx; see Anaesthetic equipment, later) or 1–2 sprays of Intubeaze (Dechra)
	Prior to placement of a nasal tube (for oxygen)	0.1–0.2 ml of 1% lidocaine solution dropped into the nostril. Do not exceed 4 mg/kg lidocaine total dose OR 1–2 drops of 0.5% proxymetacaine
	Proprietary topical local anaesthetic solutions for the eye to facilitate examination of the cornea	1–2 drops of proxymetacaine 0.5% per eye
Intrapleural analgesia	Administration of bupivacaine through a chest drain to provide analgesia of the pleural cavity where a chest drain *in situ* is causing discomfort. Bupivacaine is acidic and stings following administration via this route. If applicable, give first dose while cat anaesthetized when chest drain placed at end of surgery. NB Intrapleural bupivacaine is not appropriate for providing analgesia for chest tube placement	Administer systemic analgesia 5 minutes prior to bupivacaine. Bupivacaine 1 mg/kg diluted to a total volume of 10–15 ml. If only one side of chest affected (e.g. lateral thoracotomy) lay the cat on the affected side after administration to encourage distribution of bupivacaine to the injured area. If bilateral chest drains, divide total dose and volume between both sides. Can be repeated q8h.
Dental nerve blocks	Mandibular and maxillary nerve blocks for the lower and upper dental arcades, respectively	0.25–0.5 ml per nerve block of undiluted 0.5% bupivacaine. Safe maximum volume of undiluted solution for injection is 2 ml in a 5 kg cat
Local infiltration techniques	Examples: around cutaneous masses prior to excision; ring block around distal limb prior to procedures of the distal limb (nail removal, foot pad injuries)	1–2 mg/kg bupivacaine, depending on the vascularity of the region. Dilute 0.5% bupivacaine if a greater volume needed to allow distribution over a larger area. For example, dilute 2 ml 0.5% bupivacaine to 5 ml to inject around a 4–5 cm diameter cutaneous mass
Epidural injection of local anaesthetics	Hindlimb and pelvic procedures. This is a specialized technique and requires training before adoption in practice	1 mg/kg bupivacaine diluted to 1 ml total volume per 4.5 kg bodyweight

3.20 Examples of local anaesthetic techniques. Specialist advice is required before carrying out epidural anaesthesia/analgesia or more invasive nerve blocks, such as a brachial plexus block for surgery distal to the elbow.

(up to 6 hours), which is advantageous in the immediate postoperative period. Using a proprietary preparation of lidocaine combined with adrenaline will extend its duration of action, as the adrenaline causes vasoconstriction, decreasing the rate of absorption into the systemic circulation. This is useful to achieve a more prolonged local anaesthetic block when bupivacaine is not available.

Local anaesthetics can cause cardiovascular and CNS toxicity when absorbed at high concentrations into the systemic circulation. The recommended total dose of lidocaine for local nerve blocks, including topical application, is 4 mg/kg; maximum dose of bupivacaine is 2 mg/kg (reduce maximum dose to 1 mg/kg when injected into highly vascular areas where systemic absorption is likely to be rapid, e.g. intrapleural administration).

WARNING

Bupivacaine is more cardiotoxic than lidocaine and must never be given intravenously.

Safe use:

- Calculate the dose of local anaesthetic accurately; dilute calculated dose with NaCl 0.9% if increased volume of local anaesthetic is required for the distribution of the drug over a larger area. It is not generally necessary to dilute local anaesthetics for intranasal or topical administration.
- Check that the needle has not been inadvertently introduced into a blood vessel before injection. If blood is present in the hub of the syringe following drawback, reposition the needle and reconfirm correct needle placement.
- Do not exceed the recommended total dose of either lidocaine or bupivacaine.

Chronic pain

Chronic pain can be defined as pain that outlasts the period of tissue healing. It is maladaptive and has no evolutionary advantage to the animal and so its effective management is imperative. It is, however, extremely challenging to recognize, quantify and manage chronic pain in cats and it is likely that it is under-recognized.

Chronic pain can be broadly classified into two different types:

- **Neuropathic pain** (from damage to the nervous system itself)
- **Chronic inflammatory pain** (following chronic inflammation of tissues).

Identifying chronic pain

The key to successfully managing chronic pain is accurate identification and quantification. Changes in behaviour and demeanour are usually the best way to recognize chronic pain but are commonly very subtle and progress slowly. Cat owners are much better placed than the veterinary surgeon to recognize chronic pain in their pets, although they often require education to know what sort of signs to look out for. In older animals particularly, many signs of chronic pain are commonly attributed to normal changes associated with ageing. In the veterinary clinic, which can be an unfamiliar and stressful environment (see Chapter 1), most cats will not demonstrate subtle signs of chronic pain, and/or the signs will be indistinguishable from those of anxiety.

It is impossible to produce a comprehensive list of behaviours potentially shown by cats in chronic pain. Behavioural changes will vary depending on the severity and duration of chronic pain as well as the underlying cause. Changes that should be looked for (and the owner questioned about) include:

- Inactivity
- Hiding behaviour
- Aggression
- Depressed demeanour
- Inappetence
- Fear
- Excessive grooming or licking of a particular body part
- Increased sensitivity to touch, e.g. reluctance to be stroked over the sensitive area, or skin twitching
- Altered toileting habits
- Reluctance to play
- Reluctance to engage with the owner
- Absence of normal behaviours
- Changes in normal habits associated with reduced mobility, e.g. choosing to sleep in places at floor level rather than at a height, not coming up/down stairs, not wanting to go outside or use a catflap.

It is worth emphasizing that some owners will perceive many of these signs to be normal 'old age' changes, and so may not bring them to the veterinary surgeon's attention unless specifically questioned about them.

Common diseases likely to be associated with chronic pain are listed in Figure 3.21.

- Degenerative joint disease
- Chronic cystitis associated with feline lower urinary tract disease
- Chronic gingivitis or dental disease
- Chronic skin conditions resulting in skin inflammation and pruritus
- Chronic inflammatory ear disease
- Recurrent uveitis
- Chronic non-healing wounds
- Neoplasia e.g. squamous cell carcinoma of the nose
- Chronic inflammatory bowel disease
- Chronic pancreatitis

3.21 Common diseases likely to be associated with chronic pain.

The importance of degenerative joint disease (DJD) as a cause of chronic pain in cats is known (see Lascelles and Robertson, 2010) as well as the behavioural changes that are commonly reported by owners of cats with DJD. These may vary depending on which joints are affected, but specific behavioural changes associated with DJD include:

- Reluctance to jump up on to objects (e.g. on to a bed) or a reluctance to jump down
- Unwillingness to play
- Reduced activity
- Reduced grooming
- Aggression
- Altered toileting habits, e.g. if a litter tray has high sides which make it difficult to access, cats may stop using the litter tray altogether or may miss the litter tray
- Reduction in hunting behaviour
- Increased sleeping.

Monitoring changes in chronic pain
Owners are best placed to monitor changes in pain severity when the cat is in the home environment. Lascelles *et al.* (2007) recommended using Client Specific Outcome Measures (CSOMs) to monitor changes in the severity of pain following initiation of

analgesic therapy in cats with DJD, and the same principle can be applied to cats with any chronically painful condition. CSOMs require the owner to identify four or five activities that have been altered with the onset of DJD (or any painful condition); for example, if a cat has DJD of the hip the owner might report that the cat no longer jumps on to the owner's bed at night. The owner is then asked to record (e.g. at weekly intervals) the frequency of occurrence of this activity during treatment. A reduction in chronic pain from hip DJD should increase the frequency with which the cat jumps on to the bed. It is also important to manage the owner's expectations of a successful treatment outcome. For example, if the cat is aged, it is not reasonable to expect it to return to activity levels typical of a kitten. A more realistic expectation is to show activity levels that were present when the cat was already aged but before the onset of DJD. For a cat with recurrent cystitis the activity reported by the owner might relate to frequency of urination or number of visits to the litter tray, although other measures, in addition to analgesia, are likely to be instigated in the management of feline lower urinary tract disease. Changes in activity are easy to recognize and record but it is also helpful to try to measure changes in the emotional state of the cat caused by pain (e.g. indicated by demeanour) following initiation of treatment.

Management of chronic pain
It is important to adopt a holistic approach to the management of chronic pain and to consider non-pharmacological strategies as well as drugs (see *BSAVA Manual of Canine and Feline Rehabilitation, Supportive and Palliative Care: Case Studies in Patient Management*). For non-pharmacological strategies in DJD see Chapter 16. Many owners are very motivated to participate actively in therapeutic strategies to decrease pain in their cat.

Pharmacological management of chronic pain:
Cats with chronic pain are most likely to be managed in the home environment and there are therefore a number of important considerations:

- **Route of administration:** Oral drugs are usually required for chronic administration
- **Tolerability:** The drug needs to be palatable to maintain patient compliance. Tablets must be of a suitable size to be given orally by owners, particularly if the drug should not be given with food (see QRG 3.1)
- **Duration of action:** A requirement for frequent dosing (e.g. more than three times daily) commonly leads to poor patient and owner compliance
- **Controlled Drugs** (e.g. opioids)**:** These are not suitable for chronic administration in the home environment. As well as the legal issues surrounding dispensing to owners for administration at home, most opioids are poorly absorbed following oral administration (with the exception of buprenorphine when given via the oral transmucosal route) and therefore must be given systemically to be efficacious. Systemic administration of analgesic drugs is usually impractical for prolonged periods.

As described earlier for acute pain, it is best practice to manage chronic pain using a **multimodal approach** to drug therapy. However, this can be very difficult to achieve in individual patients because of: a lack of authorized drugs; and limited knowledge of drug efficacy, optimal drug doses and dosing regimens.

Non-steroidal anti-inflammatory drugs: NSAIDs are the drugs most commonly used for the management of chronic pain, particularly pain associated with DJD. One NSAID (meloxicam) currently holds an authorization for long-term administration for the management of pain and there is a large evidence base to support drug efficacy, dose and dosing interval.

The side effects associated with NSAID administration have been described earlier. However, decision-making is often more complex in animals with chronic pain than in those with acute pain because the incidence of concurrent disease is often high (e.g. DJD is more common in aged cats which may have concurrent kidney disease). There are also few alternative drugs suitable for the management of chronic pain in the home environment.

In some cats, decision-making around NSAID administration may depend on the outcome of a cost–benefit analysis for the individual patient. It is important to involve the owner fully in this discussion and make them aware of what other analgesic treatment options are available.

A full discussion of monitoring cats receiving NSAID therapy is beyond the scope of this book but it is important that the frequency and extent of monitoring are tailored to the individual patient. Guidelines for monitoring cats on chronic NSAID therapy are given in Figure 3.22. It is also important to involve the owner in discussions about what monitoring is required (e.g. serum biochemistry) and how frequently it

should be carried out. The following should be considered (see also guidelines on page 66 for monitoring cats with specific medical conditions, where more intensive monitoring of some parameters may be required):

- Obtain baseline values for all monitored parameters before starting NSAIDs
- Re-check 5–7 days after starting treatment; do a clinical examination and speak to the owner about potential complications of NSAID therapy. Re-check monitored variables on the basis of history and clinical examination.
- Re-measure all monitored variables 2–3 weeks after starting treatment. Acute NSAID side effects are usually seen in the first 2 weeks of therapy
- Tailor ongoing frequency of monitoring to the risk of side effects presented by the individual patient. In cats with concurrent diseases that are likely to increase the risk of side effects (e.g. chronic kidney disease) re-check monitored variables every 2–3 months. In cats that are otherwise healthy with no predisposing factors, monitoring every 6 months is usually adequate.

Other drugs: Other analgesics with different mechanisms of action are also used in the management of chronic pain in cats (Figure 3.23). Currently there are no robust data to support drug selection, doses or duration of treatment (e.g. whether tolerance or dependence develops) for chronic pain. Most treatment regimens are based on anecdotal evidence and clinical experience. Generally it is recommended to wean cats off long-term analgesic drugs slowly, by gradually reducing drug dose and/or frequency while paying careful attention to whether the cat starts to show increasing signs of pain indicating the need for additional analgesia.

Parameter	Always required	Suggested minimum	Ideal if possible
Review history with owner	✓		
Full clinical examination including blood pressure measurement wherever possible	✓		
Haematology			
Haematocrit		✓	
Complete blood count			✓
Serum biochemistry			
Total protein, albumin			✓
Urea		✓	
Creatinine		✓	
Alanine aminotransferase (ALT), alkaline phosphatase (ALP)		✓	
Aspartate aminotransferase (AST), γ-glutamyl transferase (GGT), bile acids			✓
Sodium, potassium			✓
Urinalysis			
Specific gravity		✓	
Dipstick biochemistry		✓	
Protein:creatinine ratio			✓
Sediment analysis			✓

3.22 Monitoring cats receiving chronic NSAID therapy. (Adapted from Sparkes *et al.*, 2010.)

Drug	Mechanism of action	Formulation	Dose range	Clinical notes
Tramadol	Opioid, serotonergic and noradrenergic effects	Tablets; injectable solution	1–2 mg/kg q12h orally	Tablets are bitter. Sedation can occur
Gabapentin	Voltage-gated calcium channel blocker	Capsule preparation used most commonly	5–10 mg/kg q12h orally	Generally recommended to taper off gradually if discontinued. Some commercial companies can supply cat-sized formulations
Amantadine	NMDA receptor antagonist	Tablet preparation: tablets require reformulation to allow accurate dosing in cats	3–5 mg/kg q24h orally	May be more effective when given in combination with NSAIDs or opioids
Amitriptyline	Serotonin and noradrenaline reuptake inhibitor	Tablet preparation	0.5–2 mg/kg q24h orally	Sedation may occur, start at low end of the dose range. May be useful for the management of neuropathic pain

3.23 Adjunctive analgesic drugs used for the management of chronic pain in cats. Note that none of these is authorized for this use in animals in the UK.

Although not suitable for management of pain for more than a few days, administration of **buprenorphine** by the oral transmucosal route by owners in the home environment is a useful strategy to manage ongoing pain when hospitalization is not practical (e.g. due to cost or cat temperament). Owners must be taught how to administer buprenorphine correctly by this route. Buprenorphine 20 µg/kg can be given three times daily (q8h); the doses must be drawn up into preloaded, correctly labelled syringes and capped to prevent drug contamination. The owners must be made aware of the consequences of inadvertent self-administration of buprenorphine or drug abuse, including obtaining medical advice if this should occur. It is unwise to dispense more than 3–4 days' worth of buprenorphine for a single cat to owners.

Tramadol is increasingly used to manage acute and chronic pain in cats, although no preparation is currently authorized for use in animals in the UK. Optimal oral doses and dosing intervals for tramadol have not been fully elucidated in cats, but it is recognized to provide analgesia through both opioid- and non-opioid-mediated mechanisms. It is not subject to Controlled Drug legislation and can be dispensed for oral administration at home by the owner. Reformulation into gelatine capsules is required to enable accurate administration, or some pharmacies can provide small formulations for use in cats. The major disadvantage of tramadol is that cats may find it unpalatable and bitter and so patient compliance can be poor; even reformulation into gelatine capsules does not alleviate the bitter taste, although some cats take it remarkably well. Some cats show behavioural alterations when dosed with tramadol, becoming quite 'spacey' and disorientated, although in many cases lowering the dose for the individual animal alleviates this side effect. If tolerated, tramadol is a good first-line option for chronic pain management in cats if NSAIDs are contraindicated, because it has known efficacy for acute pain management in cats and the onset of analgesic action is short after oral dosing (probably 24–48 hours).

Gabapentin is a structural analogue of γ-amino butyric acid (GABA) that was initially developed as an antiepileptic agent but more recently has been investigated for the management of both chronic (e.g. caused by DJD) and acute postoperative pain. It is often used in the management of neuropathic pain, e.g. spinal pain associated with nerve root pathology or pain following tail amputation. It appears to provide analgesia in some experimental pain models in laboratory animals although robust studies investigating analgesia in cats for acute and chronic pain are lacking. The recommended dose range for gabapentin in cats is also extremely wide; it is recommended to start with 5 mg/kg q12h and to increase up to 10 mg/kg q8h if lower doses are ineffective. Gabapentin is available in 100 mg capsules; breaking the capsule and sprinkling the correct dose on food is a practical option for administration to cats, although reformulation into gelatine capsules (this can be done by a compounding pharmacy) containing smaller amounts of gabapentin allows more accurate dosing. An oral liquid preparation is available but contains xylitol, which can be toxic to cats, so the capsule preparation should be used.

Amantadine is an NMDA receptor antagonist (similar to ketamine) and therefore is likely to have analgesic effects through a reduction in central sensitization that results from acute and chronic pain. Data in cats are limited but amantadine has been useful in dogs with osteoarthritis pain that was refractory to NSAID therapy alone (Lascelles *et al.*, 2008), so it might be useful in the management of feline DJD, particularly in combination with an NSAID. Amantadine combined with an opioid might also provide better analgesia than the opioid alone, but further studies are required.

Amitriptyline is used for the management of depression in humans but also has an analgesic action through inhibition of uptake of noradrenaline and serotonin. It is no longer recommended for the management of pain associated with interstitial cystitis in cats but may be useful for other neuropathic states. Side effects that are occasionally reported include drowsiness and excessive grooming.

Effective sedation and anaesthesia

Sedation and general anaesthesia lie at different points along a continuum from fully awake to deeply anaesthetized. Both sedation and general anaesthesia require the administration of drugs that act on the CNS to depress consciousness; the degree of CNS depression is lower with sedation than with general anaesthesia.

Risk awareness and management

Cats can be difficult to sedate and anaesthetize safely. Their small body size poses some potential problems:

- Achieving intravenous access is technically challenging
- The risk of laryngeal or tracheal trauma is high if endotracheal intubation is not done carefully
- Monitoring is challenging because of limited access to the patient
- The blood volume of cats is low, so cats are less tolerant of any surgical blood loss
- Fluid therapy must be managed carefully in the perioperative period; use a syringe driver or fluid pump
- A large surface area to volume ratio predisposes cats to hypothermia, so it is vital that body temperature is monitored regularly. Measures must be put in place to support body temperature, starting after premedication and extending throughout the entire anaesthesia and recovery period (see later).

Cats must also be approached with a calm and empathetic nature to achieve anaesthesia or sedation smoothly with the minimum distress to the cat (see Chapter 1).

Factors that increase the risk of death following anaesthesia or sedation in cats include the following.

- **Procedural urgency:** Always attempt to stabilize the cardiovascular and respiratory systems before inducing anaesthesia for emergency procedures. Balance the risk of delaying surgery against the risks of anaesthesia in an inadequately stabilized patient.
- **Health status** (Figure 3.24)**:** Cats with pre-existing disease are less resilient to the physiological effects of anaesthetics, predisposing to cardiovascular and respiratory depression.
- **Age:** Increasing age is associated with an increased risk of death independent of the relationship between increasing age and concurrent disease.
- **Major *versus* minor procedures:** Major surgical procedures carry more risk than minor surgical procedures.

- **Extremes of bodyweight:** Low bodyweight (<2 kg) exacerbates the problems of small body size. Obesity (>6 kg) is also problematical due to reduced lung function, increased likelihood of drug overdose, and increased risk of regurgitation and thus aspiration.

Sedation of cats is not safer than anaesthesia *per se*. In high-risk cats, controlled and supported general anaesthesia is usually safer than sedation. All brachycephalic cats are at risk of respiratory obstruction after sedation, so should be monitored continuously for signs of obstruction; overt respiratory obstruction is not relieved by altering head and neck position, but is best managed by induction of anaesthesia and immediate intubation. Recent data (Brodbelt, 2010) have shown that the risk of death from anaesthesia or sedation in healthy cats was 0.11% (i.e. 1 cat per 1000 anaesthesias or sedations) and in sick cats 1% (i.e. 1 cat per 100).

Key points for safe and effective anaesthesia or sedation of cats are as follows.

- Obtain a thorough history from the owner and perform a full clinical examination before anaesthesia or sedation. Carry out further evaluations based on any findings. Routine haematology and biochemistry, particularly to evaluate renal parameters and electrolytes, are recommended for senior and geriatric cats.
- Assign an ASA status to the cat (see Figure 3.24); those with ASA status ≥ 3 are at high risk.
- Prior placement of an intravenous catheter is recommended for all cats undergoing anaesthesia or prolonged (>30 minutes) sedation.
- Do not neglect premedication for general anaesthesia (see later).
- Ideally, provide oxygen to all cats that are sedated or anaesthetized. In non-intubated cats, deliver oxygen via a breathing system and facemask, or via the end of a breathing system if a facemask is not tolerated (Figure 3.25).

ASA status	Description	Examples
1	Normal healthy patient	A young adult cat presenting for ovariohysterectomy or castration
2	Patient with mild systemic disease that displays no clinical signs	A 10-year-old cat that has mildly elevated liver enzymes but is otherwise healthy
3	Patient with systemic disease that displays clinical signs; or with clinical disease that is stabilized by drug therapy	A 13-year-old cat with mildly elevated urea and creatinine that is polydipsic and polyuric
4	Patient with severe systemic disease that is a constant threat to life	A cat with hypertrophic cardiomyopathy and pleural effusion
5	Patient that is likely to die with or without surgery	A collapsed cat that is dyspnoeic and unresponsive to stimulation. A cat with a ruptured diaphragm following trauma with significant blood loss

3.24 Criteria for classification of ASA (American Society of Anesthesiologists) risk status.

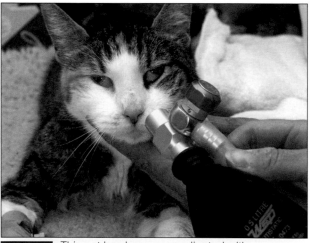

3.25 This cat has been premedicated with acepromazine and buprenorphine and is receiving oxygen, using a breathing system connected to an anaesthetic machine, immediately prior to induction of anaesthesia with intravenous propofol. Flow rates of 2–3 litres/min will increase inspired oxygen concentration and are well tolerated by most cats.

- Carry out routine monitoring with pulse oximetry in anaesthetized cats (see Figure 3.29); use in sedated cats if tolerated.
- Maintain normothermia:
  - Hypothermic cats may require active warming before premedication
  - Premedicated and sedated cats can become hypothermic rapidly; ensure a warm environmental temperature, minimize heat loss and provide active warming if necessary
  - Monitor body temperature during anaesthesia and the recovery period, and ensure that appropriate supportive measures to warm cats are implemented.
- Provide intravenous fluid therapy with a balanced crystalloid solution (e.g. Hartmann's solution) to all cats anaesthetized or sedated for >30 minutes. Adjust the rate of fluid administration:

- Sedated (3–4 ml/kg/h)
- Anaesthetized but not undergoing surgery or a procedure causing blood or fluid loss (4–5 ml/kg/h)
- Anaesthetized and undergoing surgery (6–10 ml/kg/h).

Sedation

Drugs

Using a combination of a sedative and an analgesic drug is recommended. This allows a lower dose of the sedative to be used, which may reduce the degree of cardiovascular and respiratory depression; provision of analgesia is beneficial if the cat is already in pain or the procedure is likely to cause pain. Figures 3.26 to 3.28 describe the sedative drugs available and indications for them.

Characteristics of sedation and any analgesic action	Important side effects	Onset of sedation and duration of action	Clinical notes	Sedative combinations with this drug
α-2 agonists (e.g. medetomidine, dexmedetomidine)				
Dose-dependent profound sedation and analgesia. Analgesia of shorter duration (<1 h) than sedation (2–3 h)	Decrease in heart rate and transient increase in blood pressure. Significant reduction in cardiac output. Minimal respiratory effects	Onset of sedation 15–20 min after i.m. administration. Analgesia duration: ~45 min after a 10 μg/kg dose of dexmedetomidine. Duration of sedation: 2–3 h, dependent on dose	Do not use in cats with ASA ≥3 or cardiovascular disease. Avoid in geriatric cats. Vomiting common after i.m. administration. Antagonize dexmedetomidine/medetomidine with atipamezole at end of sedation	Opioid [a] + α-2 agonist: synergistic sedative and analgesic effects; allows lower dose of α-2 agonist. Benzodiazepine + α-2 agonist: increases depth of sedation; allows lower dose of α-2 agonist. Ketamine + α-2 agonist: general anaesthesia, duration dependent on dose
Phenothiazines (e.g. acepromazine (ACP))				
Anxiolysis and moderate sedation, dependent on dose. Not considered analgesic	Peripheral vasodilation can cause hypotension in cats with cardiovascular disease or pre-existing hypotension or low normal blood pressure (systolic blood pressure <110 mmHg). Peripheral vasodilation can reduce body temperature	Onset of sedation 30–40 min. Duration of sedation 4–6 h, although sedation may not be clinically apparent >2 h after administration	Greater margin of safety with ACP compared to α-2 agonists in terms of cardiovascular effects; low doses (≤0.05 mg/kg) suitable for cats with mild to moderate cardiovascular disease	Opioid [a] + ACP will produce synergistic sedation. ACP alone can be used when minimal sedation required, e.g. chest radiography for investigation of lung disease or heart size
Benzodiazepines (e.g. midazolam, diazepam)				
Minimal or no sedation when given alone to healthy cats. Mild sedation in cats <3 months old or with severe systemic disease resulting in CNS depression. Not analgesic	Minimal effects on cardiovascular or respiratory system; useful for sedation of cats ≥ASA 3.	Onset of sedation 10–15 min i.m. Duration of sedation 1 h in healthy patients. Metabolism may be prolonged in animals with liver dysfunction	Useful combined with ketamine in cats ASA status ≥3. Use midazolam in preference to diazepam, as duration of action more predictable and injection less painful	Ketamine + benzodiazepine: provides profound sedation. α-2 agonist + benzodiazepine: provides profound sedation. Opioid + benzodiazepine: quality of sedation limited unless concurrent CNS depression. May cause excitement in healthy cats
Ketamine				
Profound sedation/ general anaesthesia in high doses. Analgesic effect poorly characterized in animals	Avoid ketamine in cats with hypertrophic cardiomyopathy as can increase heart rate and myocardial oxygen requirement. Cats may appear 'spacey' after recovery from sedation	Onset of sedation 5–10 min i.m. In combination with benzodiazepines will provide deep sedation for ~20 min. Recovery from ketamine sedation can be prolonged (1–2 h)	Do not use alone for sedation due to likelihood of CNS excitation and muscle rigidity. Even in combination with a sedative, individual cats can show marked excitation. If this occurs: do not handle the cat; leave in quiet environment where risk of injury reduced (e.g. well padded cage). Use a different sedative for that cat in the future. Anecdotally, excitation reactions more commonly reported in oriental breeds. Do not give atipamezole to reverse α-2 agonist until 30 min after ketamine administration	Midazolam + ketamine: ideal for deep sedation. α-2 agonist + ketamine: causes general anaesthesia, dependent on dose

3.26 Characteristics of drugs used for sedation and/or premedication in cats. [a] Use: methadone if moderate to severe pain is anticipated; buprenorphine for mild pain (or moderate pain with a multimodal analgesia protocol); butorphanol for non-painful or very mildly painful procedures. (continues) ▶

Technique	Advantages	Disadvantages
'Hot hands', i.e. latex gloves filled with warm water	Quick to set up. Cheap. Do not require specialist equipment. Portable	If water is too hot will burn the patient. Temperature not controlled. Cool down over time; therefore need refilling or replacing. Not very effective at warming a patient that is already hypothermic. Claws may puncture
Traditional electrically heated mat	Cheap to buy. Can be placed under a patient on the operating table and covered with a cloth pad to prevent burns	Heating of pad uneven; leads to 'hot spots' that can cause burns. Cannot use in conscious cats due to risk of electrocution. No means by which temperature can be controlled
Forced warm air heating device (e.g. Bair Hugger)	Very effective at warming hypothermic patients. Can be used during anaesthesia and recovery period. Temperature can be controlled	Can be impractical for some types of surgery due to blanket limiting access to cat. Blankets are disposable and cannot be reused. Can disrupt laminar air flow and increase risk of airborne contamination of surgical environment
Heated blankets (e.g. ThermAssure)	Even heating of fabric; multiple temperature sensors provide accurate controlled heating. Do not disrupt laminar flow in operating theatres. Puncture of blanket will not result in electrical shock due to isolated low-voltage current. Very effective at warming hypothermic cats	Type of surgery and required access can limit how much of patient can be exposed to blanket and thus warming. Expensive

3.30 Advantages and disadvantages of techniques used to support body temperature during sedation or anaesthesia.

Prolonging sedation

The drugs listed in Figure 3.26 can be re-administered *once* in order to prolong the duration of sedation, but it is difficult to avoid drug accumulation or prevent overdose. If prolonged sedation (>30 min) is required, general anaesthesia should be considered; alternatively, an intravenous catheter can be placed after initial sedation and low doses (1–2 mg/kg i.v.) of alfaxalone or propofol given to effect. *Note: alfaxalone is not authorized for sedation.*

Deepening sedation

If deeper sedation is required, a second dose of the same drug combination is unlikely to work because the cat is usually already agitated and anxious. Rescheduling the procedure for a different day may be better, or the following can be tried:

- Administer a low dose of alfaxalone or propofol intravenously
- If acepromazine (ACP) was administered initially, then a low dose of an α-2 agonist can be given afterwards, but only in cats rated ASA 1 or 2
- Administration of alfaxalone alone or of ketamine combined with midazolam will further deepen sedation in cats that have been given ACP or an α-2 agonist; but the cat must be monitored carefully as anaesthesia may be induced.

Improving the quality of sedation

- Give sedative drugs intramuscularly rather than subcutaneously.
- Allow adequate time for sedation to occur before disturbing the cat.
- Leave the cat in a quiet environment with minimal audible and visual stimulation.

Anaesthetic equipment

Equipment for induction and intubation

- **Catheters and needles:** Ensure appropriate sizes are available:
  - Intravenous catheters: 22 G 1 inch and 24 G ³/₄ inch
  - Needles: 23 G 1 inch and 1¼ inch, 25 G 5/8 inch needles

- **Laryngoscope:** Use a laryngoscope with a short straight fibreoptic blade.
- **Endotracheal tubes (ETTs):** Two types of ETT are commonly used: red rubber or softer PVC tubes. Use PVC tubes to minimize the likelihood of tracheal trauma.
  - Size:
    - A 3.5 mm internal diameter (ID) tube (Figure 3.31) is suitable for small cats (2–3 kg bodyweight).
    - Many 4–6 kg cats can be intubated with tubes ranging from 4.5 to 5.5 ID.
    - Very narrow ETTs (e.g. 2–2.5 mm ID) can obstruct easily with respiratory secretions.
  - *Length:* If the ETT is too long, there is a risk of 'one lung' intubation, so the length of the ETT should be measured against the neck of the cat from the entrance to the mouth to the thoracic inlet; the tip of the ETT should not extend past the thoracic inlet.
  - *Cuffed versus uncuffed:*
    - Both cuffed and uncuffed ETTs can be used in cats >4 kg. Only uncuffed tubes should be used in smaller cats, as they allow use of a larger diameter tube that is less likely to obstruct.

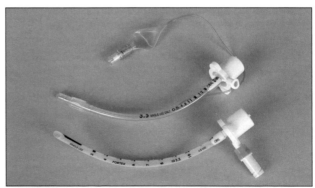

3.31 PVC endotracheal tubes with an internal diameter (ID) of 3.5 mm; one tube has a cuff while the other does not. The connector at the end of the tube allows a sampling line to be attached directly into the breathing system to sample airway gases for sidestream capnometry. Care must be taken when inflating cuffs of PVC tubes as overinflation can still lead to tracheal damage.

– Cuffed tubes provide a better seal in the airway reducing the risk of aspiration (e.g. during dental procedures) but *red rubber tubes with inflated cuffs (Figure 3.32) should not be used* as they can cause tracheal necrosis due to their high-pressure low-volume cuffs; the low-pressure, high-volume cuffed PVC tubes should be used, but note that overinflation of PVC tube cuffs can still cause tracheal damage.

- **Local anaesthetic for laryngeal desensitization:** A proprietary product containing lidocaine (e.g. Intubeaze; 1–2 sprays on the larynx) may be used. Alternatively, 0.1–0.2 ml lidocaine hydrochloride 1% can be drawn up into a 1 ml syringe, attached to an intravenous catheter sheath, and applied to the larynx; divide the total volume between right and left sides of the larynx. Do not use the spray preparation of xylocaine manufactured by Astra Zeneca for human use, as it causes severe laryngeal oedema and dyspnoea in cats and fatalities are commonly reported after its use (Fisher, 2010).

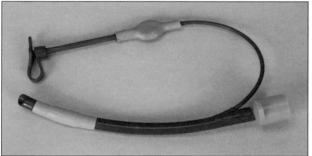

3.32 A red rubber tube with a cuff. **Do NOT use this type of tube for intubating cats as the high-pressure low-volume cuff can cause tracheal damage.**

Intubation technique

Atraumatic placement of an endotracheal tube is illustrated in Figure 3.33.

1 Ensure that the cat is adequately anaesthetized before attempting intubation; otherwise laryngeal spasm may result. The head of the cat must be positioned correctly to facilitate intubation using a laryngoscope.

2 Extend the cat's tongue gently out in front of its mouth using one hand, while holding the handle of the laryngoscope in your other hand. Place the tip of the blade of the laryngoscope at the base of the tongue just in front of, but not touching, the epiglottis, and depress the blade ventrally. This action will allow visualization of the larynx.

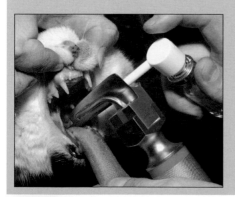

3.33 Placing an endotracheal tube.

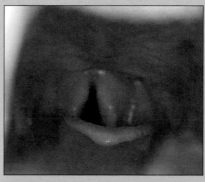

View of the larynx. The tip of the epiglottis is visible ventrally in the midline; the laryngeal opening is the orifice in the midline caudal to the epiglottis.

3 Once the laryngoscope blade is in position and the tongue extended out of the mouth so that it is not obstructing the view of the larynx, your hand will be free to hold the bottle of Intubeaze (or syringe containing lidocaine). Apply local anaesthetic to the larynx to desensitize it; wait at least 30 seconds before intubation.

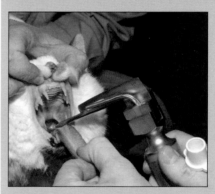

4 Hold the ETT in the other hand to the laryngoscope, with the tip of the tube just in front of the larynx, and visualize opening and closing of the larynx during normal respiration.

5 Advance the ETT quickly and gently through the larynx when the vocal folds are open (during inspiration). Aim the tube ventrally to prevent inadvertent intubation of the oesophagus.

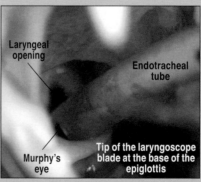

The Murphy's eye at the tip of the tube is to allow a passageway for airflow should the lumen of the tube be obstructed by being positioned directly against the wall of the trachea.

Laryngeal opening

Endotracheal tube

Murphy's eye

Tip of the laryngoscope blade at the base of the epiglottis

6 Attach the ETT to the T-piece circuit and administer oxygen ± gaseous anaesthetic as required.

7 Inflate the cuff if present; always inflate the cuff carefully to prevent overinflation. To inflate the cuff safely, ask an assistant to occlude the expiratory limb on the T-piece circuit while gently squeezing the reservoir bag, and listen at the mouth of the cat for a leak around the ETT (gas can be heard during delivery of the breath). If a leak is present, gradually inflate the cuff with air until a leak can no longer be detected when subsequent breaths are delivered by the assistant. Be sure to release the occlusion of the expiratory limb on the circuit between each breath. If an uncuffed tube is used for a procedure with a high risk of aspiration, such as a dental procedure, the back of the pharynx can be packed, for example, with a surgical swab with a piece of nylon suture attached; the packing can be quickly removed at the end of anaesthesia

Troubleshooting: If it is **not possible to pass** the ETT through the larynx after one or two attempts and *the cat is breathing normally*:

1. Stop trying to intubate the cat; allow the cat to breathe oxygen via a facemask and anaesthetic circuit for 30–60 seconds.
2. Check the depth of anaesthesia. Administer a low dose of induction agent intravenously to effect if the cat has a brisk eye reflex or is swallowing during intubation.
3. Once the cat is well oxygenated, calmly attempt to intubate the cat again. Reapply lidocaine to desensitize the larynx if more than 3 minutes have elapsed since the first application.
4. Use a smaller diameter tube if intubation is difficult; it can always be replaced with a larger diameter tube once the airway is secure. Alternatively, intubate the trachea using a 5 Fr urinary catheter; then immediately slide a larger ETT over the urinary catheter into the laryngeal opening and remove the catheter from the trachea. This technique often allows a larger diameter ETT to be placed than would otherwise be possible (e.g. 5 mm ID rather than 3.5–4 mm ID), ensuring maintenance of a secure airway.

If **laryngeal spasm** occurs (the larynx remains closed) and the cat becomes dyspnoeic, do not panic but call for help. Establish an airway by gently advancing a 5–6 Fr urinary catheter through the larynx after further application of lidocaine (stop and give oxygen via a facemask every 15–20 seconds if airway catheter insertion is not immediately possible). Once the airway catheter is in place, attach it to the breathing system via a syringe case and give oxygen. Monitor haemoglobin saturation with oxygen using a pulse oximeter. Replace the urinary catheter with a narrow ETT after 5–10 minutes once oxygenation is adequate via the urinary catheter (SpO_2 is >95%).

Airway secretions can frequently obscure the laryngeal opening, severely hindering attempts at endotracheal intubation and also contributing to reduced oxygenation due to airway obstruction. If secretions are problematic, apply gentle suction to the back of the pharynx to clear the secretions using either a hand-operated vacuum pump and a suction catheter or a syringe and 5–6 Fr urinary catheter, if a suction pump is not available.

PRACTICAL TIP

It is useful to have suction apparatus on standby when preparing to intubate cats with known airway, oesophageal or oral cavity disease, so that intervention to clear any secretions can be implemented promptly.

Requirements during maintenance phase

- **Anaesthetic breathing system:** Use a system with low dead space and low resistance to respiration; an Ayres T-piece with a Jackson–Rees modification (addition of a reservoir bag; Figure 3.34) is suitable for all cats, or an Ayres T-piece with a reservoir bag and an adjustable pressure-limiting (APL) valve to facilitate scavenging from

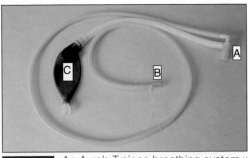

3.34 An Ayre's T-piece breathing system with a Jackson–Rees modification (the reservoir bag, C). The reservoir bag allows manual IPPV should respiratory support be required during anaesthesia. A connects to the ETT in the patient; B connects to the common gas outlet of the anaesthetic machine to supply fresh gases. The reservoir bag is to be connected to a scavenging system. Take care that the outlet of the reservoir bag does not become obstructed by twisting at this connection. Always check that the bag is emptying adequately; excessive bag inflation indicates that outflow from the bag is obstructed and this rapidly becomes very dangerous for the patient, as it causes increased expiratory pressure.

the system. Every practice should have at least one Ayres T-piece circuit (with either modification) available.

- **Ensure that a qualified veterinary nurse trained in monitoring anaesthesia, or a veterinary surgeon, monitors anaesthesia at all times.** This requires continuous or very frequent monitoring of pulse rate and quality, and observation of respiration.
- **Use appropriately sized monitoring equipment and have appropriate equipment to maintain body temperature during anaesthesia (>37.0°C)** (see Figure 3.30).
  - Oesophageal temperature probes are useful for continuous monitoring of body temperature during anaesthesia but are usually only available as part of a multiparameter monitoring system
  - Oesophageal stethoscopes can be useful to monitor heart rate (HR) during anaesthesia (see later)
  - Pulse oximeter for continuous measurement of SpO_2 (see Figure 3.29).
- **Ensure appropriate equipment to allow controlled administration of fluid therapy during anaesthesia** (see QRG 4.1.3).

Requirements during recovery from anaesthesia

- **Warm and quiet environment away from dogs.**
- **Preventing hypothermia** in the recovery period is vital (Figure 3.35). Ensure that the environmental temperature is warm and the cat is placed where it is not vulnerable to cooling from air conditioning units or fans. Place the cat on warm comfortable bedding for recovery and use appropriate aids to maintain body temperature (see Figure 3.30).
- **Continuous monitoring.** Sixty per cent of anaesthetic deaths occur in the first 3 hours of recovery. All cats should be monitored continuously until they are extubated, able to maintain sternal recumbency, and normothermic. Extubation should occur when the cat has regained a swallowing reflex. However, this point

can be difficult to determine because cats rarely start to swallow during recovery. *Do not move the ETT in the trachea to stimulate swallowing, as this can cause laryngeal trauma.* If not seen to swallow, most cats can be extubated when they are able to lift their head. Delaying extubation too long can stimulate coughing or laryngeal spasm.

- **Supplemental oxygen** can be given via a facemask (Figure 3.35).

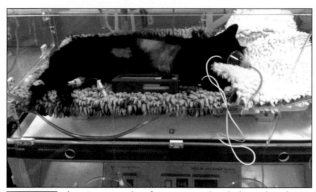

3.35 A cat recovering from anaesthesia in an incubator to maintain body temperature. The cat is also receiving supplemental oxygen via a facemask, and a pulse oximeter is being used to measure SpO_2 via a probe placed on the tongue. Intravenous fluid therapy is being delivered via an indwelling catheter in the medial saphenous vein.

General anaesthesia procedures

Different techniques exist for induction and maintenance of anaesthesia (Figure 3.36). Balanced anaesthesia is imperative and usually includes:

- Premedication
- Good intraoperative analgesia (see above)
- Use of different drugs for induction and maintenance of anaesthesia rather than a large dose of a single agent, to reduce the likelihood of adverse cardiovascular and respiratory side effects.

Premedication

Premedication provides anxiolysis and sedation, reduces doses of induction and maintenance agents required, can contribute to intraoperative sedation and analgesia so that depth of anaesthesia is less volatile, and can smooth recovery from anaesthesia. Premedication drugs are similar to those used for sedation (see Figure 3.26). Factors affecting choice include:

- ASA status
- Cat's temperament
- Invasiveness of the procedure and required duration of anaesthesia
- Pain (pre-existing pain and that caused by the procedure).

Technique	Advantages	Limitations	Clinical use
Intravenous induction of anaesthesia; maintenance with a volatile agent. For example: induction with propofol or alfaxalone; and maintenance with isoflurane or sevoflurane	Intravenous induction is rapid and stress-free; intravenous agent will provide short-term background sedation to facilitate transition to volatile agent. Maintenance phase can be extended without significant prolongation of recovery period. Depth of anaesthesia easy to control with a volatile agent	Requires i.v. access, which may be problematic in some cats. Requires equipment for volatile agent maintenance phase. Requires delivery of volatile agent via respiratory tract – problematic during bronchoscopy or examination of upper respiratory system	Optimal technique for induction and maintenance of anaesthesia in cats with ASA status ≥3. Use this technique if duration of anaesthesia expected to be >30–40 mins or unpredictable
Volatile agent induction; volatile agent maintenance. For example: induction and maintenance with isoflurane; or induction with sevoflurane and maintenance with isoflurane	Recovery from anaesthesia very quick, dependent on expiration of volatile agent. Does not require i.v. access for induction	Mask or chamber induction with volatile agents is stressful and unpleasant for most cats unless very sick (and systemically depressed) or highly sedated/premedicated	Use sevoflurane for mask or chamber induction rather than isoflurane because the smell of sevoflurane (sweet) is less aversive than isoflurane (pungent) and induction of anaesthesia will be more rapid. Can be a useful technique for cats <3 months of age. Can be useful when a very short duration of anaesthesia is required
Induction and maintenance of anaesthesia using an intravenous anaesthetic agent. For example: induction and maintenance with alfaxalone or propofol	Does not require delivery of anaesthetic gases via respiratory tract. Prevents environmental pollution with waste gases. Useful for short procedures	Requires i.v. access, which may be problematic in some cats. Difficult to adjust depth of anaesthesia. As the duration of anaesthesia increases, the duration of recovery is also likely to increase	Provide supplemental oxygen by facemask or nasal/tracheal catheter. Place an i.v. catheter. CRI infusion of anaesthetic drug preferred to incremental bolus doses
Total injectable anaesthesia using *intramuscular* medetomidine (or dexmedetomidine), ketamine + butorphanol. (Replace butorphanol with buprenorphine 20 μg/kg for a longer duration of analgesia)	Does not require i.v. access. Does not require anaesthetic machine. Useful for short procedures. Medetomidine (or dexmedetomidine) reversible with atipamezole to shorten recovery time; wait until 30 min after ketamine administration before giving atipamezole. With currently available formulations, volume of atipamezole required is half the volume of medetomidine injected, but check formulations	Difficult to adjust depth of anaesthesia. In cats that are not intubated ventilation cannot be supported by IPPV. Recovery from anaesthesia can be prolonged, particularly if top-up doses of the injectable agents are given	Provide supplemental oxygen via ETT or facemask; routinely intubate cats unless procedure very short (<10–15 min); brachycephalic cats should be intubated routinely. Consider placement of i.v. catheter in some cases – established i.v. access is useful if unexpected complications arise. Useful for procedures of short and predictable duration. Do not use in cats with ASA status ≥3. Best reserved for young healthy cats undergoing surgery of predictable duration

3.36 Advantages and limitations of commonly used anaesthesia techniques.

Figures 3.37 and 3.38 provide recommendations for premedication combinations for cats of different ASA status and undergoing different procedures. Continuous observation is required for high-risk patients (ASA ≥3) and brachycephalic cats that may encounter breathing difficulties when premedicated. See Figure 3.30 for measures to support body temperature.

ASA status	Premedication protocols	Clinical notes
1	(Medetomidine (10–20 µg/kg) or dexmedetomidine (5–10 µg/kg)) + buprenorphine (20 µg/kg) i.m.	Gives profound reliable sedation. Significant drug-sparing effect on subsequent induction and maintenance anaesthesia drugs. α-2 agonist can be reversed with atipamezole at end of anaesthesia to shorten recovery period
	ACP (0.05 mg/kg) + (buprenorphine (20 µg/kg) or methadone (0.3–0.5 mg/kg)) i.m.	Sedation with ACP is less profound than α-2 agonist-mediated sedation. Buprenorphine can be replaced with methadone (0.5 mg/kg i.m.) when more intense analgesia is required
2	As for ASA status 1, but generally avoid α-2 agonists if there is any evidence of CVS compromise	As for ASA status 1
3	ACP (0.03 mg/kg) + (buprenorphine (20 µg/kg) or methadone (0.3–0.5 mg/kg)) i.m.	Avoid ACP in cats with pre-existing hypotension or low normal blood pressure (systolic blood pressure <110 mmHg). ACP + opioid can be used in cats with HCM, causing minimal or no effect on cardiovascular function. An opioid alone can be used in cats with clinically significant disease
	Midazolam (0.3 mg/kg) + ketamine (5 mg/kg) i.m. **OR** Midazolam (0.3 mg/kg) + ketamine (2.5 mg/kg) i.v.	Avoid ketamine in cats with hypertrophic cardiomyopathy
4	Midazolam (0.3 mg/kg) + ketamine (5 mg/kg) i.m. **OR** Midazolam (0.3 mg/kg) + ketamine (2.5 mg/kg) i.v.	Avoid ketamine in cats with HCM
	Opioid (butorphanol 0.3–0.4 mg/kg, buprenorphine 20 µg/kg or methadone 0.3–05 mg/kg) i.m.	Opioids alone can provide effective sedation in cats that are systemically ill with CNS depression
5	Opioid (butorphanol 0.3–0.4 mg/kg, buprenorphine 20 µg/kg or methadone 0.3–05 mg/kg) i.m. is usually sufficient	In animals that are systemically very depressed a distinct premedication phase may not be required
	Midazolam (0.3 mg/kg) + methadone (0.3–0.5 mg/kg) i.m.	In animals that are systemically very depressed, a distinct premedication phase may not be required. Another option is to give midazolam (0.3 mg/kg i.v.) during induction of anaesthesia with alfaxalone or propofol to reduce the dose of induction agent required; give 1 mg/kg alfaxalone or propofol, administer midazolam and give further induction agent to effect. Administer an opioid to ensure adequate perioperative analgesia

3.37   Premedication drug recommendations for cats of different ASA status.

Condition	Premedication protocol	Clinical notes
Chronic kidney disease	ACP 0.03–0.05 mg/kg + (buprenorphine 20 µg/kg or methadone 0.3–0.5 mg/kg) i.m.	α-2 agonists may be required in cats that are very difficult to handle: (medetomidine 5 µg/kg or dexmedetomidine 2.5 µg/kg) i.m. + an opioid (doses as for combination with ACP). Ideally establish intravenous fluid therapy before premedication
Hyperthyroidism with concurrent cardiovascular system changes	ACP 0.03–0.05 mg/kg + (buprenorphine 20 µg/kg or methadone 0.3–0.5 mg/kg) i.m. **OR** (Medetomidine 5–10 µg/kg or dexmedetomidine 2.5–5 µg/kg) + (buprenorphine 20 µg/kg or methadone 0.5 mg/kg) i.m.	Consider use of α-2 agonists carefully; use will depend on temperament of cat. α-2 agonists useful in cats that are very difficult to handle such that inadequate sedation following premedication will cause significant stress during induction
Hypertrophic cardiomyopathy	ACP 0.03–0.05 mg/kg + (butorphanol 0.3 mg/kg or buprenorphine 20 µg/kg or methadone 0.3–0.5 mg/kg) i.m. **OR** α-2 agonist combinations as described above	Avoid ketamine in cats with hypertrophic cardiomyopathy. Choose opioid depending on level of pain expected to be caused by procedure. Considerations for α-2 agonists as above
Diaphragmatic rupture	ACP 0.03–0.05 mg/kg + methadone 0.3–0.5 mg/kg i.m. **OR** Midazolam 0.3 mg/kg + ketamine 5 mg/kg i.m.	Constant monitoring after premedication is essential
Collapsed cat following trauma	A distinct premedication phase is usually unnecessary	Administer midazolam 0.3 mg/kg i.v. during induction with propofol or alfaxalone. Provide analgesia with an opioid i.v. or i.m. after induction. Choice of opioid determined by expected severity of pain
Feral aggressive cat of unknown health status	Midazolam 0.3 mg/kg + ketamine 5 mg/kg i.m.	
Suspected urethral obstruction	ACP 0.03–0.05 mg/kg + (buprenorphine 20 µg/kg or methadone 0.3–0.5 mg/kg) i.m.	If possible measure plasma K+ before sedation and stabilize at <5.5 mmol/l before drug administration; or monitor ECG for arrhythmias and/or pulse rate and quality
Liver dysfunction	Midazolam 0.3 mg/kg + ketamine 5 mg/kg i.m.	Avoid ketamine + midazolam, and ACP, in cats with hepatic encephalopathy. Use methadone 0.3–0.5 mg/kg or buprenorphine 20 µg/kg alone
Significant anaemia (PCV <20%)	Midazolam 0.3 mg/kg + ketamine 5 mg/kg i.m.	Avoid ACP in cats with moderate to severe anaemia. Provide supplemental oxygen by facemask

3.38   Premedication recommendations for cats with common clinical conditions.

Induction

Different methods of induction (injectable, inhalation or combinations) are described in Figure 3.36. Alfaxalone and propofol are the two injectable drugs suitable for induction of anaesthesia in cats.

- **Alfaxalone:** Solubilized in a cyclodextrin that is not associated with histamine release. The solution does not contain an antimicrobial or preservative but the medium is less likely to support bacterial growth than are propofol lipid solutions, which do not contain a preservative. Open bottles should be discarded at the end of each day.
- **Propofol:** In the lipid preparation, propofol is solubilized in a mixture of soya bean oil and egg phosphatide. The solution does not contain any antimicrobial or preservative and the lipid medium supports bacterial growth. Thus open bottles of propofol should be discarded after use. PropoFlo Plus is a new lipid preparation of propofol that contains benzyl alcohol as a preservative; it has a 28-day shelf life once the bottle is opened but should not be used for maintenance of anaesthesia (see later).

Alfaxalone and propofol are very similar: both cause respiratory depression and can lead to apnoea if injected quickly intravenously *(always administer slowly over 60 seconds)*; and both are predominantly metabolized by the liver with a short duration of action after single dose administration. However differences between them to note include:

- Cardiovascular effects: Both cause hypotension, but with alfaxalone this is usually associated with a concurrent increase in heart rate (do not automatically confuse this with inadequate depth of anaesthesia); whereas with propofol the heart rate remains stable (in fact bradycardia can occur, so use alfaxalone in cats with pre-existing bradycardia). There is some evidence that alfaxalone is more cardiovascularly stable than propofol, although the clinical significance is currently unknown
- Propofol is associated with pain on injection in a small minority of cats.

Tips for safe and smooth induction

- Premedicate the cat (see Figures 3.37 and 3.38) and keep it in a quiet, calm and warm environment.
- Place an intravenous catheter before induction of anaesthesia.
- Pre-oxygenate cats that are ASA ≥3 for 1–2 minutes using either a facemask or delivery via the end of the anaesthetic breathing system (see Figure 3.25). *Stop the administration of oxygen if it causes distress to the cat.*
- Adjust the dose of alfaxalone or propofol according to the depth of sedation after premedication. Well sedated cats require 1–2 mg/kg of propofol or alfaxalone, but doses up to 5–7 mg/kg may be required in unsedated or

anxious/fear-aggressive animals. If using these higher doses, give 3–4 mg/kg first, over 60 seconds, and re-evaluate depth of anaesthesia/sedation before further administration.
- Monitor the cat (pulse rate and quality and observe respiration) during induction of anaesthesia in order to evaluate the cardiovascular and respiratory systems. If possible, record an ECG during induction in cats with cardiovascular disease at a high risk of arrhythmias (see QRG 4.1.4).

Maintenance

Volatile agents: Isoflurane is currently the only volatile agent authorized for cats that is readily available; sevoflurane is currently not authorized for administration to cats but can be used instead of isoflurane under the prescribing cascade system (in the UK) if the properties of sevoflurane compared to those of isoflurane justify its administration to an individual patient.

Both sevoflurane and isoflurane cause dose-dependent cardiovascular and respiratory depression. Neither has analgesic properties and both are minimally metabolized by the liver. Induction and recovery from anaesthesia are quicker with sevoflurane than with isoflurane, but recovery time is heavily influenced by the concurrent administration of injectable drugs for premedication, induction and/or analgesia. Sevoflurane may be preferred over isoflurane if anaesthesia is being induced with a volatile agent (isoflurane has a pungent smell), or if a quick recovery from a short duration of anaesthesia without concurrent administration of injectable agents is desired.

Intravenous agents:

- **Alfaxalone:** Authorized for maintenance of anaesthesia in cats, either by repeated intravenous boluses of 1–2 mg/kg given over 30 seconds or by CRI (0.1–0.3 mg/kg/min). Maintenance of anaesthesia for >60 min is not recommended due to drug accumulation and a prolonged recovery.
- **Propofol:** Widely used for maintenance of anaesthesia in cats, either by CRI (0.1–0.3 mg/kg/min) or by intermittent bolus dosing (1–2 mg/kg over 30 seconds). Maintenance of anaesthesia for >30 min is not recommended, as recovery time can be prolonged. *Propofol preparations containing benzyl alcohol preservative (e.g. PropoFlo Plus, Abbott Animal Health) should not be used to maintain anaesthesia in cats either by repeated bolus injection or CRI, due to the risk of benzyl alcohol toxicity.*

Triple combination intramuscular anaesthesia

The combination of ketamine + medetomidine + butorphanol, mixed in the same syringe, is authorized for intramuscular injection for induction and maintenance of anaesthesia in cats. See Figure 3.51 for dose rates; these doses are also applicable to adult cats. Butorphanol can be substituted by buprenorphine 20 µg/kg to provide a longer duration of analgesia. See Figure 3.36 for further discussion of this technique. Reversal of medetomidine with atipamezole is possible.

Recommendations for monitoring during general anaesthesia

Monitoring equipment allows continuous monitoring of physiological variables. The anaesthetist (veterinary nurse under the supervision of a veterinary surgeon, or veterinary surgeon) must be able to interpret the clinical significance of generated data and the limitations of the equipment. Manual monitoring (e.g. pulse quality, pulse rate, respiratory rate and effort, mucous membrane colour and depth of anaesthesia) should not be neglected, even if monitoring equipment is being used. An anaesthetic record must be prepared to show drug administration, timing of events (e.g. start of surgery) and physiological parameters; an example is shown in Figure 3.39.

Anaesthetic Record-Langford Veterinary Services Ltd

3.39 An example of an anaesthetic record. This form allows patient details to be recorded as well as information about premedication (drug, dose, route of administration, time of administration), induction agents, and other drugs given during anaesthesia and fluid therapy. The graphical format for recording changes in physiological variables facilitates early detection of changes. (Courtesy of Langford Veterinary Services)

Three tiers of monitoring, depending on the ASA status and the procedure (invasiveness and duration), exist:

- **Tier 1:** Essential monitoring that should be carried out in all anaesthetized cats:
  - Depth of anaesthesia
  - Pulse rate and pulse quality (manually). Palpation of a more peripheral pulse (i.e. the metatarsal or metacarpal rather than the femoral pulse) facilitates the early detection of changes in pulse quality likely to be indicative of hypotension.
  - Respiration rate and quality (observation)
  - Body temperature
  - Pulse oximetry: haemoglobin saturation with oxygen (SpO_2).
- **Tier 2:** Monitoring *additional* to Tier 1 that should be carried out in cats with ASA status ≥3, or during prolonged anaesthesia (>60 min) or during invasive procedures (e.g. those likely to cause cardiovascular or respiratory compromise or significant blood loss of >10% blood volume):
  - Electrocardiography (see later)
  - Non-invasive blood pressure monitoring using Doppler (see QRG 5.18.1) or oscillometric technique
  - Capnometry (end-tidal CO_2 concentration; capnography) if available.
- **Tier 3:** Monitoring additional to Tiers 1 and 2 that can be carried out in certain situations as indicated:
  - ***Blood glucose concentration:*** In cats <3 months of age or cats with diabetes mellitus. Diabetic cats are usually given half their standard insulin dose on the morning of any pre-planned surgery, to balance the effects of starvation for surgery. Ideally, take the first blood glucose measurement before premedication to obtain a baseline concentration (this can be done by conventional blood sampling or from the ear vein (see QRG 14.2)); otherwise measure after premedication. Repeat after induction of anaesthesia. During anaesthesia, adjust the frequency of measurement according to stability of the blood glucose concentration; e.g. if stable and within acceptable limits (compared to baseline) repeat measurements every 30 minutes. Supplement glucose if the concentration is <3 mmol/l (see QRG 4.5.1). Severe hyperglycaemia (>30 mmol/l) necessitating soluble insulin treatment during anaesthesia is very rare.
  - ***Urine output:*** in cats with disturbances in blood volume, acute kidney injury or cardiovascular dysfunction. This requires placement of a urinary catheter and connection to a closed collection system (see Chapter 4.11). Drain the bladder following placement of the urinary catheter and measure urine production over the next 30–60 minutes. This will allow the rate of urine production to be estimated; urine production should be at least 1 ml/kg/h.

Monitoring depth of anaesthesia

Anaesthetic depth should be assessed at least every 5 minutes to maintain an adequate depth for the procedure and to prevent overdose (and ensuing cardiovascular and respiratory depression).

PRACTICAL TIP

Different measures should be used in combination to make decisions regarding depth of anaesthesia; do not rely on use of one sign in isolation.

- **Crude indicators:**
  - Eye position: With most anaesthetic agents, in awake or very lightly sedated cats the eye is central and a blink reflex (elicited by gently tapping the medial canthus of the eye) is present. As depth of anaesthesia increases, the eye rotates downwards so that only the white sclera is visible, and the blink reflex disappears (Figure 3.40); this depth is usually suitable to carry out surgery. The eye will rotate upwards to a central position as anaesthesia deepens further. Very deep and very light anaesthesia give the same eye position but can be differentiated by the presence or absence of a blink reflex. *Always check the position of both eyes as they can look different.* Following administration of ketamine the eye remains central with no blink reflex, therefore eye position is a less useful guide to depth of anaesthesia.
  - Jaw tone: Relaxes as depth of anaesthesia increases; serial assessment of jaw tone can be helpful.
  - Evidence of body movement: Abolished at an adequate depth of anaesthesia for surgery.

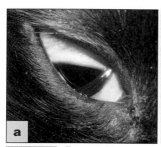 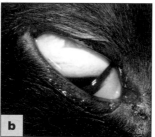

3.40 Eye position and depth of anaesthesia. **(a)** Ventromedial rotation of the eye at a light to moderate depth of anaesthesia with isoflurane. The blink reflex had been abolished. **(b)** Further ventromedial rotation of the eye as depth of anaesthesia increases. Surgery is usually possible when both eyes show this degree of ventromedial rotation and the blink reflex is abolished. However, eye position alone should not be relied upon; a combination of signs (e.g. eye position, blink reflex, heart and respiratory rates) should be used.

- **Sensitive measures:**
  - Drug administration: Consider the doses of anaesthetic agents given or the concentration of delivered volatile agent to interpret information about anaesthetic depth; e.g. if a cat is receiving 3% isoflurane via an Ayres T-piece breathing system it is likely to be deeply anaesthetized.
  - Heart rate and respiratory rate: Generally decrease with increasing depth of anaesthesia. Sudden increases usually indicate lightening of anaesthesia but may be associated with other physiological changes such as pain. Sudden blood loss will cause an increase in heart rate. Severe hypoxia will cause an unexpected increase in respiratory rate.

Monitoring the cardiovascular system

Pulse rate and quality: Cats' arteries are smaller in diameter than those of most dogs, so it can be challenging to locate and palpate peripheral pulses, particularly if the cat is hypotensive. The easiest sites at which to feel the pulse on cats are the femoral, sublingual and metatarsal arteries (Figure 3.41). Palpation of a more peripheral pulse facilitates early detection of hypotension via a decrease in the strength of the pulse; practice is helpful to gain confidence with pulse palpation.

- Heart rates usually vary between 100 and 160 beats per minute (bpm) in anaesthetized cats; heart rates at the low end of this range are expected following medetomidine (without ketamine).

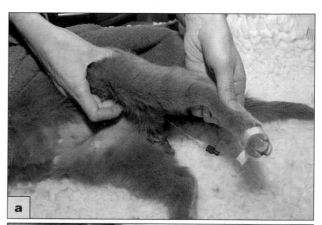

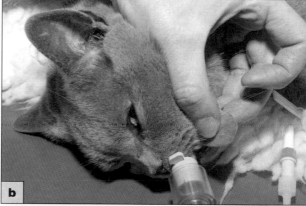

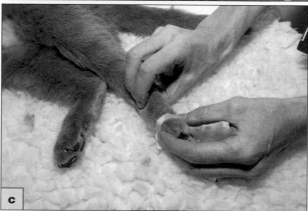

3.41 Pulse palpation. **(a)** Femoral: in this image the pulse is being palpated on the medial aspect of the right thigh caudal to the femur. **(b)** Sublingual artery. The tongue is gently extended and the fingertips used to palpate the artery as it runs on the ventral midline of the tongue. Pressure should be gentle; excessive pressure will occlude the vessel so that the pulse is no longer palpable. **(c)** Metatarsal artery, running craniomedial to the hock. The left hand of the anaesthetist is holding the limb in gentle extension at the tip of the toes. Overextension of the limb would make the metatarsal artery very difficult to palpate.

- The most common causes of changes in heart rate are: excessively deep anaesthesia (heart rate low), or inadequate anaesthesia or analgesia (heart rate high). The depth of anaesthesia should be checked, and adjusted if appropriate; or additional analgesia may be provided if necessary.
- If heart rate is too low (<70–80 bpm) at an appropriate anaesthetic depth, administration of an anticholinergic should be considered (e.g. atropine 0.03–0.04 mg/kg i.m. or 0.01 mg/kg slowly i.v. over 2 minutes, waiting at least 5 minutes after administration to see peak effects).
- If heart rate is too high (160–200 bpm) at an appropriate depth of anaesthesia and analgesia, blood pressure should be checked, as hypotension is often accompanied by an increase in heart rate (although the cardiovascular effects of some anaesthetic drugs might prevent this). If blood pressure is within the normal range and there are no arrhythmias, management is rarely required for this level of heart rate. If blood pressure is low (SBP <90 mmHg) and the peripheral pulse is weak, treatment for hypotension is required (see later).

Heart rate monitoring: Small or medium-sized oesophageal stethoscopes are inexpensive and provide an easy and reliable way to monitor heart rate continuously.

1. Measure how far to insert the stethoscope (its tip should lie over the base of the heart; at about the level of the 6th rib).
2. Gently insert the lubricated tip of the stethoscope into the back of the mouth and thread it into the oesophagus until at the required depth.
3. If heart and breath sounds cannot be heard, gently advance the stethoscope cranially and caudally in the oesophagus until sounds are audible.

When using an oesophageal stethoscope pulse quality should also be assessed frequently to evaluate cardiac output and pulse rate. Heart rate should be the same as the pulse rate; if the heart rate is higher, ECG monitoring is required (see below and QRG 4.1.4). Abnormally fast or slow heart rates should prompt action as described for pulse rates above.

Pulse oximetry: Pulse oximeters record SpO_2 and are essential during anaesthesia; every practice should have at least one portable pulse oximeter. Reduced SpO_2 is a common endpoint for many physiological disturbances that cause hypoxaemia. A veterinary pulse oximeter should be used, capable of detecting high heart rates (up to 300 bpm) with a small clip sensor (probe). Large sensors (e.g. human fingertip sensors) are too big for cats as they compress the tissue and prevent blood flow so that SpO_2 cannot be measured. The tongue is usually the most reliable site for sensor placement (see Figure 3.29). If the tongue cannot be used (e.g. dental procedure) the sensor may be placed on a toe, ear pinna (Figure 3.42) or skin flap. Reliable readings are more likely from unpigmented and hairless sites. Many multiparameter monitors also include a pulse oximeter sensor.

SpO_2 should always be >95%. Pulse oximeters rarely give erroneously high readings. Low readings should be investigated immediately:

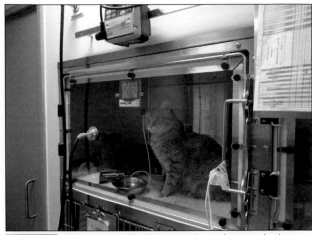

3.42 Many cats will tolerate pulse oximetry via the ear pinna, and this site can be very effective if the pinnae are unpigmented and relatively unhairy. This cat is awake and receiving oxygen supplementation in an oxygen cage with a covered front.

- Check that the sensor probe has not been detached from the tissue; if it has, re-place it. Alternatively, the sensor probe may have compressed the tissue so that no blood flow through the tissue is detected; if so, change the position or site of the probe
- Check pulse quality and/or blood pressure and act accordingly. If the cat is hypotensive, no pulse may be detectable by the oximeter; an alarm is usually heard when saturation falls to <90% (see QRG 4.1.1).
- If the cat is intubated and connected to an anaesthetic machine and T-piece, check the oxygen supply is turned on and the cat is connected to the breathing system. Provide supplemental oxygen by facemask to cats that are not intubated
- Check the cat is breathing spontaneously by looking at its respiration rate and pattern; support reduced ventilation with intermittment positive pressure ventilation (IPPV) if required (intubate the cat if necessary)
- Check the placement of the ETT in intubated cats to confirm it is in the trachea; this can be achieved quickly using a laryngoscope, as the larynx will be visible and not obstructed by the ETT if it has been inadvertently placed in the oesophagus
- Check cardiovascular function (heart rate and pulse quality); provide or adjust intravenous fluid therapy if necessary.
- Checking mucous membrane colour is *not* helpful in the early detection of low haemoglobin saturation with oxygen. Saturation must be very low before cyanosis of the mucous membranes is clinically detectable.

Electrocardiography: Continuous ECG recording is useful in cats at risk of cardiac arrhythmias during anaesthesia. A lead II ECG is usually adequate, and can be recorded as described in QRG 4.1.4. Under anaesthesia, adhesive tape (e.g. micropore) can be used to secure the electrodes firmly to the pads and decrease electrical noise in the ECG signal (Figure 3.43).

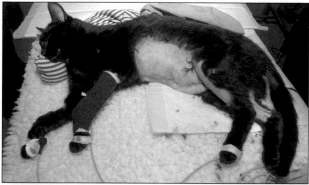

3.43 ECG monitoring via electrodes placed on the metacarpal/metatarsal pads of the left and right forelimbs and right hindlimb. For the purposes of monitoring heart rhythm during anaesthesia the precise electrode configuration is not important. For example, if surgery were being carried out on the right forelimb, the electrodes could be placed on the left forelimb metacarpal pad and right and left hindlimb metatarsal pads. On the right forelimb it can be seen that the gel pad of the electrode is positioned against the metacarpal pad; the ECG lead clips directly to the electrode via a metal pin.

Blood pressure measurement: Blood pressure should be measured indirectly using either a Doppler or oscillometric technique. The two techniques are compared in Figure 3.44 and the Doppler technique is further described in QRG 5.18.1.

- Systolic blood pressure should be >110 mmHg and mean arterial blood pressure >65 mmHg during anaesthesia.
- Hypertension is very rarely encountered; if SAP is >160 mmHg potential underlying causes (e.g.

Oscillometric technique	Doppler technique
Requires placement of a single cuff over a superficial artery so access easier during anaesthesia: ■ Over coccygeal artery, with cuff placed 1 cm distal to base of tail and artery arrow on cuff positioned along ventral midline ■ Over median artery, with cuff placed on proximal thoracic limb, between elbow and carpal pad, and artery arrow over medial surface of limb ■ Over cranial tibial artery, with cuff placed on pelvic limb proximal to the hock and artery arrow facing cranially	Requires location and fixation of Doppler probe over artery distal to cuff position, such that arterial pulse is clearly audible. Forelimb usual but alternatives are ventral tail coccygeal artery (cuff placed at base of tail) or just proximal to metatarsal pad on hindlimb (cuff placed between hock and tarsal pad)
Allows measurement of systolic, mean and diastolic arterial blood pressure	Allows measurement of systolic arterial pressure only
Measurement is automatic and can be carried out at predetermined time intervals, e.g. every 5 minutes. This is helpful during complex anaesthesia	Measurement is not automatic. It can be difficult to measure blood pressure frequently if anaesthesia is complex or the patient unstable
	Method is more accurate, particularly during hypotension

3.44 Comparison of blood pressure measurement techniques during anaesthesia. Both methods use a cuff that is 40% the width of the circumference of the limb at the site of cuff placement (cuffs 2–4 cm wide are good to stock in the practice).

inadequate anaesthesia and pain) should be investigated.

- Hypotension (SBP <90 mmHg) is more commonly seen. It is often accompanied by an increase in heart rate (although the cardiovascular effects of some anaesthetic drugs might prevent this). If encountered:
  - Check depth of anaesthesia as excess depth is the most likely cause of the hypotension; reduce anaesthetic depth as required. Intraoperative opioids can reduce the requirement for isoflurane and help support blood pressure
  - Consider fluid balance. Has there been significant (>10% of circulating blood volume) blood loss? If not already administering a crystalloid solution at 10 ml/kg/h, start administration at this rate. Consider administration of a bolus of crystalloid (5–10 ml/kg aliquot over 5 min), or/and then a colloid bolus (2–5 ml/kg i.v. over 5–10 min) if the SBP fails to increase to ≥90 mmHg or is severely low (<60 mmHg) (see Chapter 4.1). The rate at which it is safe to administer a fluid bolus depends on the underlying reason for the hypotension. If it is caused by blood loss, administer a bolus at the upper end of the volume and infusion rate. Reassess blood pressure every 5 minutes.
  - Positive inotropes (e.g. dopamine) can be administered to support blood pressure if optimization of fluid balance and depth of anaesthesia fail to correct hypotension. Most positive inotropes should be given by CRI and are very potent drugs; therefore they should only be used in combination with continuous monitoring of blood pressure, heart rate and ECG. Hypotension can usually be managed with fluid therapy.

Body temperature

Monitoring body temperature is essential in cats to prevent hypo- or hyperthermia. An oesophageal temperature probe (Figure 3.45) allows continuous recording of body temperature; the probe should be

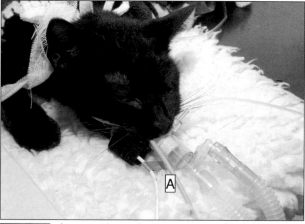

3.45 An oesophageal temperature probe (A) has been placed in this cat. The tip of the probe lies in the distal oesophagus (approximately level with the heart base). The probe has a thermocouple at the distal end, and is connected to a multi-parameter monitor that gives a continuous reading of body temperature.

inserted to the level of the thoracic inlet. Rectal thermometers commonly give falsely low readings due to the presence of faeces or gas in the rectum but may be used if an oesophageal probe is not available.

- Maintain body temperature between 37 and 38.5°C during anaesthesia.
- If body temperature is outside this range actively warm (see Figure 3.30) or cool (rarely required) the cat.

Capnometry

Measurement of end-tidal carbon dioxide concentration provides information about both cardiovascular and respiratory function (Figure 3.46). Although capnometry modules for multiparameter monitors are expensive, the information provided greatly assists decision-making as it concerns both adequacy of respiration (is the cat hyper- or hypoventilating; is the cat re-breathing?) and cardiovascular system function (has cardiac output increased or decreased?). For a more detailed explanation of capnometry see the *BSAVA Manual of Canine and Feline Anaesthesia and Analgesia.*

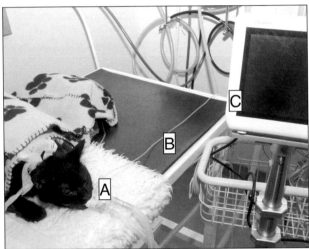

3.46 Sidestream capnometry. The sampling line delivering airway gases from the respiratory system to the capnometer is connected to the endotracheal tube via a low dead space connector (A). The sampling line (B) is connected to the capnometer module of the multiparameter monitor and produces a continuous capnogram trace (C) showing changes in end-tidal CO_2 concentration during inspiration and expiration.

Fluid therapy for surgical haemorrhage

The blood volume of the cat (6.6–8% bodyweight) should be calculated before the start of invasive procedures, so that any blood loss can be calculated as a percentage of total blood volume.

- **Blood loss of >10% blood volume** should be managed aggressively by increasing the rate of fluid administration (to 15–20 ml/kg/h) or by administration of a colloid solution (bolus of 2–5 ml/kg over 5–10 minutes, to a maximum of 20 ml/kg/24h). When administering crystalloids rapidly, the total volume of fluid given must be monitored carefully; in extreme cases rates up to 50–60 ml/kg/h for a maximum of 20 minutes are acceptable.

- **Blood loss >20% blood volume** may be an indication for a blood transfusion (see QRG 20.2) depending on ASA status, haemoglobin concentration or PCV, rate of blood loss and clinical status of the cat. In the majority of cats, support of blood volume with any fluid type (a crystalloid or colloid) is more important than replacement of blood with a blood transfusion. Decision-making about the requirement for a blood transfusion can be made, commonly after the end of anaesthesia, once deficits in blood volume have been corrected).

Routine measurement of PCV before anaesthesia is recommended in cats with ASA status ≥3 or if blood loss is expected to be moderate to severe during surgery. PCV frequently drops by around 5% after induction of anaesthesia, and this fall must be taken into consideration when determining any drop in PCV due to blood loss. Rechecking PCV after induction of anaesthesia before the start of surgery is helpful. During prolonged surgery with continuous intravenous fluid administration, haemorrhage will cause the PCV to fall, and serial monitoring of PCV during anaesthesia is useful to aid decision-making about fluid therapy in the perioperative period.

It is difficult to identify a critical PCV to recommend as a threshold for a blood transfusion:

- PCV of 15–20% is usually well tolerated by cats
- If PCV falls to <15% consideration should be given as to whether a blood transfusion is appropriate.

For cats recovering from anaesthesia with a PCV <20%, supplemental oxygen should be provided and the cat kept as calm as possible with minimal shivering (maintain normothermia). These strategies help ensure adequate oxygen delivery to tissues despite a low haemoglobin concentration.

Cardiopulmonary resuscitation

Cardiopulmonary arrest is relatively uncommon in anaesthetized patients, but to increase the chance of successful CPR the following should be in place.

- Practice CPR with the vets and nurses you work with. Create arrest scenarios and practise how you would manage them; if you only carry out CPR in an emergency, the chances of success are low.
- Careful monitoring of the patient during anaesthesia enables early detection of complications, hopefully preventing the requirement for CPR.
- CPR is a team event; make sure that you call for help early. A minimum of three people is required; ideally four people are needed.
- Assign roles to people so that everyone knows what they are doing:
  - Leader: one person must take overall responsibility for leading the resuscitation and directing what the team is doing; the leader will monitor patient response to interventions.
  - Dedicate one person to carry out chest compressions; switch this person regularly because the task quickly becomes tiring,

although this is less of a problem with cats than dogs.

- Dedicate one person to airway maintenance and IPPV.
- Ideally, a fourth person can administer resuscitation drugs.

■ A readily accessible crash box with all equipment and drugs required for CPR. This should be ready at all times and should contain the contents listed in Figure 3.47; drug doses (Figure 3.48) are prepared in clearly labelled syringes and stored in the crash box.

Item	Notes
Laryngoscope	
Cuffed and uncuffed ETTs	2–5 mm internal diameter
Gauze	To tie the ETT in place
Syringes	1 ml, 2.5 ml
Needles	21 G, 23 G
Intravenous catheters	18 G, 20 G, 22 G
Intraosseous catheters or bone marrow needles	In case it is not possible to obtain intravenous access
5 Fr urinary catheter	For administration of drugs via the ETT
Drugs: adrenaline (1:1000 solution), vasopressin, atropine, lidocaine	It is useful to have at least one syringe of all of these drugs drawn up ready for rapid administration in the event of an arrest. Volumes for cats are low; therefore prepare diluted doses so that injectate volume is between 0.2 and 1.0 ml. The drugs should be clearly labelled and dated, and changed regularly when they become out of date (at least every 28 days)
Dose chart	Dose chart (see Figure 3.48) indicates the dose and volume of each drug to be administered to a 5 kg cat; scale doses up or down for smaller or larger cats. Halve the dose for cats that are <3 kg; give 1.5 times the dose for cats that are 6–7 kg bodyweight
Guide to CPR	Flow chart indicating the CPR protocol, that can be rapidly read and followed (for example see Figure 3.49)

3.47 Contents of a crash box.

Basic life support

This is the most important phase of CPR and involves:

■ Establishing an airway to ventilate the patient
■ Initiating chest compressions to support the circulation.

CPR guidelines have changed recently and it is now recognized that *circulatory support is more important than ventilation*; priority should be given to carrying out chest compressions at sufficient frequency to maintain cardiac output. Do not stop chest compressions to ventilate the patient, and ensure that the chest is allowed to recoil fully between each compression. Push hard and push fast.

Figure 3.49 shows how to perform basic life support.

Advanced life support

Figure 3.49 also shows how to perform advanced life support. Use of open chest massage and electrical defibrillation can follow (if appropriate and available).

Routes of drug administration

■ Peripheral intravenous catheter: Follow with a ~10 ml intravenous fluid bolus and raise the extremity to promote distribution of the drug to the central circulation.
■ Intraosseous: Drugs are rapidly absorbed from the bone marrow cavity so rapid placement of an intraosseous catheter or bone marrow needle is the next best alternative if intravenous catheterization is problematic.
■ Via the ETT (intratracheal): Adrenaline, atropine, vasopressin and lidocaine (Figure 3.48) can be given via this route; this delivers the drug to the lung alveoli, where it is rapidly absorbed into the pulmonary circulation. It is useful to have doses suitable for intratracheal administration drawn up in the crash box, as well as doses prepared for intravenous administration but mark each *very* clearly.

Medication	Indication	Dose	Volume for a 5 kg cat	Comments
Adrenaline (epinephrine) (1:1000)	To increase coronary and cerebral perfusion pressure during CPR	Initially: 0.01 mg/kg i.v. or i.o. OR 0.03–0.1 mg/kg i.t. Increase dose to 0.1 mg/kg i.v. if 2–3 initial doses unsuccessful	Initial dose: 0.05 ml i.v. or i.o. OR 0.15–0.5 ml i.t. Increased dose: 0.5 ml i.v.	Administer repeat doses q3–5min. Can alternate with vasopressin (if available) if first dose unsuccessful
Vasopressin (ADH) (20 IU/ml)	To increase coronary and cerebral perfusion pressure during CPR	0.2–0.8 IU/kg i.v. or i.o. OR 0.4–1.2 IU/kg i.t.	0.05–0.2 ml i.v. or i.o OR 0.1–0.3 ml i.t.	Repeat q3–5min or alternate with adrenaline
Atropine (600 µg/ml)	To treat vagal-induced asystole (usually preceded by bradycardia)	0.04 mg/kg i.v. or i.o OR 0.08–0.1 mg/kg i.t.	0.33 ml i.v. or i.o. OR 0.9 ml i.t.	Can repeat q3–5min up to a maximum of 3 doses
Lidocaine (1% solution, 10 mg/ml)	To manage ventricular arrhythmias	0.2 mg/kg i.v., i.o or i.t.	0.1 ml i.v., i.o or i.t.	Use cautiously; only administer for diagnosis of ventricular arrhythmia refractory to support of circulation and ventilation by CPR

3.48 Dose rates for emergency drugs during CPR. i.o. = intraosseous; i.t. = intratracheal. For intratracheal use, dilute drug with sterile water (absorbed better than in 0.9% NaCl) to a volume of 5–10 ml to facilitate distribution and deliver via a 5 Fr urinary catheter (ensure of sufficient length so drug not distributed within lumen of ETT). Higher doses of drugs (3–10 times the intravenous dose of adrenaline; 2–2.5 times for other drugs) are required intratracheally to attain adequate plasma concentrations.

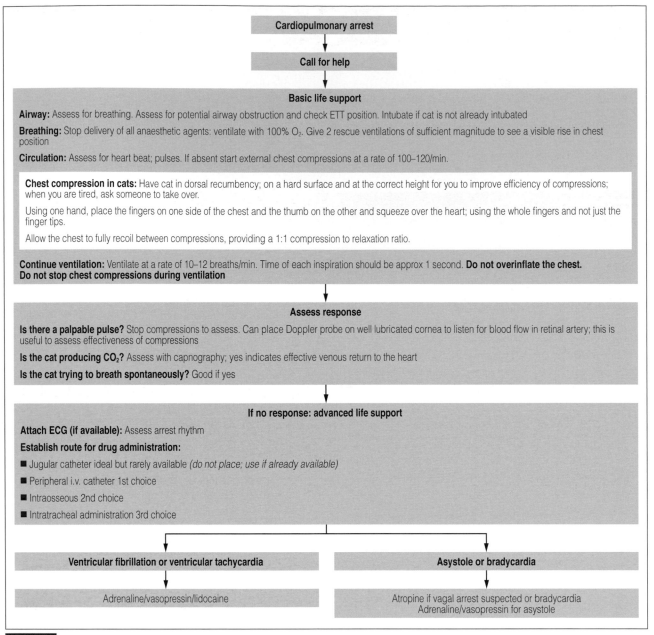

Cardiopulmonary arrest

↓

Call for help

↓

Basic life support

Airway: Assess for breathing. Assess for potential airway obstruction and check ETT position. Intubate if cat is not already intubated

Breathing: Stop delivery of all anaesthetic agents: ventilate with 100% O_2. Give 2 rescue ventilations of sufficient magnitude to see a visible rise in chest position

Circulation: Assess for heart beat; pulses. If absent start external chest compressions at a rate of 100–120/min.

> **Chest compression in cats:** Have cat in dorsal recumbency; on a hard surface and at the correct height for you to improve efficiency of compressions; when you are tired, ask someone to take over.
>
> Using one hand, place the fingers on one side of the chest and the thumb on the other and squeeze over the heart; using the whole fingers and not just the finger tips.
>
> Allow the chest to fully recoil between compressions, providing a 1:1 compression to relaxation ratio.

Continue ventilation: Ventilate at a rate of 10–12 breaths/min. Time of each inspiration should be approx 1 second. **Do not overinflate the chest. Do not stop chest compressions during ventilation**

↓

Assess response

Is there a palpable pulse? Stop compressions to assess. Can place Doppler probe on well lubricated cornea to listen for blood flow in retinal artery; this is useful to assess effectiveness of compressions

Is the cat producing CO_2? Assess with capnography; yes indicates effective venous return to the heart

Is the cat trying to breath spontaneously? Good if yes

↓

If no response: advanced life support

Attach ECG (if available): Assess arrest rhythm

Establish route for drug administration:

- Jugular catheter ideal but rarely available *(do not place; use if already available)*
- Peripheral i.v. catheter 1st choice
- Intraosseous 2nd choice
- Intratracheal administration 3rd choice

Ventricular fibrillation or ventricular tachycardia	**Asystole or bradycardia**
Adrenaline/vasopressin/lidocaine	Atropine if vagal arrest suspected or bradycardia Adrenaline/vasopressin for asystole

3.49 An example of a flow chart for carrying out CPR (assuming that no defibrillator is available).

Fluid therapy during CPR

Cats that were normovolaemic before arrest should not be given excessive volumes of intravenous fluids; a 10 ml/kg bolus of crystalloids or 2–3 ml/kg of a colloid solution (e.g. hetastarch) can be given.

Special considerations

Considerations and recommendations for anaesthesia of cats with specific disease conditions or health status are given in Figure 3.50.

Considerations	Recommendations
Senior and geriatric cats	
High incidence of concurrent disease	Haematology and biochemistry tests before anaesthesia to identify concurrent disease. Ensure clinical examination and history are thorough
More susceptible to physiological derangements caused by anaesthesia due to reduced homeostatic mechanisms	Avoid α-2 agonists; use anaesthetic drugs that have minimal effects on cardiovascular system. Monitor cardiovascular/respiratory systems and body temperature carefully. Provide routine i.v. fluid therapy in geriatric cats
More likely to become hypothermic during anaesthesia	Ensure body temperature is supported from premedication until recovery
More likely to show signs of distress during recovery due to reduced ability to cope with new and strange environments	Provide quiet stress-free recovery area to reduce anxiety and distress

3.50 Considerations and recommendations for anaesthesia of cats with specific disease conditions or health status. (continues) ▶

Considerations	Recommendations
Chronic kidney disease	
Many of these cats are also geriatric	See above
Maintenance of renal perfusion during anaesthesia is very important to prevent renal ischaemia	Provide i.v. fluid therapy throughout anaesthesia until cat is able to drink normally and regulate its own fluid balance. Correct dehydration before premedication if at all possible
Elevated urea and creatinine can decrease myocardial contractility and cause metabolic acidosis	Avoid α-2 agonists
	Do not give NSAIDs until fully recovered from anaesthesia and normotensive. Then consider whether NSAID appropriate for each patient individually
Urethral obstruction	
Likely to present with elevated plasma urea, creatinine and potassium	Measure plasma urea, creatinine and potassium before anaesthesia. Do not proceed with anaesthesia unless plasma potassium within normal limits
Potential to be dehydrated depending on duration of obstruction	Provide i.v. fluid therapy before induction of anaesthesia concurrent with cystocentesis to reduce volume of urine in the bladder
Relief of the obstruction by flushing the urethra is painful	Provide analgesia with opioids. Avoid NSAIDs until: obstruction relieved; cat normotensive and able to regulate fluid balance; and renal function re-checked. Do not give NSAIDs if evidence to suggest acute kidney injury
Cats with this condition can be overweight	Monitor and support respiration with IPPV if required. Maintain anaesthesia with volatile agents, as duration of anaesthesia is unpredictable
Diaphragmatic rupture (Consider referral for treatment if inexperienced in managing these cases)	
May be concurrent pulmonary or myocardial damage associated with the trauma	Take a chest radiograph during assessment of patient. This will inform about concurrent damage, particularly degree of pulmonary compromise. Provide oxygen support using technique that does not cause additional stress to the cat. Monitor ECG, pulse quality and blood pressure (arrhythmias not uncommon following myocardial trauma)
Commonly hypovolaemic due to blood loss	Establish i.v. access and provide appropriate fluid therapy
Respiration will be impaired, particularly if abdominal contents have entered chest cavity. Pulmonary compromise might be lateralized depending on the injury, e.g. right lung might be more compromised than left	Maintain cat in sternal recumbency until intubated and IPPV initiated. Elevating forelimbs and thorax can help push abdominal contents from the chest cavity back into the abdomen and improve respiratory function. Maintain IPPV throughout anaesthesia
Surgery is invasive. Perioperative period painful	Provide analgesia with methadone (0.5 mg/kg i.m.). Delay NSAID administration until fully recovered from anaesthesia and normotensive
Caesarean section	
Drugs that cross blood–brain barrier will also cross placenta and have effects on the kittens	Use short-acting drugs for induction of anaesthesia and volatile agents for maintenance. A distinct premedication phase may not be necessary depending on demeanour of the cat. Premedicate with opioids and a low dose of a α-2 agonist in cats that are otherwise healthy (e.g. buprenorphine 20 µg/kg and medetomidine 5 µg/kg i.m.). Avoid midazolam + ketamine as has been shown to increase kitten mortality
Cat is likely to be distressed and anxious	Handle carefully and gently to reduce distress. Ensure environment for induction of anaesthesia is quiet and stress-free
Cardiovascular function compromised due to weight of gravid uterus on vena cava when cat in dorsal recumbency. Manipulation of uterus during surgery is likely to have significant haemodynamic consequences	Tilt cat slightly to the left when in dorsal recumbency to reduce pressure of uterus on vena cava. Provide i.v. fluid therapy and monitor cardiovascular parameters carefully
Rapid recovery from anaesthesia is desirable to allow dam to start mothering and feeding the kittens	Avoid administration of long-acting agents such as ketamine and ACP. α-2 agonists can be reversed at the end of anaesthesia with atipamezole to hasten recovery
Surgery is painful, but systemically acting analgesic drugs administered perioperatively are likely to be excreted in the milk	Give a single dose of NSAID at the end of anaesthesia when cat fully recovered and normotensive. Provide perioperative analgesia with buprenorphine (20 µg/kg i.m. or i.v.) for at least 48 hours after surgery and then reassess for pain frequently. Continue with buprenorphine if necessary
The kittens need care after delivery (see also Chapter 15)	Ensure adequate staff are available to care for kittens. Provide a warm oxygenated environment for kittens once dry and breathing adequately. Ensure naloxone and atipamezole available for sublingual administration to kittens that appear sleepy and non-responsive.

3.50 (continued) Considerations and recommendations for anaesthesia of cats with specific disease conditions or health status. (continues) ▶

Considerations	Recommendations
Hyperthyroid cats for thyroidectomy	
May have concurrent hypertrophic cardiomyopathy (HCM) and elevated heart rate	Fully assess cardiovascular status before surgery. If possible render cats euthyroid prior to surgery via oral medication. If heart rate remains high, consider a β-1 antagonist (e.g. esmolol, propanolol) to reduce heart rate prior to surgery
Cats are often difficult to handle due to temperament	Adequate sedation prior to induction of anaesthesia is essential. Avoid ketamine if cat has concurrent HCM. Consider use of α-2 agonists for premedication in very excitable and anxious cats
At risk of catecholamine-induced arrhythmias; metabolic rate is increased	Although preoxygenation is desirable, reducing stress during induction of anaesthesia is of paramount importance
Cats likely to be thin	Adopt measures to prevent hypothermia
Surgical site is adjacent to major blood vessels and nerves of the autonomic nervous system	Monitor cardiovascular system carefully during anaesthesia; ECG is useful. If arrhythmias arise as result of surgical manipulation (e.g. bradycardia due to stimulation of the vagal nerve) the veterinary surgeon should stop what they are doing to allow heart rate/rhythm to normalize. Manage pharmacologically with atropine (0.02–0.04 mg/kg i.m. or 0.01 mg/kg i.v.) if appropriate
Derangements in plasma calcium can occur 24–72 hours after surgery	Monitor plasma calcium concentration after surgery

3.50 (continued) Considerations and recommendations for anaesthesia of cats with specific disease conditions or health status.

General anaesthesia of kittens

General anaesthesia for neutering is the most likely reason to anaesthetize kittens. There are a number of specific physiological considerations associated with anaesthesia of kittens.

- Establishing intravenous access may be challenging. Ensure good sedation via adequate premedication before inducing anaesthesia to facilitate intravenous catheter placement (see Figure 3.37). Avoid α-2 agonists in kittens <6 weeks of age.
- The very small body size is challenging; use appropriate anaesthetic equipment and monitoring devices.
- Metabolic rate is significantly higher in kittens; provide oxygen throughout anaesthesia (see below). Cardiac output is more dependent on heart rate than in adults; combining ketamine with medetomidine will reduce the likelihood of bradycardia after α-2 agonist administration.
- Liver immaturity means that the effects of anaesthetic drugs can be prolonged. In very young kittens (<6 weeks) consider induction of anaesthesia with sevoflurane (but see earlier regarding authorization status).
- Otherwise, use short-acting intravenous agents such as propofol and alfaxalone for induction. Maintain anaesthesia with sevoflurane.
- Immaturity of the sympathetic nervous system reduces the ability of the cardiovascular system to maintain normotension during blood loss and anaesthesia.
- Total blood volume is low (~100–120 ml in a 1.5 kg kitten) so blood loss >10 ml can be clinically significant.
- Drug-induced respiratory depression is more likely to be clinically significant and produce hypoxia. Support respiration with IPPV if necessary. If an ETT <2 mm ID (uncuffed) is likely to be necessary,

do not intubate but provide oxygen (± volatile agent) via a tight-fitting facemask.
- Thermoregulation is impaired compared to adults, so minimize heat loss and support body temperature (see Figure 3.30).
- Kittens are at a higher risk of hypoglycaemia; starve for a maximum of 3 hours prior to anaesthesia and offer food as soon as fully recovered. Measure blood glucose concentration before (prior to or after premedication) and during anaesthesia, and administer glucose intravenously if hypoglycaemic (see QRG 4.5.1). Check blood glucose concentration in kittens that do not recover quickly after anaesthesia.

Recommended protocols for castration and ovariohysterectomy: If kittens presented for pre-pubertal neutering (see Chapter 2 and QRGs 2.2 to 2.4) originate from a shelter they may be unused to handling. In any case, obtaining intravenous access can be challenging in very small patients, even when well sedated. Practically, adoption of a total injectable intramuscular technique (Figure 3.51) ensures stress-free induction and predictable recovery. A 1 ml syringe is used to facilitate accurate dosing and a 25 G needle used to minimize pain on injection. Incorporation of midazolam and buprenorphine into the anaesthesia protocol allows lower doses of medetomidine or dex-medetomidine to be used, and the opioid provides postoperative analgesia. Intubation is recommended in both males and females. Although castration is a short procedure, use of a total injectable anaesthesia technique results in the anaesthesia duration being similar for castration and ovariohysterectomy. Mede-tomidine can be reversed with atipamezole at the end of anaesthesia, waiting at least 30 minutes after ketamine administration before reversal. Meloxicam is authorized for injection in kittens older than 6 weeks and administration will provide 24 hours of analgesia.

Drugs and doses	Route	Clinical notes
(Medetomidine 80 μg/kg OR dexmedetomidine 40 μg/kg) + ketamine 5 mg/kg + buprenorphine [a] 20 μg/kg	Intramuscular	Can combine all drugs in the same syringe. Reverse medetomidine with atipamezole; delay administration until 30 min after ketamine
Medetomidine 600 μg/m² + ketamine 60 mg/m² + midazolam 3 mg/m² + buprenorphine [a] 180 μg/m²	Intramuscular	'Quad' protocol recommended by Joyce and Yates (2011). Dosing by body surface area takes account of metabolic body size. Midazolam reduces the likelihood of excitation by ketamine. Reverse medetomidine with atipamezole at 10% of volume of the previously administered medetomidine, not less than 20 mins after administration of the quad combination. Although waiting at least 30 mins after ketamine administration before giving atipamezole is mentioned elsewhere in this chapter, experience suggests that in the 'quad' protocol 20 mins is an adequate time to wait

Bodyweight (kg)	Volume (in ml) of *each* drug
0.5	0.04
1.0	0.06
1.5	0.08
2.0	0.1
2.5	0.12

3.51 Anaesthesia protocols for prepubertal castration or ovariohysterectomy in kittens. [a] The authorized alternative uses butorphanol at 0.4 mg/kg instead of buprenorphine.

References and further reading

Boothe DM (1990) Drug therapy in cats: mechanisms and avoidance of adverse drug reactions. *Journal of the American Veterinary Medical Association* **196**, 1297–1305

Boothe DM (2001) Principles of antimicrobial therapy. In: *Small Animal Clinical Pharmacology and Therapeutics*, ed. DM Boothe, pp. 125–149. WB Saunders, Philadelphia

Boothe DM and Mealey KA (2001) Glucocorticoid therapy in the dog and cat. In: *Small Animal Clinical Pharmacology and Therapeutics*, ed. DM Boothe, pp. 313–329. WB Saunders, Philadelphia

Brodbelt D (2010) Feline anaesthetic deaths in veterinary practice. *Topics in Companion Animal Medicine* **25**, 189–194

BSAVA Guide to the Use of Medicines. Available online at www.bsava.com

Day MJ (2008) Immunomodulatory therapy. In: *Small Animal Clinical Pharmacology*, 2nd edn, ed. JE Maddison *et al.*, pp. 270–286. Elsevier, Edinburgh

Fisher J (2010) Use of Xylocaine spray in cats. *Veterinary Record* **167**, 500. [letter]

Giguére S, Prescott JF, Baggott JD, Walker RD and Dowling PM (2006) *Antimicrobial Therapy in Veterinary Medicine*, 4th edn. Blackwell, Iowa

Joyce A and Yates D (2011) Help stop teenage pregnancy! Early-age neutering in cats. *Journal of Feline Medicine and Surgery* **13**, 3–10

Lascelles BD, Gaynor JS, Smith ES *et al.* (2008) Amantadine in a multi-modal analgesic regimen for alleviation of refractory osteoarthritis pain in dogs. *Journal of Veterinary Internal Medicine* **22**, 53–59

Lascelles BD, Hansen BD, Roe S *et al.* (2007) Evaluation of client-specific outcome measures and activity monitoring to measure pain relief in cats with osteoarthritis. *Journal of Veterinary Internal Medicine* **21**, 410–416

Lascelles BD and Robertson SA (2010) DJD-associated pain in cats: what can we do to promote patient comfort? *Journal of Feline Medicine and Surgery* **12**, 300–312

Lindley S and Watson P (2010) *BSAVA Manual of Canine and Feline Rehabilitation, Supportive and Palliative Care: Case Studies in Patient Management.* BSAVA Publications, Gloucester

Maddison JE (2006) Special considerations related to drug use in cats. In: *Problem-based Feline Medicine*, ed. J Rand, pp. 1342–1350. Elsevier Saunders, Edinburgh

Maddison JE and Page SW (2008) Adverse drug reactions. In: *Small Animal Clinical Pharmacology*, 2nd edn, ed. JE Maddison *et al.*, pp. 41–58. Elsevier, Edinburgh

Maddison JE, Watson ADJ and Elliott J (2008) Antibacterial drugs. In: *Small Animal Clinical Pharmacology*, 2nd edn, ed. JE Maddison *et al.*, pp. 148–185. Elsevier, Edinburgh

Page SW and Maddison JE (2008) Principles of clinical pharmacology. In: *Small Animal Clinical Pharmacology*, 2nd edn, ed. JE Maddison *et al.*, pp. 1–26. Elsevier, Edinburgh

Pascoe PJ, Ilkiw JE and Frischmeyer KJ (2006) The effect of the duration of propofol administration on recovery from anaesthesia in cats. *Veterinary Anaesthesia and Analgesia* **33**, 2–7

Robertson SA and Taylor PM (2004) Pain management in cats – past, present and future. Part 2. Treatment of pain – clinical pharmacology. *Journal of Feline Medicine and Surgery* **6**, 321–333

Seymour C and Duke-Novakovski T (2010) *BSAVA Manual of Canine and Feline Anaesthesia and Analgesia*, 2nd edn. BSAVA Publications, Gloucester

Sparkes AH, Heiene R, Lascelles BD *et al.* (2010) ISFM and AAFP consensus guidelines: long term use of NSAIDs in cats. *Journal of Feline Medicine and Surgery* **12**, 521–538

Taylor PM and Robertson SA (2004) Pain management in cats – past, present and future. Part 1. The cat is unique. *Journal of Feline Medicine and Surgery* **6**, 313–320

Woodward T (2008) Pain management and regional anaesthesia for the dental patient. *Topics in Companion Animal Medicine* **23**, 106–114

QRG 3.1 Giving oral medications to cats

by Martha Cannon

Getting cats to take oral medications is famously difficult and there are no 'quick fixes' that will change that. However, finding ways to help clients to medicate their cat will have a huge impact on the success or otherwise of your treatment plan, and being seen to make efforts to help your client to medicate their cat will often leave a lasting positive impression and help to build a relationship of trust. *For more tips and tricks on cat-friendly medicines and medicating cats see the FAB Guides to Cat Friendly Practice available at www.fabcats.org*

- Take the time to demonstrate to owners how to dose cats – or ask your practice nurse(s) to do it for you.
- Use all the gadgets that you can:
  - Pill givers – with a soft rubber end to reduce risk of injury

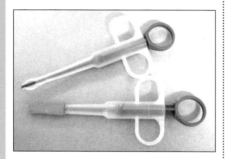

  - Gelatine capsules: available from veterinary wholesalers in a variety of sizes, e.g.:
    - Size 1 (approx 2 cm length, 0.5 ml capacity) – suitable for giving several compatible medications at the same time
    - Size 3 (approx 1.5 cm length, 0.3 ml capacity), useful for masking bitter-tasting tablets

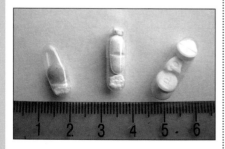

  - Pill crushers
    - Crushing a tablet into a powder and then mixing the powder with water produces a liquid formulation which, for some cats, will be easier to give than a tablet

- Ensure that the tablet is suitable for crushing, e.g. not enteric-coated; contact the manufacturer for advice if required
- Owners should wear gloves to crush tablets, and should take care to avoid breathing in the crushed powder

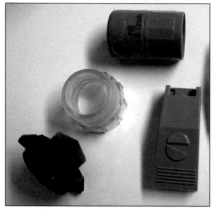

Pill crushers and pill splitters

- Where an unauthorized medication is required, human formulations are often of inappropriate size for cats:
  - Pill cutters (see above, right) can be of value to owners where tablets need to be divided to achieve an appropriate dose for the cat
  - Commercial companies (e.g. Summit Veterinary Pharmaceuticals) can supply a range of 'off-licence' products in 'cat-friendly' doses, e.g. metronidazole, amlodipine, cisapride, tramadol
  - Alternatively, formulating pharmacies can re-compound medications into more appropriate sizes for cats (e.g. Nova Laboratories; The Specials Laboratory).
- Encourage owners to explore the use of pill pockets or soft treats in which to hide tablets, e.g. Vivitreats (Intervet), RCW Mobility Support tablets, soft or processed cheeses, meat paté, cooked chicken or ham
- Chilling strongly flavoured liquids or tablets in the fridge prior to dosing may reduce their flavour and make them easier to hide in strong-tasting food.
- Tablets and capsules frequently lodge in the oesophagus. Some drugs (e.g. some formulations of doxycycline and clindamycin) are

irritant and can cause oesophagitis and oesophageal strictures and must always be given with water or food to encourage complete swallowing into the stomach.
- Even if it is not inherently irritant, a lodged tablet or capsule will be uncomfortable and may make the cat less amenable to dosing next time.
  - Lubricate capsules with oil or butter
  - Wash all tablets or capsules down with food or water. If the owners opt to wash the tablet down with water, supply an empty 5 ml syringe with the medication to encourage them to follow your advice.
- Choose your medication carefully:
  - Consider the size, shape and palatability of the product you prescribe:
    - If it has an FAB 'easy to give' logo you can be sure it will be a reasonably cat-friendly product.

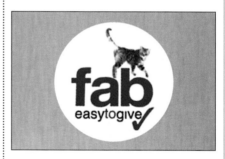

    - Go for smaller, oval tablets where possible
    - Use 'palatable' formulations where possible
    - Liquid oral preparations may be easier to administer in some cats
  - Discuss the available alternatives with the client and let them have a say in which formulation you prescribe
- Ask owners to call you (or your nurse) if they are having difficulty administering the medication.

All images © Martha Cannon.

Collapse

Angie Hibbert

Collapse is defined as a failure to maintain a normal supported posture with or without loss of consciousness. Three types of presentation are typically associated with collapse:

- An acute emergency presentation
- An episodic event
- Apparent collapse, whereby the patient is recumbent but unable or reluctant to stand or walk.

Many disease processes may lead to a patient collapsing (Figure 4.1.1); therefore a logical approach is necessary to reach a diagnosis. It is helpful to consider whether collapse may be due to an abnormality in:

- The provision of oxygen and metabolic substrates (e.g. glucose, potassium, sodium, calcium) to the central and peripheral nervous systems or musculoskeletal system
- The local environment of the central (CNS) and peripheral (PNS) nervous systems and muscles (e.g. hypoxia, acidosis, electrolyte disturbances and toxins)
- The structure and function of the brain, upper motor neurons, motor unit (peripheral nerve, neuromuscular junction and muscle), bones or joints.

Cause	Typical form of collapse		
	Acute	Episodic	Apparent
Cardiovascular disease			
Congestive heart failure (CHF) due to cardiomyopathy	•		
Arrhythmia	•	•	
Pericardial disease causing tamponade	•		
Arterial thromboembolism	•		
Shock: ■ Hypovolaemic – inadequate circulatory volume ■ Distributive – inappropriate vascular tone, vasodilation and impaired local microcirculation ■ Obstructive – mechanical interference to venous return and ventricular filling ■ Cardiogenic – failure to maintain cardiac output	•		
Respiratory disease			
Pleural effusion, e.g. CHF, pyothorax, haemothorax	•		
Asthma	•	•	
Pneumothorax	•		
Airway obstruction; foreign body, tumour, laryngeal paralysis	•		
Diaphragmatic rupture	•		
Haematological disease			
Severe anaemia: ■ Regenerative – – Haemorrhage: internal (e.g. rodenticide toxicity, urinary or gastrointestinal tract), systemic amyloidosis); external (e.g. trauma) – Haemolysis: immune-mediated – primary or secondary; incompatible transfusion; neonatal isoerythrolysis ■ Non-regenerative – bone marrow disorder; FeLV infection	•		
Hyperviscosity; erythrocytosis, hyperproteinaemia	•		
Methaemoglobinaemia (e.g. paracetamol toxicity); carboxyhaemoglobinaemia (e.g. smoke inhalation)	•		

4.1.1 Causes of collapse in the cat. (See relevant chapters for more details on these conditions.) (continues) ▶

Cause	Typical form of collapse		
	Acute	**Episodic**	**Apparent**
Metabolic disorders			
Hypoglycaemia	•		
Hypokalaemia, hyperkalaemia	•		
Hyponatraemia, hypernatraemia	•		
Hypocalcaemia	•		
Hypercalcaemia	•		•
Hepatic encephalopathy	•	•	
Uraemic encephalopathy	•		
Endocrine disease			
Diabetic ketoacidosis	•		
Phaeochromocytoma	•	•	
Thyroid storm due to acute thyrotoxicosis ± concurrent disease (signs may include tachypnoea, dyspnoea, tachycardia, muscle weakness, paresis/paralysis, hyperthermia ± hypertensive complications)	•		
Gastrointestinal and pancreatic disease			
GI perforation and peritonitis	•		
Acute pancreatitis and associated metabolic complications	•		
GI obstruction	•		
CNS disease – brain and upper motor neurons			
Seizures	•	•	
Central vestibular disease	•		
Brain and spinal neoplasia	•		
Narcolepsy/cataplexy	•	•	
Ischaemic myelopathy	•		
Head trauma	•		
Peripheral nervous system and musculoskeletal disease			
Peripheral vestibular disease	•		•
Polymyopathy (e.g. hypokalaemic myopathy of Burmese cats, _Toxoplasma gondii_ myositis)		•	•
Polyneuropathy (e.g. diabetic, inherited hyperchylomicronaemia)			•
Myasthenia gravis	•		•
Intervertebral disc disease	•		•
Severe orthopaedic pain; fractures	•		•
Toxins and drugs			
Organophosphates and carbamate insecticides, permethrin, ethylene glycol, paracetamol, lilies, rodenticides	•		
Hypotensive drugs (e.g. beta-blockers, calcium channel blockers, alpha-2 agonists, phenothiazines, diuretics)	•		
Miscellaneous			
Sepsis; systemic inflammatory response syndrome (SIRS)	•		
Anaphylaxis	•		
Severe pain	•		•

4.1.1   (continued) Causes of collapse in the cat. (See relevant chapters for more details on these conditions.)

Acute emergency presentation

Initial approach

An assistant (if available) should obtain owner consent and a key history, to allow the veterinary surgeon to focus on initial assessment and to begin stabilization of the patient.

1. Perform initial survey examination

- Immediately assess:
  - **A** – is the airway patent?
  - **B** – is the patient breathing?
  - **C** – is there circulation? First palpate for peripheral pulses (metatarsal or metacarpal artery); if not detectable assess femoral arterial pulses; if undetectable check for cardiac apex beat.
    - **If 'no' to any of the above, intubate the trachea and begin cardiopulmonary resuscitation (CPR)** (see Chapter 3); otherwise continue to preliminary examination.
- Preliminary examination:
  - Respiratory system:
    - Assess breathing rate, pattern and effort
    - Any upper respiratory tract noise, wheezes, pulmonary crackles, or loss of lung sounds over the thorax?
    - See Chapter 4.2 for further discussion of respiratory patterns and management

- Cardiovascular system:
  - Assess:
    - Mucous membrane colour (e.g. pallor due to vasoconstriction as a result of shock or anaemia)
    - Capillary refill time (CRT)
    - Peripheral and femoral artery pulse quality and rate (auscultate heart simultaneously to detect pulse deficits; see QRG 1.5)
    - Mucous membrane hydration
  - Any heart murmur, gallop, arrhythmia, or muffled heart sounds (see QRG 1.5)?
- Neurological system:
  - Assess mentation (see Chapter 5.24)
  - If the cat is conscious, assess ability to ambulate and pedal withdrawal response (see QRG 1.6)
- Abdominal palpation:
  - Check for ascites (see Chapter 5.1), bladder size, organomegaly and abdominal pain
- Rectal temperature:
  - Hypothermia <37°C.
2. **Place an intravenous catheter** (see QRG 4.1.1) – for fluid therapy and drug administration.
3. **Administer flow-by oxygen** (see QRG 4.2.2).
4. **Obtain blood for an emergency database:**
- Collect blood into EDTA and heparin tubes
  - PCV, total solids, urea, glucose, calcium, potassium, sodium, chloride
  - Blood smear examination
  - Acid–base and lactate, if available.
5. **Assess systolic blood pressure** (see QRG 5.18.1). The aims of hypotension treatment are summarized in QRG 4.1.2.
6. **Obtain/review the key history:**
- Any known trauma?
- Any known toxin exposure? (see Chapter 4.9)
- Any home administration of human drugs by owner?
- Any prior clinical signs especially relating to respiratory, cardiac, neurological or gastrointestinal disease?
- Any current known medical or surgical disease?
- Any current or recent medication?

Formulating the stabilization plan

On the basis of the initial assessment, it is important to decide whether the cat is showing any signs of life-threatening cardiac or respiratory disease (e.g. dyspnoea, cyanosis, heart murmur, gallop sounds, arrhythmias, pulmonary crackles, muffled heart sounds due to pleural effusions or loss of femoral pulses) and/or shock (Figure 4.1.2).

- Poor peripheral pulse quality – initially bounding progressing to difficult to palpate, thready
- Prolonged capillary refill time (>2 seconds)
- Pallor
- Hypothermia (rectal temperature <37°C)
- Tachycardia or bradycardia. Bradycardia is a unique feature of shock in cats, particularly associated with septic shock
- Cold extremities
- Obtunded mentation

4.1.2 Clinical features of shock. Note that the rapid CRT and congested appearance of mucous membranes in septic shock seen in dogs is NOT typically seen in cats.

Acute collapse is frequently associated with shock. The aim in all cases of shock is to provide treatment that will rapidly increase oxygen delivery to the vital organs.

Where cardiorespiratory disease is the primary problem, increased oxygen delivery is achieved by provision of supplemental oxygen (see QRG 4.2.2) together with treatment of the underlying cardiac cause (e.g. diuresis ± thoracocentesis in CHF; see Chapter 9) or respiratory cause (e.g. administering a bronchodilator in an asthmatic crisis; see Chapter 10).

Stabilization

1. **Fluid resuscitation and warming.**

> **WARNING**
>
> Fluid resuscitation (see below) is the first step in addressing all causes of shock except when cardiac disease is the underlying problem, as *fluids are contraindicated in cardiogenic shock due to congestive heart failure*.

- An initial bolus of crystalloids (5–10 ml/kg of lactated Ringer's over 5–15 min) should be administered whilst a more detailed physical examination is performed and results of the emergency database are interpreted; the speed of administration of fluid depends on the degree and rate of onset of hypovolaemia (see box overleaf).
- Concurrent active warming is important if the cat is hypothermic since the vascular response is blunted until core temperature rises. Use of a warm air device (e.g. Bair Hugger) or incubator is ideal, along with wrapping the extremities (bubble wrap or light bandage) and minimizing the use of surgical spirit and clipping to prevent further heat loss. The heat should be directed primarily at the trunk. If heat mats are used, the cat should be placed on a soft bed on top of the mat and covered over. Intravenous fluids should also be gently warmed.
- Following the first fluid bolus, parameters of perfusion should be reassessed (pulse quality, heart and pulse rate, CRT, mucous membrane colour, systolic blood pressure and mentation).
  - If the patient is still showing signs of shock, a second crystalloid bolus is administered over 5–15 minutes. Aliquots can be repeated up to a total dose of 40–60 ml/kg (equivalent to the blood volume of a cat).
  - If marked hypoproteinaemia is identified or hypotension persists, colloids (e.g. hydroxyethylstarch) can be given (2–4 ml/kg over 5–15 minutes).
  - If severe anaemia is identified, whole blood or haemoglobin glutamer (Oxyglobin; if available) should be administered to provide oxygen-carrying support.

Particular care should be exercised if the patient has pulmonary disease, is actively bleeding or has a history of head trauma. If the patient is actively bleeding, a lower target for systolic blood pressure is used during fluid resuscitation (90 mmHg *versus* 100 mmHg); higher levels could exacerbate haemorrhage.

Low-volume fluid resuscitation using hypertonic saline may be more appropriate for patients with head trauma, provided the patient is not dehydrated or hypernatraemic.

Frequent reassessment of cardiorespiratory parameters is essential during and after fluid resuscitation. Aliquots of fluid are given, as opposed to a total shock dose, to titrate volume replacement to effect and prevent volume overload. Cats are more prone than dogs to the development of pulmonary oedema and pleural effusion with volume overload. Risk factors for volume overload include hypothermia, occult cardiac disease, pre-existing pulmonary disease (e.g. aspiration pneumonia), SIRS/sepsis, renal failure, acidosis, hypocalcaemia, hypoalbuminaemia, administration of colloids (especially haemoglobin-based oxygen-carrying solutions) and severe anaemia. The absence of a heart murmur does not exclude occult cardiac disease.

Fluid resuscitation

Crystalloid: 1st choice: 5–10 ml/kg aliquots; bolus over 5–15 min[a] up to total dose 40–60 ml/kg. If two or three boluses have been given and blood pressure remains <90 mmHg ± hypoproteinaemia, move to colloids.

Colloids:

- Hydroxyethylstarch: 2–4 ml/kg aliquots; bolus over 5–15 min[a] to total dose 10 ml/kg.
- Hypertonic saline[b] if low-volume resuscitation indicated (e.g. head trauma): 2–3 ml/kg bolus over 5–10 min, followed by conservative rates of crystalloids.

Whole blood or Oxyglobin: if anaemic (see Chapter 20).

Whole blood (or plasma, ideally, if available) **± vitamin K1:** if anaemia due to coagulopathy (see QRG 20.2 and Chapter 4.9).

[a] Speed of administration depends on degree and speed of onset of hypovolaemia (e.g. more rapid for severe acute haemorrhage than for less acute gastrointestinal losses)
[b] Contraindicated if severely dehydrated or hypernatraemic

---

2. **Address life-threatening electrolyte, glucose and acid–base abnormalities.**
- Hypocalcaemia (see QRG 4.4.1)
- Hypoglycaemia (see QRG 4.5.1)
- Hyperkalaemia (see QRG 4.11.1):
  - Typically reduces with fluid resuscitation
- Metabolic acidosis (pH <7.1):
  - Typically improves with treatment of shock, provided the cat has normal renal function
  - Sodium bicarbonate administration rarely required, associated with risk of causing paradoxical cerebral acidosis and hypocalcaemia
- Hyponatraemia and hypernatraemia:
  - *It is essential that derangements of sodium are not collected too rapidly, to prevent neuronal damage. The presence of hypo- or hypernatraemia may change the choice of crystalloid fluid used for initial fluid resuscitation in hypovolaemic patients.*
  - Careful monitoring required; consider referral for management if close monitoring is not available
  - Aim to change Na+ at a rate of ≤0.5 mmol/l/h; for initial volume expansion use a fluid that has a similar sodium concentration to the patient (± 6 mmol/l)
  - Hypernatraemia (Na+ >162 mmol/l): 0.9% NaCl used for initial volume expansion, then provide maintenance fluids as 0.45% NaCl or 5% dextrose (to correct free water deficit), monitoring Na+ levels every 1–2 hours, adjusting fluid type to ensure Na+ dropping at ≤0.5 mmol/l/h
  - Hyponatraemia (Na+ <149 mmol/l): use lactated Ringer's for initial volume expansion. Continue with isotonic crystalloids (0.9% NaCl or lactated Ringer's) for replacement and maintenance fluid requirements, monitoring Na+ levels every 1–2 hours, adjusting fluid type to ensure Na+ increasing at ≤0.5 mmol/l/h
  - Further information regarding correction of hypo- or hypernatraemia can be obtained from the *BSAVA Manual of Emergency and Critical Care*

3. **Address congestive heart failure or primary respiratory disease** if signs consistent with these (see Chapters 9 and 10).
4. **Consider possible triggers for any arrhythmia identified,** e.g. hypoxia, electrolyte and acid–base derangements, drug therapy, intrathoracic drains, pain, or conditions causing high vagal tone (ocular, gastrointestinal or respiratory tract).
5. **Address any analgesia requirements** – short-acting opioids are preferable (see Chapter 3); avoid NSAIDs.

Continued patient evaluation
To search for the underlying cause of collapse:

- Carry out a complete full physical examination (remember to look for clues of trauma, e.g. contused skin, scuffed nails, hip/mandible luxation)
- Set-up ancillary monitoring equipment (as available):
  - Pulse oximetry (see Chapter 3)
    - Hypoxaemia if SpO2 <95%
    - Consider whether oxygen supplementation method is adequate
  - ECG (see QRG 4.1.4)
  - Urinary catheter to measure urine output (if acute kidney injury or signs of severe shock). This may be possible without sedation in a collapsed cat if a gentle technique is used, but if it is not tolerated catheter placement may need to be delayed until the cat has been stabilized and can receive a short-acting sedative (e.g. propofol to effect). In the interim the size of the bladder should be repeatedly assessed (by palpation or ultrasonography) to check for urine production
- Reassess perfusion parameters – heart and pulse rate, peripheral pulse quality, CRT, mucous membrane colour, systolic blood pressure, mentation

- Perform additional diagnostic tests as appropriate once the patient's cardiovascular status is stable, for example:
  - Complete blood count with differential
  - Serum biochemistry
  - Neurological and orthopaedic examination
  - Imaging
  - Echocardiography
  - Thyroxine concentration
  - Feline pancreatic lipase immunoassay, cobalamin and folate
  - Holter ECG monitoring if available (referral may be indicated for continuous ECG monitoring).

Episodic collapse

This may be due to syncope, pre-syncope, seizure activity or episodic neuromuscular or musculoskeletal weakness (see Figure 4.1.1). Observing the event, or a video recording of it, is extremely helpful to be able to direct investigations appropriately. Consideration of the following features is important when obtaining a description of the event from the owner:

- Any pattern to episodes – time of day, activity, feeding?
  - Syncope or collapse associated with neuromuscular disease could be induced by activity/exercise
  - Hepatic encephalopathy is less commonly associated with the immediate postprandial period in cats than in dogs
- Any premonitory signs?
  - Altered behaviour (e.g. agitation, vocalization) may be a prequel to seizure activity
- Duration and frequency of collapse episodes:
  - Syncope is usually short in duration, lasting <10 seconds
  - Duration of seizure activity is highly variable. Partial seizure activity often lasts for only a few seconds whereas status epilepticus is prolonged generalized seizure activity lasting >2–5 minutes (see Chapter 4.7)
  - Increasing frequency of collapse events may indicate progression of the underlying disease process
- Body posture, limb tone and activity during episode
  - Syncope is typically associated with recumbency and flaccid limb tone
  - Generalized seizures are usually manifested by falling into recumbency, tonic–clonic limb activity ± autonomic signs (urination, defecation, hypersalivation)
- Is the cat conscious, i.e. responsive, during the episode?
  - Loss of consciousness occurs with syncope and generalized seizures
  - Consciousness is retained in neuromuscular and musculoskeletal collapse
- Any loss of urinary or faecal continence, any ptyalism?
  - These are autonomic signs that may be associated with collapse episodes in generalized seizures
  - Persistent urinary or faecal incontinence could be a feature of neuromuscular disease
  - Ptyalism is a unique feature of hepatic encephalopathy in cats
- Mucous membrane colour during the episode:
  - Is there any cyanosis or pallor that could indicate cardiorespiratory disease?
- Behaviour immediately following the episode:
  - Neurological deficits including abnormal behaviour may persist for hours to a few days in cats post-ictally
- Is the cat normal between episodes?
  - Structural diseases more often have persistent abnormalities between episodes of collapse; e.g. a cat with seizures due to a brain tumour may have neurological deficits, including altered mentation and cranial nerve and proprioceptive deficits, between seizures and beyond the post-ictal period.

Apparent collapse or ambulatory disorders

These may be due to weakness, pain or dysfunction associated with the motor unit (peripheral nerves, neuromuscular junction and muscles), bones or joints (see Figure 4.1.1). There is no directly associated loss of consciousness, but complications (e.g. aspiration pneumonia) could cause malaise and reduced consciousness.

When to refer

Cases should be referred after stabilization if:

- An underlying cause cannot be identified and addressed rapidly
- 24-hour nursing and/or monitoring care is not available for acutely presented patients
- Spinal or neurological disease is suspected (referral for advanced diagnostics, e.g. MRI, cerebrospinal fluid testing, electromyography).

References and further reading

Benitah N (2010) Electrolyte disorders: Sodium. In: *Textbook of Veterinary Internal Medicine*, ed. S Ettinger and E Feldman, pp. 299–303. Elsevier Saunders, St. Louis

Costello M (2010) Shock. In: *Feline Emergency and Critical Care Medicine*, ed. K Drobatz and M Costello, pp. 23–30. Wiley-Blackwell, Iowa

Fletcher DJ, Boller M, Brainard BM *et al.* (2012) RECOVER evidence and knowledge gap analysis on veterinary CPR. Part 7: Clinical guidelines. *Journal of Veterinary Emergency and Critical Care* **22**(S1), 102–131

Pachtinger G (2010) Fluid therapy. In: *Feline Emergency and Critical Care Medicine*, ed. K Drobatz and M Costello, pp. 77–86. Wiley-Blackwell, Iowa

Stepien RL and Boswood A (2007) Cardiovascular emergencies. In: *BSAVA Manual of Canine and Feline Emergency Care, 2nd edn*, ed. LG King and A Boag, pp. 57—84. BSAVA Publications, Gloucester

Wray J (2005) Differential diagnosis of collapse in the dog. *In Practice* **27**, 16–28, 62–69, 128–135. [This text is based on the dog but the approach to diagnosis is well described to help with investigation of feline cases]

QRG 4.1.1 Intravenous catheterization
by Samantha Taylor

Indications

- Provision of intravenous fluids for the management of fluid loss (e.g. dehydration, hypovolaemia) or poor perfusion (e.g. sepsis, hypotension)
- Provision of intravenous medication (e.g. anaesthetic agents, chemotherapeutics)
- Provision of blood products in the management of anaemia
- Access for repeat blood sampling (NB central venous catheterization preferred, see *BSAVA Guide to Procedures in Small Animal Practice*)

WARNING

Significantly hypertonic solutions should not be administered via a peripheral vein (including cephalic and medial saphenous veins).

Choice of site

- Catheterization of the **cephalic vein** is technically simple but cephalic catheters should be replaced every 3 days and this can be difficult to maintain in patients requiring longer-term intravenous fluid therapy. A multi-access port can be attached to allow provision of more than one type of fluid at the same time.
- An alternative site for catheterization is the **medial saphenous vein**, into which a longer length, larger bore 'long-stay' catheter can be fed and maintained for longer periods (usually around 7–10 days, although these can safely be used for longer if there is no patient discomfort, no indication of thrombophlebitis and the catheter is patent). This type of catheter is well tolerated, less prone to becoming dislodged and facilitates higher-rate fluid therapy. This type of catheter is indicated in critical patients requiring fluid therapy for more than 48 hours, for example in cats with pancreatitis, diabetic ketoacidosis or hepatic lipidosis. A multi-access port can be attached to allow provision of more than one type of fluid at the same time.

Placement of a cephalic catheter

Equipment

- Over-the-needle catheters are recommended, with 22 G suitable for most adult cats, and 24 G for kittens/small cats.
- Small, quiet clippers are recommended.

- T connectors are useful to allow connection of a giving set without disturbing the catheter and to facilitate injection of other drugs via the bung. All connectors should be flushed with saline or heparinized saline (5–10 IU/ml) prior to connection to avoid air embolization when flushed.
- Tape and bandaging material should be prepared, as catheters should be secured with tape and covered with bandage material to prevent patient interference and contamination. Highly adhesive tape (e.g. zinc oxide) that is difficult to remove is not desirable, as this can cause patient distress when the catheter is removed, and can tighten in time and cause discomfort. Thin tape with adhesive that dissolves with surgical spirit is easier to remove. If using more adherent material, it should be placed over the top of thinner tape rather than directly on to skin.
- Swabs moistened with chlorhexidine and surgical spirit are also required, for preparation of the skin before catheter placement.

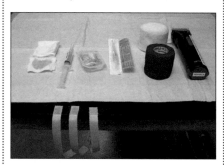

Patient preparation and restraint

- The cat should be restrained correctly and comfortably by an assistant, causing minimum distress (see QRG 1.2).
- If the patient is receiving analgesia (e.g. a hospitalized cat receiving buprenorphine) then it is helpful to time catheter placement *following* administration of the analgesic.
- The area over the cephalic vein in the region of the mid-radius should be clipped (including fur on the palmar side of the limb in longhaired cats to avoid problems when securing with tape). Turning on the clippers with them held behind your back allows the cat to become familiar with the noise before starting to clip on the limb itself.
- Following hair removal, the area should be prepared aseptically by wiping over the area with the swabs moistened in chlorhexidine solution followed by surgical spirit. Do not over-wet the whole site, e.g. by spraying spirit, as the tape will then not stick.

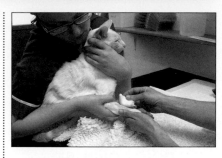

If a cat is very sensitive to catheter placement and jumps when the catheter needle enters the skin, local anaesthesia can be used:

- Following clipping, local anaesthetic cream (such as EMLA cream 5% lidocaine/prilocaine) can be applied and covered with an occlusive dressing and left for a minimum of 30 minutes prior to catheter placement
- Anecdotally, spraying the area with local anaesthetic spray (such as used for laryngeal anaesthesia at intubation) and leaving for 5–10 minutes can reduce pain on catheterization.

Procedure

1 Stabilize the vein by gently stretching the overlying skin with the hand not being used to hold the catheter (left hand in photo). Introduce the tip of the needle (bevel up) into the vein at the distal end of the clipped area (to allow further attempts more proximally if needed). Keep the catheter horizontal in line with the vein to prevent puncturing the deep wall of the vein. Blood should be seen in the hub of the catheter; at this point advance both needle and catheter slowly for about 1 mm to ensure it is within the vein. (NB 'Cut down' techniques are rarely required and may cause patient discomfort and increase complications. If required, e.g. for a patient that is severely hypovolaemic or has very thick skin, then meticulous aseptic technique is required.)

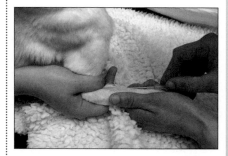

2 With the hand holding the needle/catheter (right hand in photo below), hold the needle still and with the index finger slowly advance the catheter off the needle and into the vein until the hub abuts the skin. Note that the ▶

QRG 4.1.1 continued

needle should not be replaced into the catheter if placement fails, as this risks catheter damage and catheter embolization. If failure occurs, a new catheter should be used and catheterization reattempted.

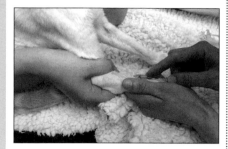

3 The assistant should adjust their grip to occlude the vein just above the catheter and the needle can then be removed. (Some clinicians prefer to secure the catheter with the needle in place, but this may risk the needle damaging the catheter/vein during tape placement.)

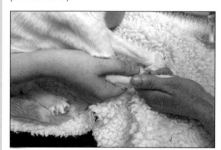

4 The bung or T connector is then attached securely to the catheter and the catheter is held in place with tape. Generally the tape is positioned first underneath the hub, then around the limb and over the hub, taking care to avoid the catheter becoming dislodged. This can be aided by holding the end of the bung (as shown), keeping the catheter from slipping distally out of the vein.

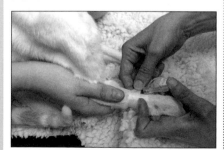

5 A second piece of tape can be placed over the catheter where it is attached to the bung/T connector. Once secured in position the catheter should be flushed with heparinized saline (1–2 ml is usually plenty) to confirm the position within the vein. No swelling dorsal to the catheter should be noted and the patient should not resent this injection. The assistant may feel the fluid passing proximally within the vein.

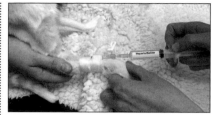

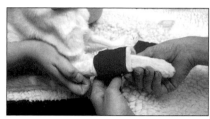

6 The catheter/T connector is covered with a layer of soft bandage followed by a self-adhesive wrap-type bandage, leaving the bung/T connector accessible.

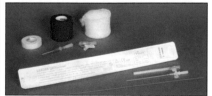

WARNING

Avoid including the paw in the bandage as cats dislike their paws being bandaged and this could result in them interfering with the bandage more, and being less ambulatory. Swelling of the paw is also more likely to go unnoticed.

PRACTICAL TIP

It is good practice to use a set colour of bandage when an intravenous catheter is in place, and a different colour when there is not an intravenous catheter in place. This makes it obvious to all staff whether the cat has an intravenous catheter in place or not.

Placement of a medial saphenous long-stay catheter

Equipment

Equipment is as for cephalic catheterization (above) plus a long-stay catheter. Available from major suppliers, these 18 G, 10 cm soft plastic catheters are suitable for most cats. (NB Human arterial catheters are useful for this procedure and come with a catheter, introducer and guidewire.)

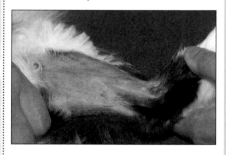

Leadercath from Vygon, long-stay catheter shown alongside guidewire and introducer that come as a set. The author prefers to use a 22 G over-the-needle short intravenous catheter as an introducer.

Patient preparation and restraint

- This type of catheter can be placed in some conscious patients, but sedation/anaesthesia may be required for others. Two assistants may be needed for conscious patients (see QRG 1.2).

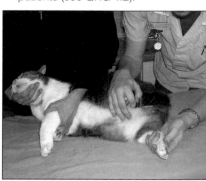

- The skin overlying the medial saphenous vein proximal to the hock is clipped and aseptically prepared as for cephalic catheterization. Sterile gloves should be worn and draping the area may be considered.

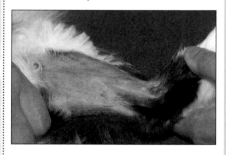

Procedure

1 The assistant occludes and 'raises' the medial saphenous vein by applying pressure into the groin proximal to the clipped area.

2 Catheterize the vein mid-way between the hock and stifle with the short intravenous catheter (or introducer) and remove the needle. (NB Ensure the catheter is not placed close to the hock, to avoid the catheter or the attached connector dislodging when the hock is flexed.) Place the guidewire through the catheter and gently feed into the vein approximately 2 cm from the skin insertion site, as shown. Then carefully remove the catheter over the top of the guidewire, leaving the guidewire in the vein.

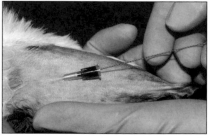

▶

QRG 4.1.3 *continued*

Considerations

When approaching a patient requiring fluid therapy there are many considerations, and administration of an arbitrary fluid rate is not ideal. The following should be considered.

What is the type and severity of the fluid volume deficit and what is the clinical effect on the patient?

A thorough physical examination is indicated, involving measurement and recording of vital parameters (including mentation, bodyweight, heart rate, respiratory rate, capillary refill time, mucous membrane colour, rectal temperature and systolic blood pressure). If blood pressure monitoring is not available, an assessment of peripheral pulse quality should be made. Further tests may be indicated prior to fluid therapy, e.g. PCV, total solids, urine specific gravity. *If the patient is in shock then emergency aggressive fluid resuscitation is needed.*

Hypovolaemic patients have different clinical signs to dehydrated patients (see earlier) and require different treatment. The severity of the deficit should be estimated. In dehydrated patients the level of dehydration should be estimated in percentage terms (see Chapter 5.11). Calculating the deficit allows accurate replacement.

What is the type of fluid deficit and therefore replacement fluid required?

Replacement of the missing fluid is appropriate. In addition, it is necessary to take into account any electrolyte and acid–base abnormalities that may need correction (e.g. hypokalaemia; see QRG 4.6.1).

- The majority of patients with fluid deficits will be treated with crystalloid fluids.
- Colloids are indicated in patients with low oncotic pressure (e.g. hypoalbuminaemia) or as part of management of hypotension.
- Blood products should be given to cats with haemorrhage; low-volume resuscitation using hypertonic saline can be considered in certain patients (e.g. head trauma, pulmonary haemorrhage).

How will the fluid be given?

The route of administration depends on the severity and duration of fluid loss/deficit.

- The majority of cases require intravenous fluid therapy, which allows rapid intravascular volume expansion and distribution of water and electrolytes.
- Subcutaneous fluid administration (see QRG 13.2) is indicated for management of chronic, mild dehydration and maintenance fluid therapy, particularly for cats with chronic kidney disease.
- The oral route is the most physiological but is not suitable for cats with gastrointestinal disease, electrolyte abnormalities or moderate/severe fluid deficits or ongoing losses.
- In some cases, water given via a naso-oesophageal feeding tube (see QRG 5.5.2) can manage mild fluid deficits and ongoing losses (e.g. due to anorexia).

At what rate should the fluids be given?

The clinical assessment will indicate the need for emergency resuscitation or replacement of deficits over a longer period.

- An arbitrary rate – in multiples of maintenance – will not allow accurate fluid therapy, and risks either over-supplementation or failure to administer adequate volumes.
- A 'shock fluid rate' has traditionally been calculated for hypovolaemic patients (or patients with other types of shock) but the use of bolus doses of fluids, followed by reassessment and repeat boluses, can avoid complications and allow more accurate fluid therapy. Administration of 5–10 ml/kg of crystalloid fluids intravenously over 5–15 minutes, repeated according to response, is appropriate (see QRG 4.1.2).
- A rate can be calculated for dehydrated patients following calculation of the deficit, addition of maintenance requirements and ongoing losses (see Chapter 5.11).

Accurate fluid therapy requires the use of infusion pumps or syringe drivers. If these are not available, then using paediatric burettes can avoid overhydration; the bolus doses of fluid can be administered intravenously via a syringe manually, whilst timing administration.

How will response to fluid therapy be monitored?

Fluid requirements in an individual patient will change with time and disease progression, so patients receiving fluid therapy should be regularly reassessed and their fluid therapy adjusted as required.

Endpoints should be decided prior to commencing fluid therapy, based on initial physical examination or biochemical abnormalities. For example, in a hypovolaemic cat, normalization of heart rate and systolic blood pressure abnormalities are endpoints, to be followed by recalculation of fluid requirements with consideration of ongoing fluid losses and maintenance requirements.

Dehydrated patients will respond more slowly to treatment but regular assessment of level of dehydration with physical examination and assessment of other parameters (e.g. PCV, urine specific gravity, plasma or serum urea) is recommended. Measurement of central venous pressure is useful but rarely available in general practice.

What ongoing losses and maintenance requirements will the patient have?

Once initial fluid deficits are corrected, then ongoing losses should be considered.

- Measurement of urine output can be useful to calculate 'ins and outs', particularly in patients with acute kidney injury.
- A rough estimate of losses through vomiting and diarrhoea should be made (e.g. 4 ml/kg per episode of vomiting or diarrhoea).
- Maintenance requirements are approximated at 40–60 ml/kg/day or around 2 ml/kg/h but this should be adjusted according to regular reassessment of volume status.

What complications may be encountered?

Overhydration can occur if fluid is administered too rapidly or in too great a volume. Signs of overhydration include:

- Serous nasal discharge
- Chemosis
- Tachycardia
- Crackles on thoracic auscultation
- Cough
- Tachypnoea
- Hypertension
- Effusions (ascites, pleural effusion).

Certain patients are at increased risk of overhydration, including cats with pre-existing (can be occult) cardiac or renal abnormalities; regular monitoring reduces the risk.

Catheter complications may occur but are avoided with correct catheter care (see QRG 4.1.1).

QRG 4.1.4 Recording and interpreting an electrocardiogram
by Luca Ferasin

Recording an ECG

Patient preparation

The patient should be unsedated but sufficiently relaxed. Excitement, body movements and muscle tremors are likely to cause artefacts that make the ECG interpretation more laborious. In order to compare the recorded values with the available standard references, ECG recording should be performed with the patient in right lateral recumbency. However, ECG is most commonly recorded to assess the heart rhythm, which is not affected by body position.

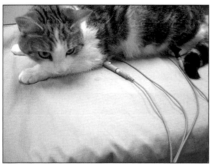

ECG recording in right lateral recumbency.

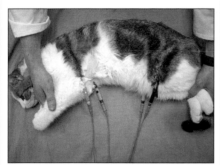

ECG recording in sternal recumbency.

Lead attachment

Non-traumatic alligator or other clips can be attached to the skin. Alcohol can be applied before or after attachment, to maintain electrical contact with the skin.

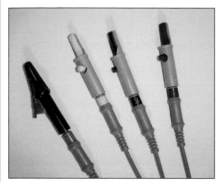

Plastic colour-coded alligator clips.

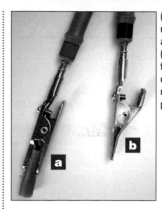

(a) Standard metal alligator clip; (b) filed and flattened clip to reduce skin pinching.

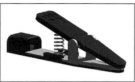

Comfy Clips. (Courtesy of East Anglia Cardiology Ltd)

Alternatively, the ECG clips can be attached to the animal's hair rather than its skin, using a small quantity of ultrasound gel applied between the skin at the base of the hair and the clip; additional alcohol is not generally required.

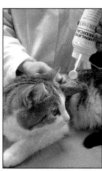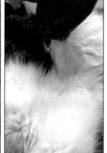

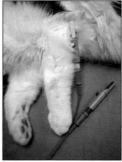

Attaching clips to the hair.

Disposable pre-gelled self-adhesive electrodes (applied to the footpad of the patient), to which clips are attached, can also be used.

All three methods described above have been validated and can be used interchangeably in a clinical setting. However, a wandering ECG baseline may be observed in approximately one third of cats when using the self-adhesive pad recording system.

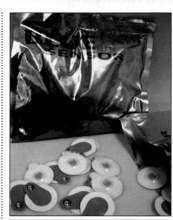

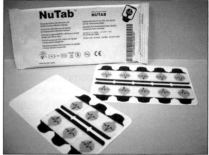

A variety of disposable pre-gelled self-adhesive electrodes are available.

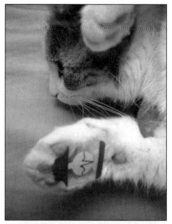

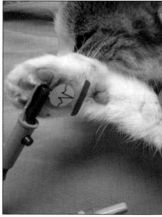

Clips can be attached to pre-gelled self-adhesive electrodes.

patients for an increase in heart rate after terbutaline administration, as this can indicate that the drug has had a physiological effect (although note that other causes of increased heart rate exist); terbutaline can be repeated after 30–60 minutes if necessary. In refractory cases adrenaline or atropine can be used as bronchodilators, but these are rarely required.

- If respiratory distress is severe or does not resolve promptly following administration of a bronchodilator, a short-acting anti-inflammatory dose of steroid (hydrocortisone 2 mg/kg i.v. or dexamethasone sodium phosphate 0.1–0.2 mg/kg i.v.) can also be given.

Pulmonary parenchymal disease

- Cardiogenic pulmonary oedema should be considered in the presence of any gallop rhythms, heart murmurs or arrhythmias. An initial 2 mg/kg dose of furosemide should be given (i.v. if access, otherwise i.m.); if pulmonary oedema is present, the cat's respiratory rate and effort will often begin to reduce within 30–60 minutes. A second dose (1 mg/kg) can be repeated after 30–60 minutes if an inadequate response is seen. Topical glyceryl trinitrate (nitroglycerine) may also be used to increase systemic venous dilation, provided the cat is not markedly hypotensive (systolic BP should be >100 mmHg before using glyceryl trinitrate).
- Pneumonia is treated with broad-spectrum antibiotics (e.g. amoxicillin/clavulanate i.v. initially), nebulization and coupage, intravenous fluid therapy and nutritional support.
- Pulmonary haemorrhage due to coagulopathy is treated with a transfusion of whole blood (or ideally plasma if available) for replacement of clotting factors ± vitamin K1, rest and continued oxygen therapy. Blood typing (see QRG 20.1) is essential before performing a transfusion.
- Pulmonary contusions following thoracic trauma are treated with cage rest and opioid analgesia (e.g. buprenorphine, methadone).

Pleural space disease

- Pleural effusion: initial treatment requires thoracocentesis (see QRG 4.2.4), unless the cause is ongoing haemorrhage (compare the PCV of the effusion *versus* a venous sample; similar levels will be measured if the cat is actively bleeding into the thorax). For other types of effusions, thoracocentesis should be followed by a search for the inciting cause, dependent upon the nature of the effusion.
- Pneumothorax: initial treatment requires thoracocentesis. An indwelling thoracic drain (see

QRGs 4.2.5 and 4.2.6) may be required if there is rapid recurrence of air accumulation.

- Space-occupying lesion: determination of the nature of the lesion is needed to direct specific therapy. In the interim, maintain the cat with oxygen, minimize interventions and consider judicious use of sedative agents (e.g. butorphanol).

Thoracic wall disease

- Diaphragmatic rupture is an indication for surgery; referral is advised if experience in management of diaphragmatic ruptures is not available in the practice.
- Flail chest is treated supportively (oxygen and analgesia); rarely, surgical stabilization of the isolated fragment is required (if the patient cannot maintain oxygenation or remains in pain).

When to consider referral

In many cases of dyspnoea, tachypnoea or hyperpnoea, a diagnosis can be rapidly reached with tests widely available in first opinion practice. Referral should be considered:

- For patients requiring endoscopic examination of the nasopharynx, trachea and lower respiratory tract
- If intrathoracic tissue sampling is indicated
- If a patient is refractory to treatment
- Where a definitive diagnosis remains elusive
- If the required monitoring or nursing care is not available
- If more advanced surgery is required.

Measures to stabilize the cat prior to travelling to a referral centre are essential.

References and further reading

Beatty J and Barrs V (2010) Pleural effusion in the cat: a practical approach to determining aetiology. *Journal of Feline Medicine and Surgery* **12**, 693–707

Crowe D (2008) Oxygen therapy. In: *Kirk's Current Veterinary Therapy XIV*, ed. JD Bonagura and DC Twedt, pp. 596–603. Elsevier Saunders, St. Louis

Good JM and King LG (2010) Clinical approach to respiratory distress. In: *BSAVA Manual of Canine and Feline Cardiorespiratory Medicine, 2nd edn*, ed. V Luis Fuentes et al., pp. 1–10. BSAVA Publications, Gloucester

Mawby D (2005) Dyspnoea and tachypnoea. In: *Textbook of Veterinary Internal Medicine, 6th edn*, ed. S Ettinger and M Feldman, pp. 192–195. Elsevier Saunders, St. Louis

Sigrist NE, Adamik KN, Doherr MG et al. (2011) Evaluation of respiratory parameters at presentation as clinical indicators of the respiratory localisation in dogs and cats with respiratory distress. *Journal of Veterinary Emergency and Critical Care* **21**, 13–23

Swift S, Dukes-McEwan J, Fonfara S et al. (2009) Aetiology and outcome in 90 cats presenting with dyspnoea in a referral population. *Journal of Small Animal Practice* **50**, 466–473

QRG 4.2.1 Immediate management of severe dyspnoea

by Angie Hibbert

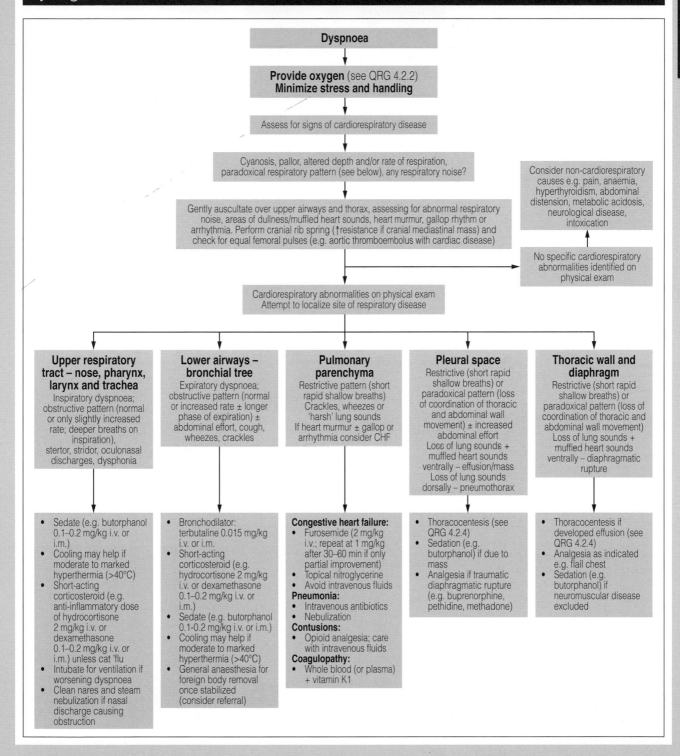

Dyspnoea

↓

Provide oxygen (see QRG 4.2.2)
Minimize stress and handling

↓

Assess for signs of cardiorespiratory disease

↓

Cyanosis, pallor, altered depth and/or rate of respiration, paradoxical respiratory pattern (see below), any respiratory noise?

↓

Gently auscultate over upper airways and thorax, assessing for abnormal respiratory noise, areas of dullness/muffled heart sounds, heart murmur, gallop rhythm or arrhythmia. Perform cranial rib spring (↑resistance if cranial mediastinal mass) and check for equal femoral pulses (e.g. aortic thromboembolus with cardiac disease)

→ No specific cardiorespiratory abnormalities identified on physical exam

→ Consider non-cardiorespiratory causes e.g. pain, anaemia, hyperthyroidism, abdominal distension, metabolic acidosis, neurological disease, intoxication

Cardiorespiratory abnormalities on physical exam
Attempt to localize site of respiratory disease

Upper respiratory tract – nose, pharynx, larynx and trachea
Inspiratory dyspnoea; obstructive pattern (normal or only slightly increased rate; deeper breaths on inspiration), stertor, stridor, oculonasal discharges, dysphonia

- Sedate (e.g. butorphanol 0.1–0.2 mg/kg i.v. or i.m.)
- Cooling may help if moderate to marked hyperthermia (>40°C)
- Short-acting corticosteroid (e.g. anti-inflammatory dose of hydrocortisone 2 mg/kg i.v. or dexamethasone 0.1–0.2 mg/kg i.v. or i.m.) unless cat 'flu
- Intubate for ventilation if worsening dyspnoea
- Clean nares and steam nebulization if nasal discharge causing obstruction

Lower airways – bronchial tree
Expiratory dyspnoea; obstructive pattern (normal or increased rate ± longer phase of expiration) ± abdominal effort, cough, wheezes, crackles

- Bronchodilator: terbutaline 0.015 mg/kg i.v. or i.m.
- Short-acting corticosteroid (e.g. hydrocortisone 2 mg/kg i.v. or dexamethasone 0.1–0.2 mg/kg i.v. or i.m.)
- Sedate (e.g. butorphanol 0.1–0.2 mg/kg i.v. or i.m.)
- Cooling may help if moderate to marked hyperthermia (>40°C)
- General anaesthesia for foreign body removal once stabilized (consider referral)

Pulmonary parenchyma
Restrictive pattern (short rapid shallow breaths) Crackles, wheezes or 'harsh' lung sounds If heart murmur ± gallop or arrhythmia consider CHF

Congestive heart failure:
- Furosemide (2 mg/kg i.v.; repeat at 1 mg/kg after 30–60 min if only partial improvement)
- Topical nitroglycerine
- Avoid intravenous fluids

Pneumonia:
- Intravenous antibiotics
- Nebulization

Contusions:
- Opioid analgesia; care with intravenous fluids

Coagulopathy:
- Whole blood (or plasma) + vitamin K1

Pleural space
Restrictive (short rapid shallow breaths) or paradoxical pattern (loss of coordination of thoracic and abdominal wall movement) ± increased abdominal effort
Loss of lung sounds + muffled heart sounds ventrally – effusion/mass
Loss of lung sounds dorsally – pneumothorax

- Thoracocentesis (see QRG 4.2.4)
- Sedation (e.g. butorphanol) if due to mass
- Analgesia if traumatic diaphragmatic rupture (e.g. buprenorphine, pethidine, methadone)

Thoracic wall and diaphragm
Restrictive (short rapid shallow breaths) or paradoxical pattern (loss of coordination of thoracic and abdominal wall movement)
Loss of lung sounds + muffled heart sounds ventrally – diaphragmatic rupture

- Thoracocentesis if developed effusion (see QRG 4.2.4)
- Analgesia as indicated e.g. flail chest
- Sedation (e.g. butorphanol) if neuromuscular disease excluded

QRG 4.2.2 Oxygen therapy
by Angie Hibbert

Indications

- Dyspnoea, shock, collapse
- Hypoxaemia: pulse oximetry SpO_2 <95%
- Increased demand for oxygen, e.g. seizuring
- Pre-oxygenation before induction of anaesthesia (see Chapter 3)

WARNING

- ***Minimal restraint and gentle handling is essential in the dyspnoeic cat; excessive handling or restraint could tip a fragile patient into a cardiorespiratory arrest.***
- 100% oxygen supplementation for 12–24 hours can induce respiratory epithelial damage; this level is rarely achieved, however, unless a patient is intubated for ventilation.

Monitoring

- Respiratory rate and effort
- Mucous membrane colour
- SpO_2 (if tolerated; using phalanx or pinna in conscious patients) – aim for SpO_2 >95%. NB. Severe anaemia, administration of a haemoglobin-based oxygen carrier (e.g. Oxyglobin), peripheral vasoconstriction and skin pigmentation may all prevent a reliable reading from being obtained by pulse oximetry. Hypoxaemia may also arise due to methaemo-globinaemia (may see a characteristic chocolate-brown colour to the mucous membranes and blood; arises due to paracetamol toxicity) and carboxyhaemoglobinaemia (may see injected red mucous membranes; due to carbon monoxide poisoning with smoke inhalation); pulse oximetry is unreliable in these scenarios as the pulse oximeter cannot differentiate the haemoglobin compounds (e.g. methaemogloblin from oxyhaemoglobin)

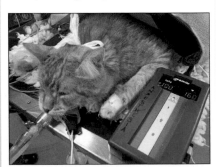

Placement of pulse oximeter probe on the tongue – suitable for anaesthetized, heavily sedated or comatose patients.

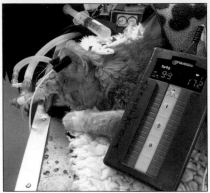

Placement of pulse oximeter probe upon the pinna – suitable for conscious patients; may not work if skin pigmented.

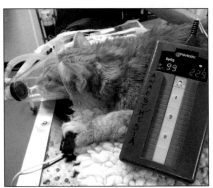

Placement of pulse oximeter probe across the phalangeal pad – suitable for conscious patients; may not work if skin pigmented or in larger cats.

Methods

In extremis, if none of the methods detailed below is effective, and treatment for an underlying cause has been started, consideration should be given to intubation for ventilation with 100% oxygen under heavy sedation or anaesthesia.

The advantages and disadvantages of the techniques illustrated are noted in the table opposite.

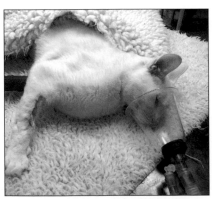

Flow-by oxygen delivery with a facemask.

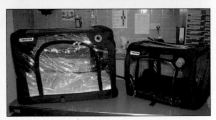

Oxygen tents.

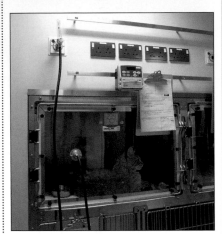

Oxygen cage.

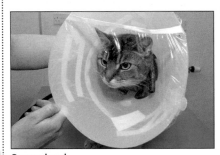

Oxygen hood.

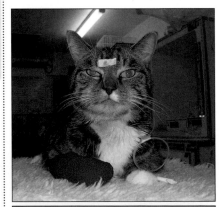

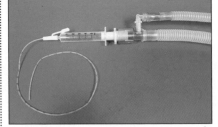

Nasal catheter.

▶

QRG 4.2.2 *continued*

Oxygen supplementation equipment and set-up	Flow rate	Advantages	Disadvantages
Flow-by ± facemask			
Connect breathing system or tubing to oxygen cylinder. Attach clear facemask and hold over nose or in proximity to face; if mask is poorly tolerated try with tubing only	2–3 litres/min	Quick to set up. Suitable for immediate supplementation during triage. Equipment readily available. Suitable for preoxygenation before anaesthetic induction	Poorly tolerated by some cats. Short-term unless patient is unconscious or recumbent, as restraint required. Wastes oxygen. Risk of carbon dioxide accumulation if tight-fitting mask applied
Oxygen tent/cage			
Specially designed chambers (e.g. Kruuse) and cage doors are available. Alternatively, cover front of a cage with clear plastic and run oxygen tubing through front. Second-hand paediatric incubators work well	3–10 litres/min depending on cage size	Allows hands-off approach without restraint, minimizing stress. Suitable for conscious dyspnoeic patients on immediate arrival. Suitable for preoxygenation before anaesthetic induction	Delay in reaching increased inspired oxygen concentrations. Difficult to maintain oxygen levels if patient requires intervention and hands-on monitoring. High flow rates required. Risk of hyperthermia; monitor for overheating
Oxygen hood			
Cover the bottom 80% of the front of an Elizabethan collar with cling film; place on cat. Run oxygen tubing through the back of the collar	0.5–1 litres/min	Allows hands-off approach without restraint, minimizing stress. Suitable for conscious dyspnoeic patients on immediate arrival. Cheap	May not be tolerated by some patients. Risk of hyperthermia and carbon dioxide accumulation – risk reduced by leaving gap at the top of the front of the collar as shown
Nasal catheter			
Instil local anaesthetic (e.g. proxymetacaine) into nares; wait 1–2 minutes. Take a 4-6 Fr soft feeding tube catheter and measure to level of medial canthus. Apply sterile lubricant and insert tube via ventral meatus to level of medial canthus. Secure in place to hair with tape and spot of super glue. Nasal catheter can be connected to a T-piece using a 5 ml syringe and ET tube connector	50–100 ml/kg/min; slowly increase flow rate to desired level over 3–5 minutes. A gradual increase is generally well tolerated, reducing the risk of inducing sneezing and dislodging the catheter	Highly effective. If tolerated, can apply two catheters to maximize oxygen supplementation	Insertion can be stressful – **do not attempt if the cat struggles.** Often poorly tolerated. Contraindicated if coagulopathy, nasal disease or raised intracranial pressure. Oxygen should be humidified if possible to prevent nasal mucosa irritation

QRG 4.2.3 Emergency thoracic radiography

by Esther Barrett

Is thoracic radiography really necessary?

- The dyspnoeic cat should be approached as a genuine emergency, with a real risk that the stress of attempting to obtain a thoracic radiograph could precipitate rapid decompensation, or even death.
- Non-specific supportive treatment, such as cage rest and oxygen supplementation, may lead to enough improvement in the cat's clinical status to allow thoracic radiography to be performed more safely.
- If there is a strong clinical suspicion of pleural fluid, then thoracocentesis (see QRG 4.2.4) is indicated *prior* to radiography. If required, placing an ultrasound transducer with a small contact area (e.g. sector or microconvex) into the ventral aspect of the intercostal spaces should allow quick non-invasive confirmation of the presence of pleural fluid prior to thoracocentesis.

Alternative radiographic techniques to minimize patient stress

Should a thoracic radiograph be considered essential in a severely dyspnoeic patient, it may be necessary to compromise on positioning and employ suboptimal or non-standard views, keeping any restraint to an absolute minimum.

WARNING

- VD views are generally contraindicated in dyspnoeic patients.
- Manual restraint of the patient for radiography is unlikely to reduce patient stress significantly and should only be considered in very exceptional circumstances.

In the UK, the 1999 Ionising Radiation Regulations (IRR99) state that all radiation exposures to members of staff are to be restricted to as low as is reasonably practicable (Regulation 8), usually by using a combination of written procedures (which form part of the Local Rules) and physical protection. The Guidance Notes for the Safe Use of Ionising Radiations in Veterinary Practice (BVA, 2002) advise that:

i. Manual restraint should only be used in exceptional circumstances where there are good clinical reasons why the patient cannot be restrained by any other means
ii. Manual restraint should only be permitted if the X-ray machine is fitted with a light beam diaphragm
iii. No part of the handler's body is allowed within the primary beam, even if covered by lead.

▶

QRG 4.2.3 *continued*

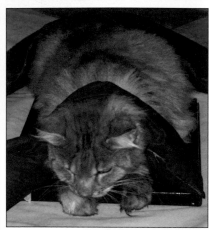

Obtaining a DV view of a dyspnoeic cat using minimal restraint.

■ A screening DV view can be obtained by placing the X-ray cassette or imaging plate, and then the cat, in an open cat carrier, as shown below. A radiolucent cover (e.g. an incontinence pad) makes the patient feel more secure and less inclined to escape. Remember not to close the lid, or the wire grid will be superimposed on the image!

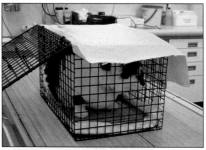

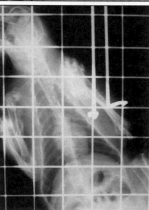

Obtaining an image with the cat in a carrier. Do not close the lid, or the grid will form part of the image. (Courtesy of Paul Mahoney)

■ Try to avoid restraining a severely dyspnoeic cat in lateral recumbency. It may be possible to use a horizontal X-ray beam to obtain a lateral view in a cooperative cat positioned in sternal recumbency, although the information gained may be limited by the inevitable superimposition of the forelimbs on to the cranial thorax.

NB The use of a horizontal X-ray beam increases the potential radiation hazard, and may not be permitted by the Local Rules governing the use of ionizing radiation.

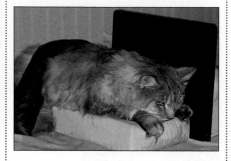

■ Remember that although many of the common causes of dyspnoea involve the lower airways and thoracic structures, upper airway and extrathoracic disease is also possible, and in some cases it may also be necessary to obtain nasal, upper airway and/or abdominal radiographs.

Interpreting the emergency thoracic radiograph

Accurate interpretation of any radiograph requires a consistent logical approach, evaluating the Roentgen signs – size, shape, number, opacity and margination – of each and every structure included on the image (see *BSAVA Manual of Canine and Feline Thoracic Imaging* for full details). Areas to evaluate on every thoracic radiograph include:

■ Trachea and lower airways
■ Heart and major vessels
■ Lung parenchyma
■ Mediastinum
■ Pleural space
■ Thoracic boundaries (with particular attention to the diaphragm and the ribs in a possible trauma patient).

PRACTICAL TIP

In the acutely dyspnoeic cat, where a rapid diagnosis is needed, it is useful to have a shortlist of likely differentials and their typical radiographic appearance.

The typical radiographic appearance of common thoracic abnormalities identified in the acutely dyspnoeic feline patient are shown below. This list is not exhaustive and does not include abnormalities of the upper respiratory tract or non-respiratory causes of dyspnoea, which should also be considered. **Note that not all the radiographic features described are necessarily present in the example images shown.**

Once a preliminary diagnosis has been made and any urgent treatment initiated, it is important that emergency radiographs are reviewed – both to evaluate radiographic quality and to look for any findings that may have been missed. Image quality is often compromised by the limited options for safe positioning of the dyspnoeic patient, and it may be appropriate to retake radiographs and/or to image additional areas once the cat's condition has stabilized.

Pleural effusion

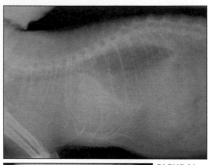

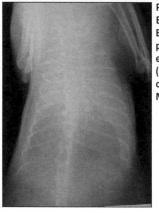

PLEURAL EFFUSION. Bilateral pleural effusion. (Courtesy of Paul Mahoney)

Lateral view:
■ Loss of clear cardiac silhouette and diaphragmatic line, especially ventrally
■ 'Scalloping' of ventral lung lobes highlighted by fluid opacity in ventral thorax, with widening of fissures between lung lobes
■ Retraction of caudodorsal lungs from thoracolumbar spine, highlighted by fluid opacity around lung margins
■ May be tracheal elevation.

DV view:
■ Separation of lung margins from thoracic wall by a fluid opacity. Although usually bilateral, changes can be unilateral or even localized around one lung lobe
■ Soft tissue (fluid) widening of fissures between lung lobes
■ Loss of clear cardiac silhouette
■ Apparent widening of mediastinum.

NB: A small volume of pleural fluid may be difficult to recognize on the DV view, seen only as a vague, usually generalized, haziness of the lung fields due to superimposed fluid, with mild widening of the mediastinum where fluid collects ventrally.
▶

QRG 4.2.3 *continued*

Feline lower airway disease

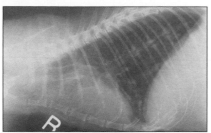

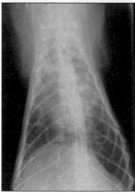

FELINE LOWER AIRWAY DISEASE.
Hyperinflation and increased bronchial markings, together with cranial bronchiectasis in a cat with asthma. The asymmetrical appearance of the diaphragm on the DV view is probably an artefact due to partial collapse of the right lung from the patient lying in right lateral recumbency. Old fractures of left ribs 8–11 can be seen on both views. (Courtesy of University of Bristol)

Lateral and DV views:
- Hyperinflation of lung fields, resulting in increased distance between heart and diaphragm, and sometimes an exaggerated funnel shape to the thorax on the lateral view
  - Occasionally with concurrent lung lobe collapse (most frequently right middle lobe) due to mucous plugs in the bronchi
- Flattening and possible 'tenting' of the diaphragm seen on the DV view; with a caudally positioned flattened diaphragm, seen on the lateral view, often intersecting with the spine caudal to T13
- Increased bronchial markings seen as thickened 'tramlines' and 'doughnuts', often visible in the peripheral lung fields
  - Occasionally with dilatation of the lower airways, consistent with bronchiectasis.

Pulmonary oedema

Lateral and DV views:
- Areas of increased opacity within lung fields, with loss of normal bronchovascular markings
  - Increased opacity is caused by fluid accumulating both within alveoli (alveolar infiltrate) and within connective tissues of the lung (interstitial infiltrate)

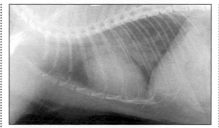

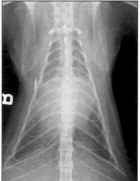

PULMONARY OEDEMA. Patchy areas of increased opacity are seen around the hilus and within the caudal lung fields, together with marked cardiomegaly. The diagnosis was cardiogenic oedema. (Courtesy of University of Liverpool)

- Air-filled bronchi often highlighted by soft tissue opacity of flooded alveoli, resulting in air bronchograms
- Variable distribution, often patchy and asymmetrical (in contrast to perihilar oedema typically seen in dogs), affecting several different areas of the lung fields
- Cardiogenic oedema most likely:
  - Look for evidence of cardiomegaly and vascular congestion.

Non-cardiogenic oedema is rare in cats but is occasionally seen due to electrocution or upper airway obstruction. Radiographically, non-cardiogenic oedema is recognized as increased lung opacity and appears similar to cardiogenic oedema. In mild cases, the changes are typically peripheral, progressing to a more diffuse distribution in more severe cases.

Mediastinal mass

Lateral view:
- Soft tissue opacity occupying cranial thorax
- Elevation of trachea to run almost parallel to thoracic spine (normal feline trachea is approximately 10–20 degrees to thoracic spine).

DV view:
- Soft tissue widening of mediastinum, with trachea often deviated to the right.

General:
- Caudal displacement of cardiac silhouette and lung lobes
- May be hyperinflation of the caudal lung lobes
- May be pleural fluid.

Most mediastinal masses in the cat are cranioventral.

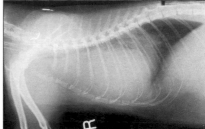

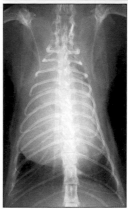

MEDIASTINAL MASS. A large soft tissue mass fills the cranial thorax, displacing the trachea dorsally and the heart and lungs caudally. (Courtesy of University of Bristol)

Pneumothorax

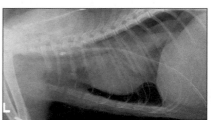

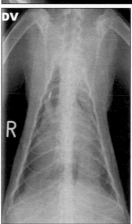

PNEUMOTHORAX. Bilateral pneumothorax, with marked increase in the opacity of the collapsed lung lobes. A chest drain is seen on the lateral view. (Courtesy of University of Bristol)

Lateral view:
- Retraction of ventral and caudodorsal lung margins from thoracic wall, highlighted by surrounding gas lucency with no airway markings visible
- Apparent lifting of the cardiac silhouette from the sternum
- Without any superimposed lung, the aorta is often clearly visible in the caudodorsal thorax
- Increased opacity of the relatively collapsed lung lobes, typically seen as triangular opacities retracted towards the hilus.

▶

QRG 4.2.3 *continued*

DV view:

- Retraction of lateral lung margins from thoracic wall and diaphragm, highlighted by peripheral gas lucency with no airway markings visible
  - Usually bilateral
- Increased opacity of the relatively collapsed lung lobes, which retract towards the hilus.

General:

- Look for evidence of concurrent thoracic and more distant trauma:
  - Pulmonary contusions (patchy localized areas of increased lung opacity)
  - Pneumomediastinum (streaks of gas opacity highlighting external walls of trachea, oesophagus ± major mediastinal vessels)
  - Subcutaneous emphysema (streaks and bubbles of gas opacity within peripheral soft tissues)
  - Fractures – especially ribs, pelvis, limbs

- Look for evidence of a tension pneumothorax (air enters pleural space on inspiration but cannot escape on expiration, resulting in dangerously increased intrapleural pressure):
  - Markedly flattened diaphragm, ribs perpendicular to spine, widening of intercostal spaces
  - Marked collapse of lung lobes, which appear very radiopaque
  - Rapid refilling after removal of the air.

Diaphragmatic rupture

Lateral and DV views:

- Loss of part or all of the clear diaphragmatic line
- Increased, often heterogenous, opacity within the thorax
- Normal cardiac silhouette often obscured
- Evaluate cranial abdomen for displaced or 'missing' organs
- Look for evidence of concurrent trauma, e.g. rib fractures.

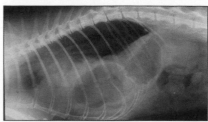

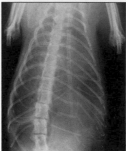

DIAPHRAGMATIC RUPTURE. The stomach is identified in the right ventral thorax as a well defined gas-filled viscus, with the heart displaced craniodorsally and to the left. Several rib fractures can be seen. (Courtesy of University of Bristol)

QRG 4.2.4 Thoracocentesis
by Angie Hibbert

Indications

- To relieve dyspnoea
- To obtain samples of pleural fluid for diagnostic purposes: cytology, protein analysis and microbial culture

> Drainage should be via the mid-dorsal third of the thorax for a pneumothorax, and via the ventral third, at the level of the costochondral junction, for pleural effusions.

Contraindications

- Ongoing haemorrhage into pleural space, e.g. haemothorax due to coagulopathy or trauma
- Small volume effusion

Possible complications

These are rare but may include:

- Pulmonary laceration and pneumothorax
- Haemorrhage
- Iatrogenic infection
- Pulmonary re-expansion injury, leading to devopment of pulmonary oedema.

Patient preparation

- Quiet room with minimal people, activity and noise. Non-slip surface – placing the cat on a warm

comfortable bed can encourage it to settle in sternal recumbency more easily.
- Gentle minimal restraint. Sternal recumbency.
- The coat is clipped over the cranial to mid thorax on both sides. (NB The cat in the photo has had its abdomen clipped previously for another procedure.)
- Provide supplemental flow-by oxygen (see QRG 4.2.2); remove the facemask if this distresses the cat.
- Sedation is rarely required provided a quiet room and gentle approach is used. If the patient is uncooperative, sedation with butorphanol 0.1–0.2 mg/kg i.v. or i.m. is usually effective.
- If the cat is stable enough to wait, EMLA cream can be applied over the 7–8th intercostal space at the intended insertion point 20 minutes in advance; however, this is not routinely required.
- Aseptically prepare the skin with chlorhexidine or povidone–iodine followed by surgical spirit.

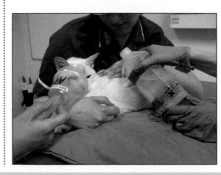

Equipment

- 21 G ¾–1 inch needle (as shown) or 19–23 G ¾–1 inch butterfly catheter
- T-port
- 3-way tap
- Syringe (10 or 20 ml)
- Sterile gloves
- Collection pots (EDTA for cytology, plain tubes for protein measurement and microbial culture)
- Sterile swabs, antiseptic and surgical spirit for skin preparation (not shown)
- Clippers (not shown)
- Breathing system (T-piece + mask) and anaesthetic trolley for delivery of supplemental oxygen (not shown)

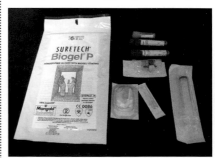

Procedure

1 Put on sterile gloves and then attach the needle to the T-port, 3-way tap and syringe; the 3-way tap should be closed to the syringe. ▶

QRG 4.2.4 *continued*

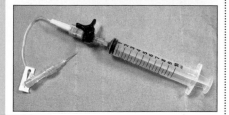

2 Identify the 7–8th intercostal space by counting forward from the most caudal intercostal space (the 12th usually, as most cats have 13 ribs).

3 Gently insert the needle through the skin and intercostal muscles at the cranial aspect of the rib, to avoid damage to the intercostal blood vessels and nerve, which run caudal to the rib.

4 As soon as the pleural cavity is entered, direct the tip of the needle ventrally (or laterally as shown below, where the needle is pointing caudally and laterally), to lie parallel to the thoracic wall, to minimize the risk of pulmonary laceration. The needle should be inserted fully to the hub once inside the pleural cavity.

5 An assistant should open the 3-way tap. Apply suction to the syringe for drainage of the fluid or air.

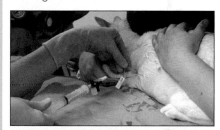

6 Collect an initial fluid sample for cytology (EDTA tube and/or direct smear), microbial culture and protein measurement (plain sterile collection pots).

PRACTICAL TIP

Fluid may be pocketed; redirection of the needle may facilitate further fluid collection.

- If frank bloody fluid is initially aspirated, consider whether this is due to a haemothorax, iatrogenic haemorrhage or a haemorrhagic effusion. Withdraw the needle and assess whether the sample clots; if it does, it is probably iatrogenic haemorrhage from an intercostal or pleural vessel (rather than due to cardiac penetration, since cardiac aspiration is very rare; if the myocardium is accidently penetrated the needle may be felt moving rhythmically with cardiac contractions).
- Fluid from a haemothorax (e.g. due to coagulopathy or trauma) or haemorrhagic effusion would not be expected to clot.
- Running a manual PCV on the sample and comparing it to the patient's PCV is useful to differentiate whether the fluid is due to a haemothorax or haemorrhagic effusion; the PCV of a haemorrhagic effusion will be lower than the patient's PCV whereas recent or ongoing haemorrhage in a haemothorax will have a similar PCV to the blood (± platelets present on a smear).
- In a haemothorax, thoracocentesis is only ever performed if significant dyspnoea persists despite oxygen supplementation and fluid support,

since erythrocytes will be resorbed from the pleural space. If necessary, the smallest volume required to alleviate dyspnoea is drained.

7 Continue drainage by applying suction when the 3-way tap is open to the pleural space.

8 Fluid can then be expelled from the syringe into a collecting dish, by closing off the 3-way tap to the pleural space. Keep a note of how many syringes are filled (or measure the total volume at the end); the volume collected may vary from a few ml up to 300 ml, and drainage of even small volumes (e.g. 50–60 ml) may relieve dyspnoea.

9 Continue drainage until a negative vacuum is achieved when applying suction to the syringe (do not use more than 2 ml of negative suction, as this could risk pulmonary trauma).

10 Close off the 3-way tap and withdraw the needle from the thorax.

11 Assess whether drainage from the contralateral side is required, by auscultation or ultrasonography (a conscious dorsoventral radiograph might be taken if it is not clear whether residual fluid or air remains, but only if dyspnoea has been relieved and the cat remains calm). In most cases drainage from one side of the thorax is adequate unless fluid is highly pocketed or viscous.

12 Thoracic radiography should be performed after drainage, provided the patient is stable, to look for an inciting cause of a pneumothorax or pleural effusion (see QRG 4.2.3).

QRG 4.2.5 Inserting a chest drain
by Geraldine Hunt

Indications

- Pneumothorax
- Pyothorax
- Haemothorax
- Chylothorax

Chest drains are usually placed in patients requiring repeated drainage of fluid or air from the pleural space by thoracocentesis (see QRG 4.2.4); they reduce the risk of injury to the thoracic viscera but do not eliminate it.

Equipment

- Lidocaine 2% (no more than 4 mg/kg or 1 ml per 5 kg cat) in a syringe with 23 G needle for local anaesthesia if tube placement to be done conscious or under sedation (although general

anaesthesia usually preferred)
- Fenestrated drape
- No. 15 scalpel blade
- 3 metric (USP 2/0) monofilament non-absorbable skin suture
- 16 Fr chest tube approximately 9 or 10 inches in length (silicone or PVC: e.g. Mila, Argyle, Covidien) with trochar (12 and 14 Fr are alternative sizes)
- 3-way stopcock
- Chest tube – Luer-lock connector

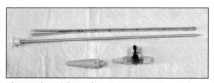

Chest tube with trochar, Luer connector and stopcock.

Tubes are placed bilaterally if there is a bilateral effusion and the material is tenacious (e.g. with pyothorax). One chest tube is usually sufficient if air or non-tenacious fluid, such as chyle, is being drained, as such fluid will usually move easily from one hemithorax to the other. If bilateral chest tube placement is required, the above items need to be duplicated.

Patient preparation

In critically ill patients, it may be possible to place a chest tube with the patient conscious or sedated, using local anaesthetic, but general anesthesia is usually necessary to reduce movement and associated trauma and contamination. Pre-oxygenate the ▶

QRG 4.2.5 *continued*

patient for 5 minutes before anaesthesia (see QRG 4.2.2).

Thoracocentesis is *not* obligatory before placement of a chest drain, but careful consideration should be made as to whether drainage of a pleural effusion (e.g. under mild sedation) would improve the respiratory function of the cat so that subsequent general anaesthesia, if required, for chest drain placement would be safer. If the cat is stable and dyspnoea is not marked (e.g. due to previous diagnostic and/or therapeutic thoracocentesis), chest drain placement can proceed without preceding pleural effusion drainage.

■ Clip the thoracic wall from the 3rd to 13th rib dorsal to the ventral midline – on one or both sides depending on how many tubes are going to be placed.
■ Prepare the skin for sterile surgery and apply a fenestrated drape (not shown in photos). Introduction of bacteria and other debris should be minimized by using a sterile technique.

An area on the procedure table should also be draped to enable the tube and dissecting instruments to be placed close to the patient in a sterile manner.

Key considerations

The key elements in successful and safe chest tube insertion are to ensure that:

■ The tube enters the pleural space quickly and directly
■ Underlying structures are not damaged in the process
■ The amount of air entering the thorax during the procedure is minimized.

The tube should enter the skin at least two intercostal spaces caudal to where it punctures the chest wall, so that it tunnels under the skin before being turned medially into the chest between the ribs. Because of the cat's elongated thorax, there is a tendency to insert drains too far cranially, restricting the amount of tube within the thoracic cavity, causing the tip of the tube to protrude through the thoracic inlet, and making it harder to stabilize the drain. Therefore, the tube should enter the skin at the junction of the dorsal and middle third of the 10th intercostal space (circle) or more caudally, and tunnel forward under the skin to the 7th or 8th intercostal space (X).

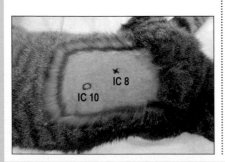

Technique

1 Have an assistant grasp the skin firmly over the lateral thorax at the 4th rib and draw the proposed skin insertion site (circle) cranial from the 10th intercostal space to the level of the 8th intercostal space; the assistant then keeps the skin in that position. If local anaesthestic is being used (because the patient is conscious or sedated), the needle attached to the syringe of lidocaine is inserted directly down through the subcutaneous tissue and intercostal muscles. A distinct pop is usually felt when the needle penetrates the pleura. The needle is withdrawn slowly and the local anaesthetic (1 ml per 5 kg cat) is infiltrated into the tissues as the needle is being withdrawn.

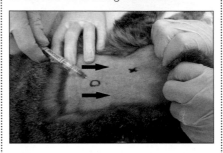

2 With the assistant maintaining the pulled skin cranially, make a small skin incision in the skin with the scalpel.

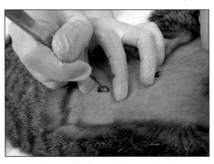

3 Insert the chest tube containing the trochar at right angles to the chest wall directly through the skin incision and the intercostal space. When the skin is released (do not do this yet though), the skin will return to its original position, thereby creating a subcutaneous valve that reduces the tendency for air to track into the thorax alongside the chest tube.

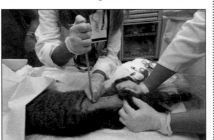

Hold the tip of the trochar during insertion to prevent it penetrating too deeply.

Alternative approach if compliance of the chest makes insertion with a trochar difficult: Most cats have a very compliant chest wall, making the use of sharp trochars difficult as the chest wall tends to collapse before the trochar penetrates the intercostal muscles. If this occurs, blunt dissection through the chest wall using haemostats or right-angled forceps may be preferable. Once a hole has been made, the chest tube can be inserted without a trochar, using the haemostats or forceps; in this case make sure that the connector with 3-way stopcock is already applied to the chest tube and that the 3-way stopcock is closed to the cat.

4 Once the chest tube has penetrated the thoracic wall, angle it so the tip is facing cranially and ventrally.

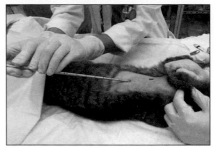

5 Advance the tube over the trochar. Directing the tip of the chest tube cranially and ventrally allows it to be fed along the ventrolateral thoracic wall.

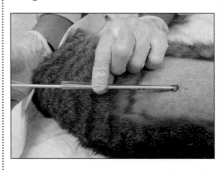

PRACTICAL TIP

Successful drainage of the thoracic cavity is contingent on having a chest tube of the appropriate size, appropriately stabilized to avoid kinking, and not protruding through the thoracic inlet; the cranial end of the tube should ideally lie in the ventral thorax, before the sternum begins rising towards the thoracic inlet, and its tip should curve gently upwards, but this exact positioning is not always possible. This tube location should be effective whether air or fluid is to be drained, and will assist with retrieval of dense flocculent material in cats with pyothorax.

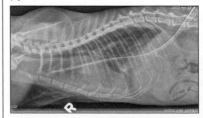

QRG 4.2.5 *continued*

6 The assistant now releases the skin fold and it retreats caudally.

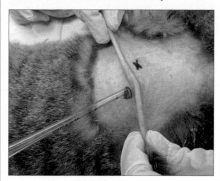

7 The release of the skin forms a valve-like seal (arrowed) between the skin entry site and where the tube passes into the intercostal musculature.

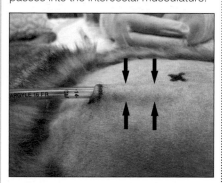

8 Use a clamping instrument or obturator to clamp the tube as soon as it has been passed into the pleural cavity and the trochar has been removed.

Alternatively, the stopper of a blood collection tube usually fits into the flared end of the tube.

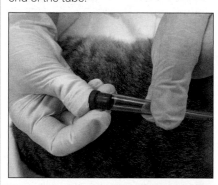

9 The connector and 3-way stopcock are then applied to the chest tube. Always read the instructions for the stopcock carefully to ensure that the 'on' and 'off' positions are not confused.

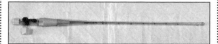

10 The stopcock should never be opened between the patient and the room. It should be maintained closed to the patient (as shown), or closed to the room when drainage is performed.

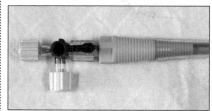

11 Stabilize the chest tube to the skin using a Chinese finger-trap suture.

■ The suture is started using a mattress or purse-string configuration (see Appendix). The suture should include a bite of the musculature deep to the subcutaneous tissue, to anchor the suture in place and avoid migration of the skin forward over the site where the tube exits the pleural space.

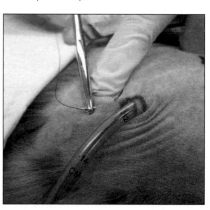

■ The suture crosses behind the drain, and a single surgeon's knot is applied each time the suture encircles the drain.

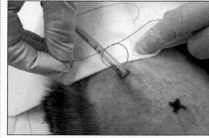

■ The suture is completed with a regular knot after passing completely around the tube at least four times (here this has been done about eight times).

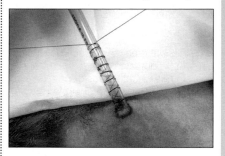

12 The tube is further secured by applying tabs of catheter tape and suturing or stapling these to the dorsum of the patient. The tube should always be covered by a light bandage (stockinette, or conforming non-adhesive wrap) and an Elizabethan collar placed to avoid trauma to the tube and possible pneumothorax. The stoma site and the 3-way tap should be managed as aseptically as possible.

Drainage

The thorax is drained either by intermittent suction using a syringe applied directly to the 3-way tap, or via intravenous fluid extension tubing. The latter is preferable in restless or uncooperative patients as there is no direct manipulation of the chest tube while drainage or lavage is being performed. If the tube is placed without kinking and adequately secured, the cat's position may be gently manipulated to encourage movement of lavage solution around the thorax, or dislodgement of fluid from pockets within the mediastinum (particularly in the caudal mediastinum around the accessory lung lobe). Further discussion of lavage and timing of chest tube removal can be found in Chapter 10.

QRG 4.2.6 Inserting a small-bore wire-guided chest drain

by Dan Lewis

Small-bore chest drain catheters, placed using a modified Seldinger technique, are reported to be associated with fewer complications compared with large-bore trochar chest drains, are easier to place given the small size of cats, and may well be more comfortable. Their placement appears less distressing than a large-bore trochar; sedation and systemic analgesia are required (see Chapter 3) but local infiltrative anaesthesia at the site of insertion is not usually necessary.

The general principles of patient preparation, asepsis and insertion site are similar to the placement of a large-bore trochar (see QRG 4.2.5), although a shorter subcutaneous tunnel (skin incision at the 9th intercostal space) before entry of the tube into the chest (at the 7th or 8th intercostal space) is adequate.

Equipment

Several proprietary kits are available (e.g. MILA, Portex, Rocket) containing the necessary equipment (except surgical drape, 3-way tap and sterile scalpel blade) for placement of sterile small-bore wire-guided chest drains using the modified Seldinger technique. The MILA 14 G 20 cm small-bore chest tube kit is shown below. This contains: two over-the-needle catheter introducers (18 G – green, used in cats; 14 G – orange, used in dogs); a 60 cm 'J-wire'/guidewire with insertion distance markings (shown coiled up in protective opaque sheathing); the small-bore chest tube with extension tubing; needle-free drainage and sealing caps; as well as extra suture wings.

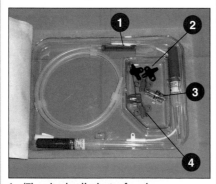

1 = 'Thumb-wheel' adapter for wire introduction. 2 = Extra suture wings.
3 = Needle-free drainage cap. 4 = Locking cover for extra suture wing.

The guidewire needs to be prepared for introduction before starting the procedure. To prepare the guidewire for introduction, withdraw it until its tip is just visible outside the blue adapter.

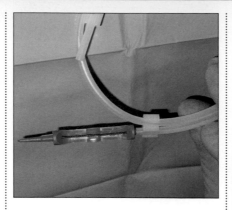

Technique

1 Make a small skin incision using a scalpel at the junction of the dorsal to middle third of the 9th intercostal space, and tunnel the 18 G over-the-needle catheter introducer subcutaneously and cranially.

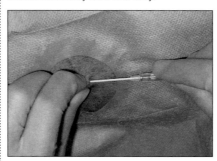

2 Insert the catheter introducer into the thoracic cavity at the 7th or 8th intercostal space; it should enter the thoracic cavity at the cranial border of the rib in order to avoid damaging the neurovascular bundle. This is achieved with minimal pressure. Once in the pleural space, advance the catheter introducer fully over the needle stylet. The stylet (shown here with transparent hub) is then removed.

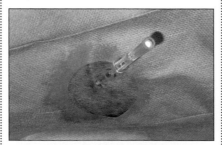

3 Immediately following removal of the stylet, thread the prepared guidewire through the green catheter introducer (the blue adapter on the end of the guidewire will seal the catheter introducer to avoid introduction of air). Advance the guidewire in a cranioventral

direction through the catheter introducer, using the thumb to thread it along the blue adapter. The wire is retained within its opaque plastic sheath, as shown, until fully advanced. *Always keep hold of the guidewire.* Continue the advancement of the guidewire for around 10–20 cm (indelible markers are present – 20 cm mark shown here with double blue stripes), or until resistance is encountered.

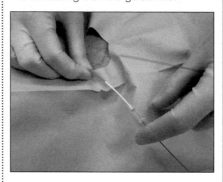

4 Remove the catheter introducer by threading it off the guidewire.

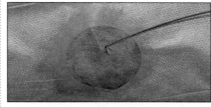

5 This leaves the guidewire *in situ*.

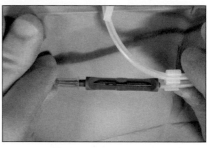

6 Advance the chest drain over the guidewire.

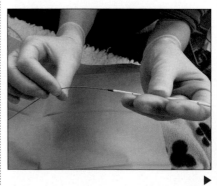

▶

QRG 4.2.6 *continued*

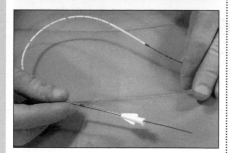

7 Continue to advance the chest drain over the guidewire, into the thoracic cavity. Distance from the most distal side hole is marked on the drain to enable correct placement of the drain, with the cranial end lying in the ventral thorax before the sternum begins rising towards the thoracic inlet. Once in place, the guidewire is removed, the needle-free cap is attached and the chest drain immediately connected to a syringe for aspiration to confirm correct placement (chest radiography can also be used to check placement if required (see Chapter 10)).

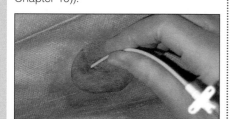

8 Secure the chest drain in place.

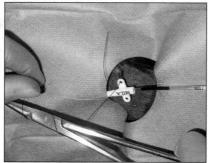

9 Attach additional suture wings to the drain and secure them in place at the proximal end of the drain if it is not inserted fully. Suture wings (provided with the kit) have here been placed over the drain at the point of entry into the thorax, and the locking cover then clipped in place over the suture wings before attaching it to the skin.

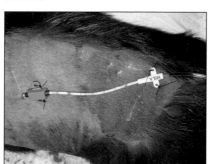

10 Attach a sterile 3-way tap to the needle-free cap.

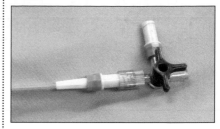

11 Cover the chest tube with a light dressing (stockinette or conforming non-adhesive wrap) and place an Elizabethan collar to avoid trauma to the tube and possible pneumothorax. The stoma site and the 3-way tap should be managed as aseptically as possible.

Drainage

For details of drainage see QRG 4.2.5.

Hypercalcaemia

Samantha Taylor

Hypercalcaemia is a relatively uncommon finding in cats. It is often associated with non-specific clinical signs (polyuria, weakness, depression, anorexia, vomiting, constipation, muscle twitching, cardiac arrhythmias), or may be detected as an incidental finding not causing any noticeable clinical signs.

Calcium is distributed in serum in three fractions: 50% free or ionized calcium (the physiologically active form); 40% protein-bound; and 10% bound to anions. Calcium homeostasis is controlled by parathyroid hormone (PTH), active vitamin D (calcitriol; $1,25(OH)_2$-vitamin D) and calcitonin, and abnormalities in this axis can result in hypercalcaemia (see *BSAVA Manual of Canine and Feline Endocrinology*).

Important considerations when measuring calcium include:

- Total serum calcium (tCa; reference range 2.3–2.5 mmol/l) is affected by alterations in serum albumin. Therefore, measurement of ionized calcium (iCa; reference range 1.2–1.32 mmol/l) is indicated to negate these effects
- Measurement of iCa requires special handling with anaerobic sample collection (avoid air alongside blood in syringe following collection) and storage (bung the syringe immediately following collection) and is most easily performed by immediate analysis with a point-of care analyser (e.g. iSTAT)
- Measurement of PTH and parathyroid hormone-related protein (PTHrp) also requires special sample handling.

Always contact the laboratory for advice prior to collecting blood samples for assay.

PRACTICAL TIP

Kittens can have calcium (and phosphate) values above the adult reference ranges as a normal finding, with no further investigation required. This finding (presumed due to skeletal growth) can persist until bone growth has slowed down at around 6 months of age.

Differential diagnosis

Common causes include:

- Artefact due to sample handling, lipaemia, haemo-concentration/hyperproteinaemia (affecting tCa)
- Hypercalcaemia of malignancy – common but less so than in dogs; lymphoma, carcinoma, multiple myeloma, sarcoma
- Idiopathic hypercalcaemia of cats – relatively common
- Chronic kidney disease (CKD) – usually elevated tCa but iCa is low
- Excessive calcium supplementation – often following thyroidectomy and treatment of resulting hypoparathyroidism.

Uncommon causes include:

- Primary hyperparathyroidism due to parathyroid neoplasia
- Hypervitaminosis D – ingestion of calciferol-containing rodenticides, topical psoriasis medication and some plants, iatrogenic oversupplementation with Vitamin D, diet-related toxicity due to contamination
- Granulomatous disease – toxoplasmosis, feline infectious peritonitis (FIP), cryptococcosis, mycobacterial disease
- Acute kidney injury (AKI) – can result in hyper- or hypocalcaemia
- Hypoadrenocorticism – very rare in cats
- Diseases causing bone destruction – metastasis, primary bone tumour, osteomyelitis.

Diagnostic approach

The diagnostic approach to hypercalcaemia is summarized in Figure 4.3.1. Points to consider include:

- Artefactual hypercalcaemia should be excluded by consultation with the laboratory and/or analysis of a second sample. Mild elevation above the reference range may be within normal variation, so check with the laboratory whether the degree of elevation is significant before embarking on extensive investigations

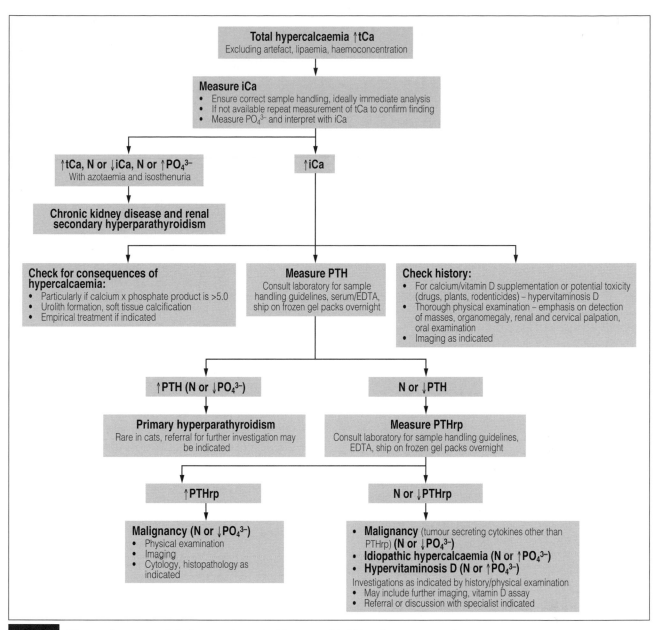

4.3.1 Diagnostic approach to hypercalcaemia. N = normal (within reference range).

- Measurement of iCa will confirm true hypercalcaemia
- Measurement of phosphate (PO_4^{3-}) is recommended, as interpretation of this alongside iCa can help narrow the differential diagnoses (Figure 4.3.2)
- Historical information should exclude oversupplementation and Vitamin D toxicity
- Full physical examination will sometimes identify a

likely cause, avoiding the need for expensive hormone assays
- As malignancy can cause hypercalcaemia, physical examination should include oral examination for masses, abdominal palpation and further imaging as indicated
- Measurement of PTH is only indicated if history, physical examination and imaging fail to identify a cause for the hypercalcaemia

Condition	tCa	iCa	PO_4^{3-}	PTH	PTHrp	1,25(OH)$_2$-vitamin D
Hypercalcaemia of malignancy	↑	↑	N or ↓	N or ↓	N or ↑	N, ↑ or ↓
Idiopathic hypercalcaemia	↑	↑	N or ↑	N or ↓	N or ↓	N, ↑ or ↓
Renal secondary hyperparathyroidism (chronic kidney disease)	↑	N or ↓	N or ↑	↑	N or ↓	N or ↓
Hypervitaminosis D	↑	↑	N or ↑	↓	N or ↓	↑
Primary hyperparathyroidism	↑	↑	N or ↓	↑	N or ↓	N or ↑

4.3.2 Changes in calcium, phosphate and related parameters expected with different conditions associated with hypercalcaemia. N = normal (within reference range).

- Primary hyperparathyroidism is rare in cats (cats usually remain relatively well, cervical parathyroid mass may be visible on ultrasonography) and can be excluded when PTH is low or low-normal
- PTHrp is produced by tumours and acts on PTH receptors, thereby causing hypercalcaemia. Other cytokines produced by tumours can also cause hypercalcaemia, via different mechanisms, so a normal PTHrp **does not** exclude neoplasia.

Hypercalcaemia and renal disease

- Elevated tCa with normal/low iCa and concurrent azotaemia, isosthenuria ± hyperphosphataemia suggests CKD as a cause of the elevated tCa.
- Hypercalcaemia of other causes can cause renal damage and secondary CKD but affected cats will have an elevated tCa **and** iCa.

Idiopathic hypercalcaemia (IHC)

This condition is common in cats and is diagnosed when no underlying cause for hypercalcaemia is found. The mechanism of the hypercalcaemia is unknown. Affected cats usually have a low to low-normal PTH. Some cats show few clinical signs whilst others exhibit signs of hypercalcaemia. Treatment includes a dietary change to a renal (or sometimes a high-fibre) diet, if appropriate, and glucocorticoids (once a malignancy has been excluded). Different cats can respond to different dietary management. The use of bisphosphonates has also been reported in the treatment of IHC. As there is limited published information on the treatment of this condition, discussion with a specialist before treatment is recommended.

Empirical treatment

Treatment of the underlying cause is desirable but supportive treatment to decrease serum calcium levels may be indicated. If hypercalcaemia exists with hyperphosphataemia then there is a risk of soft tissue calcification (significant risk if the calcium x phosphate product is >5.0). Consideration should be given to the effect of any treatment on achieving a diagnosis and prejudicing future treatment (e.g. glucocorticoids would mask lymphoma, and reduce future response to chemotherapy).

Empirical treatments include the following:

- **Fluid therapy.** Correction of dehydration is desirable, along with mild volume expansion to encourage calciuresis. Sodium chloride 0.9% with potassium supplementation (see Chapter 4.6) is indicated at 2–3 times the maintenance rate. Care to avoid overperfusion should be taken, especially if the patient has cardiac or renal insufficiency
- **Diuretics.** Furosemide promotes calciuresis; however, low doses are recommended (2–4 mg/kg i.v., s.c. or orally q8–12h) and care should be taken to avoid dehydration and hypokalaemia
- **Glucocorticoids** (e.g. suggested dose of prednisolone 0.5–1 mg/kg orally q12h). As well as treating the primary cause in cases of lymphoma, glucocorticoids lower calcium levels in hypercalcaemia of other causes. However, avoid their use before investigating the cause of the hypercalcaemia to avoid affecting diagnosis and response to further treatment in cases of lymphoma (see Chapter 21)
- **Other treatments** depend on the underlying cause and include bisphosphonates to inhibit bone resorption of calcium in the management of IHC, and calcitonin in refractory hypercalcaemia (little information available in cats; specialist advice should be sought before using these drugs).

Referral may be indicated for investigation, particularly where IHC is suspected; e.g. for thorough diagnostic imaging to investigate the possibility of lymphoma. If finances are limited empirical treatment may improve clinical signs. If further investigation is declined by owners and lymphoma is *suspected*, palliative treatment with glucocorticoids may be appropriate. If owners opt for this, they should be made aware that this will prevent detection of lymphoma and reduce responsiveness to chemotherapy should they change their mind after glucocorticoid treatment has been instigated.

Hypocalcaemia

Samantha Taylor

Hypocalcaemia is most commonly diagnosed in cats following thyroidectomy for the treatment of hyperthyroidism. When significant hypocalcaemia occurs, prompt identification, investigation and treatment are required.

Clinical signs of hypocalcaemia are usually only noted in cases of moderate to severe hypocalcaemia (total calcium (tCa) <1.5 mmol/l; ionized calcium (iCa) <1.0 mmol/l) and include agitation, seizure activity, tremors and facial rubbing.

Clinical signs can be precipitated by stimulation and therefore cats should be kept quiet with minimal handling and caution on handling while hypocalcaemia is present.

Measurement of calcium is discussed in Chapter 4.3.

Differential diagnosis

Common causes include:

- Hypoalbuminaemia – very common cause of mild reduction in tCa, not associated with clinical signs
- Acute pancreatitis
- Toxicity – ethylene glycol toxicosis most common (causing acute kidney injury); also oxalate ingestion
- Hypoparathyroidism – usually as a result of parathyroid damage following thyroidectomy (i.e. iatrogenic hypoparathyroidism); primary hypoparathyroidism is uncommon in cats
- Chronic kidney disease (CKD) – usually mildly decreased iCa, with normal to elevated tCa
- Acute kidney injury (AKI) – various causes including urinary obstruction.

Less common causes include:

- Peripartum hypocalcaemia – pregnancy, parturition, lactation
- Iatrogenic – furosemide treatment, phosphate enemas, bicarbonate infusions

- 'Spurious hypocalcaemia' – EDTA contamination of sample
- Nutritional hyperparathyroidism – seen with all-meat diets (Figure 4.4.1).

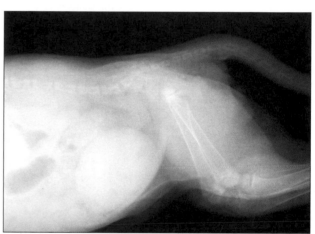

4.4.1 Lateral radiograph of a kitten with nutritional hyperparathyroidism due to feeding of a minced beef-only diet since weaning. The poor calcium content of this diet stimulates secondary hyperparathyroidism, and bone resorption occurs in response to the hypocalcaemia. The bones are very poorly mineralized and of markedly reduced radiopacity compared to normal.

Diagnostic approach

The diagnostic approach to hypocalcaemia is summarized in Figure 4.4.2.

Empirical treatment

Calcium supplementation must be carefully considered due to potential side effects and is only indicated in cases of moderate to severe hypocalcaemia that is already, or likely to become, clinically significant. See QRG 4.4.1 for details of treatment of hypocalcaemia. Referral to a specialist centre may be indicated for severe cases as close monitoring during treatment is required.

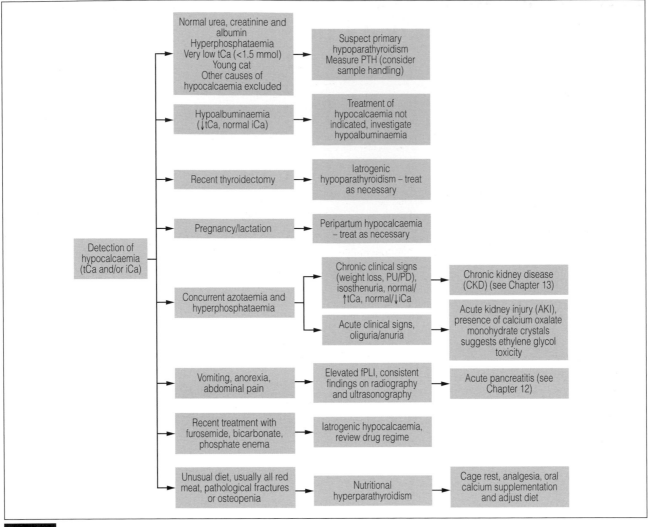

4.4.2 Diagnostic approach to the investigation of hypocalcaemia.

QRG 4.4.1 Treatment of hypocalcaemia
by Samantha Taylor

Indications

■ Mild hypocalcaemia (tCa: 1.8–2.29 mmol/l, reference range 2.3–2.5 mmol/l; iCa: 1.1–1.19 mmol/l, reference range (iSTAT) 1.20–1.32) is relatively common and usually does not require specific treatment in an otherwise clinically normal cat. Regular monitoring may be indicated. Post-thyroidectomy calcium levels should be checked at least once to twice daily for the first 3 days postoperatively.

■ Mild to moderate hypocalcaemia (tCa: 1.5–1.79 mmol/l; iCa: 1.0–1.09) in a clinically normal cat may not require treatment if the underlying cause can be addressed and/or if close monitoring of clinical signs and calcium levels is possible. However, in cases where the underlying condition cannot be treated promptly (e.g. after thyroidectomy), prophylactic treatment (subcutaneous/oral calcium plus oral vitamin D) may be indicated.

■ Moderate to severe hypocalcaemia (tCa: <1.5 mmol/l; iCa: <1.0 mmol/l) in a cat showing clinical signs requires immediate treatment (intravenous calcium if moderate to severe clinical signs are seen, or subcutaneous if milder clinical signs; followed by oral calcium and oral vitamin D).

Note that reference ranges for calcium vary depending on method and/or laboratory used.

Protocols

Parenteral calcium – indicated in acute/clinical cases

10% calcium gluconate (= 9.3 mg/ml) is used.

■ A bolus of 5–15 mg/kg (0.5–1.5 ml/kg) can be administered:
 • Slowly i.v. (over 10–20 min); monitor heart rate (ECG or auscultation) for bradycardia and slow rate of administration further if this occurs
 • OR subcutaneously, diluted 1:1 with normal saline.
 • The intravenous route is preferred, as subcutaneous administration may cause tissue irritation and skin sloughing, especially if repeated.
 ▶

QRG 4.4.1 *continued*

- If repeated bolus injections are required, consider using a continuous rate infusion (CRI) to avoid fluctuations in serum calcium level:
  - 60–90 mg/kg/day (2.5–4.0 mg/kg/h) calcium gluconate
  - For example: if fluid rate being given is 2.5 ml/kg/h:
    - For CRI at 2.5 mg/kg/h of calcium gluconate: add 50 ml of 10% calcium gluconate to 500 ml 0.9% NaCl
    - For CRI at 4 mg/kg/h of calcium gluconate: add 80 ml of 10% calcium gluconate to 500 ml 0.9% NaCl
  - **Do not add** calcium gluconate to fluids containing bicarbonate, lactate or phosphate.

Follow with oral calcium/vitamin D. May need repeated treatments depending on clinical signs and calcium levels.

Oral calcium – as maintenance or prophylactic treatment

- Calcium carbonate (preferred as best bioavailability) – approximately 200 mg/kg/day divided with food.

- OR calcium gluconate – approximately 1 g/kg/day divided with food.
- OR calcium lactate – approximately 700 mg/kg/day divided with food.
- Oral calcium is usually discontinued once vitamin D treatment is established in cases of chronic hypocalcaemia (e.g. after thyroidectomy).

Oral vitamin D – as maintenance or prophylactic treatment

- Use active forms of vitamin D if possible (calcitriol and alfacalcidol preferred)
- Start as soon as possible if chronic hypocalcaemia is predicted (e.g. after thyroidectomy)
- Calcitriol (e.g. Rocaltrol) OR alfacalcidol (e.g. One-alpha) – 20–30 ng/kg (0.02–0.03 µg/kg) q24h for 3–4 days (a higher dose of 30–60 ng/kg can be used in severe cases), decreased to 5–15 ng/kg (0.005–0.015 µg/kg) q24h for maintenance, titrated according to serum calcium (these raise serum calcium quickly over 1–4 days; takes up to 2 weeks for effects to subside once stopped)
- Dihydrotachysterol (e.g. AT10) – 0.02–0.03 mg/kg/day for 1 week; then, depending on calcium level, half this dose for maintenance treatment (raises serum calcium over 1–7 days; takes up to 3 weeks for its effect to subside once stopped)
- Capsulated formulations designed for humans – remove liquid with needle and syringe and small dose can be administered on food
- Dose can be gradually reduced (25% reduction every 2–4 weeks) according to serum calcium. If underlying cause reversible or treatable (e.g. after thyroidectomy) parathyroid function can return with time (weeks to months).

PRACTICAL TIP

- Aim to maintain serum calcium in low-normal range; ~2 mmol/l.
- In cases that are proving difficult to stabilize, further advice should be sought from a specialist.

Hypoglycaemia

Samantha Taylor

Hypoglycaemia (blood glucose <3.5 mmol/l) is most commonly diagnosed in cats following insulin overdosage in the treatment of diabetes mellitus. Significant hypoglycaemia (blood glucose <2.8 mmol/l) may result in clinical signs such as weakness, ataxia, depression, tremors, seizures and death. Prolonged hypoglycaemia can also result in long-term clinical problems such as blindness.

Correct sample handling with prompt separation of serum/heparinized plasma or use of sodium fluoride tubes is important to avoid pseudohypoglycaemia.

Differential diagnosis

Common causes include:
- Artefact – hand-held glucometers may underestimate serum glucose if not used according to manufacturer's instructions (e.g. insufficient blood on sample stick, inappropriately calibrated). Glucometers designed for feline serum are available, but *still need to be calibrated appropriately*
- Pseudohypoglycaemia – if separation of serum is delayed, red blood cell glycolysis will lower glucose in the sample. Severe leucocytosis or erythrocytosis can also result in hypoglycaemia.
- Insulin overdose – dosing error, use of incorrect syringe for insulin type, spontaneous reduction in insulin requirement, inappropriate treatment of stress hyperglycaemia
- Sepsis/systemic inflammatory response syndrome (SIRS) – or, less commonly, other severe inflammatory conditions such as FIP
- Hepatic insufficiency/failure – congenital (portosystemic shunts, glycogen storage diseases) or acquired (hepatic lipidosis, neoplasia)
- Neoplasia – non-beta cell neoplasia, including hepatoma, lymphoma
- Erythrocytosis
- Neonatal hypoglycaemia – particularly if concurrent infectious process.

Uncommon causes include:
- Insulinoma (beta cell neoplasia) – very rarely reported

- Hypoadrenocorticism – rarely reported
- Prolonged seizures
- Starvation – severe malnutrition rather than short-term anorexia, unless dealing with neonates.

Diagnostic approach

- Once artefactual hypoglycaemia has been excluded by correct sample handling and analysis, historical information will likely identify insulin overdosage in diabetic patients. Note that feline diabetic patients can recover beta cell function over time with insulin treatment, with subsequent reduction in insulin requirements.
- Serum biochemistry (including dynamic bile acids) may suggest hepatic dysfunction.
- A leucocytosis, left shift neutrophilia or consumptive neutropenia ± toxic neutrophils on haematology may indicate a septic process, while haematocrit/PCV will diagnose or exclude erythrocytosis.
- Imaging to look for a neoplastic process may be a further diagnostic step.
- Neonatal patients with mild hypoglycaemia will respond to small frequent meals, i.e. glucose levels will rise.
- Insulinoma and hypoadrenocorticism are rarely reported in cats and should be investigated only after exclusion of more common causes of hypoglycaemia.

Empirical treatment

Symptomatic hypoglycaemia requires **emergency treatment** with intravenous dextrose supplementation (see QRG 4.5.1 for details). In the home emergency situation, sugar or honey can be applied to the cat's oral mucous membranes. Severely hypoglycaemic patients following insulin overdosage may benefit from a glucagon infusion. Conscious patients with no contraindications should be fed small, frequent meals. A continuous rate infusion of dextrose may be required in some patients while the underlying cause is managed. Referral for intensive care treatment and further investigation may be appropriate in severely affected patients.

QRG 4.5.1 Treatment of hypoglycaemia
by Samantha Taylor

Indications

- **Mild asymptomatic hypoglycaemia** (3.0–3.5 mmol/l) may be managed by feeding small, frequent meals, with regular monitoring for clinical signs and frequent measurement of blood glucose.
- **Moderate/severe hypoglycaemia** (<3.0 mmol/l) will require intravenous supplementation in most cases. Continuous rate infusion (CRI) is indicated in many cases of insulin overdosage, due to the duration of action of insulin.
- Patients following **insulin overdosage** may initially be normoglycaemic or mildly hypoglycaemic but can rapidly become severely hypoglycaemic, so should be hospitalized and closely monitored.
  - Obtaining intravenous access is advisable.
  - A glucagon infusion may be used to antagonize insulin in the event of an overdose, and human pharmacies/hospitals may be willing to supply glucagon in the event of an emergency.

Note that artefactual hypoglycaemia is relatively common and correct sample handling/analysis is important.

Protocols

Oral supplementation – home treatment or mild/asymptomatic cases

- In a home emergency situation honey/sugar can be applied to mucous membranes by owners. Owners of diabetic cats may like to keep dextrose gels (from human pharmacies) at home in case of hypoglycaemia.
- Mild hypoglycaemia, such as seen in kittens, may be treated with small, frequent meals of food low in simple sugars (e.g. wet kitten food).

Parenteral supplementation – acute/clinical cases

Symptomatic cases should be treated *immediately* to avoid further deterioration and long-term complications or death.

WARNING

Crystalloid solutions containing small amounts of dextrose (5%) are NOT appropriate for emergency treatment of hypoglycaemia and may result in other electrolyte abnormalities. Glucose and dextrose are often used interchangeably in veterinary medicine. Glucose is made up of both D- and L-glucose isomers, whereas dextrose comprises just the D-glucose isomer. The L-glucose isomer cannot be metabolized by cells.

Dextrose

- **50%** (0.5 g/ml; usually 25 g in a 50 ml bottle of 50% dextrose) **dextrose diluted 1:1 with an isotonic fluid** (e.g. Hartmann's or 0.9% sodium chloride) to make a 25% dextrose solution (0.25 g/ml) – administer this **25% solution** at 0.5–1 ml/kg slowly i.v. over 5–10 minutes.
  - *This solution is hypertonic and may result in phlebitis so only administer via peripheral veins (e.g. cephalic) in emergency situations and flush with adequate amounts of heparinized saline.*
  - Ideally, to reduce the risk of phlebitis, dilute the 50% dextrose further with an isotonic fluid (1:4; to make up a **10% dextrose solution**) before giving via a peripheral vein.

Rapid clinical improvement should be noted. Re-assess blood glucose 5–10 minutes after bolus administration. A glucometer (ideally species-specific, but a human glucometer is suitable) can be used for monitoring.

- Follow the initial bolus with a dextrose saline solution CRI via a peripheral vein if ongoing hypoglycaemia is suspected, documented or anticipated (e.g. insulin overdose, sepsis). Since most of these patients need ongoing isotonic support, it is usually preferable to use a solution made up in house by adding 50% dextrose to an isotonic fluid (0.9% saline), rather than using pre-prepared 4% dextrose saline as the latter is only 0.18% saline and is therefore hypotonic.

Monitor blood glucose every 20 minutes during initial treatment.

- Depending on the blood glucose concentrations obtained, the patient can be given a 5%, 2.5% or 1.25% dextrose solution made with 0.9% saline:

Final dextrose concentration required in saline solution	Volume of 50% dextrose required	Volume of 0.9% saline required [a]
5%	50 ml	450 ml
2.5%	25 ml	475 ml
1.25%	12.5 ml	487.5 ml

[a] **Best made up in a 500 ml bag of 0.9% saline; remove volume of dextrose to be added; then add the 50% dextrose and mix well before setting up the CRI**

If the hypoglycaemia is as a result of seizuring, and/or the seizure activity continues despite correction of hypoglycaemia, additional treatment will be required for seizuring (see QRG 4.7.1).

Monitor blood glucose and serum potassium levels (± sodium and chloride levels) regularly (glucose at least hourly, electrolytes every 4 hours). Repeat boluses of 25% dextrose may be required in some cases.

In cases of **insulin overdose**, corticosteroids (e.g. dexamethasone 0.1 mg/kg i.v. or prednisolone 0.5 mg/kg orally) can be administered to antagonize insulin. One dose is usually adequate but it may be repeated q24h in cases with persistent hypoglycaemia.

Glucagon CRI – indicated for insulin overdosage and persistent hypoglycaemia despite intravenous supplementation

- 1 mg of glucagon is added to 1 litre of 0.9% saline to result in a 1000 ng/ml solution (reconstitute glucagon according to manufacturer's instructions).
- Administer glucagon via syringe driver: give 50 nanograms i.v. once, followed by 10–15 ng/kg/min i.v. (up to 40 ng/kg/min if inadequate response).

Close monitoring of blood glucose is required.

Hypokalaemia

Samantha Taylor

The majority of potassium in the body is located intracellularly (95–98%), and extracellular potassium levels are usually tightly controlled at 4–5 mmol/l.

Hypokalaemia is a common electrolyte disturbance in cats. Overt clinical signs, including skeletal muscle weakness causing a plantigrade stance and neck ventroflexion, are usually only noted at serum concentrations <3.0 mmol/l. ECG changes, including ventricular and supraventricular arrhythmias, decreased T wave amplitude and ST segment depression, may be documented. However, even mild to moderate hypokalaemia can result in inappetence and lethargy and hypokalaemia can be life-threatening if untreated.

Differential diagnosis

Common causes include:

- Inadequate potassium intake – inappetence, anorexia, low-potassium diet
- Gastrointestinal loss – vomiting and/or diarrhoea; exacerbated if metabolic alkalosis develops
- Chronic kidney disease (CKD) – usually results in mild to moderate hypokalaemia. Note that hypokalaemia may also result in further renal damage (hypokalaemic nephropathy)
- Endocrine disorders – during treatment of diabetes mellitus, particularly diabetic ketoacidosis (DKA), and with primary hyperaldosteronism (Conn's syndrome) and hyperthyroidism (mild)
- Iatrogenic – treatment with potassium-free intravenous fluids (common cause and exacerbates mild, pre-existing hypokalaemia in dehydrated/ hypovolaemic patients), furosemide treatment.

Less common causes include:

- Periodic hypokalaemia in Burmese cats – inherited condition resulting in potassium translocation into cells and episodic muscle weakness
- Polyuric phase of acute kidney injury (AKI)
- Congestive heart failure (exacerbated by use of loop diuretics)
- Hepatic failure
- Hyperadrenocorticism
- Renal tubular acidosis.

Diagnostic approach

The majority of hypokalaemic cats are presented with clinical signs indicative of the underlying disease, commonly inappetence, vomiting/diarrhoea and/or polyuria, rather than clinical signs of hypokalaemia. Exceptions include young Burmese cats with periodic hypokalaemia, cats with hyperaldosteronism and cats with moderate to severe CKD, which may have severe hypokalaemia and resultant muscle weakness.

- Hypokalaemia is frequently identified via blood tests performed during the investigation of the underlying disease.
- Serum biochemistry and urinalysis should be performed to identify cases of CKD or AKI, and to demonstrate hyperglycaemia and glucosuria in diabetic cats.
- Hyperthyroid cats with mild hypokalaemia are diagnosed via measurement of total thyroxine.
- Hyperaldosteronism may be suspected in cats with hypokalaemia and hypertension, and the diagnosis is confirmed via measurement of aldosterone and/or identification of an adrenal mass.

Hyperaldosteronism (Conn's syndrome)

This condition is most commonly caused by an aldosterone-secreting adrenal tumour (but bilateral adrenal hyperplasia is also reported). Presenting signs relate to the resultant hypokalaemia (muscle weakness) and/or hypertension (cardiac, ocular or, rarely, neurological signs). Cats with hyperaldosteronism can be severely hypokalaemic and/or have a hypokalaemia that is quite refractory to treatment. Diagnosis is via measurement of plasma aldosterone and identification of an adrenal mass. Treatment may be via adrenalectomy, or medical treatment with spironolactone (aldosterone antagonist), potassium supplementation (large amounts can be required; dose to effect) and management of hypertension (see QRG 5.18.2).

Empirical treatment

Management of hypokalaemia involves treatment of the underlying cause and potassium supplementation (see QRG 4.6.1). Many cases of hypokalaemia can be predicted and avoided. Cats receiving intravenous fluid therapy should be given balanced potassium-supplemented fluids. Serum potassium should be measured and monitored in diabetic cats during treatment, particularly cases of DKA. All cats with CKD and cats receiving loop diuretics such as furosemide can develop hypokalaemia, so monitoring and, if required, oral supplementation is appropriate. Primary hyperaldosteronism is managed surgically or medically and the latter includes oral potassium supplementation. Burmese cats with periodic hypokalaemia may require life-long high-dose oral potassium supplementation, but many cases of spontaneous recovery are reported.

QRG 4.6.1 Treatment of hypokalaemia
by Samantha Taylor

Indications

- **Mild hypokalaemia** (3.5–3.9 mmol/l; reference range 4–5 mmol/l) is common in cats with reduced potassium intake (anorexia) or increased losses via the gastrointestinal tract (vomiting/diarrhoea) or urinary tract (polyuric conditions). Supplementation is desirable if the underlying cause cannot be promptly corrected.
- Hypokalaemia can be anticipated and avoided in cats receiving **fluid therapy or loop diuretics** by supplementing with potassium.
- Cats with **chronic kidney disease** (CKD) are commonly hypokalaemic and may require supplementation.
- **Moderate to severe hypokalaemia** (<3 4 mmol/l) may require intravenous supplementation.

Protocols

Oral supplementation – mild and/or ongoing hypokalaemia in clinically stable, hydrated patients

- Dose is variable and should be adjusted according to response, with starting dose of 2–6 mmol (mEq)/cat/day in divided doses. Different oral formulations exist:
  - Tablets, powder (e.g. Tumil-K: potassium gluconate)
  - Liquid (e.g. Kaminox: potassium gluconate together with an amino acid blend and B vitamins).
- Potassium gluconate is thought to result in less gastrointestinal irritation than potassium chloride.

Parenteral potassium – moderate/severe hypokalaemia and cases requiring fluid therapy

- Potassium chloride is usually used.
- Intravenous route preferred but can be given subcutaneously with crystalloid fluids if rapid correction **not** required (concentration of potassium must not exceed 30 mmol/l to avoid tissue irritation)
- Avoid rapid intravenous administration (maximum infusion rate 0.5 mmol/kg/h).
- Dilute concentrated solutions:

Serum potassium concentration (mmol/l)	Amount of potassium (mmol) to add to 500 ml of NaCl 0.9%
<2	40
2–2.5	30
2.5–3	20
3–3.5	14
3.5–5.5	10 (considered 'maintenance supplementation')

Supplementation should be adjusted for higher infusion rates and should not exceed 0.5 mmol/kg/h.

- Consider maintenance potassium supplementation in all cats receiving fluid therapy, unless contraindicated (e.g. hyperkalaemic cats).
- In a cat that has concurrent hypophosphataemia, 25–50% of potassium requirement can be provided in the form of potassium phosphate, and 50–75% as potassium chloride.
- If the cat is extremely refractory to potassium supplementation, consider checking magnesium concentrations as hypomagnesaemia can cause refractory hypokalaemia. Advice can be sought from a specialist regarding this if suspected or found.

Seizures

Laurent Garosi

Seizure types

- A **seizure** is caused by abnormal electrical activity in the forebrain and is characterized by a sudden episode of transient neurological signs. A seizure is not a disease entity in itself but is a clinical sign generally indicative of a forebrain disorder.
- Similarly, the term **epilepsy** is not a specific disease but is used to define *recurrent* seizures.

Generalized *versus* focal (partial) seizures
Seizures can be classified into two major categories: generalized and focal (partial).

Generalized seizures affect both sides of the brain from the start of the seizure. They are characterized by having some or all of the following features:

- Peracute, lasting about 1–3 minutes, with unexpected onset and offset (except in cases of 'reflex seizures' where seizures are exclusively observed in response to specific stimuli)
- Stereotypical pattern (i.e. seizures are fairly similar in following the same pattern)
- Presence of involuntary motor activity
- Abnormal mentation and behaviour with loss of consciousness
- Autonomic signs (salivation, urination and/or defecation) are often seen.

Focal (partial) seizures are characterized by having only one specific area of the brain affected, and are more common in cats than in dogs due to the higher incidence of focal intracranial pathology in cats.
Focal (partial) seizures can be:

- **Simple partial:** consciousness is retained but motor (e.g. eyelid or orofacial twitching), sensory (e.g. growling, vocalization, tail chasing, floor licking) or autonomic (e.g. vomiting, diarrhoea, abdominal pain) signs are seen
- **Complex partial** (formerly called psychomotor seizures): consciousness is impaired or lost, and signs include bizarre stereotypical behaviour (e.g. unprovoked aggression, growling, hissing, rapid running) or repetitive motor activity. A syndrome of complex partial seizures with orofacial involvement has been described, in which cats will sit and stare and display signs of salivation, facial twitching, lip smacking, chewing or swallowing.

Intracranial *versus* extracranial
Seizures can be divided into **intracranial** (originating from inside the brain) and **extracranial** (originating from outside the brain). Intracranial epilepsy can be further separated into **primary/idiopathic**, a functional disorder in which no structural forebrain disease is present, and **secondary/symptomatic**, in which structural forebrain disease is present. Extracranial seizures are also known as **reactive epileptic seizures.**

Clinical approach

History
The first step is to obtain a thorough history, including details of seizure onset and frequency, and a description of the seizures (see above for possible signs associated with different types of seizure). Seizures are often confused with other paroxysmal events, such as syncope, vestibular attack, pain, or behavioural or paroxysmal movement disorders.

> **PRACTICAL TIP**
>
> - Video footage obtained by the owner can be of great help in differentiating a seizure event from other non-epileptic paroxysmal events.
> - The owner should also be questioned about the presence of any abnormalities in between the seizures (e.g. abnormal mentation, abnormal behaviour, visual disturbances, circling, head turn).

Compared to dogs, cats tend to experience **high seizure frequency**, whatever the underlying cause.

Neurological examination
The neurological examination (see QRG 1.6) should focus primarily on evaluating for forebrain dysfunction, by assessing for the following:

- Mental status and behaviour abnormalities
- Abnormal posture such as head turn
- Abnormal gait pattern such as propulsive (moving) circling
- Postural reaction abnormalities
- Decreased/absent menace response
- Decreased response to nasal stimulation.

A completely normal neurological examination would be compatible with primary/idiopathic epilepsy, as one of the features of primary/idiopathic epilepsy is the absence of neurological deficits in the inter-ictal period.

Secondary/symptomatic epileptic patients often have inter-ictal abnormalities on neurological examination due to their structural brain disease; these are usually consistent with unilateral brain dysfunction. However, they may also have a normal neurological examination if the causative structural lesion is located in a 'clinically silent' area of the forebrain such as the olfactory lobe. During the early stages of a slowly enlarging mass in such a region, seizures may be the only clinical signs but, with time, other neurological deficits related to the site of the mass will develop.

Diffuse and symmetrical forebrain abnormalities on neurological examination should prompt consideration of an extracranial cause (reactive epileptic seizures) but, occasionally, extracranial disease may also wax and wane, resulting in a normal neurological examination. Structural intracranial disease (secondary/symptomatic seizures) can occasionally cause diffuse and symmetrical forebrain abnormalities on examination.

The presence of neurological abnormalities in the inter-ictal period would usually *exclude* primary/idiopathic epilepsy from the differential diagnoses *but* there are two exceptions to this:

- Depression of forebrain activity occurs during the period immediately following a seizure (so-called **post-ictal depression**). During this period subtle neurological deficits, including conscious proprioceptive deficits, may be evident. Post-ictal depression lasts a variable amount of time; most cats return to normal a few hours following the seizure episode although it can take up to a few days in some cases
- Neurological deficits may also result after severe or prolonged seizures, due to **hypoxic injury** and/or the so-called **excitotoxicity phenomenon** (nerve cell damage after excessive stimulation by neurotransmitters during a seizure). Sequential neurological examinations at 2–3-day intervals are recommended if in doubt about the origin of the neurological deficits (i.e. post-ictal *versus* relating to potential underlying structural intracranial (secondary/symptomatic) or extracranial (reactive epileptic) seizures). With post-ictal neurological deficits, gradual improvement would be expected over several days, with resolution within a week in the majority of cases.

Differential diagnoses

Seizures indicate a forebrain disorder. Their causes are extensive (Figure 4.7.1) and, as described above, may be extracranial or intracranial in nature.

Disease mechanisms (VITAMIND)	Specific diseases
Vascular	Ischaemic stroke; hypertension; polycythaemia; high-grade atrioventricular dysfunction
Inflammatory/ Infectious	**Infectious encephalitis (*Toxoplasma*, bacterial, FIP, *Cryptococcus*, blastomycosis, FIV, aberrant parasitic migration, FeLV);** meningoencephalitis of unknown aetiology (presumed immune-mediated); hippocampal necrosis
Trauma	**Head injury – may be chronic response to earlier trauma**
Toxic	Lead; organophosphate; ethylene glycol
Anomalous	Hydrocephalus
Metabolic	Hepatic encephalopathy; hypoglycaemia; hypocalcaemia; hyperthyroidism; renal encephalopathy
Idiopathic	Primary epilepsy
Neoplastic	**Primary or metastatic brain tumour**
Nutritional	Thiamine deficiency
Degenerative	Lysosomal storage disease

4.7.1 Differential diagnoses for seizures. Common causes in cats are shown in bold.

Extracranial causes of seizures may originate from outside the body (toxic disorder) or inside the body (e.g. hypoglycaemia, portosystemic shunt (Figure 4.7.2)). Intracranial causes of seizures can be primary/idiopathic in type, or secondary/symptomatic

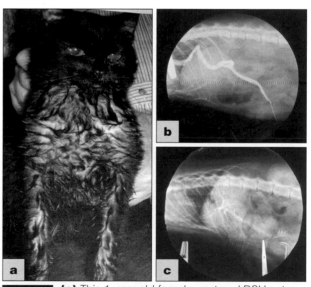

4.7.2 **(a)** This 1-year-old female neutered DSH cat was presented for investigations for seizures and tremors. She had also experienced episodes of reduced mentation, alternating with episodes of aggression, and periods of being apparently normal. Extreme hypersalivation also occurred frequently, as can be seen in this photo. Portosystemic shunt (PSS) is an important differential diagnosis for seizures in a young cat, and is particularly likely when other consistent clinical signs are present (e.g. hypersalivation, periods of aggression), as in this case. Diagnosis was confirmed by demonstrating elevated postprandial bile acids and identification of the PSS on ultrasound scanning. Management options are medical management (low-protein diet, lactulose and antibiotics, together with anti-epileptic treatment if required) or surgical management. **(b)** A portovenogram demonstrating a single portocaval shunt. **(c)** Portovenogram following complete ligation of the shunting vessel.

if structural forebrain disease is present (Figures 4.7.3 and 4.7.4). Primary/idiopathic epilepsy is considered to be less common in cats than in dogs and therefore more extensive neurological investigation should be considered earlier in cats.

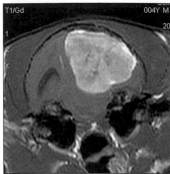

4.7.3 Transverse T1-weighted contrast-enhanced MR image of an 11-year-old cat with a large left-sided meningioma causing seizures and left forebrain signs (obtundation, compulsive circling to the left, right-sided postural reaction deficit and right-sided menace response deficit with normal pupillary light reflex). The owner reported that the cat had been 'slowing down' over the last 6 months and had started to circle to the left one week prior to presentation. Surgical treatment of meningioma in cats can carry a very good prognosis. Surgery (rostrotentorial craniectomy) was carried out successfully on this cat and resulted in resolution of the neurological signs and cessation of seizures. The cat was reported still to be 'free' of neurological signs 2 years later.

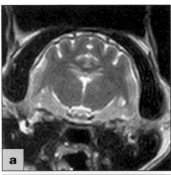

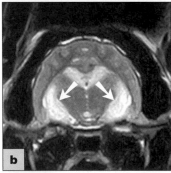

4.7.4 Transverse T2-weighted MR images of **(a)** a normal cat; and **(b)** a 3-year-old DSH cat presented because of acute onset of behavioural changes and severe cluster of complex partial seizures that had started 24 hours before referral (complex partial seizures with orofacial involvement). There is marked bilateral hyperintensity (arrowed) within the hippocampus, suggestive of feline hippocampal necrosis (limbic encephalitis). The cat was treated symptomatically with anti-epileptic medications (oral phenobarbital initially as sole therapy, then oral levetiracetam added). Unfortunately the cat was euthanased 3 months later due to persistent behavioural changes and poor seizure control.

Diagnostic approach

Baseline blood work, including a complete blood count, biochemistry profile (ensuring blood glucose, sodium, potassium, chloride, calcium and phosphate are included), total T4 (in senior and geriatric cats) and dynamic (pre- and postprandial) bile acids, plus blood pressure measurement and urinalysis, should be performed in all cats with seizures to rule out systemic/metabolic causes.

Investigation of intracranial causes involves the use of advanced imaging of the brain (MRI or CT) (Figure 4.7.5) and cerebrospinal fluid (CSF) analysis.

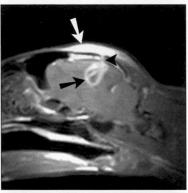

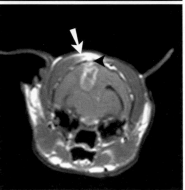

4.7.5 Sagittal and transverse T1-weighted contrast-enhanced MR images of a cat with a right-sided brain abscess (black arrow) secondary to a bite wound; the cat was presented with seizures and right forebrain signs (severe obtundation, circling to the right, left-sided postural reaction deficits and left-sided menace response deficit with normal pupillary light reflex). Note the calvarial defect (black arrowheads) and contrast enhancement of the right temporalis muscle (white arrows) at the site of the bite. The abscess was drained surgically via craniectomy followed by a 2-week course of oral antibiotic. The cat regained normal neurological examination within 2 days of surgery and remained normal after that.

Specialist advice should be sought and/or the cat referred for further evaluation where investigation of intracranial disease is indicated. The prognosis for many intracranial diseases can be good with appropriate treatment, and so further evaluation should not be discouraged if there are no financial limitations. CSF sampling is indicated if the imaging is normal or suggestive of intracranial disease and the cat is believed to have normal intracranial pressure (ICP), but if there is any indication of raised ICP (e.g. suspicion of a space-occupying mass or evidence of brain herniation), a CSF tap is contraindicated; in such cases a CSF tap should not be performed prior to advanced imaging.

If finances are limited

If the cat has no abnormal inter-ictal signs and no abnormalities on neurological examination, once systemic/metabolic causes have been excluded, it is not unreasonable to start management (as below) without having performed advanced imaging if finances are limited. However, the owners should be warned that intracranial disease cannot be excluded and that clinical signs may progress.

In cases with evidence of intracranial disease where finances limit further investigation, managing the seizures alone can maintain quality of life for a reasonable period of time in some cases (e.g. meningiomas are the most common brain neoplasms in cats and are usually very slow growing). However, owners should be advised that the treatment is only palliative and that clinical signs will progress. In this situation, euthanasia should be considered once a good quality of life is no longer sustainable.

The diagnosis of primary/idiopathic epilepsy is a diagnosis of exclusion, after elimination of extracranial causes and structural forebrain disorder. There is, to date, no definitive diagnostic test to confirm the diagnosis of primary epilepsy.

Management

Unless primary/idiopathic epilepsy is considered to be the main differential for seizure activity, specific treatment of the underlying cause of the seizures is essential rather than purely symptomatic treatment for the seizures themselves. The success of treatment of the underlying cause will determine the need for any symptomatic seizure therapy.

> All cats presented whilst seizuring should be treated symptomatically (see QRG 4.7.1) alongside initial investigation.

The aim of any anti-epileptic treatment is to 'control' the seizures by reducing their frequency, intensity and severity, with minimum side effects, rather than totally abolishing them. Owners should be advised appropriately to ensure that their expectations are realistic from the outset. Whether to start anti-epileptic treatment is still a subject of controversy. Cats with a single seizure, or isolated seizures separated by long periods of time (more than a month), do not require treatment.

Treatment is indicated when:

- The first seizure(s) is/are life-threatening:
  - Status epilepticus: seizure activity lasting 5 minutes or more, or multiple seizures without recovery in between
  - Severe clusters: a cluster is two or more seizures within 24 hours, between which the cat regains consciousness

- Multiple seizures are observed over a few days
- Seizures occur more than once a month and/or owner objects to their frequency
- The seizures are becoming more frequent or more severe
- An underlying progressive intracranial disorder has been identified as the cause of the seizures.

Commonly used anti-epileptics in cats are:

- Phenobarbital (3 mg/kg orally q12h), most commonly used (see below)
- Levetiracetam (10–20 mg/kg orally q8h)
- Zonisamide (5–10 mg/kg orally q24h)
- Pregabalin (4–10 mg/kg orally q8–12h).

Phenobarbital is the first choice of many clinicians for cats with seizures; the other agents listed above can be used in addition to phenobarbital or as alternatives but consultation with a specialist is advised.

In dogs, repeated phenobarbital administrations are known to alter estimated steady state serum concentration as a consequence of enzyme induction. This results in the need to increase oral dosage progressively with time in order to maintain steady state therapeutic level. This phenomenon of enzyme evinduction following repeat administration of phenobarbital is negligible in cats. The elimination half-life is stable at around 34–43 hours and therefore drug concentrations of phenobarbital are not expected to decrease in cats receiving long-term therapy without changing dosage.

In cats, monitoring the serum level of phenobarbital is mainly justified shortly after the onset of treatment (10–15 days after starting treatment, when steady state levels are reached, or if seizure control is inadequate). Recommended therapeutic ranges have not been properly defined in cats but are considered to be similar to the recommended range in dogs (20–35 µg/ml). Cats should not be considered as refractory to treatment until serum phenobarbital concentrations reach 35 µg/ml, unless unacceptable side effects persist.

Side effects of phenobarbital in cats include: sedation, ataxia, polyphagia, weight gain, neutropenia, thrombocytopenia, severe cutaneous eruptions and marked lymphadenopathy (pseudolymphoma). Hepatotoxicity, a common side effect in dogs, has not been reported in cats.

The author does not recommend the use of oral bromide in cats due to the high incidence of lower airway side effects in this species – in particular, clinical (coughing and/or dyspnoea) and radiographic signs similar to feline asthma that can be refractory to treatment and even fatal, despite ceasing bromide therapy.

Specialist advice should be sought for management of cases that appear refractory to phenobarbital treatment.

QRG 4.7.1 Emergency management of the seizuring cat
by Laurent Garosi

Systemic stabilization

All cats with status epilepticus (SE) or cluster seizures should be treated as emergencies. Whilst stopping the seizures is the ultimate aim, it is essential to maintain a patent airway, support proper breathing patterns and oxygenation, provide circulatory support, and maintain body temperature (see Chapter 3 for a description of CPR). All these measures are paramount, since the combination of circulatory collapse, organ hypoperfusion, and energy depletion that may occur due to SE can lead to severe, irreversible renal, cardiac and hepatic organ failure.

Stopping seizure activity

1 Place an intravenous catheter if possible (see QRG 4.1.1).

2 Give an intravenous bolus of diazepam (0.5–1.0 mg/kg) or midazolam (0.06–0.3 mg/kg) as first-line emergency therapy. If intravenous access is not available, diazepam can be given rectally and midazolam can be given intramuscularly at same dosage.

3 Obtain a blood sample for an emergency database (see later).

4 If the bolus is successful in stopping seizure activity but additional seizures occur, additional boluses or a continuous rate infusion (CRI) may be administered. CRI of diazepam at 0.5–2 mg/kg/h or midazolam at 0.2 mg/kg/h diluted in 5% dextrose in water (D5W) in a volume corresponding to the maintenance requirements (50 ml/kg/day), is used to maintain a seizure-free state. An infusion pump or syringe driver must be used for accuracy.

WARNING

- Concerns regarding aqueous solubility, formation of deposits and adsorption on to PVC tubing have been raised with diazepam.
- Compatibility should be checked before combining diazepam with any other medication or intravenous fluid, as formation of precipitates is common (e.g. with calcium-containing fluids). **Never administer diazepam if a precipitate forms.**
- If diazepam is used, the administration set should be protected from light by covering it with a bag or bandaging, and changed every 2 hours. Use of midazolam in lieu of diazepam circumvents many of these concerns; however, it is far more expensive. ▶

WARNING *continued*

- Careful monitoring of heart rate, blood pressure and respiratory rates, as well as diligent nursing care, is needed while cats are being treated with diazepam or midazolam infusions, due to their cardiorespiratory depressant effects.

5 Once the cat has been seizure-free for approximately 6 hours, the infusion should be slowly tapered by 25% every 6 hours to avoid potential withdrawal-induced seizure activity, while carefully monitoring for additional seizure activity.

6 If diazepam or midazolam is unsuccessful in stopping seizure activity, other options include phenobarbital and/or propofol:

- Phenobarbital can be used as an initial intravenous bolus dose of 3 mg/kg. The effect is not immediate but can take 15–25 minutes, so overdosing needs to be avoided and its use needs to be considered early in a patient presenting in SE or cluster seizures. Using phenobarbital as an emergency drug is useful when it is the chosen maintenance drug (see main chapter). Phenobarbital can also be used at an intravenous loading dose of 18 mg/kg. However, it is recommended to administer smaller boluses (2–4 mg/kg) to avoid excessive sedation, repeating every 20–30 minutes, to effect but not exceeding 18 mg/kg over 24 hours.
- A CRI of propofol can be considered as an alternative to phenobarbital, or if phenobarbital fails to control the seizures. Propofol is very successful in quickly stopping seizure activity when diazepam has failed to achieve this. An initial intravenous bolus of 1–4 mg/kg can be used to effect, followed by a CRI at 0.1–0.4 mg/kg/min titrated to effect. Once the cat has been seizure-free for approximately 6 hours, the infusion should be slowly tapered, by 25% every 6 hours, to avoid potential withdrawal-induced seizure activity. In addition to causing apnoea, propofol is also a cardiovascular depressant, so this too requires careful monitoring. Propofol is a phenol and thus capable of causing oxidative injury to the cat's erythrocytes, resulting in Heinz body formation and possible haemolytic anaemia, although this is rarely clinically significant following seizure management.

PRACTICAL TIP

Recovery from phenobarbital and propofol anaesthesia may include paddling movements of the limbs, which should not be confused with recurrent seizure activity. Differentiation can be achieved by turning the cat into a different recumbency: motor activity caused by anaesthesia will be expected to stop, while an epileptic seizure cannot be stopped.

7 All the above agents, though useful emergency drugs, cause sedation of varying degrees, which is undesirable. Intravenous levetiracetam is a viable alternative to phenobarbital and/or propofol that does not cause sedation. Side effects have not been noted in cats. Levetiracetam can be administered in 20 mg/kg intravenous boluses. Its intravenous use may be effective for 8 hours, at which time it can be repeated if necessary. Levetiracetam is not a veterinary authorized drug and is expensive, so is unlikely to be on the shelf in most veterinary clinics, though it may be possible to obtain on prescription from a chemist or local hospital if urgent need arises.

Maintaining the cat seizure-free

Once the seizures stop, institution of a maintenance anti-epileptic treatment (phenobarbital 3 mg/kg q12h orally (or i.m. if oral intake is not possible due to excessive sedation)) is critical to prevent seizure recurrence. In a cat already receiving phenobarbital, oral phenobarbital dosage can be increased by 25–30% if serum level is below or in the lower half of the therapeutic range. See main chapter for discussion of longer-term management.

Underlying conditions

Alongside initial management of the seizures, investigations should begin for treatable underlying causes. Initial investigations should include an emergency database (PCV, total solids, blood glucose and electrolytes) and blood pressure assessment. Hypoglycaemia should be treated if severe (blood glucose <3.0 mmol/l) (see QRG 4.5.1). The cat's medical history should be reviewed, including potential toxin exposure and possibility of trauma. Further investigations (see main chapter) are only considered when SE is controlled and the cat is systemically stable.

Sudden-onset blindness

Natasha Mitchell

Sudden-onset blindness is a veterinary emergency. Typically the affected cat is anxious and disorientated, with changes in behaviour such as bumping into things, walking in a crouched position and showing a reluctance to jump. There may also be a change to the appearance of the eyes, such as dilated pupils, tapetal hyper-reflectivity (Figure 4.8.1) or a colour change.

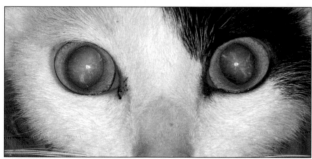

4.8.1 Tapetal hyper-reflectivity and moderately dilated pupils in a young cat with retinal degeneration of unknown cause.

Sudden-onset blindness usually occurs as a result of a systemic condition (see below) that affects both eyes. However, a cat with vision in one eye could become suddenly blind as a result of a primary ocular condition affecting the visual eye.

Cats that become blind gradually adapt very well; the owner may suddenly notice poor vision due to a change of environment and think that the onset was more rapid than it was. The more common causes of *gradual*-onset blindness are summarized in Figure 4.8.2.

- Uveitis: immune-mediated, or secondary to infectious disease, trauma or cataracts
- Glaucoma: secondary to chronic uveitis, trauma or neoplasia
- Cataracts: secondary to chronic uveitis, trauma or *Encephalitozoon cuniculi* infection
- Neoplasia – primary: melanoma; may lead to secondary glaucoma
- Retinal degeneration: e.g. due to taurine deficiency
- Progressive retinal atrophy: inherited retinal degenerations, such as retinal degeneration of the Abyssinian or Somali cat (can also affect other breeds) and rod–cone dysplasia of the Abyssinian and Somali cat

4.8.2 Causes of *gradual*-onset blindness, which may, however, be noticed suddenly.

Causes

A variety of ophthalmic, neurological and systemic diseases can cause sudden-onset vision loss in cats. The more common causes are noted below.

- **Systemic hypertension:** This is the most common cause of blindness in cats (see Chapter 5.18). The hypertensive cat typically presents with sudden-onset blindness and widely dilated pupils, and there may be hyphaema (Figure 4.8.3 and see Chapter 5.19). If the fundus can be seen, there may be multifocal retinal haemorrhages, oedema and/or detachment.

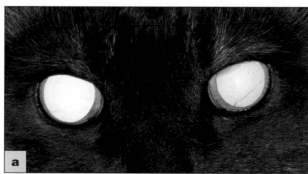

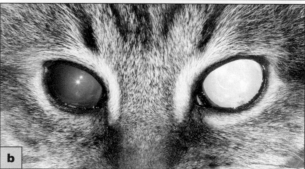

4.8.3 **(a)** Dilated pupils, tapetal hyper-reflectivity in the right eye and a visibly detached retina in the vitreous chamber of the left eye in a hypertensive cat. A fold in the retina can be seen at the dorsal aspect of the left pupil, and the blood vessels within the retina are visible as they are in a forward position, just behind the lens. Vessels are never visible unaided in a normal eye. **(b)** Hyphaema in the right eye, and mydriasis and tapetal hyper-reflectivity in the left eye of a hypertensive cat.

- **Trauma:** Blunt trauma may occur as a result of road traffic accidents. Sharp, penetrating trauma may occur due to cat claw injury, foreign bodies or gunshot pellets (Figure 4.8.4). Trauma can result in globe rupture, retinal detachment, hyphaema, lens luxation or cataract, and may lead to secondary glaucoma or phacoclastic (release of immunogenic lens protein when the lens capsule is damaged) uveitis.
- **Uveitis:** Uveitis is inflammation of the uveal tract, and presents with conjunctival hyperaemia, corneal oedema, keratic precipitates, aqueous flare and miosis (see Chapter 8). Chronic uveitis can lead to cataracts or glaucoma, both of which may cause eventual blindness.
- **Corneal ulceration and endophthalmitis:** Corneal ulcers that are not successfully treated may result in blindness due to corneal scarring or the consequences of severe intraocular inflammation or infection. This may occur with feline herpesvirus-1 (FHV) infection in kittens.
- **Toxic retinal degeneration:** This has been reported after administration of enrofloxacin in cats (Gelatt *et al.*, 2001). Although rare, sudden-onset blindness with mydriasis has been reported after accidental overdose, prolonged treatment or through an apparent idiosyncratic adverse reaction. Blindness can be temporary if the drug is withdrawn quickly but vision can also deteriorate further with time. Retinal degeneration occurs that is not immediately obvious but becomes more noticeable after a few weeks (Figure 4.8.5).
- **Neurological disease:** Central blindness may be caused by inflammatory, neoplastic (e.g. lymphoma, meningioma), or vascular disease anywhere along the afferent arm of the visual pathway. There may be no visible ocular changes, with normal pupillary light reflexes, clear ocular media and normal fundus appearance. Neurological symptoms, such as abnormal behaviour, seizures, circling, incoordination, head tilt, vestibular ataxia or nystagmus, can be suggestive of central blindness.
- **Central anoxia/hypoxia:** Reduced blood or oxygen supply to the visual cortex during general anaesthesia may affect vision temporarily or permanently. If vision does not return in 48–72 hours, the blindness is likely to be permanent. Affected cats have fixed dilated pupils after recovering from anaesthesia and tend to be quite distressed by their sudden blindness. Fortunately, this complication is uncommon.

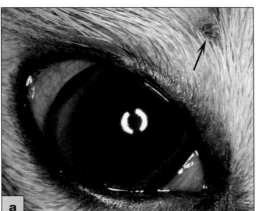
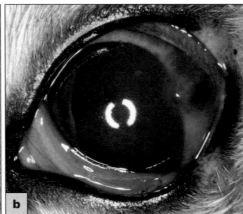
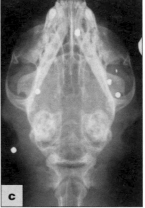

4.8.4 **(a)** The right eye of a cat which went missing for a week and returned blind and lame. There is conjunctival hyperaemia, and hyphaema, and the pupil was quite dilated. There is a small skin wound above the medial canthus (arrow). **(b)** The left eye of the same cat. There is depigmentation and alopecia of the lateral canthus, indicating a healing wound, and conjunctival hyperaemia. The lateral aspect of the cornea has neovascularization around a black corneal wound. The pupil is dilated, and difficult to see in detail because of a diffuse haziness in the anterior chamber caused by resolving hyphaema. There are reflections on the cornea, both medially and laterally, from the hand holding the eyelids open when the photograph was taken. **(c)** A radiograph shows several gunshot pellets; additional pellets were shown on thoracic and abdominal radiographs.

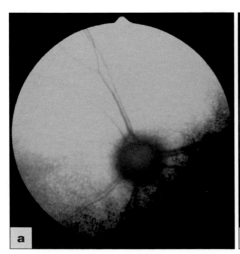
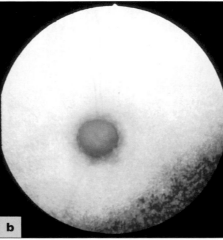

4.8.5 Fundus photographs of a cat that had received 20 mg/kg enrofloxacin orally q24h for 5 days, and presented suddenly blind. **(a)** One week after blindness; the fundus looks relatively normal with some mild tapetal hyper-reflectivity visible dorsal to the optic disc. **(b)** Five weeks later there is much more advanced retinal degeneration, with more pronounced tapetal hyper-reflectivity, very marked retinal blood vessel attenuation, and a very pale optic disc due to the loss of vascularization. (Courtesy of David Gould)

- **Complication of enucleation:** The feline optic nerve is short, and excessive traction or twisting of the globe during enucleation can damage the contralateral optic nerve via the optic chiasm. This can cause blindness in the remaining eye, and thus much care must be taken during surgery (see QRG 8.1).

Assessing the blind cat

The appropriate work-up depends on the presenting signs but includes taking a full history along with a thorough ocular (see QRG 1.3), neurological (see QRG 1.6) and physical examination. This may reveal the cause or may lead to further diagnostic tests being indicated.

- If glaucoma is suspected, the intraocular pressure should be measured by tonometry.
- Ultrasonography should be performed on eyes with hyphaema to assess for retinal detachment or intraocular masses (see Chapter 5.19). If the fundus appears normal, the cat may be referred for an electroretinogram.
- Advanced imaging may be required if neurological disease is suspected (see Chapter 17).

Caring for a blind cat

Visually impaired cats can cope very well and lead happy fulfilled lives. Cats with sudden-onset blindness are initially disorientated and confused, but they usually adapt quickly when provided with a safe and predictable environment. They are able to compensate with their other senses, and quickly become familiar with the layout of the home.

When to refer

Given the wide range of causes of sudden-onset blindness, if the cause (e.g. systemic hypertension) is not readily apparent, rapid referral is recommended as early intervention can reverse vision loss in some cases.

References and further reading

Gelatt KN, Van Der Woerdt A, Ketring KL et al. (2001) Enrofloxacin-associated retinal degeneration in cats. *Veterinary Ophthalmology* **4**, 99–106
Mitchell N (2008) *Caring for a Blind Cat*. Cat Professional, UK

- **Maintain body temperature:** Seizure activity may cause hyperthermia. In severe cases (>41°C) initial cooling may be required but once seizures are controlled warming measures are likely to be required.
- **Intravenous lipid emulsion therapy:** If available, use of an intravenous lipid emulsion may have benefit in improving recovery rates and survival rates. There are currently very few published data regarding this treatment option but anecdotally it holds great promise, and extrapolation from its use in humans and experimentally suggests it to be both safe and effective. It appears that infusion of the lipid emulsion helps to bind lipophilic toxins such as permethrin, reducing their toxic effect until they are cleared from the circulation.
  - The currently recommended dosing protocol is to use a 20% lipid emulsion (e.g. Intralipid). This can be administered through a standard peripheral intravenous cannula but should not be given mixed with any other fluids or drugs – placement of a separate cannula is therefore recommended.
  - Administer an initial bolus of 1.5 ml/kg over 5–15 minutes, followed by an infusion of 0.25 ml/kg/min for 1–2 hours.
  - If signs of toxicity return after a few hours a blood sample should be assessed for visible evidence of lipaemia. If lipaemia has resolved a repeat dose of lipid emulsion can be administered.
  - The lipid emulsion is a good medium for bacterial growth. Strict aseptic technique is required during cannula placement and administration of the emulsion. Unused emulsion must be discarded within 24 hours of opening.
- **Supportive care**: Intravenous fluids and good nursing care are required until seizures have abated and the cat has recovered a normal appetite. In severe cases assisted feeding may be required.

Prognosis

In most cases the prognosis is good as long as the problem is recognized early and treated aggressively. Seizures and body tremors usually resolve within 48–72 hours but residual ear tremors and facial twitching may persist for up to a week.

Ethylene glycol

Ethylene glycol is a common component of antifreeze. It is metabolized to highly oxidative byproducts that are toxic to cats and can cause:

- Metabolic acidosis
- Renal tubular necrosis
- Calcium oxalate nephroliths and uroliths.

Accidental ingestion of even small amounts, such as from grooming contaminated fur, can be damaging. Ethylene glycol has a sweet innocuous flavour that is easily disguised in food and it has been implicated in a number of cases of malicious poisoning of cats.

Clinical signs

- Immediate signs of toxicity include acute-onset vomiting and a dull demeanour.
- Within 1 hour signs progress to include ataxia, hyperpnoea, tachycardia, polyuria, polydipsia and depression.
- Within 12–24 hours metabolic acidosis develops, and signs include dehydration, vomiting, uraemia and haematuria. Renomegaly may be palpable. Oxalate crystals may be seen in the urine (see QRG 4.11.3)
- Within 1–3 days oliguric acute kidney injury (AKI) develops. Signs include vomiting, anorexia, depression, hypothermia and eventually coma.

The severity of signs is dose-dependent. If only a small quantity of ethylene glycol has been ingested the immediate signs of toxicity may resolve without treatment, but oliguric AKI may still develop a few days later.

Diagnosis

An initial presumptive diagnosis is based on clinical signs and known or suspected contact with the toxin. Early detection of ethylene glycol in the plasma can also be achieved using commercially available diagnostic test strips. Changes in serum biochemistry and urinalysis develop later in the course of disease, by which time the window of opportunity for effective treatment will have passed.

Treatment

Absorption of ethylene glycol and metabolism to toxic byproducts is very rapid. **Immediate treatment (within 3 hours of ingestion) is required to try to prevent fatal AKI.**

- **Reduce further absorption:** Gastrointestinal absorption of ethylene glycol is very rapid. If the cat is presented within 3 hours of ingesting ethylene glycol it may be helpful to induce vomiting and administer activated charcoal (see Figure 4.9.3), but in most cases this will no longer be helpful.
- **Fluid therapy:** Aggressive use of intravenous fluids will help to counter the acute kidney injury and metabolic acidosis. Additional use of sodium bicarbonate may be required to counter metabolic acidosis but this is not without risk, and specialist advice should be sought (see also *BSAVA Manual of Canine and Feline Emergency and Critical Care*).
- **Fomepizole** (4-methylpyrazole) is an effective antidote if given within 3 hours of ingestion of ethylene glycol. The required dose is higher in cats than in dogs: 125 mg/kg initially, then 31.25 mg/kg at 12, 24, and 36 hours, has been effective in preventing AKI. Administer by slow intravenous injection, over 15–20 minutes. Heavy sedation may occur, so close monitoring and supportive treatment are required. The sedative effect may persist for around 12 hours after ceasing treatment.
- **Ethanol:** If fomepizole is not available or is unaffordable, an intravenous infusion of ethanol can be started within the first 3 hours after intoxication to divert alcohol dehydrogenase from metabolizing ethylene glycol to its toxic byproducts. However, ethanol infusion may increase acidosis and worsen CNS depression.

- For dilute ethanol solutions (5–7%; 50–70 mg/ml) give 600 mg/kg ethanol i.v. over 15–20 minutes then use a constant rate infusion of 100 mg/kg/h for 36–48 hours.
- If using a 20% ethanol solution (200 mg/ml), give 5.0 ml/kg i.v. over 15–20 minutes, then repeat the dose q6h for five treatments, then q8h for four treatments.
- **Monitor urine output** to identify anuria or oliguria.

Prognosis

The damage caused by ethylene glycol is dose-dependent but the prognosis is guarded at best. Onset of irreversible renal damage is rapid; early aggressive treatment is required but may not be successful in preventing this. If treatment is not started within 3 hours of ingestion and/or anuric AKI develops, the cat is very unlikely to survive and euthanasia should be considered.

Non-steroidal anti-inflammatory drugs

Cats are vulnerable to adverse effects from overdosing or inappropriate use of NSAIDs (see Chapter 3 for appropriate drug use). The major adverse effects are gastric ulceration and AKI, which is a particular risk in cats with low renal perfusion, for example due to dehydration or hypotension. Therefore:

- NSAIDs should only be used in metabolically healthy cats
- Precautions should be taken to maintain hydration at all times, and to maintain blood pressure, particularly during anaesthesia
- Oral preparations should be given with food and must be withheld if the cat is inappetent.

Clinical signs of gastric ulceration include inappetence, depression, anterior abdominal pain and vomiting. Haematemesis may occur but is not an invariable sign. If presented early after accidental overdose, initial treatment is with induction of vomiting and administration of activated charcoal (see Figure 4.9.3). Thereafter, treatment is with antacids (cimetidine, ranitidine, famotidine or omeprazole) and sucralfate. Misoprostol (a prostaglandin analogue), if available, at a dose of 2–5 µg/kg orally q8h may also be useful in preventing these adverse effects of NSAID overdose, but should not be used in pregnant animals nor handled by personnel who may be pregnant.

AKI is mostly associated with subcutaneous injection of NSAIDs in cats with renal compromise or prior to general anaesthesia. Signs develop within 24–48 hours and, if not treated aggressively, damage may progress and lead to irreversible chronic kidney disease. Treatment is as for AKI due to lily ingestion (see earlier).

Paracetamol

Cats are relatively deficient in the enzyme glucuronyl transferase, which is required for metabolism of paracetamol. **The toxic dose in cats is approximately 50 mg/kg and toxicity can result from a single dose.**

Clinical signs

- Clinical signs include weakness, dullness, inappetence, hypersalivation, vomiting, facial oedema, tachypnoea and tachycardia.
- Pallor with cyanosis and/or muddy brown mucous membranes develops within 1–4 hours. Blood has a characteristic brown colour (Figure 4.9.4) due to methaemoglobinaemia. There may be urine discoloration due to methaemoglobinuria.
- Within 12–24 hours there is increased formation of Heinz bodies in red blood cells (see QRG 5.4.2), leading to haemolytic anaemia that may persist for up to 7 days.
- Liver failure develops within days, evidenced by increases in serum ALT, ALP and bile acids.

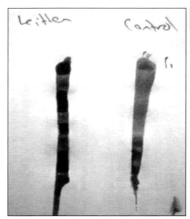

4.9.4

Paracetamol toxicity causes brown discoloration of the blood, due to methaemoglobinaemia. (© Martha Cannon)

Treatment

The aims of treatment are: to replenish glutathione; to convert methaemoglobin back to haemoglobin; and to prevent or treat hepatic necrosis.

- **Decontamination:** If the cat is presented within 2–3 hours of ingestion, induce vomiting and administer activated charcoal (see Figure 4.9.3).
- **Acetylcysteine** increases synthesis and availability of glutathione.
  - A 5% solution of acetylcysteine is given orally at an initial loading dose of 140 mg/kg and then at 70 mg/kg q4h for three to five treatments and for as long as visual evidence of methaemoglobinaemia persists.
  - Intravenous use may be necessary in severe cases; a bacteriostatic filter should be used during administration.
- **Cimetidine** inhibits cytochrome P450, limiting the metabolism of paracetamol into its toxic metabolites.
  - Dose: 5–10 mg/kg orally, i.m. or i.v. q6–8h.
  - **NB:** Ranitidine and famotidine do not have this effect.
- **Vitamin C** may help to reduce methaemoglobin back to haemoglobin.
  - Dose: 30 mg/kg q6–12h orally or i.v.
- **S-Adenosylmethionine** has been shown experimentally to be hepatoprotective when given prior to a single dose of paracetamol. It is safe to use in cats and may provide some extra benefit when given in addition to the treatments outlined above.
- **NB:** Methylene Blue is **not** safe for use in cats and should **not** be used.

1. Assess the respiratory rate and rhythm, and address any dyspnoea present (see Chapter 4.2).
2. Perform a neurological examination prior to anaesthetizing and manipulating patients for multiple radiographic views. If a spinal injury is suspected, the patient should be strapped to a board in lateral recumbency (a regular kitchen chopping board works well for cats) and lateral radiographs taken before the patient is rolled into dorsal or sternal recumbency. Palpate the musculoskeletal system carefully for swelling, crepitus and instability.
3. Take radiographs of injured limbs (lateral and craniocaudal projections), making sure to include the joint both proximal and distal to a site of suspected fracture. It is not uncommon for the hip joint to be luxated on the same side as a femoral or tibial fracture, for instance.
4. Radiograph the pelvis and evaluate the sacroiliac joints in both the lateral and dorsoventral projection.
5. Take lateral and dorsoventral radiographs of the thorax for pulmonary contusion (Figure 4.10.1), pneumothorax or diaphragmatic rupture. Thoracic wall injuries can also occur, but because the cat's chest wall is so compliant, intrathoracic injuries tend to occur earlier and to be more severe than rib or sternal fractures.

Uroabdomen

Uroabdomen is an emergency, requiring quick diagnosis and treatment. Causes of uroabdomen include:

- Rupture of the kidney
- Rupture of the ureter
- Bladder rupture
- Urethral rupture.

The most likely cause of uroabdomen in a cat that has suffered blunt abdominal trauma is rupture of the urinary bladder. Bladder rupture can also be caused by trauma resulting from abdominal palpation of an abnormal bladder, and prolonged uncorrected urethral obstruction (see QRG 4.11.2).

The cat must be quickly diagnosed by monitoring urine output (as this will be <1–2 ml/kg/h), serum biochemistry (elevated urea, creatinine, potassium concentrations), imaging (abdominal radiography may reveal loss of serosal detail and/or absence of urinary bladder, and abdominal ultrasonography may reveal an effusion and/or absence of the bladder) and abdominocentesis (see QRG 5.1.1). A urinary contrast study can be performed to delineate the level of urine leakage (see QRG 5.21.1). A water-soluble iodinated contrast agent suitable for intravenous injection (e.g. iohexol) should be used, due to the potential for leakage into the peritoneal cavity. Chapter 5.1 gives further details on uroabdomen.

It is important to stabilize the cat as much as possible before surgery for bladder rupture repair is undertaken, to minimize the risks of anaesthesia; fluid therapy should be administered for the azotaemia and the hyperkalaemia should be corrected (see QRG 4.11.1). Additionally, placement of a urethral catheter before surgery can be helpful in decreasing further leakage of urine into the abdomen. Therapeutic abdominocentesis (see QRG 5.1.1) should be

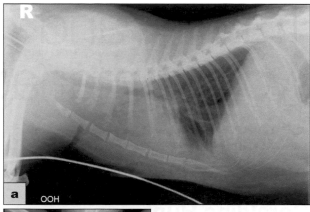

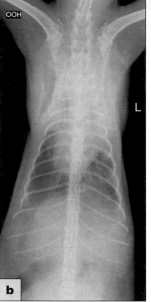

4.10.1 Lateral and dorsoventral radiographs of the thorax of a 4-year-old cat with tachypnoea 24 hours after a road traffic accident. **(a)** A small volume of pleural fluid is present, most evident caudoventrally. Air bronchograms extend into the cranial lung lobes indicating consolidation – essentially an alveolar infiltrate that can reflect pulmonary haemorrhage (such as contusion due to trauma) or pulmonary oedema, neoplasia or pneumonia. Some subcutaneous gas is evident over the cranial thorax. The diaphragmatic line appears to be intact. No skeletal injuries are evident. **(b)** There is consolidation of the right and left cranial lung lobes, and small volumes of pleural fluid bilaterally. A large pocket of subcutaneous gas is superimposed over the right scapula. Suspected pulmonary contusions and pleural effusion secondary to trauma were diagnosed. Treatment included oxygen therapy, cage rest and analgesia (methadone in this case). (Courtesy of Langford Veterinary Services, University of Bristol)

performed to remove as much urine from the abdomen as possible. Note that some small bladder defects can heal with conservative management only (i.e. without surgical repair), which may be a consideration if finances are limited. Repeat urinary contrast radiography can be performed after a few days of conservative management, to assess whether the defect has healed.

Animal attack

Injuries may range from a few bite wounds, leading to cellulitis and abscess formation, to major multi-trauma with penetration of body cavities, widespread devitalization of soft tissues and fractures. Each case must be carefully evaluated in its own right.

Bite wounds from dogs and other carnivores often produce small skin wounds, with much more severe injury to the underlying soft tissues as a result of the canine teeth raking the underlying tissues. This may result in severe damage to the thoracic wall, puncture of intra-abdominal organs, or tearing of musculature. Damage may often be particularly severe around the rump, thighs and inguinal area if the cat was trying to escape at the time it was being mauled. Initial management should focus on emergency stabilization and pain relief.

1. Palpate pulses in each limb to assess whether the major arteries have been disrupted due to trauma or thrombosis. If Doppler is available, this could also be used to assess blood flow (see QRG 5.18.1). If circulation to the limb is compromised, the limb and patient should be closely monitored. Emergency amputation should be considered if signs of sepsis appear (e.g. bradycardia or tachycardia, hypothermia, hypotension not responding to fluid administration) due to tissue necrosis.
2. Assess the integrity of the abdominal wall and the bladder by palpation (plus imaging). Is an abdominal rupture or ruptured bladder present? See QRGs 4.10.1 and 4.10.2 for repair of abdominal and bladder ruptures.
3. Take lateral and dorsoventral radiographic views of the thorax, looking for abnormalities such as pneumothorax, haemothorax or diaphragmatic rupture. Perform abdominal ultrasonography if injuries have been sustained to that area, looking for peritoneal fluid accumulation and integrity of the bladder.
4. Once the patient has been stabilized and assessed, musculoskeletal injuries should be evaluated with further radiographs. It can be difficult to obtain a good assessment of the degree of muscular injury in a non-ambulatory patient. The limbs and torso should be palpated and joint stability assessed.
5. Clean open wounds and either close them or apply absorbent, wet-to-dry bandages (see Wound management, below). Assess sites that have sustained severe injuries at least twice daily for evidence of necrosis or infection, such as purulent discharge, grey or black tissues or foul smell. Evaluate the cat regularly for signs of impending sepsis, (e.g. bradycardia or tachycardia, hypothermia, poor peripheral pulses); the presence of a large amount of necrosing muscle can quickly lead to abscess formation or even gangrene. Severely traumatized hindlimbs will sometimes need to be amputated due to progressive signs of infection or devitalization, and this may not become apparent until some days after the injury. Immediate placement of drains in damaged, but not yet infected, sites is controversial. This author prefers to monitor the area and be prepared for immediate exploration, debridement or drainage when it becomes obvious which tissue is likely to survive and which is becoming necrotic.
6. Give a broad-spectrum antibiotic with activity against oral flora (such as amoxicillin/clavulanate), as the wound sites will be contaminated at the time of presentation and the risk of infection is high.

Falling from a height

Classic injuries associated with 'high-rise syndrome' include pulmonary contusion (see Figure 4.10.1), pneumothorax, traumatic cleft palate and facial fractures, and other orthopaedic injuries. Blunt-force trauma involves a large portion of the body, with particular focus on the sternum, muzzle and limbs, if the cat falls in an upright position. Bladder rupture is also possible (see QRG 4.10.2 for repair). The basic principles of emergency stabilization and assessment are similar to those described above. See Chapter 16 for orthopaedic treatment.

Penetrating injuries

A case can always be made for immediate surgical exploration following penetrating injury to a body cavity. Minimally invasive surgery (laparoscopy) has made this simpler and with less impact for human patients but is rarely feasible in first-opinion small animal practice.

Practically speaking, many penetrating injuries do not damage the internal viscera and patients can recover with conservative management of rest with appropriate analgesia. Air pellets are commonly seen but do not need to be removed unless they are obviously associated with an abscess or have penetrated the lumen of a structure such as the nasal cavity or bladder.

A patient with a projectile injury (e.g. gunshot wound) to the thorax should at least have thoracic radiography performed. If pleural fluid or air is minimal, the patient responds to resuscitative attempts and its condition remains stable, thoracic exploration is probably not needed. The exception is a dog bite injury (see above), where exploration, debridement and stabilization of the thoracic wall is usually indicated due to the high likelihood of severe subcutaneous trauma.

Projectile (gunshot) injuries to the abdomen should undergo surgical exploration, as it is likely that the gastrointestinal tract has been perforated; quick diagnosis and closure is then highly likely to eliminate the risk of septic peritonitis. Referral to a specialist should be considered early in the patient's management if the attending veterinarian is not an experienced surgeon.

Decision-making in wound management

Wounds come in many shapes and sizes and, depending on their aetiology, require different treatment. The most important factors to consider when deciding how to manage a given wound are:

- Is the wound clean, contaminated or infected?
- Does it contain necrotic tissue or debris that will need to be debrided over the coming days?
- Does it communicate with a body cavity or joint?
- Does it contain healthy granulation tissue that is trying to contract?
- Is eventual closure likely to require migration of epithelium across granulation tissue that has covered a wound bed?
- Is motion or tension putting a lot of strain on the healing tissues?

More information on 'open' and 'closed' wound management can be found in the *BSAVA Manual of Canine and Feline Wound Management and Reconstruction*.

There are thousands of products available to assist with management of wounds in their various stages; the most critical decision that must be made prior to treatment is therefore, 'What is the goal of wound management at this point?'. Some wounds require simple management; others require a sequence of management techniques, dictated by the various stages of wound healing.

- **Is the wound actively bleeding?**
  - Place an absorbent pressure bandage (such as a combined cotton and gauze dressing) or perform surgical haemostasis.
  - It may be necessary to cauterize or ligate bleeding vessels with absorbable suture material.
- **Is the wound a simple laceration?**
  - Flush the wound with copious amounts of sterile saline and close routinely.
  - Do not place a drain unless obvious infection is present.
- **Is the wound penetrating a body cavity?**
  - Explore the wound, flush and debride as indicated.
  - Close the wound to restore integrity of the body cavity.
    - Wounds involving joints may be treated using open wound management, as long as further contamination of the joint is avoided. These wounds will often require some form of external stabilization, as the support structures around the joint have probably been compromised. External skeletal fixators are often helpful in that they stabilize the region but still allow for open wound management.
  - Seeking the advice of an experienced surgeon is recommended.
- **Does the wound contain potentially devitalized tissue and debris?**
  - These wounds are usually highly effusive, so use a dressing capable of absorbing moisture. A wet-to-dry dressing is recommended (although alginates, sugar or vacuum-assisted wound closure are also effective). A wet-to-dry dressing is created by soaking a regular absorbent dressing with sterile saline or chlorhexidine diluted in saline (according to the manufacturer's instructions) and allowing it to dry out slowly.
  - Check the wound every 12–24 hours and debride necrotic tissue or debris as indicated (Figures 4.10.2 to 4.10.5).
- **Does the wound mainly comprise healthy granulation tissue?** (See Figure 4.10.6)
  - Either close primarily, or use a dressing designed to facilitate granulation tissue growth, contraction and epithelialization. Honey, silver-impregnated dressings, silver sulfadiazine ointment and absorbent hydrocellular foam dressings (Figure 4.10.7) are all equally effective.
  - Dressing changes can take place every 48 hours.

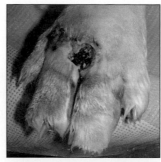

4.10.2 This actively necrotic wound with purulent discharge should be treated as an open wound. The initial goal is debridement. A dressing (gauze squares or other absorbent material) is applied and allowed to dry out, so that dead tissue will be removed when the inner layer of the dressing is changed.

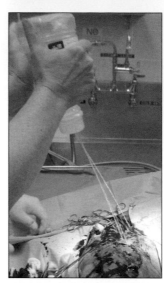

4.10.3 Debridement using a saline jet. Purulent discharge, tissue debris and other contaminants are removed by high-pressure saline jets, created in this case by fenestrating the lid of a saline bottle with a 22 G needle. Alternatively, a syringe can be filled with saline which is then injected through a 22 G needle.

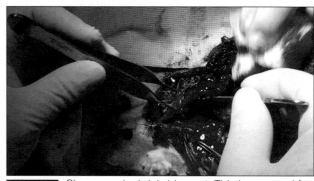

4.10.4 Sharp surgical debridement. This is reserved for cases where it is obvious which tissues will survive and which are necrotic. Debridement should be performed with scissors or a scalpel, the aim being to sharply cut back necrotic or infected tissue until healthy, bleeding tissue is reached. Scraping is not appropriate, as it damages otherwise healthy tissue.

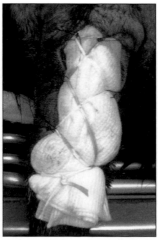

4.10.5 A tie-over dressing for an effusive wound (shown here on a dog but a similar approach is used for a cat). Sutures of 3.5 metric (0 USP) polypropylene are placed in the skin surrounding the wound. Nylon tape is passed through these anchoring sutures and tied over an absorbent dressing to hold it in place. The dressing is changed every 12–24 hours, depending on how quickly strikethrough of wound exudate is noticed on the exterior.

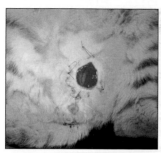

4.10.6 This wound has been treated with a tie-over wet-to-dry dressing. The wound has passed its inflammatory phase and is now less effusive; it is thus ready for a less aggressive form of wound management, such as a non-adherent dressing using honey or paraffin gauze.

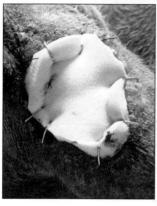

4.10.7 A polyurethane foam dressing has been stapled to the wound edges to hold it in place (shown here on a dog). This is appropriate for granulating wounds with a small amount of discharge, where the main aim is to keep the wound moist while preventing environmental contamination and self-trauma. This type of dressing need only be changed every 72 hours.

■ **Is epithelium trying to cross the wound bed?**
  • This is usually only the case for partial-thickness burns, or full-thickness burns treated with artificial skin substitutes.
  • Use an occlusive dressing that maintains sterility.
  • Wounds like this are rare in small animal practice and advice from a specialist with experience in burn wounds should be sought.
■ **Is this a chronic healing wound with contracting granulation tissue?**
  • Wound management may simply consist of leaving the wound open, cleaning once daily with dilute saline solution and allowing contraction to occur. This is a practical solution for some patients and clients for whom regular bandage changes are not feasible for financial or practical reasons.

Antibiotics and antiseptics

Antibiotics are indicated perioperatively for contaminated wounds or those involving joints or body cavities. Systemic antibiotics active against normal skin and oral flora (for bite wounds) should be continued in the patient with actively necrosing or obviously infected wounds. The most common example is amoxicillin/clavulanate (12–20 mg/kg orally q8–12h). Systemic antibiotics are not indicated for patients with healthy granulation tissue, as the main issue is surface contamination rather than tissue infection. In these patients, the veterinary surgeon may choose to apply silver sulfadiazine lotion to the dressing itself to reduce bacterial growth between dressing changes.

Topical management of microbial contamination includes the use of bactericidal or bacteriostatic products such as silver, honey or antimicrobial creams such as silver sulfadiazine. Chlorhexidine diluted in saline according to the manufacturer's instructions (usually diluted to 0.01% or 1:10,000) can be used to soak dressings (thereby creating a wet-to-dry dressing) and will reduce contamination with *Pseudomonas*.

It is important to remember that all antibiotic and antiseptic products have a potential to delay wound healing. A clear indication of microbial contamination, such as smell or discoloration, must therefore be present each time the dressing is changed, before the decision is made to use such products.

> **PRACTICAL TIP**
>
> Owners of pets with complex or necrotic wounds must always be warned that the wound management process can be lengthy and expensive, and will go on for as long as the wound takes to heal. This can take some weeks, and there is always a chance that reconstructive surgery may be required at the end.

General health of the patient

It is important to make sure the patient is systemically healthy. Other systemic problems that might interfere with wound healing, such as hyperadrenocorticism, diabetes mellitus or renal disease, should be addressed. It should also be ensured that the patient is receiving adequate nutrition, especially in the first few days after injury.

Non-healing wounds

If wound healing is slower than expected, or fails, despite adequate initial management, the following possible causes of non-healing wounds should be considered:

■ Infection with:
  • *Nocardia* or *Actinomyces*
  • Mycobacterial species
  • Resistant bacteria, e.g. L-form bacteria (wall-less forms of bacteria; these usually respond to doxycycline treatment), meticillin-resistant *Staphylococcus aureus* (MRSA)
  • Retroviruses (FeLV and/or FIV)
  • Fungi, e.g. dermatophytosis, sporotrichosis (in parts of the world where this is prevalent)
■ Neoplastic disease, e.g. squamous cell carcinoma, fibrosarcoma
■ Foreign bodies.

It is advisable to contact a diagnostic laboratory and/or a specialist for advice on sample requirements for further diagnostics and management. Samples for culture and sensitivity are likely to be required at an early stage of diagnostic investigation, and biopsy (for histopathology and culture) may be required if initial diagnostic investigation is unrewarding.

Further reading

Williams J and Moores A (2009) *BSAVA Manual of Canine and Feline Wound Management and Reconstruction*, 2nd edn. BSAVA Publications, Gloucester

QRG 4.10.1 Abdominal rupture and hernia management

by Geraldine Hunt

Abdominal ruptures may occur at any location around the abdomen, depending on the traumatic event. Herniation of viscera may occur secondary to abdominal rupture.

Terminology

A true hernia contains three main components: the hernia contents (viscera); the hernial ring (tissues surrounding the defect through which the viscera has herniated); and a hernial sac (thickened peritoneum covering the herniated viscera). In the case of herniation following trauma, the hernial sac is absent because the peritoneum is usually torn at the time of rupture. It is still helpful to assess the visceral contents and the defect through which they have exited the abdomen to aid the decision-making as to whether to perform surgery, and the local tissues available for repair.

- The term 'hernial ring' should only be applied to a defect caused by non-traumatic processes where the abdominal viscera exit the abdomen within a covering of peritoneum (the hernial sac), e.g. umbilical hernia.
- The term 'rupture' is more appropriate than hernia for the traumatic events seen commonly in small animal practice, whereby viscera exit the abdomen through a traumatic rent in the body wall or the diaphragm, e.g. diaphragmatic rupture, abdominal rupture. The act of viscera moving out of the abdomen through an abnormal orifice is nonetheless termed 'herniation'.
- For the purposes of this QRG, the term hernia will be used to describe the entire lesion, including herniated organs, and the term rupture will be used to describe a traumatic defect in the abdominal wall. If there is no clinical evidence to suggest that the defect was traumatic in origin, the term hernia will be used.

Injuries that can result in abdominal rupture

- Blunt-force trauma tends to result in muscles being pulled from skeletal attachments, e.g. separation of the dorsal abdominal musculature from its epaxial attachments to the spine; prepubic rupture and separation of the rectus abdominus muscles from the pubis; or radial tearing of the diaphragm from its costal attachments.

- Patients with pelvic trauma may experience herniation between the fractured bones of the ilium or pubis, and these fractures can sometimes be accompanied by trauma to the abdominal viscera. Avulsion of the ileum from the ileocolic junction, or of the ureters from the renal pelvis or bladder can be encountered. Colonic or urethral perforation may be present in cases with pelvic fractures.
- Penetrating injuries to the abdomen (e.g. dog bites) may result in an abdominal wall defect anywhere and should be evaluated on a case-by-case basis.

Assessing the defect

The size of the abdominal wall deficit cannot be determined by the amount of herniated viscera, as the entire small intestine is capable of herniating through a 1 cm diameter defect over a period of time. Abdominal ultrasonography can be useful in determining what organs have herniated through an abdominal rupture, and may assist with the diagnosis of some intra-abdominal trauma, but it is not as specific as surgical exploration. Advice from a specialist can be sought regarding the investigation and management, and possible referral, of cats where the extent of an injury is not clear and/or techniques such as ultrasonography are not readily available for thorough investigation.

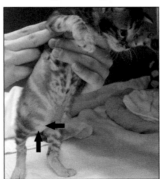

Kitten with abdominal wall rupture (arrows) and herniated bowel identified by ultrasonography. This otherwise healthy kitten presented for evaluation of a traumatic abdominal rupture. There was no evidence of damage to the abdominal viscera but it was considered an emergency due to the large amount of viscera present within the hernia and an inability to reduce it, suggesting a very small rupture.

Traumatic hernias

Penetrating injury to the abdomen is always considered an indication for surgical exploration.

Patients experiencing blunt-force trauma to the abdomen should be evaluated for:

- Bladder rupture – by palpation, radiography, ultrasonography, abdominocentesis (see QRG 5.1.1), urinary tract contrast studies (see QRG 5.21.1)
- Diaphragmatic rupture – by thoracic auscultation and radiography, and ultrasonography
- Orthopaedic injuries – by radiography.
- If none of these is found, patients may be treated conservatively, although complete evaluation of the abdominal viscera may not be possible without abdominal exploration. Surgical exploration is indicated if the patient remains haemodynamically unstable, deteriorates again after initial stabilization, or develops an abdominal effusion.

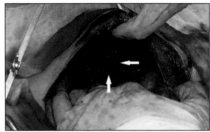

Large dorsal hernia (arrowed) following rupture of the left cranial abdominal wall viewed from within the abdomen. (The patient's head is to the left.) This hernia could only be properly evaluated with an exploratory laparotomy, followed by dissection dorsally between the ventral skin incision and the body wall, revealing its true extent.

Non-traumatic hernias

Non-traumatic hernias should be classified as reducible or non-reducible, and the presence of intestines, spleen or other organs should be assessed using ultrasonography or radiography. Palpation may be misleading, as indurated fat can feel like intestinal loops. Surgery is always indicated for a non-reducible hernia containing intestinal loops, due to the risk of strangulation.

A reducible hernia containing fat is less urgent, and will often only cause aesthetic problems. However, large long-standing reducible hernias, which may cause the overlying skin to stretch and ulcerate, with a risk of eventration, should also be repaired.

Considerations regarding timing of surgery

- A large abdominal wall defect may be less of a surgical emergency than a small defect, as incarceration and ▶

QRG 4.10.1 *continued*

strangulation of the hernia contents may be more likely with a small hernial ring.

- Diaphragmatic rupture should be treated as soon as the patient has been appropriately stabilized and anaesthesia can be performed safely. Diaphragmatic rupture repair is not performed routinely in first-opinion practice (referral to a specialist can be considered), unless there are veterinary surgeons within the practice who are experienced with both soft tissue surgery and anaesthesia in such cases.
- With other traumatic ruptures, in which there is no evidence of injury to the abdominal viscera, there can be some benefit to delaying the repair. Torn abdominal musculature is usually bruised and friable, and it can be difficult to determine whether it is viable. Traumatized muscle with marginal vascularity will not hold sutures well and dehiscence is likely. Waiting 2–3 days for the tissues to either recover their vascularity (become pink again) or declare themselves as necrotic (pale/blackened) may result in a more secure repair with better chance of healing.

Preparations for surgery

- Think about how you will anchor sutures if the muscle has been pulled away from a bony attachment. Have a pin and wire set or drill available to make anchor holes in bone. If there is a large muscle defect, it may be necessary to use a local muscle flap or prosthetic mesh to close the defect, and advice from a specialist or experienced colleague is advisable.
- Familiarize yourself with local anatomy, as abdominal ruptures occurring around the natural hiatuses from the abdomen (inguinal ring, femoral triangle, oesophageal hiatus) will contain neurovascular structures that must be preserved when closing the defect. Repair of a dorsal body wall defect involves reattachment of the abdominal muscles to the epaxial muscles around the spine.
- Ensure you have the equipment and experience to perform artificial or manual ventilation if the thoracic cavity is opened.

Equipment

- Atraumatic forceps
- Metzenbaum scissors

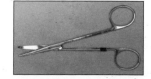

- Abdominal retractors (e.g. baby Balfour retractors)

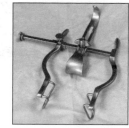

- Kirschner wire set and chuck for drilling bone tunnels in pubis if appropriate

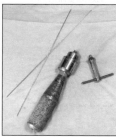

- Malleable retractor for retracting viscera
- 3 and 2 metric (2/0 and 3/0 USP) polydioxanone suture material

Procedure

1 Prepare the patient for a full exploratory laparotomy (from mid-sternum to pubis). Extend the clip and skin preparation down the affected side of the abdomen in case it is necessary to use a dual approach, where a lateral skin incision is also made to approach the rupture from both its external and peritoneal aspects.

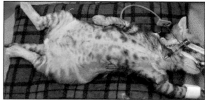

Kitten being prepared for hernia repair. A jugular catheter (optional; usually performed in specialist centres only) has been inserted to allow fluid administration intraoperatively due to the kitten's small size; alternatively, the intraosseous route (using the trochanteric fossa of the proximal femur) can be used if cephalic vein cannulation is not possible.

2 Identify the hernial ring and gently retract the viscera from the hernia. This may necessitate enlargement of the incision with scissors (not shown).

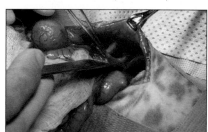

The right (at top) linea alba is being retracted using atraumatic Babcock forceps. DeBakey forceps are being used to manipulate the delicate muscle of the rupture in the abdominal wall and a ribbon (malleable) retractor is being used to gently retract the viscera. (The kitten's head is to the right.)

3 Close the rupture with single interrupted sutures of 3 or 2 metric (2/0 or 3/0 USP) monofilament absorbable material. Secure bites of muscle and fascia should be taken, avoiding retroperitoneal structures such as the ureters and deep circumflex iliac arteries (paired structures that arise from the caudal aorta and travel laterally and into the caudal abdominal wall just cranial to the ilium).

In general, the best philosophy for repair of hernias or ruptures is to coax the tissues to come together and stabilize them in a way that best assists healing. There has been much debate about the type of suture material that should be used. Some surgeons believe that using a highly inflammatory suture such as gut would strengthen the repair. Others recommend using a non-absorbable suture as it maintains its strength for a long time. This author believes that the type of suture material is of little importance in the long term as the success or otherwise of repair will depend on whether the tissues heal back together. Monofilament absorbable sutures of 3 or 2 metric (2/0 or 3/0 USP) are appropriate for cats. A 3 metric (2/0) suture might be used to re-attach muscle to bone but is much stiffer and stronger than required for direct muscle-to-muscle apposition.

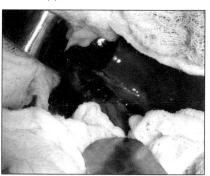

Rupture closed with single interrupted sutures.

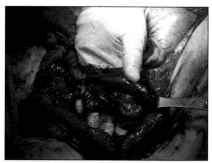

Large dorsal hernia. The linea alba incision is dorsal and the surgeon has slipped their fingers down along the outside of the abdominal wall and in through the traumatic defect in the body wall. This rupture should be repaired in layers. The internal layer (transversus abdominus muscle) should be sutured to the ventral muscles of the spine without impinging on the retroperitoneal structures such as the ureter. The internal and external abdominal oblique muscles should be sutured to the lateral epaxial (spinal) muscles and the lumbar fascia.

QRG 4.10.2 Bladder rupture repair
by Geraldine Hunt

See section on Uroabdomen in main chapter for further information on stabilization of a patient with uroabdomen before undertaking bladder rupture repair.

Equipment

- Basic surgical kit
- 3 Fr urinary catheter of any type
- 500 ml sterile saline
- 20 ml syringe and 25 G needle
- Delicate forceps (e.g. DeBakey)
- Laparotomy sponges
- Surgical suction

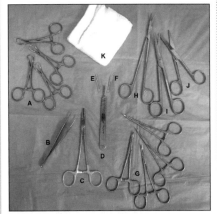

Basic surgical kit. A = towel clamps; B = Brown–Adson thumb forceps; C = needle-holders; D = No. 3 scalpel handle; E = No. 15 scalpel blade; F = No. 10 scalpel blade; G = mosquito forceps; H = Metzenbaum scissors; I = Mayo scissors; J = Blunt–sharp suture scissors; K = gauze surgical swabs.

Patient preparation

Prepare the cat for a ventral midline laparotomy and place a urethral catheter if possible when placement has not already been required for medical stabilization.

Procedure

1 Make an incision from the xiphoid to the pubis to enable thorough abdominal exploration.

2 Inspect the entire urinary tract, from the kidneys to the pelvic urethra, to identify any obvious tears or haematomas suggesting focal trauma.

3 Sharply divide the median and lateral ligaments of the bladder to allow investigation of the dorsal and ventral surfaces of the bladder. Bladder tears often occur towards the trigone, and the caudal ureters and trigone should be evaluated to ensure that the ureters are intact.

4 Once the area of rupture has been identified, exteriorize the bladder and pack the abdomen with moistened surgical sponges. Place full-thickness stay sutures at the apex of the bladder and on either side of the rupture.

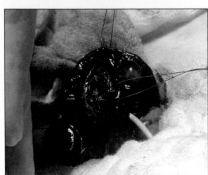

Rupture of the bladder in a cat with feline idiopathic cystitis. The blue catheter is a cystostomy tube that had been placed following the original episode of obstruction, before bladder rupture occurred (the cystostomy tube did not prevent rupture in this case, due to its occlusion). The three stay sutures are visible. The apex of the bladder is towards the top of the photograph and the rupture has occurred on the ventral aspect of the bladder. Debris within the bladder is consistent with urinary crystal formation, and fibrinous inflammation of the bladder mucosa.

5 Resect obviously pale or grey devitalized and bruised tissue or shredded/torn wound edges with scissors, until healthy pink tissue that bleeds from its cut edges can be seen.

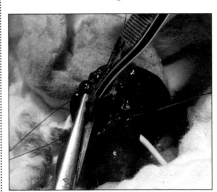

6 Check the patency of the ureters by palpating them and observing whether urine appears in the bladder.

7 Pass the 3 Fr urinary catheter from the bladder into the urethra to check its patency. If a catheter has been placed prior to surgery, this catheter should be removed and catheterization repeated in an anterograde manner (from the cystostomy site down the urethra) to confirm bidirectional patency of the urethra. If it is not possible to catheterize the urethra, a urethrogram will need to be taken (see QRG 5.21.1), and consideration given to referring the patient for further investigation and/or a salvage procedure such as perineal or prepubic urethrostomy.

8 Close the bladder in one layer using full-thickness single interrupted sutures of an absorbable monofilament suture such as polydioxanone or poliglecaprone (1.5 or 2 metric; USP 3/0 or 4/0). The bladder edge should be grasped gently with forceps and held with the mucosa *inverted* while the suture is being placed.

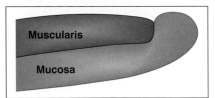

The mucosa everts when the bladder wall is excised.

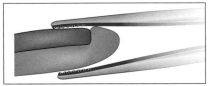

Incorrect way to hold bladder for suturing. Grasping the cut edge directly across the everted mucosa would cause it to evert again once the sutures were placed and tightened.

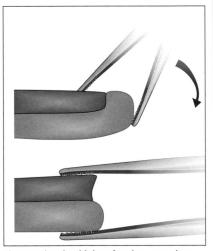

The cut edge should therefore be grasped at right angles. The forceps are then rotated to ensure that mucosal eversion is reduced, prior to placing the sutures, so that there is no eversion of mucosa when the suture is tightened.

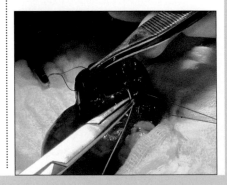

QRG 4.10.2 *continued*

9 Ensure that no eversion of the mucosa occurs when the suture is tightened.

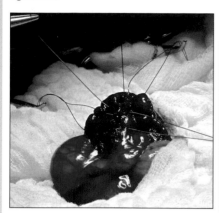

10 Test for leaks by instilling warm saline and observing for any leakage from the suture sites or other parts of the bladder. If leakage is observed, full-thickness single interrupted sutures should be placed at the site of leakage until there is no further leakage.

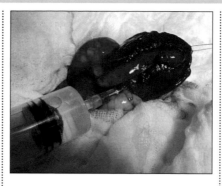

11 Lavage the abdomen vigorously using at least 500 ml of warm sterile saline with suctioning.

12 Close the laparotomy incision routinely.

Postoperative care

- Maintenance of a urinary catheter is optional and would only be recommended if increased urethral resistance were expected (e.g. following an episode of urethral obstruction). The catheter is maintained for 24–48 hours. The patient must wear an Elizabethan collar for this time and appropriate analgesia must be given.
- Antibiotics should not be given while the urinary catheter is in place, unless a severe systemically compromising UTI is present, as antibiotic-resistant bacterial strains will develop that are then extremely difficult to eradicate.
- The urine should be evaluated microscopically following catheter removal and culture performed on the urine (and the tip of the removed urinary catheter if available).
- Tube cystostomy should only be contemplated if the rupture occurred secondary to an unresolved urethral obstruction such as urethral neoplasia, or severe urethral spasm that requires time for institution of management (e.g. medication with spasmolytics and behavioural therapy).

Unsuccessful catheterization

If a urinary catheter cannot be passed relatively quickly and the bladder is extremely distended, decompressive cystocentesis (see QRG 4.11.4) can be performed before reattempting urethral catheterization. In cases where a urinary catheter cannot be passed despite prolonged attempts, an emergency urethrostomy or a temporary tube cystostomy may be required. Referral may be required for this, or advice sought from a specialist. Tube cystostomy is preferred to multiple cystocenteses; it allows the cat to be stabilized and urethral relaxants given for a later repeated attempt at catheterization or, if that fails, possible surgical correction. An alternative to an emergency urethrostomy or temporary tube cystostomy is placement of a urinary pigtail catheter.

Urinary pigtail catheters

Pigtail catheters provide a straightforward means of placing a cystostomy tube non-surgically but under general anaesthesia, being inserted into the bladder using an approach similar to that for cystocentesis. They can be used in situations where urinary diversion is required but a urethral catheter cannot be passed, e.g. in cats with calculi, urethral/trigone tumours or urethral rupture (Figure 4.11.2). Referral or consultation with a specialist is recommended before using this technique.

> ### WARNING
>
> **Perineal urethrostomy** is a salvage procedure that should not be undertaken lightly: unless the obstruction is in the penis it will not help and in the long term it risks recurrent urinary tract infections and stricture formation.

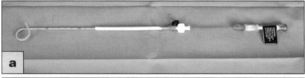

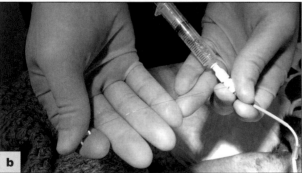

4.11.2 **(a)** A pigtail catheter. Pigtail catheters contain a stylet to allow insertion directly through the body and bladder wall. After placement the stylet is removed. There is a locking loop (a small string) that is then pulled to lock and secure the pigtail loop within the bladder. **(b)** Urine has been aspirated into this syringe, which has been attached to the end of a pigtail catheter which has been inserted into the bladder; the urine confirms the catheter's placement in the bladder. Pulling the locking loop as shown secures the pigtail loop in the bladder. This cat had a urethral rupture due to a road traffic accident, and the pigtail catheter allowed urinary diversion. (Courtesy of The Feline Centre, Langford Veterinary Services, University of Bristol) (continues) ▶

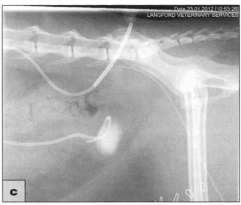

4.11.2 (continued) **(c)** This lateral abdominal radiograph shows the pigtail catheter with its end in the bladder. The bladder contains some positive contrast material but there is moderate loss of serosal detail in the caudal abdomen due to uroabdomen. Additionally a urethral catheter is seen caudally, superimposed over the thighs and bladder neck and ending at the level of the ventral aspect of L7, thus not following a normal urethral path due to the urethral rupture which was confirmed by a positive contrast urethrogram (not shown here). Staples are present due to a previous laparotomy. (Courtesy of The Feline Centre, Langford Veterinary Services, University of Bristol)

Relief without catheterization

For cases of known urethral spasm, *and where systemic biochemical changes are absent or mild*, a protocol has been published (Cooper *et al.,* 2010) that avoids urethral catheterization. This may be considered in cases where owners are unwilling to consent to general anaesthesia or catheterization and/or have limited funds, **but the welfare of the patient must be considered at all times to avoid suffering as a result of the obstruction.** It can be very difficult, without attempting urinary catheterization, to know that urethral spasm is the cause of obstruction, especially on first presentation. This protocol involves:

- Giving acepromazine (0.25 mg/cat i.m. or 2.5 mg/cat orally q8h) with buprenorphine (0.075 mg/cat sublingually q8h) and medetomidine (0.1 mg/cat i.m. q24h)
- Performing decompressive cystocentesis (see QRG 4.11.4)
- Giving subcutaneous fluids as needed
- Placing the cat in a quiet, dark environment to minimize stress.

Treatment success was defined as spontaneous urination within 72 hours and the protocol was effective in 11 of 15 cases.

References and further reading

Bass M, Howard J, Gerber B *et al.* (2005) Retrospective study of indications for and outcome of perineal urethrostomy in cats. *Journal of Small Animal Practice* **46**, 227–231

Cooper ES, Owers TJ, Chew DJ *et al.* (2010) A protocol for managing urethral obstruction in male cats without urethral catheterization. *Journal of the American Veterinary Medical Association* **237**, 1261–1266

Lee JA and Drobatz KJ (2003) Characterization of the clinical characteristics, electrolytes, acid–base, and renal parameters in male cats with urethral obstruction. *Journal of Veterinary Emergency and Critical Care* **13**, 227–233

Straeter-Knowlen IM, Marks SL, Rishniw M *et al.* (1995) Urethral pressure response to smooth and skeletal muscle relaxants in anesthetized, adult male cats with naturally acquired urethral obstruction. *American Journal of Veterinary Research* **56**, 919–923

QRG 4.11.1 Approach to hyperkalaemia
by Angie Hibbert

Potassium levels >5.5 mmol/l are consistent with hyperkalaemia. Note: Contamination of samples with potassium EDTA will lead to artefactual hyperkalaemia.

Causes

Common causes include:

- Urethral obstruction
- Urinary tract trauma – e.g. bladder rupture
- Bilateral ureteral obstruction
- Acute kidney injury (AKI).

Less common causes include:

- Iatrogenic hyperkalaemia – e.g. excessive potassium supplementation in intravenous fluids
- Diabetic ketoacidosis
- Acute tumour lysis syndrome
- Reperfusion injury
- Gastrointestinal disease – with marked dehydration or tract perforation. Note: if associated with inappetence, gastrointestinal disease usually causes *hypo*kalaemia
- Hypoadrenocorticism
- Effusions (e.g. chylothorax following repeat drainage, peritoneal, pericardial).

Consequences

The most significant and life-threatening effects are changes in cardiac conduction, usually seen when potassium levels are >7–8 mmol/l (however acid–base status and calcium levels may influence the level of potassium at which cardiac effects are seen).

The following ECG changes occur sequentially with increasing levels of potassium:

1. Peaked T waves seen
2. Reduced R wave amplitude, prolonged P–R interval and reduced QT interval
3. P waves reduce in amplitude, widen and then become absent – 'atrial standstill'
4. Widening of the QRS complex and bradycardia
5. Ventricular fibrillation, asystole and cardiac arrest.

Treatment

Ideally an ECG is recorded to obtain a baseline rhythm, which can be monitored during treatment. If electrocardiography is not available, the heart and pulse rate should be closely monitored for the development of bradycardia and arrhythmias. All drugs that increase potassium levels should be discontinued, e.g. ACE inhibitors, spironolactone, NSAIDs.

Begin intravenous fluid therapy with 0.9% NaCl or lactated Ringer's. If K^+ >6 mmol/l, administer initial 5 ml/kg bolus over 5–15 min; repeat according to response, ensuring there is urine production. Monitor for signs of volume overload (e.g tachypnoea, heart murmur, gallop rhythm)

> In most cases fluid therapy will significantly reduce K^+ by addressing hypovolaemia (see Chapter 4.1), increasing renal perfusion for excretion of K^+ and by dilution. ***Fluid therapy is the primary method of reducing hyperkalaemia***

Address underlying cause where possible, e.g. establish urinary outflow if urethral obstruction or bladder rupture

> Sedation or anaesthesia should not be performed until K^+ levels have reduced and the ECG shows a sinus rhythm again; careful cystocentesis may be required initially for stabilization in cats with urethral obstruction. Gentle placement of a urinary catheter may be tolerated in collapsed cats

If severe hyperkalaemia (K^+ >7–8 mmol/l) and/or ECG abnormalities, give calcium gluconate: 50–100 mg/kg (0.5–1 ml/kg of a 10% solution) i.v. slowly over 10 min; reduce rate of administration if heart rate slows (i.e. aim to deliver total dose over 20 min)

> Calcium gluconate is cardioprotective through increasing the myocardial membrane threshold potential; *it does not reduce potassium levels and hence is an adjunctive treatment only*. Effects last for ~30–60 mins. Can cause bradyarrhythmias. NB Hypocalcaemia may develop in cats with urethral obstruction once hyperkalaemia and acidaemia occur and this exacerbates cardiac instability

If severe hyperkalaemia and/or ECG abnormalities persist despite aggressive fluid therapy, administer:

- Glucose alone: 0.5 g/kg bolus (i.e. give 2 ml/kg of a 25% dextrose solution slowly i.v. over 5–10 min; make a 25% solution by diluting 50% dextrose in an equal volume of saline for administration). Follow with a 2.5% CRI (25 ml of 50% dextrose in 475 ml isotonic fluid) until hyperkalaemia resolves (see QRG 4.5.1)

OR

- Regular (soluble) insulin (0.25–0.5 IU/kg) with glucose: initially administer a bolus of 1–2 g of glucose per unit of insulin (the 25% dextrose solution described above contains 0.25 g glucose/ml), then follow with glucose supplemented in lactated Ringer's or saline as 2.5 or 5% CRI, as required, to maintain glucose levels >3.5 mmol/l (see QRG 4.5.1)

> Insulin will cause K^+ to move intracellularly, thus restoring normal blood levels. To prevent hypoglycaemia, glucose must also be given. The onset of action is usually within 30 min. Glucose levels need to be monitored for 12–24 hours following insulin administration

If severe ECG abnormalities persist despite aggressive fluid therapy, and there is a metabolic acidosis, sodium bicarbonate can be used: 1–3 mmol/kg i.v. over 20–30 mins (1 mmol/ml sodium bicarbonate is present in an 8.4% solution); do not exceed 4 mmol/kg. Effects may last several hours

> Sodium bicarbonate will cause K^+ to move intracellularly *and should only be given when acid–base and calcium levels can be measured*. Risk of causing paradoxical cerebral acidosis (if given too fast) and hypocalcaemia. Contraindicated if there is hypocalcaemia or alkalosis. Treatment with sodium bicarbonate is rarely required

QRG 4.11.2 Relief of urethral obstruction in a tomcat

by Danièlle Gunn-Moore

1 Anaesthetize the cat (the author prefers this to heavy sedation as it ensures the urethra is fully relaxed). The anaesthetic used depends on personal choice and the degree of renal compromise (see Chapter 3).

2 Perform a digital rectal examination to feel for stones, trauma or neoplasia before trying to unblock the urethra. Ideally, also take a plain radiograph to confirm the presence of any radiodense uroliths.

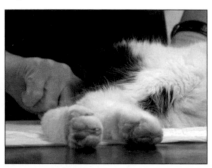

3 Clip and aseptically prepare the perineum.

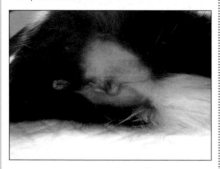

4 Select a catheter, ideally an open-ended, urethral catheter. See main chapter and Figure 4.11.1 for discussion of catheter options.

5 Where possible, catheterize the bladder without first performing cystocentesis, as cystocentesis carries a risk (albeit very small) of uroabdomen. However, if the obstruction is proving difficult to relieve, emptying the bladder helps restore renal perfusion and can make catheterization easier. In this situation decompressive cystocentesis is used rather than the routine cystocentesis technique (see QRG 4.11.4).

6 Fully extrude the cat's penis by pressing on its base, and examine it for signs of trauma, swelling or inflammation. Small uroliths or tightly packed sediment can become lodged in the tip of the penis and can be massaged out with gentle manipulation.

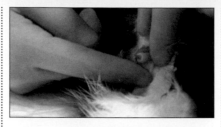

7 Measure the catheter length (to L6) maintaining sterility; Mila EZGO shown here as catheter will be left *in situ* after unblocking.

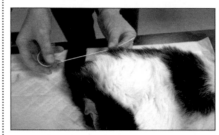

8 Lubricate the catheter with sterile lubricant and insert it into the penis.

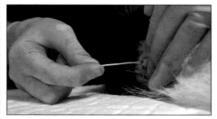

9 Once the catheter reaches the base of the penis, let go of the penis. Hold the prepuce and pull it caudally and dorsally to straighten the urethra fully.

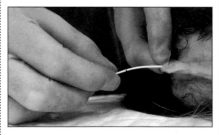

10 Gently advance the catheter into the bladder whilst flushing with sterile saline. This acts to distend the urethra and to flush obstructing material either back along the catheter and out of the penis or into the bladder.

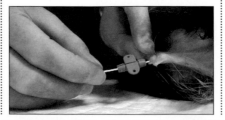

If having problems passing the catheter:

- Ensure there is a good depth of anaesthesia
- Ensure there is adequate analgesia
- Check that the urethra is fully straightened
- Try a different catheter
- Be patient and keep flushing
- Consider using sterile lubricating jelly diluted with saline (to reduce viscosity) to flush
- Consider use of local analgesia; lidocaine can be added to the lubricating jelly.

Retrograde hydropulsion

During voiding hydropulsion, the urethra is massaged per rectum and the urethra proximal to the obstruction is compressed by digital pressure. Saline flushing via a urinary catheter helps to dilate the urethra around the obstruction, helped by the increased back pressure due to digital compression.

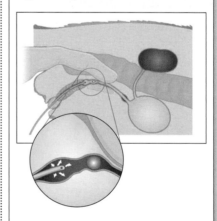

The digital pressure on the urethra is then released suddenly, hopefully allowing the obstructing material (e.g. a urolith) to be flushed into the bladder.

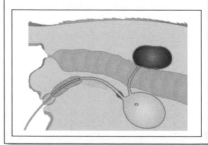

QRG 4.11.2 *continued*

11 Once the catheter has been advanced into the bladder, the bladder should be emptied, then flushed with warmed saline (to remove sediment etc.) until the flush is clear. The bladder should be left empty.

12 If the catheter is to be left *in situ* (see text) attach the wings to the catheter (if not already attached) and fix them using sutures.

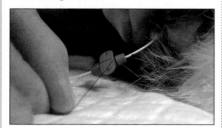

13 Secure the catheter to the cat by suturing the wings of the catheter to the perineum.

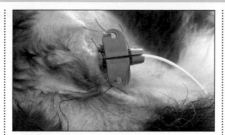

14 Attach a sterile extension line and closed-collection system. Tape the collection system to the tail so that tension is removed from the prepuce. The sutures should not be under tension once the catheter is attached to the tail.

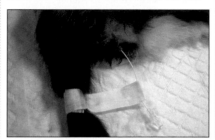

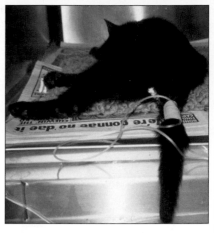

15 Fit an Elizabethan collar to prevent removal of the urinary catheter by the cat.

QRG 4.11.3 Urinalysis
by Kathleen Tennant

Urine samples

Collection methods

- Cystocentesis (see QRG 4.11.4) samples are best used for culture; if this is not possible a catheter sample can be used for culture if collected aseptically but this carries a risk of contamination (see below). In some individuals, especially the potentially immunosuppressed, the possibility of urinary tract infection (UTI) without inflammation should be considered at the time of sampling, and cystocentesis is preferred.
- Cystocentesis or catheter samples are suitable for sediment analysis, specific gravity (USG) and dipstick examination.
- Free-catch samples are generally suitable for dipstick and specific gravity, and are of limited use for sediment examination. They are not suitable for culture.

Collection tubes

- Urine for sediment and dipstick examination should be collected into a sterile universal container.
- Urine for cytology should be collected into EDTA; this is especially useful when neoplasia is suspected, or ordinary sediment is inconclusive regarding cells or bacteria.
- Urine for culture: If there is no significant time delay between urine collection and culture (i.e. urine undergoes culture on the same working day), a sterile universal collection pot is adequate. The importance of a delay will vary depending on collection technique, storage and original bacterial load. If a delay is anticipated (e.g. requirement to post the urine to a laboratory for culture), the urine should be collected into boric acid preservative to maintain bacterial numbers at representative fresh sample levels; this preservative effect, however, is not maintained beyond 72 hours. NB Boric acid samples are NOT suitable for sediment or dipstick examination.
- Order of preference for filling of urine collection tubes in new cases is:
  1. Plain sterile universal (majority of sample volume)
  2. Boric acid
  3. EDTA (small sample often adequate).

Storage

- For accurate assessment, samples should be stored at room temperature and analysed within 1–2 hours of collection.
- Storage periods of longer than 1–2 hours following collection without refrigeration *may* allow the urine to have the same original number and form of crystals but there will be a detrimental effect on cellular and bacterial elements.
- The effects of dehydration and degradation on samples left at room temperature for long periods are difficult to predict.

Specific gravity

- Urine specific gravity should be measured by a refractometer for accuracy.
- Healthy cats can concentrate urine to a high degree, and USG of 1.035 to >1.050 is usual.
- The presence of glucose in urine due to diabetes mellitus or stress-induced glycosuria may slightly elevate USG.

Dipstick analysis

- Leucocyte and nitrite panels should not be used; they are neither as specific nor as sensitive as sediment examination and culture for UTIs.
- Blood:
  - Blood detection panels do not reliably distinguish between whole blood, haemoglobin and myoglobin
  - A small amount of blood is expected in samples collected by cystocentesis.
- Bilirubin is always abnormal in feline urine, as there is no renal conjugation for excretion.
- Protein:
  - Urine protein panels are most sensitive to albumin
  - Small amounts of blood contamination that do not cause a visible colour change grossly do not significantly affect protein levels.
- Urobilinogen elevations may be seen in cholestatic hepatic or post-hepatic disease, but complete obstruction ▶

QRG 4.11.3 *continued*

of the gall bladder or biliary tract for a period of time may result in a decrease.

- pH:
  - Urine pH is normally slightly acidic, due to dietary animal proteins
  - pH varies a great deal, both with storage of the sample and with bacterial activity
  - Physiological factors such as hyperventilation in anxious cats may increase urinary pH
  - Single dipstick values showing a neutral or slightly alkaline value should not be the sole basis for a change in diet or therapy, as normal fluctuations occur according to diet, activity and interfering substances
  - Persistent, reliable trends alongside other urinary and clinical examination findings allow the use of pH as an adjunct to other findings. For example, a consistently high pH in a cat with struvite (magnesium ammonium phosphate) crystals in fresh urine and a history of distal urinary tract obstruction is worthy of note
  - Multi-use pH meters are more accurate than dipsticks.

Urine sediment

Preparation

1 Centrifuge 5 ml of urine in a lidded container at 1500 rpm for 5 minutes and discard the supernatant to leave approximately 0.5 ml at the bottom.

2 Add a drop of sediment stain if desired. This should be taken account of when determining cellularity.

3 Flick the side of the sample tube with your finger to resuspend the sediment, and place a single drop of the resuspended sediment on a glass slide under a coverslip or in a commercial graticule grid.

4 Lower the microscope condenser to sharpen detail and examine under a X40 objective lens (overall magnification X400).

Interpretation

Cells

- Erythrocytes and leucocytes present at <5 per X40 objective field are unremarkable. Higher numbers indicate haemorrhage and inflammation, respectively. Leucocytes in sediment have a granular, rounded appearance.
- Occasional renal epithelial cells and transitional cells are unremarkable.
- Squamous epithelial cells from the distal urethra or body surface may be noted in free-catch samples.

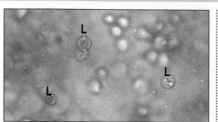

Leucocytes (L) in sediment: KovaStain; original magnification X400. At this magnification, leucocytes take up sediment stains to give a lightly granular appearance in a rounded outline. Leucocytes are around 2–2.5 times the size of erythrocytes. The background cells, which are out of focus, are a mixture of leucocytes and erythrocytes but full identification is not possible without focusing.

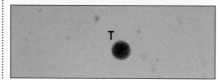

Transitional epithelial cell (T) in sediment: KovaStain; original magnification X400. These cells are larger than neutrophils and have a granular appearance with most sediment stains. They may occur singly, as here, or in aggregates or sheets. The degree of nuclear detail with sediment stain is inadequate to assess criteria of malignancy – a cytology preparation from urine collected into EDTA is required.

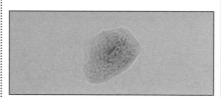

Squamous epithelial cell in sediment: KovaStain; original magnification X400. These are seen frequently in free-catch samples and are either from the distal urethra or the external skin. These large cells are often angular, and small nuclei may be noted.

Casts

Casts are tubular structures formed by mucoprotein in the tubules.

- Low numbers of proteinaceous (hyaline) or granular casts are unremarkable.
- High numbers may be seen in response to renal insult such as hypoperfusion or toxins.

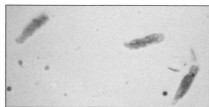

Coarse granular casts in sediment: KovaStain; original magnification X400. These casts are proteinaceous and have a stippled, grainy appearance to their interior structure. While low levels are unremarkable, higher numbers may be associated with an insult (e.g. toxic, hypoxic) to renal tubules. No numerical values exist to define what constitutes low, medium and high numbers of casts; this is a subjective assessment.

Crystals

- Crystals can occur in normal individuals – most frequently struvite or calcium oxalate dihydrate – but may be significant in some individuals with FLUTD or urolithiasis.
- Struvite and calcium oxalate dihydrate crystals may also form in urine that has been refrigerated; thus refrigerated samples may contain crystals not present *in vivo*.

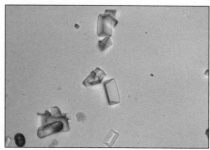

Struvite (magnesium ammonium phosphate or 'triple phosphate') crystals in sediment: KovaStain; original magnification X400. These elongated crystals may vary in size but are recognizable by their 'coffin lid' structure.

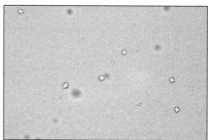

Calcium oxalate dihydrate crystals in sediment: KovaStain; original magnification X400. Square crystals with lines intersecting from the corners are the most frequent form, but aggregates may occur to give a more complex shape.

- Calcium oxalate monohydrate crystals may be seen in ethylene glycol toxicity or hypercalcaemia.

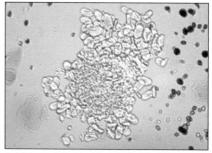

Calcium oxalate monohydrate crystals in sediment: KovaStain; original magnification X400. There are different forms of calcium oxalate monohydrate; the most common flat hexagonal form is illustrated here. There are also small slightly elongated ovoid shapes and 'bow tie' forms.

- Ammonium biurate crystals are uncommon but occasionally noted in cats with hepatic dysfunction.
- Bilirubin crystals are always abnormal and may be present due to pre-hepatic, hepatic or post-hepatic bilirubin increases in blood. ▶

QRG 4.11.3 *continued*

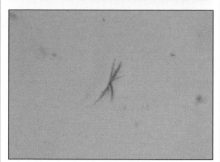

Bilirubin crystals in sediment: KovaStain; original magnification X400. Bilirubin has a golden coloration and most usually forms thin, needle-like crystals which bunch together to form a structure resembling a bundle of twigs tied in the middle.

- Amorphous material is not uncommon in very concentrated samples.
- Some drugs may give rise to unusual crystal formation.

Bacteria

Bacteria may be noted in sediment as rounded or rod shapes and are most easily recognized when motile. They may be noted with or without a host inflammatory response (neutrophils). They are often easier to appreciate in cytology preparations (see below).

Other findings

Lipid droplets from normal renal epithelial turnover are a normal finding.

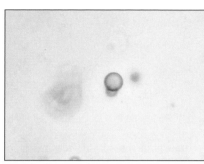

Lipid droplets in sediment: KovaStain; original magnification X400. Lipid droplets like these float above the plane of the rest of the sample and are always clear. They vary in size and have no internal structure.

Cytology

Cytology may be more useful for assessment of cellular elements, but may miss crystals or casts.

1 Place a drop of urine collected into EDTA on a slide and allow the liquid to evaporate.

2 Stain the air-dried smear with a commercial rapid stain (e.g. Diff-Quik) or Giemsa.

3 Examine under oil immersion (X500 or X1000 final magnification).

Bacteria are also often easier to appreciate in cytology preparations.

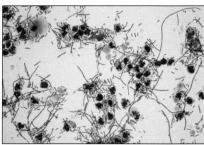

Bacteria and leucocytes in a cytology preparation: modified Wright's stain; original magnification X500. All the nucleated cells here are poorly preserved neutrophils. They are surrounded by very high numbers of a monomorphic population of bacteria. This would be compatible with the presence of a UTI if urine had been collected by cystocentesis.

QRG 4.11.4 Cystocentesis
by Margie Scherk

Indications

- To collect urine for analysis. Cystocentesis is specifically required to collect urine for culture; direct collection from the bladder prevents contamination of urine with debris, bacteria and cells from the lower urogenital tract (urethra, prostate, vagina) and the perineal region
- For temporary decompression of the bladder prior to placement of a urethral catheter in a cat with urethral obstruction

Contraindications

- Inadequate bladder volume or excessive body fat such that the bladder cannot be palpated or immobilized manually
- Patient resistance to restraint; this is usually not insurmountable and gentle restraint is usually adequate
- Recent cystotomy

Equipment

- 5–6 or 10–12 ml syringe (depending on size of bladder; 5 and 10 ml syringes shown)
- 23 or 25 G 1½-inch hypodermic needle

- Surgical spirit ± swab
- Sterile plain tube(s) to transport the sample; separate plain tubes may be required for urinalysis and culture
- EDTA tube if sample needed for cytology
- Tube with boric acid preservative (not shown) can be used if urine culture not possible within same working day

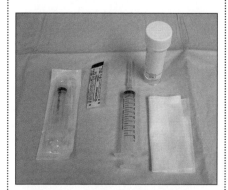

For decompressive cystocentesis:

- 20 ml syringe attached to an intravenous extension set and 23 or 25 G 1½-inch hypodermic needle via a 3-way stopcock
- Kidney dish for collection of urine
- Sample pot(s) for urine submission or analysis
- Swab with surgical spirit

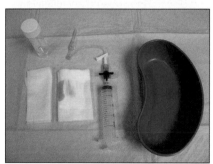

Patient preparation and positioning for cystocentesis in a conscious cat for collection of a urine sample

- Cystocentesis may be performed with the cat either standing or lying in lateral recumbency. The position chosen depends mainly on the preference of the clinician and of the patient for restraint.
- The surface the cat is standing or lying on should not be cold or slippery.

▶

QUICK REFERENCE GUIDES

QRG 4.11.4 *continued*

- The room should be quiet and calm with only a few people present.
- Use the least amount of gentle restraint possible.
- The hair can be shaved but since this often adds stress for the patient, it is usually not performed
- A small amount of surgical spirit (with or without a swab) is applied over the site of needle insertion.

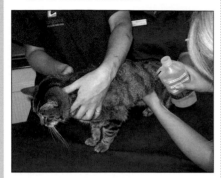

Patient preparation and positioning for decompressive cystocentesis

In cases of urinary obstruction, decompressive cystocentesis may be performed under sedation or anaesthesia before urethral catheterization (see QRG 4.11.2), with the cat in lateral recumbency. If used, sedation or anaesthesia must be appropriate for the metabolic state of the patient (see Chapter 3).

Technique

1 Position your hand around the bladder. Move your thumb over the bladder, palpating it from caudal to cranial and back, so that you are confident in its position and size.

2 Once you feel comfortable palpating the bladder, you can immobilize it with your thumb.

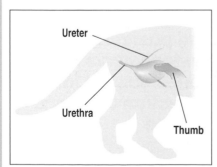

Clinician preference varies but usually the thumb is positioned at the cranial pole of the bladder, so that the bladder is immobilized caudal to the thumb, as shown here. Alternatively, you can position your thumb at the caudal extremity of the bladder, stabilizing it cranial to your thumb.

3 Insert the needle in a caudal direction (so that the layers of the bladder wall will help to seal the puncture) through the ventral or ventrolateral side of the bladder (to avoid the dorsal-lying ureters and major abdominal blood vessels).

- Aim to insert the needle a short distance (a few centimetres but will depend on degree of bladder fill) cranial to the junction of the bladder and the urethra.
- If the needle is inserted too far cranially, at the apex of the bladder, as urine is withdrawn and the bladder gets smaller it may move off the needle.
- By using a 25 G needle and not applying excessive pressure to the bladder during collection, you reduce the chance of urine leakage.

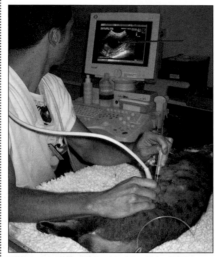

Ultrasonography of the bladder, if available, can be used to direct cystocentesis. The needle can be seen entering the black anechoic urine within the bladder (arrowed).

4 Once the needle is in the bladder, apply negative pressure to the syringe to collect the urine.

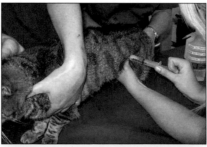

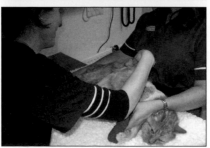

If decompressive cystocentesis is being performed (not shown): leaving the needle in the bladder, use the 3-way

stopcock to empty urine from the syringe into the kidney dish before re-aspirating from the bladder. Continue until almost all of the urine has been removed.

5 Continue to stabilize the bladder until you withdraw the needle from the abdomen.

6 If urine is not obtained:

- Do not redirect the needle as there is a risk that a bowel loop may have been penetrated, which would cause subsequent contamination of the bladder, abdominal/peritoneal cavity and urine specimen
- Use a new needle for subsequent attempts.

PRACTICAL TIPS

- Through repeated practice and visualization (imagining where the bladder is inside the abdomen), locating the bladder by palpation becomes easy in all but the most overweight cats. In these, the bladder must be quite full to be able to identify its outline and immobilize it. Practice palpation on every cat you examine, sedate or anaesthetize. Using the location and size seen on a radiograph, should one be taken, will also help improve confidence and skill.
- The bladder contracts circumferentially when emptied, and sediment will fall due to gravity. Sediment yield may be improved by gently agitating the bladder with the immobilizing hand just before inserting the needle.

Potential complications

- If a swirl of blood enters the hub of the syringe during collection, discontinue collection and make a note of the blood (iatrogenic haematuria) in the cat's medical record. This bleeding is extremely unlikely to result in problems. Iatrogenic haematuria is commonly seen in cystocentesis samples and is differentiated from true haematuria by comparison with a voided urine sample collected by free catch 1–2 days later.
- Very rarely a vasovagal response is seen immediately following cystocentesis; vomiting and hypotensive collapse occur. Treat with standard intravenous supportive fluids (see QRG 4.1.3), oxygen, atropine if severe bradycardia (≤60 bpm) occurs, and quiet; patients recover within an hour.
- Very rarely, an overdistended and traumatized bladder (e.g. urethral obstruction >1 day) will rupture during cystocentesis. Surgical repair is then required (see QRG 4.10.2).

All photographs courtesy of The Feline Centre, Langford Veterinary Services, University of Bristol.

Abdominal effusion

Myra Forster-van Hijfte

The equilibrium of fluid within the body is determined by Starling's principle, which states that hydrostatic pressure, oncotic pressure and blood vessel integrity determine the way in which fluids move within the body. An abdominal effusion or free abdominal fluid develops when one or more of these three determinants is abnormal; which factor is changed determines the type of fluid present. The presence of free urine or bile in the abdomen is generally caused by rupture of the urinary or biliary tract, either due to direct trauma or secondary to disease (e.g. unresolved urethral obstruction or neutrophilic cholangitis/cholelithiasis with bile duct blockage).

> Although many people use the terms 'ascites' and 'free abdominal fluid' interchangeably, ascites is defined as an accumulation of serous fluid in the peritoneal cavity and is usually reserved for transudates arising from liver or heart disease. In this chapter the term 'free abdominal fluid' will be used.

Clinical presentation

The clinical presentation depends on the amount of free fluid present in the abdomen and the underlying cause of fluid accumulation.

Diagnostic approach

History and initial physical examination

A thorough history and physical examination may provide clues regarding the underlying cause of the free fluid:

- Have the clinical signs developed acutely (e.g. recent trauma) or more chronically (e.g. some neoplastic causes)?
- Has there been any history of trauma (e.g. to cause bladder rupture)?
- Is there evidence of concurrent pleural effusion? (Bicavity effusions are mostly likely to occur with feline infectious peritonitis, neoplasia and cardiac disease.)

It is difficult to detect small amounts of abdominal fluid on physical examination, although the organs (especially the intestinal loops) may seem to 'slide' more easily on abdominal palpation. Ultrasonography can be particularly useful (Figure 5.1.1).

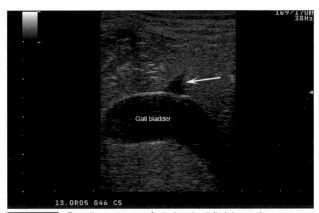

5.1.1 Small amounts of abdominal fluid can be seen with ultrasound examination. The liver lobes are separated by a small amount of free fluid (arrowed) within the abdomen, just ventral to the gall bladder. (Courtesy of North Downs Specialist Referrals.)

If the amount of free fluid is more substantial, a pot-bellied appearance may be seen. There is often a positive fluid thrill (place one hand on either side of the abdomen; tapping the hand on one side will generate a wave-like effect through the fluid that is felt in the hand on the opposite side). Large amounts of fluid make it more difficult to palpate individual abdominal organs and determine changes in their shape and size.

Other reasons for abdominal enlargement should be excluded, e.g. obesity, pregnancy, organ enlargement, constipation. Imaging can help differentiate some of these.

Blood and urine tests

Ideally, full biochemical (including sodium, potassium and calcium) and haematology profiles and urinalysis allow assessment of the general health of the cat and may also point towards involvement of a particular body system. FeLV and FIV testing should be performed if possible, although the prevalence of these infections within the UK is low.

Initial urinalysis (see QRG 4.11.3) should include specific gravity, dipstick and sediment examination (can be done at an external laboratory or in-house); dipstick examination may give a clue to excessive urine protein loss in cases that have a peripheral hypoproteinaemia discovered on serum biochemistry.

Abdominal fluid analysis

It is of paramount importance to obtain a sample of fluid for analysis by abdominocentesis (see QRG 5.1.1).

Initial fluid analysis should include macroscopic appearance, specific gravity, quantitative protein analysis and cell count (Figure 5.1.2). Cytology should also be performed. If haemorrhagic in appearance, PCV should be measured and compared to that of the peripheral blood.

Once the fluid type is determined the diagnostic approach is geared towards finding the underlying cause (Figure 5.1.3).

Further investigations

Further details on the diagnostic approach for **transudates**, **modified transudates** and **exudates** are shown in Figures 5.1.4 to 5.1.6.

Fluid type	Appearance	Specific gravity	Total protein	Cell count/cytology	Notes
Transudate	Clear, colourless to pale yellow	<1.017	< 25 g/l	<1000 cells/µl ($<1 \times 10^9$/l)	With time, pure transudates can become modified
Modified transudate	Clear, pale yellow	1.015–1.025	25–50 g/l	1000–7000 cells/µl ($1–7 \times 10^9$/l)	
Exudate	Usually turbid, purulent or serosanguineous	>1.025	>30 g/l	>5000 cells/µl ($>5 \times 10^9$/l) Septic or non-septic depending on whether bacteria are present	
Chyle	Turbid, milky	>1.025	>25 g/l	1000–7000 cells/µl ($1–7 \times 10^9$/l) Small lymphocytes	Effusion TG > serum TG; effusion cholesterol:TG ratio <1
Urine	Yellow, usually clear	Depends on renal function	N/A	N/A	As urine Cr >> serum Cr, in uroabdomen effusion Cr >> serum Cr. Also effusion K^+ >> serum K^+, although this equilibrates a lot faster than creatinine (see Chapter 5.7)
Bile	Orange-yellow to green. Can be turbid	>1.025	>30 g/l	>5000 cells/µl ($>5 \times 10^9$/l) Bilirubin crystals within macrophages	Effusion bilirubin > serum bilirubin
Blood	Serosanguineous to haemorrhagic	>1.025	>30 g/l	>1000 cells/µl ($>1 \times 10^9$/l) but depends on peripheral count	Recent haemorrhage (coagulopathy, trauma) gives effusion with features similar to blood (e.g. similar PCV ± platelets present) but fluid does not clot. Chronic haemorrhage suggested by erythrophagocytosis and lack of platelets. Iatrogenic haemorrhage (inadvertent aspiration of abdominal blood vessel) will clot. Haemorrhagic effusions have lower PCV (often much lower despite their bloody appearance) than patient's blood

5.1.2 Classification of abdominal fluid types. Cr = creatinine; K^+ = potassium; TG = triglycerides.

Fluid type	Causes
Transudate	Hypoproteinaemia. Portal hypertension. Right-sided heart failure
Modified transudate	Right-sided heart failure. Portal hypertension. Inflammatory disease (e.g. pancreatitis, lymphocytic cholangitis). Infectious (occasionally FIP effusions may be modified transudates). Neoplastic disease
Exudate	Inflammatory (e.g. pancreatitis, lymphocytic cholangitis, septic peritonitis). Infectious (including FIP but this is a low cellular exudate). Neoplastic disease
Chyle	Neoplasia. Lymphatic disease. Trauma. Right-sided heart failure. Steatitis
Urine	Trauma. Rupture of a 'diseased' urinary tract
Bile	Trauma. Rupture of a 'diseased' biliary tract
Blood	Trauma. Blood vessel rupture. Neoplasia. Coagulopathy. Systemic amyloidosis

5.1.3 Causes of free abdominal fluid.

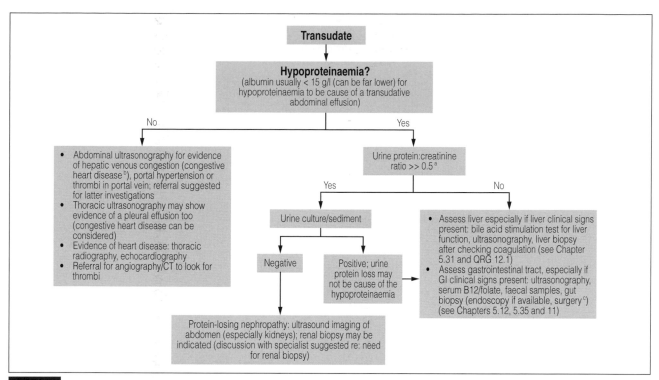

5.1.4 Diagnostic approach when the abdominal effusion is a transudate.

[a] Initial urine dipstick examination may indicate significant protein loss in the urine. Interpretation of urine dipstick protein must take into account concentration of urine. For example, a 1+ dipstick protein in very concentrated urine (USG>1.050) is less likely to indicate significant proteinuria than a 1+ dipstick protein in less concentrated urine (e.g. USG 1.020). Ultimately, the urine protein:creatinine ratio (UPC ratio; requested on submitted urine sample) gives the clearest indication as to whether there is significant proteinuria and should always be obtained if proteinuria is suspected. To cause hypoproteinaemia and subsequent free abdominal fluid, urine protein loss must be significant (UPC ratio >5 typically and often >10; normal is ≤0.4). A sediment examination will need to be done concurrently to rule out significant inflammation or infection within the urinary tract, as this will also cause proteinuria.

[b] In cats it is extremely rare to develop an abdominal effusion alone if the underlying cause is cardiac failure. Cats will often develop pleural effusion or pulmonary oedema before developing an abdominal effusion.

[c] Specialist advice should be sought if gastrointestinal biopsy specimens are to be obtained during surgery in a hypoalbuminaemic cat, due to the potential increased risk of complications.

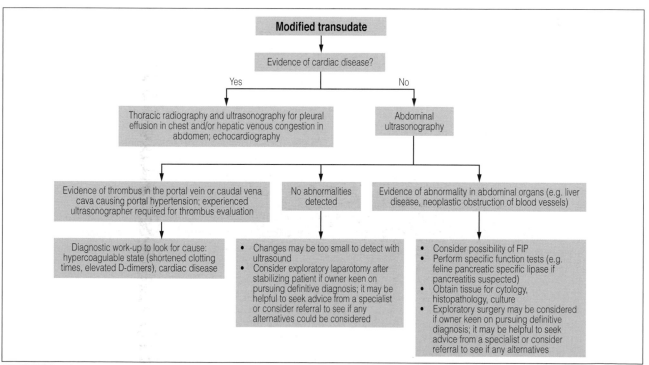

5.1.5 Diagnostic approach when the abdominal effusion is a modified transudate. In the feline patient it is extremely rare to develop an abdominal effusion alone if the underlying cause is cardiac failure. Cats will often develop pleural effusion or pulmonary oedema before developing an abdominal effusion.

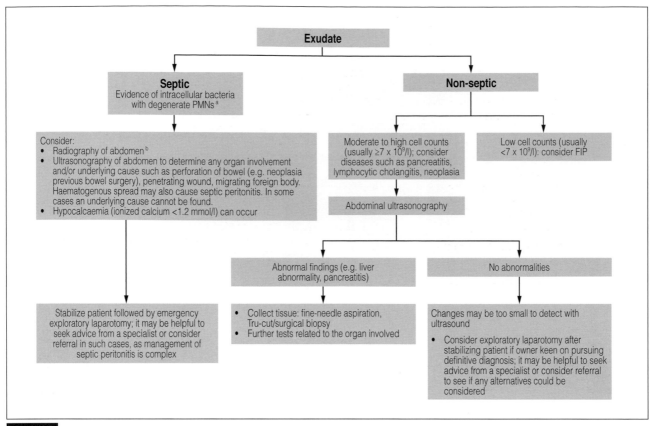

5.1.6   Diagnostic approach when the abdominal effusion is an exudate. PMNs = polymorphonuclear leucocytes.

[a] When only extracellular bacteria are observed on cytology, the clinician needs to consider whether external contamination during sampling is responsible. If bacteria are intracellular, however, this signifies the presence of a septic peritonitis. Degenerative changes in neutrophils also raise suspicion of a septic peritonitis. Fluid should be submitted for bacterial culture (both aerobic and anaerobic) and susceptibility testing.
[b] Radiography is usually not helpful if there is a significant amount of free abdominal fluid, as the loss of serosal detail precludes any meaningful interpretation. Free gas in the abdomen is an indication of either intestinal perforation or an infection with gas-forming bacteria, such as some clostridial species.

Bile or urine effusion

The patient needs to be treated with urgency. Initially it needs to be stabilized by addressing abnormalities such as hypovolaemia, hypothermia, any electrolyte abnormalities (e.g. hyperkalaemia), blood pressure abnormalities and disturbances in the acid–base balance.

- It is helpful to perform abdominal ultrasonography, where available, to evaluate relevant organs in a non-invasive way.
- If the underlying cause of any rupture has been trauma, survey radiography of the entire patient is indicated (including the thorax) to make sure no further abnormalities are present that need urgent attention.
- If the rupture is secondary to disease, surgical exploration should be used to obtain biopsy specimens as well as to repair the damage.
- Positive or double-contrast radiography of the urinary tract (see QRG 5.21.1) may be necessary to find the source of leakage of urine, as it is not always obvious on exploratory laparotomy. Note that cats with ruptured bladders may still have a palpable bladder and the ability to urinate.

Haemorrhagic effusion

The urgency of the situation depends on the degree and speed of haemorrhage. Fluid resuscitation ± blood transfusion may be necessary to stabilize the patient.

- Abdominal ultrasonography is useful to examine all organs. Further tests will be based on the abnormalities detected.
- It is important to assess coagulation status, via prothrombin (PT) and activated partial thromboplastin (APTT) times, to determine whether abnormal coagulation (e.g. hepatopathies, rodenticide toxicity, haemophilia) could be causing abdominal bleeding.
- Many cats with haemoabdomen have underlying liver disease, particularly neoplasia (although a lower percentage than in dogs) or systemic amyloidosis (which can result in sudden death due to liver rupture, particularly in Siamese and Oriental breeds).

The overall prognosis for cats with haemoabdomen is guarded.

Chylous effusion

A chylous effusion within the abdomen is usually associated with abnormalities of the lymphatic circulation, particularly traumatic rupture of a major lymph vessel or obstruction of lymphatic drainage (e.g. due to neoplasia or, rarely, infection (Sharman (2009) described obstruction due to a mass caused by an infection, which required surgery and clindamycin therapy)) or cardiac disease.

Abdominal ultrasonography can be helpful in some of these cases, but if no abnormalities are seen and the owner wishes to pursue a definitive diagnosis, further contrast studies involving the lymphatic system are indicated for which referral is necessary.

Congestive cardiac disease can also induce chylous effusions (but this is rare), so evaluation of the heart may be indicated (e.g. radiography, echocardiography; see Chapter 9).

Treatment

Treatment is directed at rectifying the underlying cause of the abdominal effusion, whilst providing supportive care. For example, treatment of any underlying protein-losing nephropathy, gut-losing enteropathy or lymphocytic cholangitis may be indicated, or surgical treatment of a severely ruptured bladder. The abdominal effusion does not usually need to be removed unless the increased pressure on the diaphragm causes breathing difficulties or the effusion is septic, bile or urine.

Reference

Sharman MJ, Goh CS, Kuipers von Lande RG and Hodgson JL (2009) Intra-abdominal actinomycetoma in a cat. *Journal of Feline Medicine and Surgery* **11**, 701–705

QRG 5.1.1 Abdominocentesis
by Myra Forster-van Hijfte

Abdominocentesis is the aspiration of free fluid from the abdominal cavity.

Indications

- Abdominocentesis should be performed if there is a strong indication that free fluid is present in the abdominal cavity. This may be based on physical examination or the detection of fluid on abdominal ultrasonography. Loss of abdominal serosal detail on abdominal radiography may also be an indication that free fluid is present.
- Abdominocentesis is performed to obtain fluid for analysis, as this may give an indication of the underlying disease process.
- Therapeutic abdominocentesis (removing a larger amount of fluid) is useful in cases that have clinical signs associated with the large volume of fluid, e.g. respiratory distress due to pressure on the diaphragm, or vomiting, general malaise and inappetence due to the marked abdominal distension in some severe cases. Therapeutic abdominocentesis will only alleviate these signs in the short term while the underlying diagnosis is pursued and appropriate treatment instigated, or for short-term palliative treatment.

Precautions

There are no major contraindications to performing abdominocentesis. Care should be taken not to aspirate inadvertently: urine from a full urinary bladder; bile from a dilated gall bladder; contents of a dilated gut loop or any large abdominal mass. Ultrasound guidance can be used to direct aspiration of the free fluid, especially if the amount of free fluid is small.

Equipment

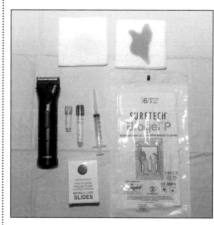

- 21–23 G 1 inch sterile needle or butterfly catheter, with a 5 ml syringe attached. For therapeutic abdominocentesis of large amounts of fluid, it is best to use a 21 G butterfly catheter attached to a 3-way tap and larger syringe (e.g. 10 or 20 ml) (not shown)
- Clippers, swabs, chlorhexidine solution, surgical spirit
- Sterile gloves
- Plain and EDTA containers for fluid collection
- Microscope slides
- Ultrasound machine if available (not shown)

Patient preparation

Depending on the temperament of the cat, manual restraint alone or mild to moderate sedation will be required. If the cat is very fractious, a short general anaesthetic may be needed. The general health status of the cat needs to be taken into account when choosing the level of sedation or anaesthesia. If a general anaesthetic is necessary, it is important for the clinician to plan this carefully and also to consider any other diagnostic tests that may be carried out under the same anaesthetic, whilst weighing the pros and cons of a longer general anaesthetic.

An area of 10 cm diameter around the umbilicus should be clipped, cleaned and prepared aseptically; in the images below the cat has been clipped extensively due to previous abdominal ultrasonography.

Technique

1 The cat is placed in lateral recumbency with the patient's feet toward the clinician. Ultrasound guidance can be used if available and if only a small amount of fluid is suspected (not shown). Before inserting the needle, the abdomen should be palpated carefully to identify any large organs that could inadvertently be aspirated rather than the free fluid. Ideally the bladder is emptied before abdominocentesis; if not, it is held to the side so that the needle can be directed away from it.

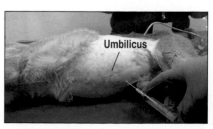
Umbilicus

▶

QRG 5.1.1 continued

2 The needle is inserted at right angles to the skin, approximately 1–2 cm caudal to the umbilicus and 1 cm ventral of the midline (linea alba). A slight 'pop' is noted as the body cavity is entered. If a moderate to large amount of fluid is present in the abdomen, the needle need not be advanced far into the abdomen; with small amounts of fluid, the needle may need to be fully inserted and ultrasound guidance, if available, is helpful in such cases.

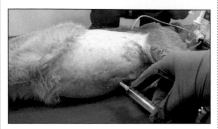

3 The fluid that is aspirated into the syringe is placed into plain (for biochemistry, culture and sensitivity) and EDTA (for cell count and cytology) collection tubes. Direct smears can also be prepared for cytology and are made by applying a drop of fluid to a microscope slide, and using the surface tension of another slide placed on top of it (see QRG 5.33.1).

4 If no fluid is obtained, the needle can be reinserted in different locations using the four-quadrant approach: approximate sites for needle insertion are shown in here by black crosses; the umbilicus is central to the four crosses. Alternatively, ultrasound guidance can be used. Note that abdominocentesis can be falsely negative if <5 ml/kg of fluid is present in the peritoneal cavity. If the amount of fluid is minimal, a diagnostic peritoneal lavage (see below) may be useful in identifying the underlying cause of the development of abdominal fluid.

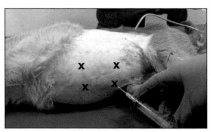

5 If no fluid is obtained, **diagnostic peritoneal lavage** can be considered:

a. Instil 20 ml/kg of warmed sterile saline into the abdomen using a 21 G 1 inch needle or catheter inserted 1–2 cm caudal to the umbilicus and 1 cm ventral of the midline (linea alba) as for abdominocentesis, stopping if any patient discomfort or respiratory difficulty is seen.
b. Remove the needle or catheter. Gently roll the cat from side to side and massage the abdomen gently for 2–3 minutes.
c. Replace the cat in lateral recumbency and repeat the abdominocentesis technique described above.

Only small amounts of fluid are typically removable by this technique, but are still worth submitting for analysis. Note that quantitative analysis of the fluid will be altered by dilution due to the peritoneal lavage.

Fluid analysis

- **Macroscopic appearance of the fluid:** assess colour, viscosity and turbidity.
- **Specific gravity:** can be measured in house using a refractometer.
- **Quantitative protein analysis;** total protein, globulin and albumin

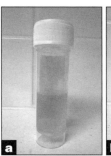
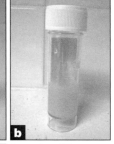
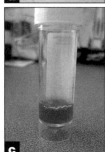

Examples of the appearance of different types of abdominal effusion. (a) Modified transudate. (b) Chyle. (c) Exudate due to feline infectious peritonitis; note the typical yellow colour. This fluid was frothy when shaken and very viscous.

concentrations. Total protein concentration can be estimated using a specific refractometer or measured by a biochemistry analyser. Albumin and globulin concentrations are measured by a biochemistry analyser.
- **Cytology:** total cell count and microscopic examination of the cells. This may be carried out in house if experience in interpretation is available. If the fluid is septic, many PMNs and intracellular bacteria may be seen and these are relatively easy to identify. However, in most circumstances cytological examination should be performed by a clinical pathologist.

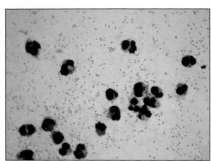

Abdominal fluid smear from a cat with septic peritonitis due to gastrointestinal tract perforation. All the cells visible are neutrophils (PMNs) and show evidence of a disrupted cellular outline and coarsened, ragged nuclear chromatin consistent with the hydropic change expected in degenerate neutrophils. Many rod-shaped bacteria are present over the whole of the smear and also within PMNs (following phagocytosis), confirming the septic nature of this effusion. (Diff-Quik stain; original magnification x 1000)

- **Culture and sensitivity testing:** samples should be submitted to a commercial laboratory.

Effusion images a and b courtesy of North Downs Specialist Referrals. Other images courtesy of The Feline Centre, Langford Veterinary Services, University of Bristol.

Abdominal masses

Myra Forster-van Hijfte

An abdominal mass is usually first detected on palpation of the abdomen during physical examination.

Tips on abdominal palpation

- Follow the principles highlighted in Chapter 1 to ensure that the cat is as relaxed as possible during examination, as this will make a significant difference to the success of abdominal palpation.
- The abdomen should always be palpated in a systematic fashion to ensure that nothing is missed, and if any aspect cannot be thoroughly examined for any reason (e.g. obesity, fractious cat, overly tense abdomen) then this should be noted, rather than recording that abdominal palpation was normal.
- Lifting the forelimbs of a cat will help when palpating the cranial abdomen, as the organs will move caudally.
- Normal abdominal structures can often be confused with abdominal masses.
- It is important to realize that in the cat the kidneys can be extremely mobile and are often palpated in the mid abdomen, rather than in the craniodorsal area of the abdomen
- Faeces within the colon can be mistaken for an abdominal mass, especially if the cat is constipated. The location and compressibility of the faecal material will often help differentiate it from a mass lesion.

Sometimes the mass may be too small to palpate, or within the confinement of an organ, and therefore not found on physical examination. Such masses are usually detected on ultrasound examination of the abdomen, either as an incidental finding, or when investigating other presenting signs. Occasionally it may be possible to deduce the likely origin of a mass from its location, mobility and relation to other organs. However, the clinician needs to be aware that it is usually not possible to determine the origin, and character (benign *versus* malignant) of the mass on the basis of physical examination alone, and further diagnostic investigations are usually required.

Clinical presentation

The clinical presentation varies, depending on the size of the mass, the organ(s) involved, and whether the mass is benign or malignant. If the mass is benign and not too large, the cat will often show no clinical signs. For example, cystic disease is a relatively common problem in the cat and usually involves either kidney and/or liver. The cysts usually do not cause any clinical signs, unless they become large and/or destroy the normal organ tissue.

The initial clinical signs caused by an abdominal mass can be very non-specific and may include a mild reduction in appetite, weight loss and lethargy. Further possible clinical presentations are:

- Mass noticed by the owner (e.g. in renal lymphoma renomegaly can be so marked that the owners notice 'a lump' when the cat is otherwise clinically well)
- Signs associated with the physical presence of a mass (e.g. if the mass causes intestinal obstruction, the cat may present with acute-onset vomiting)
- Signs associated with organ dysfunction (e.g. PU/PD or vomiting in some cases of renal lymphoma, vomiting and diarrhoea associated with intestinal mass)
- Acute signs (e.g. if the mass causes obstruction of the gastrointestinal tract).

Cats are masters of disguise but owners often report with hindsight that their cat was not entirely well, had a reduced appetite or was less active.

Diagnostic approach

A thorough history and good physical examination may narrow down a list of differential diagnoses. Further diagnostic tests are necessary to characterize whether the mass is malignant or benign, its origin, and presence of additional organ involvement and/or dysfunction, before deciding on further management of the cat.

Blood and urine tests

A full biochemical and haematology profile and full urinalysis will show the general health profile of the cat and may point towards involvement of a particular organ. The FeLV/FIV status of the cat may also be worth determining. Additional blood tests may be indicated, based on the history and physical examination or on results of the initial blood tests.

Diagnostic imaging

Radiography

In general practice radiography is readily available, and good abdominal radiographs (in two planes, dorsoventral and lateral views) may give a clue to the origin of the mass. However, radiography has only limited use. Radiographs may look normal (if the mass is very small) or they may show changes in shape, size and opacity of abdominal organs or displacement of adjacent structures by the abdominal mass. Thoracic radiography (in two planes, ventrodorsal and lateral) is essential to check the lungs for metastases and also to assess the presternal lymph node, enlargement of which can indicate an active disease process in the abdomen (neoplastic or inflammatory).

Ultrasonography

Generally of more use is abdominal ultrasonography. This will allow the clinician to determine the location and echotexture of the mass (Figures 5.2.1 to 5.2.3).

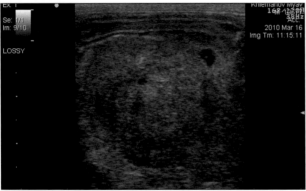

5.2.1 Ultrasound image of a cholangiocarcinoma. There is a 2 x 2.8 cm mass in the right liver lobe, hyperechoic to liver parenchyma. The duodenum is looping around the mass, which is in direct contact with the wall. This was a 13-year-old, neutered female DSH cat with a 2-month history of weight loss, reduced appetite and lethargy. (Courtesy of North Downs Specialist Referrals.)

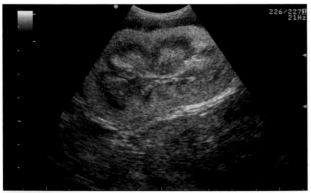

5.2.2 Ultrasound image of renal lymphoma. The kidney is enlarged, has a hyperechoic cortex and is irregular in outline. There is anechoic fluid between the renal capsule and the cortex of the kidney. This was a 4-year-old, neutered female DSH cat with a 3-week history of PU/PD, weight loss, reduced appetite and lethargy. (Courtesy of North Downs Specialist Referrals.)

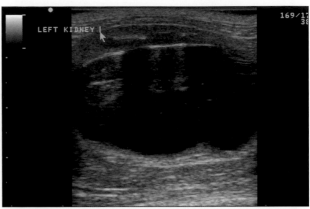

5.2.3 Ultrasound image of hydronephrosis of the left kidney. This was a 1-year-old neutered male DSH cat with a history of mild distension of the abdomen and lethargy. Following investigations an ectopic ureter was identified, which was responsible for causing secondary hydronephrosis. (Courtesy of North Downs Specialist Referrals.)

The associated lymph nodes should be assessed as well as all the other abdominal organs in order to better determine the extent of the disease process.

Cytology/histopathology

It is important to emphasize that imaging will only show the presence of abnormal tissue, but will not tell the clinician what the abnormal tissue is. Occasionally cytology may be sufficient to get a diagnosis, particularly with lymphoma, but in most cases only histopathology can provide a definitive diagnosis. Once tissue has been obtained, it is important to provide the pathologist with as many details as possible regarding history, physical examination and results of further diagnostic tests. This will help in achieving a definitive diagnosis. Culture of the tissue may also be helpful if there is an indication that the underlying disease process is caused by a bacterial infection (it is therefore good practice to keep a piece of tissue frozen in case it is needed later on rather than putting all the tissue in formalin). Special stains may also be requested on histopathology to help determine whether infection is present. Immunohistopathology may be helpful in cases of neoplasia.

Fine-needle aspiration

Obtaining tissue for cytology using fine-needle aspiration (FNA; see QRG 5.33.1) is the least invasive way to try and obtain a diagnosis. This can often be done with manual restraint and minimal sedation, depending on the precise location of the mass.

It is, however, often of low diagnostic yield. Cytology may only reveal inflammation or necrosis surrounding a primary neoplasm and there may be no exfoliation of neoplastic cells. Lymphoma is the neoplasm most readily diagnosed by fine-needle aspirate cytology. However, there may be potential for seeding of tumour cells along the needle tract, although this has not been documented in the cat in relation to the abdomen.

FNA is indicated if the mass is filled with fluid. A fluid-filled mass may represent a benign cyst, a cystic neoplasm, an abscess or haematoma. Cytology and culture of the fluid can be useful in reaching a diagnosis. The absence of neoplastic cells within the aspirate from a fluid-filled mass does not, however, exclude neoplasia. In a case of suspected lymphoma it is worth considering aspiration of the liver and spleen, in addition to the mass.

Needle-core biopsy

Tissue biopsy samples can be obtained using a Tru-cut device under ultrasound or CT guidance. This is a more invasive option than FNA and also has a higher complication rate. The cat will need either heavy sedation or general anaesthesia. Needle-core biopsy should only be performed by clinicians with training and experience in the technique, and referral may be required.

Haemostasis needs to be normal (as assessed by measurement of prothrombin (PT) and activated partial thromboplastin (APTT) times for secondary haemostasis, and platelet count (± buccal mucosal bleeding time) for primary haemostasis. The clinician also needs to ensure that the approach to the mass will not result in perforation of vessels, bile ducts, the urinary or gastrointestinal tract. It should be remembered that there is still a risk of haemorrhage despite normal coagulation, and it is important to have the option of prompt surgical intervention in case of complications. The cat needs to be kept under observation after the biopsy procedure and monitored for evidence of haemorrhage (e.g. tachycardia, pallor, weakness, reduced pulse quality). A repeat abdominal ultrasound scan a few hours after the procedure will help to determine whether there have been any complications.

The size of specimen obtained can be very small, and may not always be diagnostic.

Surgical/laparoscopic biopsy

This is the most invasive option but may be in the best interest of the cat in terms of achieving a quicker diagnosis and more complete abdominal assessment with a lower risk of complications. The decision as to whether to perform needle-core or surgical biopsy must be taken on a case-by-case basis, considering both risks and benefits. The surgical approach allows the clinician: to take samples from *all* abnormal tissues (especially if more than one organ is involved); to remove an abdominal mass; and to deal with any complications. Ideally a tissue diagnosis is made *before* the clinician embarks on removal of the abdominal mass, as this will determine the surgical plan (approach and margins).

Treatment

Further treatment depends on the histopathology/ cytology results and the general health status of the cat.

When to refer

Whether a cat with an abdominal mass benefits from referral depends very much on the equipment and expertise available to the first opinion practitioner. It is important that, during each of the stages of the diagnostic investigations, all options are considered, including the potential for complications, and that these are discussed with the owners. The decision to refer is made if this is the best option for the patient.

Alopecia

Natalie Barnard

Alopecia is the *complete* absence of hair in an area where it is normally present. The term hypotrichosis is used when there is partial hair loss or abnormal thinning of the hair coat. Alopecia is the most common reason for a dermatology consultation in the cat after pruritus, which may be associated with alopecia (see Chapter 5.26). Alopecia can be self-induced secondary to overgrooming, or can be caused by abnormalities directly affecting the hair follicle and structure of the hair itself. Alopecia may have inflammatory or non-inflammatory causes.

History

Taking a thorough history is always the starting point with dermatology patients as it provides vital information. Some points to consider with regard to alopecia are as follows.

- **Signalment.** Some alopecic conditions are breed-specific (Figure 5.3.1).
- **General health.** Some cats may have alopecic diseases that are seen as a consequence of internal disease, e.g. paraneoplastic syndromes.
- **Environment.** Infectious aetiologies (e.g. dermatophytosis) may be more likely in catteries/rescue centres.
- **In-contact animals and owners.** It is necessary to ascertain whether or not these are affected, as this narrows the differential diagnosis list considerably, e.g. dermatophytosis or pruritic ectoparasite (fleas, *Cheyletiella*) infestations.

■ Sphynx	■ Devon Rex
■ Canadian Hairless	■ Birman
■ Burmese	

5.3.1 Examples of breeds in which congenital or hereditary alopecia syndromes are recognized. In these breeds congenital alopecia, or hypotrichosis, is present at birth or shortly after. However, as hair follicle development can continue after birth, clinical signs may not be apparent until the cat is several months old. Congenital syndromes should always be considered when alopecia develops within the first year of life. There is no treatment for such conditions.

- **Dermatological history:**
  - Age of onset: a symmetrical non-inflammatory alopecia that starts when the patient is less than a year old is more suggestive of a congenital alopecia (see Figure 5.3.1); an inflammatory alopecia secondary to pruritus can start at any age
  - Progression of the disease: Does it wax and wane? Was it initially a focal disease that has now become more generalized?
  - Is there evidence of pruritus?
  - Has any medication helped? This may give important clues to the aetiology.
  - Is the cat currently on any medication? If the cat is currently receiving medication, this may alter the clinical picture.

Clinical examination

Once a thorough history has been obtained, the next step is to perform a general physical examination to ensure that there are no signs of systemic illness, followed by a dermatological examination to assess the skin lesions.

When approaching a case of alopecia in a cat the first thing that needs to be assessed is whether or not the cat is pruritic or overgrooming (see Chapter 5.26). Many clients are unaware that their cat is overgrooming and often will not perceive overgrooming as a sign of pruritus. It is very important to question the owner thoroughly; it can sometimes help for them to compare the grooming habits of the affected cat with other cats in the household. It is also useful to obtain hair pluck samples.

If it has been determined that the cat is not pruritic (see Chapter 5.26 for discussion of alopecia associated with pruritus and overgrooming), the alopecia can be assessed further. It is often useful to determine whether the pattern of alopecia is focal, multifocal or generalized. Figure 5.3.2 lists the causes of alopecia in cats and their incidence, in addition to stating their pattern of distribution. The causes of true alopecia in the cat, i.e. when the alopecia is *not* caused by pruritus, are generally uncommon to rare, with the exception of dermatophytosis.

Cause/condition	True alopecia (i.e. not caused by self-trauma)	Alopecia secondary to self-trauma	Incidence	Focal	Multifocal	Symmetrical or diffuse
Dermatophytosis	✓		Common	✓	✓	✓
Ectoparasites excluding demodicosis (e.g. fleas)		✓	Common	✓	✓	✓
Allergic skin disease		✓	Common	✓	✓	✓
Pyoderma	✓	✓	Common	✓	✓	
Demodicosis	✓		Rare	✓	✓	✓
Exfoliative dermatitis	✓	-	Rare			✓
Paraneoplastic alopecia	✓		Rare			✓
Hyperadrenocorticism	✓		Very rare			✓
Alopecia areata	✓		Very rare	✓		
Psychogenic alopecia	✓		Very rare			✓

5.3.2 Causes of alopecia in the cat, their incidence and distribution.

Diagnostic tests

Many diagnostic tests can be used to investigate alopecia (see Figure 5.3.3):

- Wood's lamp examination (see QRG 5.3.1)
- Hair pluck examination (see QRG 5.3.2)
- Coat brushing examination (see QRG 5.26.1)
- Skin scrape examination (see QRG 5.26.2)
- Fungal culture: the Mackenzie toothbrush technique is the most time- and cost-effective way of obtaining a sample for fungal culture. A sterile toothbrush is brushed over the entire cat's body, or over clinically suspicious lesions. The brush is then sent in a sealed container or bag to an external laboratory to be cultured. Fungal culture can take up to 2 weeks

- Skin biopsy (see QRG 5.3.3)
- Haematology, biochemistry, hormonal testing and diagnostic imaging – may be indicated in some cases when the patient is systemically unwell.
- Cytology can be used if there are erosions and crusting, as when investigating a pruritic cat (see QRG 5.26.3).

Differential diagnoses

Causes of alopecia include the following:

- Dermatophytosis
- Allergic skin disease (e.g. flea allergy, cutaneous adverse food reaction, atopic dermatitis)
- Congenital hypotrichosis/alopecia
- Paraneoplastic alopecia; this syndrome is rare and

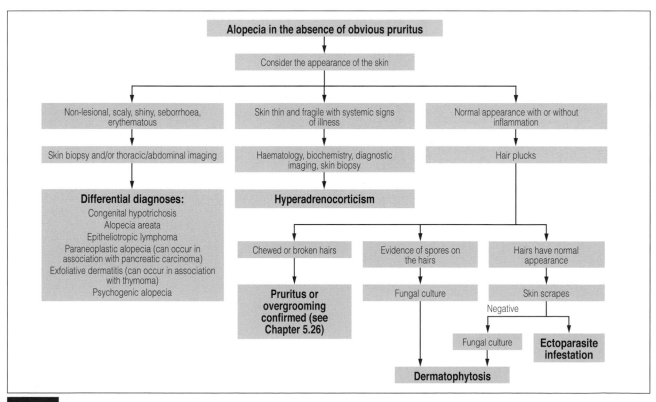

5.3.3 The diagnostic approach to alopecia.

is associated with internal malignancies such as pancreatic or liver tumours
- Epitheliotropic lymphoma
- Demodicosis
- Exfoliative dermatitis: this is a term used to describe a group of diseases in cats not associated with one aetiology. They include thymoma-associated exfoliative dermatitis, feline idiopathic mural folliculitis and feline sebaceous adenitis. Various causative factors have been identified recently. Thymoma is the most well documented of these, but other potential causes include internal malignancies, drug reactions, nutritional factors and seasonal influences. Most cases seem to be idiopathic
- Psychogenic alopecia
- Alopecia areata: this is an immune-mediated disease that targets the hair follicle
- Hyperadrenocorticism.

Treatment recommendations

Treatment of self-induced alopecia linked to pruritus is discussed in Chapter 5.26.

Where alopecia is not self-induced, if Wood's lamp examination is positive or fungal spores have been seen on a hair shaft, it is acceptable to start treatment for dermatophytosis (see Chapter 6) pending fungal culture results. All other causes of alopecia generally require skin biopsy results to confirm a diagnosis, and so only supportive care should be given pending these results. If there is evidence on cytology of infection by bacteria or yeast, this should be treated with appropriate antimicrobial therapy (see Chapter 6).

When to refer

Patients that are systemically unwell and/or have extremely fragile skin which tears easily should be referred for further investigation.

What to do if finances are limited

Hair plucks give important clues to the underlying cause of the alopecia and are cheap and easy to perform in house. They enable differentiation between: self-induced alopecia secondary to pruritus; and alopecia that is not self-induced. Most of the causes of true alopecia in cats are uncommon to rare, so the first step is to rule out pruritus and dermatophytosis before pursuing skin biopsy; biopsy is not useful in cases where alopecia is secondary to overgrooming.

QRG 5.3.1 Wood's lamp examination
by Natalie Barnard

The Wood's lamp can be a useful tool for diagnosing dermatophytosis in cats. It is important to be aware, however, that only 50% of *Microsporum canis* isolates will fluoresce with the Wood's lamp.

When using a Wood's lamp the following guidelines should be followed:

- Use the lamp in a *darkened room*
- Ensure the lamp is *warmed up for 10 minutes* before using it, by switching it on. If the lamp is not warmed up it does not emit the correct wavelength of light that causes fluorescence of the infected hairs
- Examine the *entire animal's haircoat* once the lamp is ready to use.

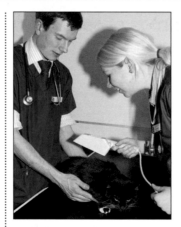

Apple green fluorescence OF THE HAIRS is a positive result. It is important that it is the hairs that fluoresce and not scale and crust.

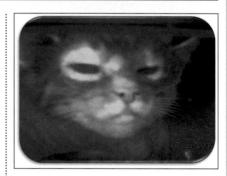

NOTE: If a Wood's lamp examination is negative, this does not exclude dermatophytosis as a cause of the patient's clinical signs. A sample should be submitted to an external laboratory for fungal culture to rule out dermatophytosis.

QRG 5.3.2 Hair plucks
by Natalie Barnard

Indications

- Evidence of alopecia or hair loss
- Crusting and scaling skin disease
- To determine whether alopecia is due to overgrooming

Equipment

- Glass microscope slides
- Pencil to label slides
- Liquid paraffin
- Artery forceps
- Coverslips
- Microscope (not shown)

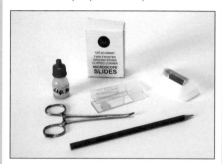

Technique

1 Label a glass slide. Place a small amount of liquid paraffin on it.

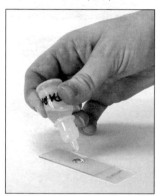

2 Using artery forceps, pluck a small number of hairs from the lesion or the area immediately adjacent to it. NB Note how easily the hair is epilated. If hairs are hard to pluck in an alopecic patient, this is more suggestive of self-induced alopecia. When hair is easily epilated, this raises the index of suspicion for paraneoplastic or immune-mediated disease.

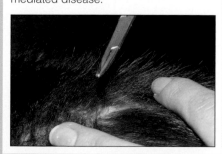

3 Place the hairs directly on to the slide into the liquid paraffin. Try to ensure that all the hairs lie in the same direction, i.e. roots together and tips together.

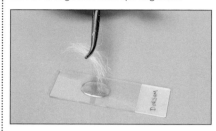

4 Place a coverslip on top of the sample.

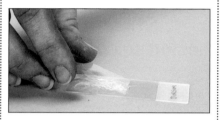

5 Examine under low power using the X4 or X10 objective. If you are not confident of finding parasites, use the X10 objective. The X4 objective (total magnification X40) will be satisfactory to examine the hair shaft itself. Examine the sample systematically, using parallel rows so that the entire slide is examined.

Examples of results

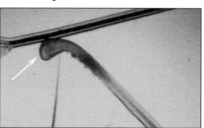

An anagen hair root at X40 original magnification. Anagen is the growing stage of the hair growth cycle. Note the rounded end of the root (arrowed).

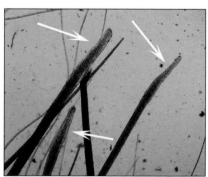

Several telogen hairs at X40 original magnification. Telogen is the resting stage of the hair growth cycle. Note that telogen hairs have pointed roots (arrowed) compared to the rounded root of anagen hairs.

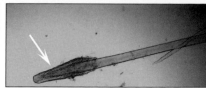

A telogen hair root at X40 original magnification. The sheath around the root is a follicular cast. Such casts can be seen in any disease affecting the hair follicles, at any stage of the hair cycle. Causes include dermatophytosis and folliculitis.

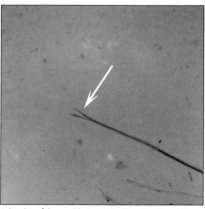

A broken/chewed hair. Note that the tip of the hair (arrowed) is frayed and broken, instead of being a finely tapered point.

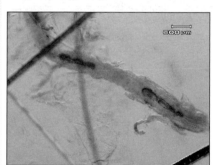

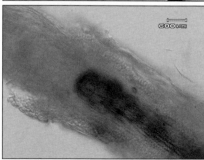

A rough or dirty-looking hair with uneven edges may be suggestive of dermatophytosis. By increasing the magnification and using the X40 objective (total magnification X400), you should be able to see the fungal spores. This hair is infected with *Microsporum canis*. The rounded ectothrix spores can be seen around the hair shaft, especially in the close-up view.

QRG 5.3.3 Skin biopsy
by Natalie Barnard

Indications

- Nodules
- Persistent ulcerated lesions
- Lesions not responding to appropriate therapy
- Unusual or atypical presentations
- Alopecia (when *not* associated with self-trauma/pruritus/overgrooming)
- Tissue culture is required

WARNING

Skin biopsy should not be carried out on patients with a coagulopathy.

Equipment

- Needle-holders
- Atraumatic forceps
- Rat-tooth forceps
- Sterile swabs
- Fine scissors
- Biopsy punches: 6 mm, 8 mm. If sampling the face or feet, a 4 mm punch may be more appropriate. The punches are disposable and should be discarded after use as they become blunt quickly

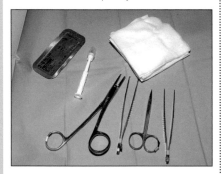

- Scalpel handle and No. 10 scalpel blade (if not using a punch)
- Suture material, e.g. 3 metric (USP 2/0) lactomer (e.g. Polysorb)
- Small artery forceps
- Pots containing formalin
- Plain pot (in case tissue is required for culture)
- Some small pieces of card (or tongue depressor) to place the samples on before placing in formalin

Patient preparation

- Skin biopsy sampling can be performed under general anaesthesia, or sedation (e.g. dexmedetomidine + butorphanol) with local anaesthesia. The choice depends on the location of the lesion to be sampled and other patient factors such as age, general health, temperament.
- If taking skin samples from the face or feet, this should always be performed under general anaesthesia.
- If using local anaesthetic, the skin should be infiltrated around the area being sampled, placing local anaesthetic into the subcutaneous tissue as well. You can move the needle gently under the skin to ensure an even distribution of the local anaesthetic. Wait 5–10 minutes for it to take effect, and check efficacy by pricking the test area gently with a 25 G needle.
- DO NOT ASEPTICALLY PREPARE THE AREA YOU WISH TO SAMPLE as this may remove vital crust and scale that could be essential for reaching the diagnosis. If hair is present, this should be gently clipped as short as possible with scissors, without removing any crust or scale or damaging the lesion

Lesion selection

Aim to sample primary or early lesions from affected areas of the skin, such as papules, pustules, vesicles and nodules. Try to avoid choosing lesions that have been excoriated or traumatized excessively. If you are sampling alopecic skin, always take at least one biopsy specimen from the centre of the most alopecic area. If sampling an ulcerated lesion, it is important to obtain a sample that spans normal and diseased tissue, as sampling just the ulcerated area will likely not yield any useful information.

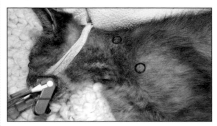

Technique using a biopsy punch

1 Place the biopsy punch on the lesion to be sampled at a 90-degree angle to the skin. Apply moderate pressure while twisting the biopsy punch in one direction. *Do not be tempted to twist the punch back and forth, as this will damage the biopsy sample.*

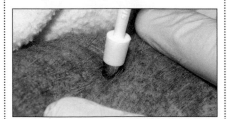

2 Once it has penetrated the full thickness of the skin, remove the punch. The sample should remain attached to the subcutaneous fat.

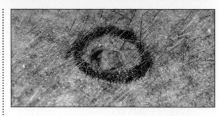

3 Using atraumatic forceps, gently grasp the sample by the deep fat. It can then be cut free from the fat.

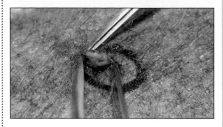

4 Because feline skin is thin, the biopsy sample should be placed on a piece of card, skin side up, to keep it flat.

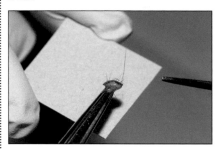

5 It can be useful to mark the direction of hair growth on the card with an arrow, as this influences the plane of sectioning by the pathologist.

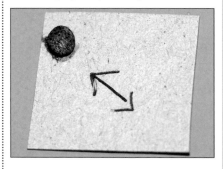

6 Wait a few minutes before dropping the piece of card and material together into a formalin pot.

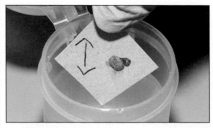

▶

QRG 5.3.3 *continued*

If a sample is required for tissue culture, it is not placed in formalin but instead is put into a sterile container with a drop of saline.

7 Once the sample has been taken the wound can be sutured. One cruciate suture or two simple interrupted sutures (see Appendix) are often sufficient.

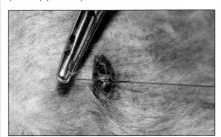

8 Submit samples for histopathology (to a specialist dermatopathologist if possible) and/or culture.

PRACTICAL TIPS

- When taking a sample from a nodular lesion or non-healing wound, it is always worth freezing a small piece of the sample in case tissue culture is required at a later date, especially in cases where mycobacterial infection is suspected.
- Remember: taking a skin biopsy is not a sterile procedure.
- To improve diagnostic yield, always submit multiple samples representative of the lesions.
- Submit a detailed history alongside your sample for the pathologist, to aid interpretation.

Excisional biopsy

This technique is preferred when sampling large lesions, nodules or ulcers. A wedge or ellipitically shaped sample can be taken using a scalpel blade. Often you aim to span normal and diseased tissue when taking this type of sample.

QRG 5.4.2 *continued*

- **Acanthocytes:** red cells with large cytoplasmic projections; may be seen as a shear injury product in association with liver disease and with lipid disorders.

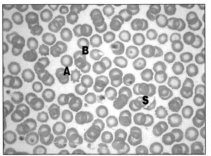

Blister cell (B), acanthocyte (A), schistocyte (S). (Modified Wright's stain; original magnification X1000)

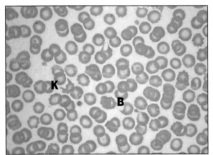

Keratocyte (K), blister cell (B). (Modified Wright's stain; original magnification X1000)

- **Ovalocytes:** elongated red cells often associated with liver disease, especially hepatic lipidosis.
- **Echinocytes:** have small 'spikes' of cytoplasm which do not disrupt the round shape of the cell; often noted as an artefact, where they may be unevenly distributed across the smear. True echinocytes may be associated with glomerulonephritis.

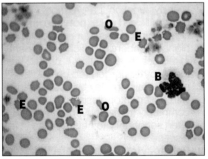

Ovalocytes (O) and echinocytes (E). Basket cells (B) are nuclear remnants of disrupted leucocytes and are usually not clinically significant. (Modified Wright's stain; original magnification X1000)

- **Heinz bodies:** rounded, clear to haemoglobin-coloured bodies; associated with oxidative injury to the red cells. Normal, healthy cats may have up to 10% of their red cells affected by small Heinz bodies; higher numbers and the presence of larger forms are considered abnormal and suggest increased oxidative damage.

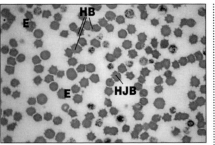

Echinocytes (E), Heinz bodies (HB) and Howell–Jolly bodies (HJB). (Modified Wright's stain; original magnification X1000)

Platelets

These are often pale-staining and may appear clear or granular. Larger platelets (**macroplatelets**), which are the same size as, or larger than, red cells, are seen in low numbers in normal cats. These may be miscounted as red cells by automated methods but will be evident on a smear (see Figure 5.4.3).

Haematological abnormalities associated with increased and decreased cell numbers

Recognized causes of increased and decreased numbers of white blood cells, red blood cells and platelets are below; the commonest causes are listed first.

Mature neutrophilia (increased number of neutrophils with normal morphology)

- Fear/excitement: increased blood pressure sweeps neutrophils situated near the blood vessel wall into the main blood flow.
- Increase in corticosteroids with long-term stress and exogenous steroid administration: corticosteroids decrease normal movement of neutrophils out of blood vessels into tissues.
- Inflammation/infection: peripheral demands result in neutrophils being recruited from bone marrow stores and more being allowed to mature and leave the marrow.
- Chronic granulocytic leukaemia: increased production independent of demand may result in extreme neutrophilia (>50 x 10^9/l); may be composed entirely of mature neutrophils but often precursors present (see below).

Neutrophilia with left shift ± toxic change

- Peripheral demand for neutrophils due to marked inflammation/infection overwhelms the normal supply of mature neutrophils. Younger precursors (bands/metamyelocytes/

myelocytes most usually) or those with dysplastic cytoplasm or nucleus begin to be released into the peripheral blood. Note: The demand may not be from a septic cause. Having more band neutrophils than mature neutrophils is termed a 'degenerative left shift' and is a poor prognostic indicator.
- Chronic granulocytic leukaemia (see above). Toxic change is generally not present.

Neutropenia

- Decreased production in bone marrow disease (e.g. crowding out of neutrophil precursors by stage 5 lymphoma, myelofibrosis, targeting of haemopoietic precursors by viruses such as FIV/FeLV/panleucopenia virus, ineffective production in myelodysplastic syndromes).
- Decreased production due to use of myelosuppressive drugs (e.g. cyclophosphamide).
- Normal marrow unable to keep up with overwhelming peripheral demand in marked inflammatory/ infectious responses. In these cases, if not already present, development of left shift and toxic change may help distinguish from failure of production.
- Drug reaction (e.g. griseofulvin, cephalosporins).
- Immune-mediated neutropenia.
- Anaphylaxis/endotoxaemia: may cause increased margination of neutrophils to the blood vessel walls.
- Chédiak–Higashi syndrome: congenital disorder seen only in blue smoke Persians; neutrophils contain abnormal granules in cytoplasm.

Monocytosis

- Inflammation/infection: monocytosis commonly accompanies neutrophilia and occurs in many of the same circumstances. Monocytosis may be more marked in cats with refractory conditions such as mycobacterial infection or foreign bodies.
- Increase in corticosteroids with long-term stress and exogenous steroid administration.
- Myelomonocytic leukaemia has been rarely reported in the cat in both acute and chronic forms.

Monocytopenia

- Most reference intervals start at zero – even where recognized, monocytopenia is of no clinical importance.

Lymphocytosis

- Has been noted as part of a mixed inflammatory response to many infectious or inflammatory stimuli, including cholangiohepatitis, immune-mediated disease, *Mycoplasma felis*, *Toxoplasma gondii*.
- Adrenaline-mediated physiological 'fight or flight' response may elevate numbers in a blood sample by redistribution.

▶

QRG 5.4.2 *continued*

- Associated with positive FIV status in some studies.
- Glucocorticoid deficiency (lymphocytosis found in 20% of cats with hypoadrenocorticism).
- Hyperthyroidism.
- Thymoma.
- Chronic lymphocytic leukaemia: high to very high numbers of small lymphocytes.
- Acute lymphoblastic leukaemia: lymphoblasts present in peripheral blood. Care should be taken not to mistake low numbers of reactive lymphocytes for early lymphoblastic leukaemia. Serial sampling and the involvement of other cell lines or organs can help distinguish these, along with more involved techniques such as immunophenotyping (seek advice from oncologist and/or clinical pathologist).
- NB Kittens have higher normal lymphocyte numbers than adults, and this may appear to be a lymphocytosis if the laboratory does not adjust its reference range accordingly.

Lymphopenia

- Corticosteroid increase: whether endogenous (long-term stress or hyperadrenocorticism) or exogenous, causes direct lysis of lymphoid cells and redistribution.
- Feline infectious peritonitis: lymphoid depletion with likely increased early apoptosis of lymphoid cells.
- FeLV, FIV, panleucopenia and other viral infections.
- Chylothorax/lymphangiectasia: loss of lymphocyte-rich fluid from the circulation.
- Immunosuppressive drugs (e.g. cyclophosphamide, melphalan, doxorubicin).

Eosinophilia

- Flea allergy.
- Gastrointestinal disease.

- Focal infection/inflammation.
- Feline asthma.
- Eosinophilic granuloma complex.
- Hypereosinophilic syndrome.
- Parasitic infections (e.g. *Aelurostrongylus*).
- Food allergy.
- Paraneoplastic: associated with lymphoma and mast cell tumours most commonly.
- Eosinophilic leukaemia: may be very difficult to distinguish from hypereosinophilic syndrome.

Eosinopenia

- Corticosteroid increase (endogenous or exogenous, as above).
- Acute inflammation.
- Often not recognized because of very low reference ranges (often start at zero).

Basophilia

- Immediate hypersensitivity reactions (e.g. secondary to arthropod bites/stings).
- Associated with some neoplasms (e.g. mast cell tumours, lymphosarcoma).
- Parasites (e.g. heartworm).

Basopenia

- Not recognized in cats.

Thrombocytosis

- Hyperthyroidism.
- Ongoing low-grade haemorrhage.
- Inflammatory/infectious diseases (e.g. pancreatitis, gastrointestinal disease).
- Neoplastic disease (e.g. lymphoma).
- Hepatic lipidosis.
- Primary erythrocytosis.
- Vascular or cardiac disease (e.g. thromboembolism).

Thrombocytopenia

- Spurious result due to *in vitro* platelet clumping – very common.
- Decreased production due to:
  - Infectious disease (e.g. panleucopenia, FeLV-related myelodysplasia)

- Drug administration (e.g. reaction to cephalosporins, direct suppression with cyclophosphamide)
- Displacement of marrow elements (e.g. stage 5 lymphoma, leukaemias, myelofibrosis)
- Endogenous abnormality within the marrow (e.g. primary myelodysplastic syndromes)
- Increased consumption (e.g. in haemorrhage, disseminated intravascular coagulation).
- Increased destruction (i.e. immune-mediated thrombocytopenia, primary or secondary).

Anaemia

- See Figure 5.4.6 for causes of feline anaemia

Erythrocytosis (also known as polycythaemia)

- Relative – due to decreased plasma volume and a relative increase in PCV (e.g. fluid loss due to diarrhoea).
- Absolute – actual increase in red blood cell mass present to cause a rise in PCV:
  - Primary (also called polycythaemia vera) – neoplastic condition (typically seen in junior to prime cats) where red blood cell production in the bone marrow is autonomously increased but erythropoietin (EPO) concentration is normal
  - Secondary – red blood cell production in the bone marrow is increased due to elevated EPO concentrations:
    - Physiologically appropriate – due to systemic hypoxia (e.g. right to left shunting congenital heart disease, chronic lung disease, high-altitude living)
    - Physiologically inappropriate – particularly seen with renal neoplasia (where local hypoxia causes a rise in EPO) or other tumours occasionally produce EPO or EPO-like substances.

QRG 5.4.3 Obtaining bone marrow samples
by Séverine Tasker

Two types of bone marrow sample are collected for diagnostic purposes: a **bone marrow cellular aspirate** provides cytological (morphological) information on individual cells, while a **bone marrow core biopsy** allows evaluation of the degree of cellularity and presence or absence of infiltration with fat or fibrous tissue. Ideally both should be collected, but sometimes presence of bone marrow disease makes sample collection difficult, and only one or the other can be obtained.

Indications

- Persistent unexplained abnormal findings on peripheral haematology: severe non-regenerative anaemia, persistent neutropenia or pancytopenia and/or abnormal blood cell morphology.
- Suspected myeloproliferative diseases.
- Staging of neoplasia.
- Unexplained hypercalcaemia.
- Unexplained increased globulin levels

(gammopathy; particularly if monoclonal).

Equipment

The equipment can be prepared before the cat is anaesthetized or while the site is being aseptically prepared. **Put on sterile gloves before the equipment is laid out, maintaining sterility of the sterile items.**

- Sterile gloves
- Sterile drape with small hole ▶

QRG 5.4.3 *continued*

- Jamshidi disposable bone marrow aspirate or biopsy needle (11 to 15 G, depending on patient size; here an 11 G 4 inch needle is used)
- Scalpel
- 20 ml syringe and 19 G needle
- 8–10 clean labelled microscope slides, laid out
- Slide holders
- Acid citrate dextrose anticoagulant (shown here in a blood transfusion collection bag; anticoagulant is not essential but allows valuable extra time for preparation of aspirate smears)
- Pot containing formalin for submission of the core biopsy sample

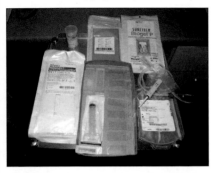

PRACTICAL TIP

Anticoagulant should be drawn up into the syringe, to coat the entire barrel, and then removed from the syringe while flushing the bone marrow needle with the stylet removed. The stylet should then be replaced back into the bone marrow needle.

Patient preparation

Routine haematology (on EDTA blood sample) should be performed on the day of bone marrow sampling (before sedation and anaesthesia is induced) so that the resultant aspirate cytology can be interpreted with knowledge of the peripheral blood counts.

The patient should undergo general anaesthesia (see Chapter 3) and should be placed in lateral recumbency. If severe anaemia is present, Oxyglobin (if available) can be given as supportive care during anaesthesia; blood transfusions should be reserved for after bone marrow collection if at all possible. If a blood transfusion is to be given (see QRG 20.2), the blood should be collected from the donor cat before anaesthesia of the patient for bone marrow collection, so that the blood is available for immediate transfusion after collection of the marrow.

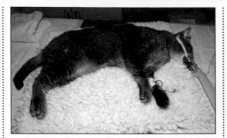

Technique

Bone marrow cellular aspirate

Bone marrow can be collected from the shaft of the humerus, by inserting the bone marrow needle into the greater tubercle of the proximal humerus and aligning with the long axis of the humerus, as shown here.

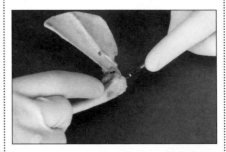

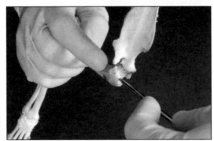

Alternative view of above photograph, to show the position of needle insertion into the proximal humerus.

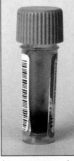 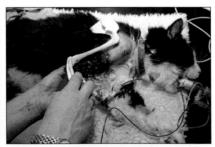

This image is for illustrative purposes only and was taken after collection of a bone marrow sample in another cat. It shows the skeletal landmarks overlying the cat's forelimb. The proximal humerus is made more accessible and laterally prominent if the elbow is pushed medially, as shown here, by an assistant during the procedure. If so, it is important that the assistant maintains the limb in the same position throughout the procedure.

1 Clip a generous area of hair around the shoulder joint of the limb, including the proximal area of the humerus, and aseptically prepare the area for sampling.

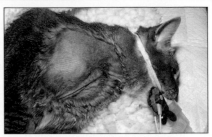

2 Whilst holding the limb as shown above, make a stab incision in the skin overlying the most prominent proximal part of the greater tubercle. The stab incision will appear not to be at the correct point when the limb is not held in position, but this is rectified when the limb is held again for insertion of the needle.

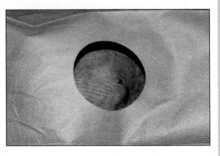

3 Again, hold the limb as shown above, and then insert the anticoagulant-flushed bone marrow needle, with the stylet in place (the stylet can be seen at the distal end of the needle; arrowed), into the humerus via the stab incision. Gradually advance the needle into the humeral marrow cavity using steady and very firm pressure with a drilling action (clockwise and anticlockwise movements). Holding the shaft of the humerus with the other hand will help you to keep the insertion along the long axis of the bone; keeping parallel to the long axis of the bone with needle insertion is very important and this should be checked frequently by eye and by feeling landmarks. Insertion of the needle can be hard work.

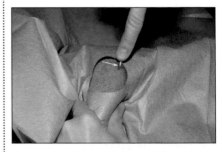

4 Stop inserting further as soon as you feel you have a good grip on the bone and the bone marrow needle feels firmly in place (you should be able to move the limb of the cat by moving the bone marrow needle). This will be around a centimetre or so into the humerus but it is based on feel rather than length.

▶

QRG 5.4.3 *continued*

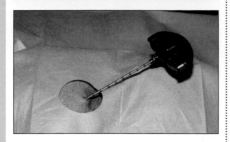

5 The stylet of the bone marrow needle is then removed and the 20 ml anticoagulated syringe is securely attached to the needle.

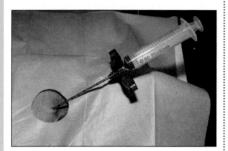

6 Rapidly and forcefully (to around the 10 ml mark on the syringe) aspirate, and look in the hub of the syringe for any visible blood-coloured liquid (arrowed), indicating the successful collection of marrow; marrow aspirate samples usually comprise <0.5 ml. Stop aspirating as soon as marrow is visible, otherwise haemodilution occurs. If marrow is not visible despite aspirating, remove the syringe, reinsert the stylet and insert the bone marrow needle a further 0.5 cm into the humerus and try aspirating again. Dry taps (where no aspirate sample can be obtained) can occur with severe marrow disease such as myelofibrosis. If this happens, it may only be possible to obtain a core sample, but another limb may be used for another attempt at obtaining an aspirate.

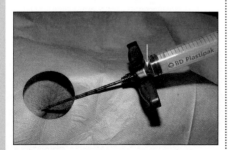

7 If marrow has been aspirated, remove the syringe from the needle and replace the stylet into the bone marrow needle while the smears are made. Apply a drop of bone marrow to each of the slides. The slides can be positioned at a slight angle, as shown here, so that any excessive blood present in the marrow samples can drain away under gravity, leaving the bone marrow spicules at the proximal top end of the slide.

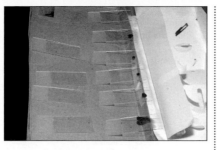

Making the aspirate smears

1 Take another microscope slide and apply it at right angles to the lower slide with the drop of bone marrow on it.

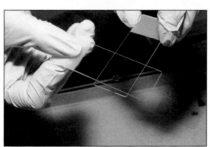

2 Make contact between the two slides so that the drop of marrow is spread (*do not apply pressure* but just use the surface tension between the two slides).

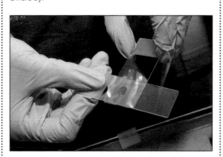

3 Slide away the second slide from the first slide to make the smear. Repeat this for each slide and then air-dry the smears by waving them in the air or using a hairdryer. Submit the smears for cytology.

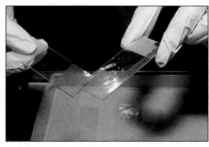

Bone marrow core biopsy

1 A bone marrow core sample can be obtained from the same site, by further insertion of the bone marrow needle, although removal of the needle and reinsertion at a different site (a slightly different insertion point on the same limb or using the contralateral limb) is sometimes required. If the same site is being used, remove the stylet and insert the bone marrow needle firmly into the shaft of the humerus with a drilling action (clockwise and anti-clockwise movements).

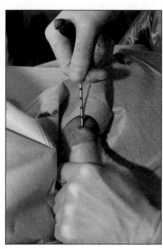

2 Continue drilling the needle into the humeral shaft (this is hard work) until it has gone in a further 1–2 cm. This drilling should fill the lumen of the bone marrow biopsy needle with a core of bone marrow.

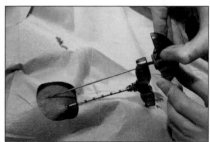

The stylet is shown adjacent to the needle, to illustrate how far the needle has been inserted.

3 Detach the bone marrow core sample from its humeral source at the distal tip of the biopsy needle by rotating and moving the handle of the bone marrow needle vigorously in different directions (circular motion, side to side, etc.), and then twisting the needle within the bone clockwise a few times and anticlockwise a few times – these movements should be done with reasonable force and conviction, otherwise the core you have collected into the lumen will be left behind as you withdraw the needle.

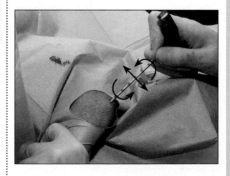

▶

QRG 5.4.3 *continued*

4 Carefully pull the bone marrow needle out from the humerus.

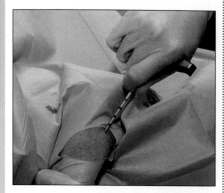

5 Use the probe provided with the bone marrow needle to push the bone marrow core sample out of the lumen of the needle; this is done by inserting the probe into the free end of the bone marrow needle, rather than the handle end, due to the tapered nature of the needle.

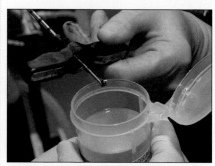

Here the probe is seen coming out of the needle lumen at the handle end to push the core sample out into the formalin pot.

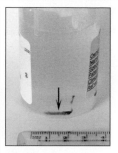

6 Submit the core biopsy sample (arrowed) for histopathology in formalin.

Postoperative care

If a blood transfusion is to be given, this can now be started and the cat is recovered from general anaesthesia. Analgesia (such as buprenorphine) should be provided postoperatively for at least 12 hours, and longer if required.

Anorexia

Samantha Taylor and Rachel Korman

Anorexia (loss of appetite for food) is a common presenting sign in feline practice. Cats are sensitive to environmental changes, and illnesses often manifest as a loss of appetite. This may be the first sign noted by an owner that their cat is unwell. As there are multiple differential diagnoses (which can occur concurrently) a logical approach with thorough history taking and physical examination are important. *It is important to distinguish a lack of ability to eat from a lack of interest in food.* Anorexia can have severe consequences for affected cats (Figure 5.5.1), complicating the diagnosis of the underlying cause and warranting prompt treatment to prevent further deterioration. Nutritional support is vital for recovery from many different diseases (see *BSAVA Manual of Rehabilitation, Supportive and Palliative Care: Case Studies in Patient Management*).

- Dehydration
- Hepatic lipidosis
- Loss of muscle, as well as loss of body fat
- Weakness
- Hypoglycaemia
- Hypokalaemia
- Suppression of the immune system and increased risk of sepsis
- Alterations in intestinal function
- Delayed wound healing and tissue repair
- Altered drug metabolism
- Reduced quality of life

5.5.1 Potential consequences of anorexia.

Diagnostic approach

Important considerations when investigating the anorexic cat include:

- Signalment: age (e.g. chronic kidney disease in older cats)
- History:
  - Home environment, including any recent changes, new additions, house moves
  - Duration of clinical signs (e.g. short history of progressive signs in neoplastic disease)
  - Concurrent clinical signs; anorexia may be the owner's primary concern but other signs such as polydipsia or gastrointestinal signs might direct the investigation

- Any medications the cat is receiving (Figure 5.5.2)
  - Dietary history, including: any recent changes in diet and amount/type of food the cat is currently eating; possibility the cat may be eating elsewhere; hunting
- Physical examination findings:
  - A thorough physical examination may identify abnormalities suggestive of the underlying cause of the anorexia. For example, jaundice in an anorexic cat will prompt investigations of the liver or for haemolytic disease
- Laboratory test results: biochemistry and haematology results may identify an underlying cause such as organ dysfunction
- Diagnostic imaging results (e.g. presence of an intestinal mass).

- Many antibiotics (e.g. penicillin, trimethoprim/sulphonamides, doxycycline)
- NSAIDs (e.g. meloxicam)
- Opioids (e.g. morphine, methadone)
- Diuretics (e.g. furosemide)
- Chemotherapeutics (e.g. vincristine, cyclophosphamide)
- Cardiac glycosides (e.g. digoxin)
- Home remedies (e.g. aloe vera)

5.5.2 Medications that can cause anorexia as a side effect.

When considering the anorexic cat it is important to distinguish the cat that **cannot eat** from the cat that **does not want to eat**. Observation of eating behaviour may be required if the owner's description is inconclusive.

- Cats may be keen to eat but have difficulty picking up, chewing or swallowing food (dysphagia) if they have oral disease (see QRG 1.4), neurological conditions, or orthopaedic conditions of the jaw (Figure 5.5.3). Full oral examination (including the frenulum) will require sedation/anaesthesia, but it should be noted that anorexic cats often have fluid deficits that require correction prior to anaesthesia. Dental disease is not always evident on preliminary oral examination, and dental radiography may be required.

- Oral foreign body (linear foreign bodies often lodge under the tongue)
- Oral neoplasia (squamous cell carcinoma for example)
- Dental disease (periodontal disease, feline tooth resorption lesions)
- Trauma to jaw/face
- Retrobulbar disorders (abscess/neoplasia)
- Neurological disorders (brainstem, cranial nerves, neuromuscular disease)

5.5.3 Causes of difficulty in eating/dysphagia.

- Observation of eating may be facilitated by a single dose of intravenous diazepam (0.2 mg/kg) which can work as an immediate appetite stimulant, allowing assessment of the cat's physical ability to eat.
- The owner can also be asked to video the cat eating at home if dysphagia is reported or suspected.
- A lack of sense of smell (anosmia) may cause anorexia and can result from nasal or, in rare cases, neurological disease. Affected cats may have signs of nasal disease (stridor, sneezing, nasal discharge) and show little interest in food. Sense of smell can be tested as part of the neurological examination by passing a noxious smell under the cat's nose, e.g. surgical spirit on a cotton wool pad.
- Nausea is a common cause of anorexia; affected

cats may initially approach food but then turn away and exhibit signs such as ptyalism, swallowing actions, and retching. Causes of nausea are numerous but commonly include intra-abdominal conditions such as gastrointestinal, liver, renal and pancreatic disease. Food aversion (see text box) can result from force-feeding a nauseous cat.

> **Food aversion**
> Food aversion is an association between food/eating (sometimes all food but more commonly a specific food fed during a period of illness) and unpleasant feelings of nausea/pain. It can occur during illness but may also be caused by force-feeding, often by well intentioned owners. Food aversion can persist despite resolution of the underlying cause of the anorexia. Affected cats strongly object to being offered the food and may require careful reintroduction of food and appetite stimulation; it is important to ensure that the original cause of the anorexia/nausea is no longer present before such treatment, and a period of assisted nutrition may be required.

The diagnostic approach is summarized in Figure 5.5.4.

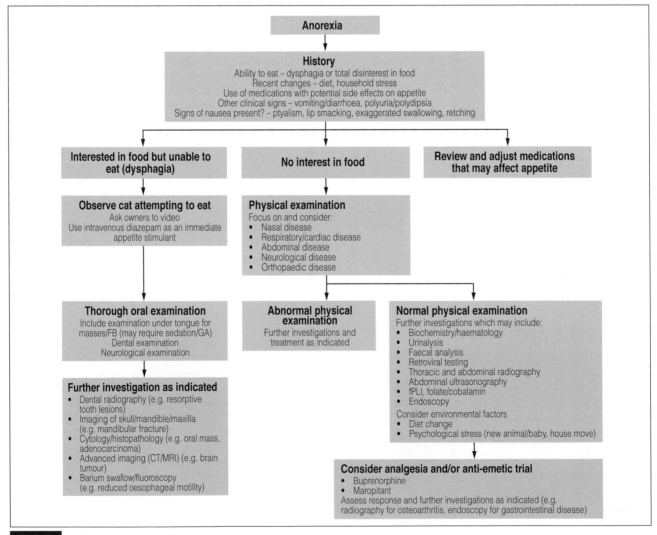

5.5.4 Diagnostic approach to the anorexic cat.

General considerations for management

With treatment of the underlying disease most cats will recover their appetite. However, it is important to improve nutrition as soon as possible to avoid complications of anorexia and to speed recovery. Considerations in the treatment of any anorexic cat include the following.

- Address and **deal with any stressors** that are identified in the cat's home environment or in the hospital if the cat is hospitalized (see Chapter 1). Examples of such stressors include: having litter trays close to food bowls; lack of food resources within the home environment due to conflict with other cats; barking dogs; too much noise and activity near the cat; presence of non-familiar cats; and being absent from owner when hospitalized. Some cats prefer human company when feeding whereas others prefer privacy (see below). If changes at home can account for the anorexia and physical examination shows no abnormalities, then methods for reducing stress should be discussed (Figure 5.5.5).
- **Fluid therapy** should be provided if there is evidence of dehydration (see QRGs 4.1.3 and 13.2).
- **Correction of any electrolyte disturbances** found is important, particularly hypokalaemia (see QRG 4.6.1).
- It is imperative that **pain**, **vomiting and nausea** are controlled prior to feeding. Sometimes analgesia and/or anti-emetic trials are indicated even if signs of nausea or pain are not overtly apparent, in case these are present and contributing to anorexia.
  - **Provision of adequate analgesia.** An *analgesia trial* can be useful when no underlying cause has been found to see whether unrecognized pain could be contributing to the anorexia. Potential therapies that can be tried are buprenorphine (0.01–0.02 mg/kg i.v., i.m., s.c. or sublingually q6h) or tramadol (2–4 mg/kg orally q8h or 1–2 mg/kg i.v. or s.c. q8h). Meloxicam (up to 0.05 mg/kg orally q24h; start with lower doses in older cats) is an alternative if renal and gut function are normal; monitoring renal parameters is advisable (see Chapter 3 for more details on analgesia).

- **Anti-emetic treatment** if nausea is suspected. An *anti-emetic trial* can be useful when no underlying cause has been found to see whether nausea could be contributing to the anorexia. Choice of agent will be determined by factors such as whether the cat is hospitalized and the ease of dosing. Potential therapies that can be tried are:
  - Mirtazapine (1.88–3.75 mg/cat (i.e. 1/8 to 1/4 of a 15 mg tablet) orally q1–3d
  - Metoclopramide (0.2–0.5 mg/kg s.c. or orally q8h, or 1–2 mg/kg i.v. over 24 hours as a constant rate infusion
  - Maropitant (1 mg/kg orally or s.c. q24h for 5 days, then resting for 2 days before repeating the course.
- Many methods can be used to **tempt cats to eat**, once stress, nausea and pain have been addressed:
  - Use different food types and textures, including both wet and dry forms of food. Favourite foods should be identified at hospital admission by talking to the owner
  - Warming food (to just above body temperature), wetting food, mashing the food to a softer texture and/or using strong-smelling foods may help increase palatability
  - Use wide shallow bowls or flat plates that avoid interfering with the cat's whiskers during feeding; talk to the owner about food bowl types to emulate the home environment as some cats prefer certain types (e.g. porcelain or glass, over plastic or metal dishes)
  - Providing physical contact and attention (coaxing) may encourage eating in some cats, so try spending time with the cat during feeding. Hand-feeding can help encourage some cats to eat, especially in a quiet relaxed location (possibly with owners in a consultation room). Other cats prefer more privacy and are more likely to eat if kept in a quiet environment with somewhere to hide; removing the cat from the hospital cage and placing it in an alternative quiet, safe environment (e.g. consultation room) may help.
- Food should not be left for long periods within the cage as this may contribute to food aversion. Offer a small quantity of one or two types of food only; if it is not eaten, remove it from the cage after 20–30 mins and offer fresh food again 1–2 hours later.
- Barriers to feeding (e.g. Elizabethan collars) may need to be removed during supervised feeding attempts such as during owner visits. Note that **food aversion** (see above) is common in hospital, particularly in cats force-fed (e.g. by syringe) or offered food during periods of nausea or pain, resulting in short-term or permanent aversion to that food.
- Prescription diets should not be introduced in the hospital environment or when the cat is inappetent. They will be less likely to accept a new diet in this situation, and furthermore it could lead to food aversion developing to the new diet; the patient should be stabilized and eating again before the new diet is introduced, usually once the cat is back home.

- Distribution of resources – availability of food, water and litter trays in accessible, quiet locations
- Other pets – new cats in the house guarding food or litter tray access; ensure the affected cat can access food without conflict
- New baby – ensure owners spend time with the cat, providing reassurance
- House moves – provide familiar beds; consider using feline pheromone products
- Food type – a recent diet change may cause anorexia in some cats who are reluctant to change flavour/texture of diet; slow introduction of new diets is recommended
- A temporary change to a strong-smelling and -tasting food may be required to renew the cat's interest in eating

5.5.5 Stressors such as the arrival of a new pet or baby, or a house move can result in reduced food intake. Management of such cases should consider these factors. See also Chapter 1.

- Always ensure accurate recording of the amount of food eaten by the cat and calculation of resting energy requirement (RER).
- **Do not delay providing enteral nutrition via a naso-oesophageal feeding tube or oesophageal feeding tube if indicated** as these are well tolerated if correctly placed (see QRGs 5.5.2 and 5.5.3) and provision of nutrition will speed recovery from illness in many cases. **Hospitalization** for assisted enteral feeding is imperative if the patient has lost 10% or more bodyweight or has been consuming less than RER (see QRG 5.5.1) for 3 or more days.

Appetite stimulants

Appetite stimulants may be useful to induce short-term appetite increases or to overcome food aversion, though underlying causes of anorexia must be addressed whenever possible, and pain and nausea must be managed prior to their use (see above). Their use is normally reserved for cases in which the cause of the anorexia has been identified; occasionally appetite stimulants are given when the cause of anorexia is not known, e.g. in cases in which chronic pancreatitis is suspected but not confirmed, trial treatment with an analgesic (typically buprenorphine) and anti-nausea/anti-emetic (mirtazapine) can be helpful. No appetite stimulant is authorized for use in cats in the UK.

- Mirtazapine (1.88–3.75 mg/cat; i.e. 1/8–1/4 of a 15 mg tablet, orally every 1–3 days) is a noradrenaline and specific serotonergic agonist with significant appetite-stimulant, anti-emetic and anti-nausea effects. Potential dose-dependent adverse effects include vocalization, drowsiness/sedation, tachycardia and hyperactivity, which may all be due to 'serotonin syndrome' caused by increased brain serotonin levels; signs will typically subside over 12–24 hours. If severe, cyproheptadine (a non-selective serotonin antagonist) may be helpful (0.2–0.5 mg/kg orally q12h). Renal and hepatic impairment may result in decreased mirtazapine clearance, and so the lower end of the dose range should be prescribed in these circumstances. The appetite stimulant effects of mirtazapine are typically seen within 30 minutes of administration. Food should be offered to coincide with this period.
- Cyproheptadine (0.2–0.5 mg/kg orally q12h) can also be a useful appetite stimulant but can take around 24 hours to be effective. It may cause mild sedation.
- Oral diazepam should be avoided, due to the possibility of an idiosyncratic reaction inducing acute hepatic necrosis. Intravenous diazepam (0.2 mg/kg) has *not* been associated with this syndrome but does result in sedation; its effects are also unpredictable and so it cannot be used in the longer term. However, intravenous diazepam, when it works in a cat, can be useful as an *immediate* appetite stimulant, e.g. to carry out swallowing studies after ingestion of a barium meal, or for observation of eating if dysphagia is suspected.

QRG 5.5.1 Enteral assisted nutrition
by Rachel Korman

Indications

- Loss of bodyweight (>10% not due to dehydration), reduced body condition score (see Chapter 1) or loss of muscle mass (e.g. over occipital crest, scapulae and hips).
- Patients that are willing but unable to eat normally (e.g. with orofacial disease).
- Any patient consuming less than their resting energy requirement (RER) for 3 days. Note that many cats will have already been anorexic for a number of days before being presented, and this time period must be taken into account when deciding when nutritional support is instigated.

$$RER_{(kcal/day)} = bodyweight_{(kg)}^{0.75} \times 70$$

Or, for cats >2 kg an estimate can be made from:

$$RER_{(kcal/day)} = (30 \times bodyweight_{(kg)}) + 70$$

For both calculations, the actual current bodyweight is used, not the patient's ideal bodyweight.

- Patients with severe malnourishment or hepatic lipidosis. Provision of adequate nutrition may result in decreased hospitalization time and improved survival.
- **Assisted enteral feeding should always be chosen over parenteral nutrition if vomiting is controlled and a functional gastrointestinal tract is present, in order to maintain gastrointestinal tract integrity.**

General considerations for tube feeding

Types of tube

Common routes are naso-oesophageal and oesophageal feeding tubes; correct placement is described in QRGs 5.5.2 and 5.5.3. Naso-oesophageal (NO) tube-feeding is often attempted first, as general anaesthesia is not required, but only thin, liquid diets can be administered. Flushing (see below) decreases the risk of blockage.

Gastrostomy tubes can be placed under endoscopic guidance or at surgery (see *BSAVA Manual of Canine and Feline Gastroenterology*).

Feeding protocols

To reduce the risk of refeeding syndrome (see below), anorexic patients should be weaned on to their full RER requirement over 3 days:

Feed 1/3 RER on Day 1; 2/3 RER on Day 2; and the entire RER on Day 3 of feeding. An example of a calculation of amounts to feed on Days 1, 2 and 3 is given at the end of this chapter.

Total food and water is split equally into 4–5 meals per day. The feline stomach capacity is approximately 40 ml/kg bodyweight. As gastric distension may result in nausea, individual feeds should not exceed 50% of this volume. Feeds of 10–15 ml/kg bodyweight are typically well tolerated.

Food should be fed at body temperature and can be warmed using a water bath. *Avoid microwave heating as this may result in uneven temperatures.* ▶

QRG 5.5.1 *continued*

Calorific density of examples of diets that can be fed via a naso-oesophageal tube

These diets are all liquid in nature when bought or made up, to enable passage via narrow NO tubes.

Diet	Calorific density
Glutalyte (Norbrook) –	0.5 kcal/ml
CliniCare Feline Liquid Diet (Abbott Animal Health)	1 kcal/ml
Royal Canin Waltham Convalescence Support Instant	1.1 kcal/ml
Fortol liquid diet (Arnolds)	1.01 kcal/ml
Enteral care high protein (Abbott Nutrition)	1 kcal/ml

Calorific density of examples of diets that can be fed via an oesophagostomy tube (or gastrostomy tube)

These diets need to be of a suitable consistency to pass down the oesophagostomy (or gastrostomy) tube; this is achieved by liquidizing them with water to convert them to a slurry. Checking that the consistency is liquid enough can be done by attempting to pass the slurry through the hub of a large syringe used to instil the food; if this can be achieved without excessive force, then they should pass through the oesophagostomy tube.

The amount of water that needs to be added will vary from diet to diet but the addition of 50 ml is a good starting point, adding further smaller increments if the consistency is still too thick. Record the amount of water that is added; this is used to calculate the resulting calorific density of the slurry. For example, adding 50 ml of water to a 156 g can of Hills a/d will generate a slurry with a calorific density of ~1 kcal/ml (as the resulting volume is 206 ml (volume of canned food + volume of water) for the total 203 kcal present in the can).

Ensure that the resulting slurry does not need to be fed at a volume of >20 ml/kg; as this comprises 50% of the feline stomach volume capacity and individual feeds should not exceed this volume (see above).

Diet	Calorific density
Hill's a/d	1.3 kcal/g
Eukanuba max calorie	2 kcal/g
Feline i/d tinned (Hill's)	1 kcal/g
Feline l/d tinned (Hill's)	1 kcal/g
Feline sensitivity control tinned (Royal Canin)	1 kcal/g
Royal Canin Waltham recovery	1 kcal/g

Water requirements

Maintenance water requirements are administered in the same number of feeds, although care should be taken to avoid gastric distension. Daily water requirements are usually *easily* met by the water provided from flushing, dilution of the food, the moisture content of the diet and/or voluntary water intake, especially once full RER is being fed. If intravenous fluid therapy at maintenance levels (2 ml/kg/h) or above is being provided to the cat with no other fluid losses, daily water provision will be adequate from this, negating the need to factor in additional water to meet daily water requirements. If the cat is receiving no water provision, other than that via the tube, it is usually adequate to subtract only the water used in the flush and any water used to dilute the food enough to allow it to be administered via the tube from the daily water requirement, to calculate the water provision required (see example calculations at the end of this QRG).

Feeding technique

- Before feeding through a naso-oesophageal or oesophagostomy tube, tube placement should be checked by aspirating from the tube with an empty 5 ml syringe. Correct placement in the distal oesophagus will be confirmed by the presence of negative suction. The pre-feeding flush should not illicit a cough; this also helps to ensure that the tube has not become dislodged into the trachea (this would be very rare after initial placement).
- If the feeding tube is in the stomach (placement too distal or with a gastrostomy tube), it is important to check – by aspiration with a syringe – whether any residual food/liquid is in the stomach before feeding; patients may also develop ileus or have delayed gastric emptying, resulting in food remaining in the stomach. If residual food/fluid is present this should be measured within the syringe; if the volume is <20% of the last feed given, the residual food is re-administered and the next feed given as usual, taking into account the residual volume to ensure gastric distension is avoided. However, if the residual volume is ≥20% of the last feed given, repeat feeding should be delayed; aspiration is re-attempted 1–2 hours later and the next feed given only when the residual volume is <20%. As NO or oesophagostomy tubes are not intentionally positioned in the stomach itself but in the distal oesophagus, aspiration of food should not occur, but the procedure should still be followed in case the tube is positioned more distally and/or there is ileus.
- The tube should be flushed with 5–10 ml of warm water before and after every feed.

- Food should be administered slowly, over about 10 minutes, particularly with wide-bore tubes where rapid syringing is easily done. Rapid administration will contribute to vomiting and nausea.
- The patient should be monitored during feeding for nausea (gulping, ptyalism, retching). Feeding should be temporarily discontinued if these develop.
- There does not appear to be any contraindication to the administration of prokinetic agents whilst enteral tubes (e.g. NO or oesophagostomy tubes) are in place and in some cases they are useful additions to help manage ileus prior to administration of food (e.g. metoclopramide 1–2 mg/kg/24 h as a CRI as described above).

Tube care

Appropriate care of enteral tubes is mandatory. Stoma sites should be checked at least once a day (see QRG 5.5.3). The tube should be flushed with warm water (approximately 5–10 ml) before and after every feed to help prevent blockage. This volume of water may be subtracted from daily water requirements (see below). If the tube becomes blocked, 3 ml of canned drink (e.g. cola or soda water) can be instilled and left for 15–20 minutes to help dislodge blockages.

Complications of tube feeding

These may include:

- Refeeding syndrome: electrolyte imbalances (particularly hyperglycaemia, hypophosphataemia, hypokalaemia) and haemolytic anaemia (secondary to hypophosphataemia) have been reported in cats following reintroduction of feeding after periods of starvation. Monitoring phosphate and potassium concentrations (daily during the first 3 days of feeding) is recommended, with supplementation of potassium chloride (see QRG 4.6.1) and potassium phosphate within intravenous fluids as required
- Aspiration pneumonia, secondary to incorrect feeding tube placement or aspiration of food secondary to vomiting or regurgitation
- Stoma site infections (e.g. oesophagostomy tubes).

Parenteral nutrition

Indications include intractable vomiting or reduced consciousness/recumbency. However, complications (e.g. catheter site infections, sepsis, metabolic derangements) are not uncommon, and most cats can be managed using enteral nutrition methods. Referral to a specialist centre is recommended if parenteral nutrition is required.

▶

QRG 5.5.1 *continued*

Example of an enteral feeding chart

Name of cat: _____ Diet chosen for enteral feeding: _____

RER = bodyweight $^{0.75}$ x 70
(kcal/day)   (kg)

Or, for cats >2 kg an estimate can be made from:
RER = (30 x bodyweight) + 70
(kcal/day)   (kg)

For both calculations, the actual current bodyweight is used, not the patient's ideal bodyweight.

Divide this total by the caloric density of the selected diet to give the total daily feed volume.

Total daily feed volume	Day 1: Feed 1/3 total Day 3 feed volume	= [ ] ml or g /day
	Day 2: Feed 2/3 total Day 3 feed volume	= [ ] ml or g /day
	Day 3: RER/caloric density of diet	= [ ] ml or g /day
Daily water requirement [a]	48 ml/kg/day (2 ml/kg/hr)	= [ ] ml/day

[a] *The flush water, the water used to dilute the food, the moisture content of the diet [b] and any fluid provided by intravenous fluid therapy must be subtracted from the daily water requirement to calculate how much additional water needs to be provided via the tube. However, daily water requirements are usually easily met by the water provided from flushing, dilution of the food, the moisture content of the diet and/or voluntary water intake, especially once full RER is being fed. If i.v. fluid therapy at maintenance levels (2 ml/kg/h) or above is being provided to the cat with no other fluid losses, daily water provision will be adequate from this, negating the need to factor in additional water to meet daily water requirements. If the cat is receiving no water provision other than that via the tube, it is usually adequate to subtract only the water used in the flush and any water used to dilute the food enough to allow it to be administered via the tube to calculate additional water requirements. See example calculations on the next page to illustrate calculation of water requirements.*

[b] *The moisture content of the diet, if calculated, is the water provided from the food (in ml); this equates to % moisture of food (~80% wet food, ~10% dried food) X grams of food fed.*

Before feeding through a naso-oesophageal or oesophagostomy tube, tube placement should checked by aspirating from the tube with an empty 5 ml syringe. Correct placement in the oesophagus will be confirmed by the presence of negative suction. The pre-feeding flush (see below) should not illicit a cough; this also helps to ensure that the tube has not become dislodged into the trachea (this would be very rare after initial placement). If the feeding tube is in the stomach (placement too distal or with a gastrostomy tube), it is important to check whether any residual food/liquid is in the stomach before feeding by aspiration with syringe; if ≥ 20% of the last feed volume is present, record this volume and reinstil what you have aspirated. Then delay feeding until residual food/liquid volume aspirated is < 20% of the last feed (check every 1 to 2 hours).

Flush the tube with 5–10 ml of warm water, before and after every feed.

Food should be fed at **body temperature**.

Total food and water is **split equally into 4–5 meals**.

Day and date	Bodyweight (kg) Record daily to ensure changes are noted	Time of feed	Food (as made up, in ml)	Water (ml)	Flush (5 ml pre- and post-feeding; total ml)	Comments Any residual food on aspiration (record volume), any complications noted during feeding e.g. swallowing, licking lips possibly suggesting nausea?

QRG 5.5.1 *continued*

Example calculations for enteral feeding

Consider a 5 kg cat, that is *not* receiving intravenous fluid therapy *nor* ingesting any voluntary water, commencing feeding with Royal Canin Waltham Convalescence support instant feed via a naso-oesophageal tube. The following calculations are given precisely, to allow the reader to derive the origin of calculations. In practice, precise measurements to the nearest decimal point are not required, and rounding up to the nearest whole millilitre is sufficient. Many cats will voluntarily drink or be given intravenous fluid therapy; in these cases, the amount of water provided by these means should be subtracted from those given below.

RER estimation =   (30 x bodyweight) + 70   = (30 x 5) + 70 = **220 kcal/day**
(kcal/day)   (kg)

Dividing this RER total by the caloric density of the selected diet gives the total daily feed volume.

The 50 g sachet of Royal Canin Waltham Convalescence support instant has directions to add 150 ml of water to it to give 200 ml of ready-to-use feed (this can be kept in the fridge for up to 24 hours); this has an energy density of 1.1 kcal/ml, as indicated by the manufacturer.

Total daily feed volume	= RER/caloric density of diet	= 220/1.1 = **200 ml/day**
	Day 1: Feed 1/3 total daily feed volume	= **66.7 ml/day**
	Day 2: Feed 2/3 total daily feed volume	= **133 ml/day**
	Day 3: RER/caloric density of diet	= **200 ml/day**
Daily water requirement	48 ml/kg/day	= **240 ml/day**

As mentioned above, 150 ml of water are added to the 50 g sachet to make the diet into a liquid form with a total volume of 200 ml. Additionally a 50 g sachet (moisture content 4%) provides (4/100 x 50) = 2 ml of water as part of the moisture content of the diet [a]. So for each 50 g sachet used and made up, 152 ml of water is provided; this equates to 152/200 = 0.76 ml of water per ml of reformulated diet fed.

Day 1: 51 (66.7 x 0.76) ml of water is provided by the diet, so 189 ml of additional water is needed to meet daily water requirements. As 50 ml water is provided in the flush, an extra 139 ml of water is required over 5 feeds = 27.8 ml water per feed.

Day 2: 101 (133 x 0.76) ml of water is provided by the diet, so 139 ml of additional water is needed to meet daily requirements. As 50 ml water is provided in the flush, an extra 89 ml of water is required over 5 feeds = 17.8 ml water per feed.

Day 3: 152 (200 x 0.76) ml of water is provided by the diet, so 88 ml of additional water is needed to meet daily requirements. As 50 ml water is provided in the flush, an extra 38 ml of water is required over 5 feeds = 7.6 ml water per feed.

[a] The water content of a dry or powdered diet is largely negligible and could be omitted from these calculations but is included to remind the reader to consider the moisture content of the diet. This volume will be far higher for a canned diet which has a moisture content of say 80% (e.g. a 156 g can of Hills a/d has a moisture content of 80/100 x 156 = 124.8 ml) and so should always be included if liquidized canned diets are being fed via an oesophagostomy tube in patients where additional fluid is not being given or consumed.

Day and date	Bodyweight (kg)	Time of feed	Food (as made up, in ml)	Water (ml)	Flush (5 ml pre- and post-feeding; total ml)	Comments
Day 1 3 Dec 12 MON	5 kg	0800	13.3	27.8	10	
		1200	13.3	27.8	10	
		1600	13.3	27.8	10	
		2000	13.3	27.8	10	
		2400	13.3	27.8	10	
Day 2 4 Dec 12 TUES	5 kg	0800	26.6	17.8	10	
		1200	26.6	17.8	10	
		1600	26.6	17.8	10	
		2000	26.6	17.8	10	
		2400	26.6	17.8	10	
Day 3 5 Dec 12 WEDS	5 kg	0800	40	7.6	10	
		1200	40	7.6	10	
		1600	40	7.6	10	
		2000	40	7.6	10	
		2400	40	7.6	10	

QRG 5.5.2 Placement of a naso-oesophageal feeding tube

by Rachel Korman

Indications

- Hospitalized patients when enteral assisted feeding is required for a short-term period, of up to one week
- Enteral assisted feeding should be considered in any cat with inadequate daily caloric intake for 3 days or longer

Contraindications

- Persistent vomiting
- Absent gag reflex
- Nasopharyngeal disease (NB risk *versus* benefit needs to be considered in the individual patient; for example, in cases of upper respiratory tract infection that require very short-term enteral feeding, a naso-oesophageal (NO) tube may still be appropriate, whereas in a cat with a nasal tumour it may be inappropriate)
- Head trauma
- Oesophageal disease
- Only liquid diets can be administered via NO tubes due to their narrow bore. Alternative wet food diets must be blended and administered via a wider-bore tube, e.g. oesophagostomy tube (see QRG 5.5.3)

Equipment

- Feeding tube (3–5 Fr, 40–75 cm, soft, polyvinyl or silicone feeding tubes are ideal). The largest bore tube possible is preferable to allow easier instillation of viscous liquids
- Proxymetacaine 0.5% (local anaesthetic)
- Lubricating jelly
- Empty 5 ml syringe
- 5 ml syringe containing sterile water for injection
- 1 cm wide Micropore tape or sticking plaster, including two pieces each 3 cm long, tissue glue or 'superglue'
- Elizabethan collar
- Permanent marker pen
- Gloves may be worn but are not essential

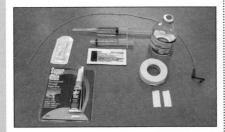

Patient preparation

- Quiet room with minimal people.
- Non-slip surface (NB Cats will be more inclined to sit down and relax if placed on bedding rather than directly on to the table surface).
- Gentle minimal restraint.
- Sedation is rarely required for this procedure.

Technique

1 Apply local anaesthetic to the nostril. Either nostril can be used, but if right-handed it is generally easier to place the NO tube into the cat's left nostril. One whole vial of proxymetacaine is instilled into the nostril; allow 1–2 minutes for it to take effect (some will inevitably be sneezed out but the rest is still effective).

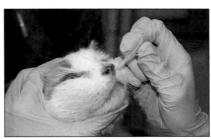

2 Measure the feeding tube from the nostril to the level of the 9th rib (the tube end should sit in the distal oesophagus, not the stomach) by counting back from the last (13th) rib. Mark the tube at the required length using butterfly tape applied 1 cm distal to this (or permanent marker pen at the required length).

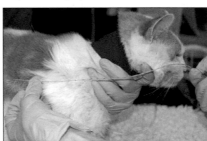

3 Apply lubricant jelly to the first centimetre of the tube. The head should be restrained and raised slightly.

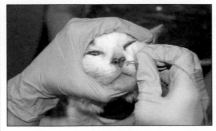

4 Insert the tube gently (but initially rapidly for the first 3–4 cm to avoid it being sneezed out) into the nostril, directing ventrally and medially. It may be easier for the person placing the tube to hold the cat's head, with the assistant restraining the cat to prevent backward movement. If the cat reacts excessively to insertion, more local anaesthetic may be instilled. The first 3–4 cm of the tube is hardest to insert, as the cat is likely to react the most. Once this section of tubing is passed, most cats tolerate it well.

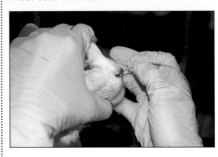

5 Insert the remainder of the tube slowly (up to the mark or tape), watching for signs of swallowing (indicating the tube is correctly in the oesophagus) and coughing or discomfort (indicating the tube may have been inserted into the trachea). In the latter case, the tube should be immediately removed and reinserted.

6 Check the tube is correctly in place by performing at least two of the three following steps. Ensure the handler keeps the cat gently restrained to avoid it removing the NO tube.

a. Attach the empty 5 ml syringe to the tube and apply suction. If the tube is within the trachea, significant amounts (complete syringe-full) of air will be readily withdrawn. If this occurs the tube should be immediately removed. If suction creates a vacuum (arrowed), meaning that no air can be sucked into the tube, it should be in the oesophagus.

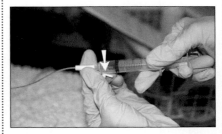

b. Attach the syringe containing the 5 ml of sterile water for injection and slowly flush it down the tube, watching the cat for signs of coughing, restlessness and/or tachypnoea. If any of these signs occurs, flushing should be stopped and the tube removed and reinserted. ▶

QUICK REFERENCE GUIDES

QRG 5.5.2 *continued*

c. Inject 3 ml of air whilst auscultating the left abdomen; borborygmi in the stomach will be heard if the NO tube is correctly placed.

Tube placement should be reassessed using these methods, prior to administration of each feed.

7 Place two butterfly tapes on to the tube, approximately 1 and 3 cm from the nostril (one may already be positioned if you have used this as a marker for tube length during insertion). Apply a thin layer of glue to each tape; bend the tube up and around the dorsal aspect of the cat's nose and head and press it on to the hair; *the aim is for the glue to contact the hair, not the skin.* Great care should be taken when applying the glue to ensure that it does not come into contact with the eyes or nasal planum and that the eyes and whiskers are not interfered with by the eventual tube position.

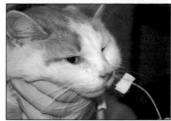
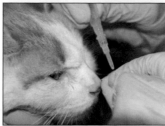
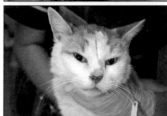

8 Place an Elizabethan collar to prevent the cat displacing the tube. Cats prefer soft collars to rigid, plastic ones. Place this whilst the cat is still being restrained to avoid risk of NO tube removal by the cat. The remaining length of the tube can be coiled and taped inside the Elizabethan collar.

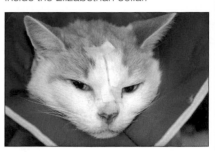

9 Tube placement should be checked and the tube flushed prior to feeding. Radiographic confirmation of placement is recommended if unsure of tube positioning to reduce the risk associated with inappropriate tube placement (e.g. aspiration pneumonia). See QRG 5.5.1 for details of administering foods.

QRG 5.5.3 Placement of an oesophagostomy feeding tube
by Rachel Korman

Indications

- When assisted enteral feeding is required for longer periods (1–2 weeks or more)
- When feeding via the mouth or nose is not possible
- To aid owner compliance for long-term tablet administration
- Inability to prehend food normally (e.g. mandibular fracture)
- Administration of more viscous diets (e.g. wet formula prescription diets) that cannot be administered via a naso-oesophageal tube
- Placement of an oesophageal feeding tube should be considered if general anaesthesia is required for other procedures
- Enteral assisted feeding should be considered in any cat with inadequate daily caloric intake for 3 days or longer

Contraindications

- Oesophageal disorders (e.g. oesophagitis)
- Persistent vomiting
- Absent gag reflex
- Conditions precluding general anaesthesia

Complications

These are uncommon but include:

- Cellulitis/infection at stoma site
- Improper placement (e.g. aspiration pneumonia)
- Perforation of jugular vein, carotid artery or recurrent laryngeal nerve neuropraxia
- Vomiting of the tube into the oral cavity.

Equipment

- Feeding tube (12–16 Fr, soft, polyvinyl feeding tubes are ideal). Avoid red rubber tubing as this material can become friable *in situ*. Avoid widening feeding tube exit holes by cutting, as sections of tubing may break and be lost; instead they may be widened by stretching with forceps but most feeding tubes have sufficient holes for most viscous liquids or blended food with water
- Permanent marker
- Sterile gloves
- Curved artery forceps
- Scalpel blade
- Suture material (e.g. 3 metric (2/0 USP) non-absorbable) with needle
- Dressing materials (e.g. Primapore adhesive dressing, Soffban non-adhesive bandage, Vetwrap)
- Elizabethan collar
- Specific oesophageal tube applicators are not required

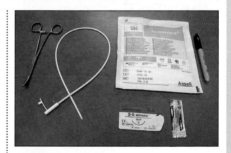

Patient preparation

- General anaesthesia and endotracheal intubation.
- Right lateral recumbency.
- Clipping and aseptic skin preparation on the lateral cervical area from the angle of the mandible to the thoracic inlet.
- The position of the jugular vein should be noted prior to tube placement to avoid jugular vein perforation. ▶

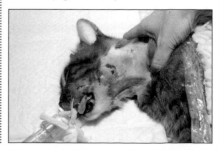

QRG 5.5.3 *continued*

Technique

1 The end of the oesophagostomy tube will lie within the distal oesophagus. After removing the tube from its packaging using sterile gloves (not shown in this image), hold the tube above the cat (to maintain sterility) and hold the distal tip of the tube at the level of the 8th–9th rib (identified by counting back from the last (13th) rib). Mark the tube with permanent marker at the point where it reaches the proposed exit point on the left lateral side of the cervical area.

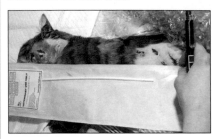

2 An assistant places the curved artery forceps into the mouth of the cat and manoeuvres them down the oesophagus to the mid-cervical region. The forceps tips are then angled laterally, pressing the oesophagus against the skin; tenting of the skin is visible (black arrow). The jugular vein should again be raised to aid its visualization and ensure it is avoided during tube placement.

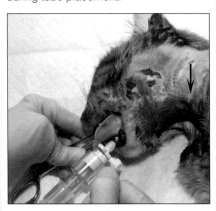

3 Identify the forceps tips by palpation and make a small (0.3–0.5 cm) incision through the skin and oesophagus on to the forceps. The incision is made down on to the metal of the forceps whilst the assistant maintains the position of the forceps, to ensure the incision is as small as possible while big enough to let the feeding tube through.

WARNING

In trauma cases, this incision site should avoid traumatic wounds or areas of questionable tissue viability that may affect formation of a clean stoma site.

4 Gently manipulate the forceps through the skin until the tips are visible. Open the forceps slightly and grasp the distal end of the oesophagostomy tube.

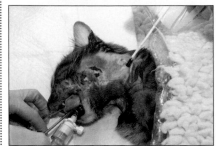

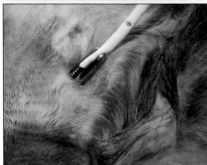

5 Close the forceps and pull both them and the tube back through the skin, up the proximal oesophagus and out of the mouth. Take care to ensure that the tube is not completely pulled through; the larger end (with port) must remain exiting the lateral cervical area, so ensure that this end is held.

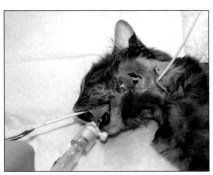

6 The forceps are released and are no longer required. Redirect the distal end of the tube exiting the mouth back into the mouth and oropharynx and manoeuvre it back down into the oesophagus (easily done using the index finger). Sterile lubricant gel can be applied to the distal end of the tube to facilitate this.

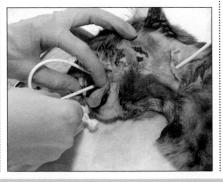

7 Once the tube passes the incision site, a gentle flip is felt as the tube straightens. It is now easily moved within the oesophagus. The tube should now be correctly positioned as determined by the premeasured mark.

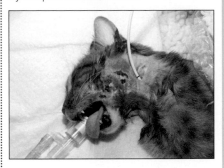

8 Correct tube placement (in the caudal oesophagus, just cranial to the stomach, level with the 8th or 9th rib) should be confirmed by lateral thoracic radiography prior to suturing the tube in place.

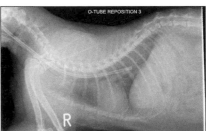

This right lateral chest radiograph shows the tube end positioned in the caudal oesophagus, just proximal to the 8th rib. (An endotracheal tube is also positioned just proximal to the 2nd rib.) There is a mild generalized interstitial pattern in the lung fields, particularly dorsally, which was attributed to underinflation/ exposure factors. On this radiograph there is also evidence of shoulder and elbow osteoarthritis, with osteophytes present caudal to the shoulder joint and cranial to the elbow joint of the more caudally positioned forelimb.

9 The tube is then sutured in place using either a purse-string suture at the entrance site or a small stay suture through the skin. Either technique is then followed by a Chinese finger-trap suture around the tube to prevent its migration.

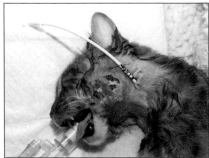

10 The stoma should be cleaned with an iodine solution (5%) following tube placement and an iodine-impregnated swab (e.g. Iodoflex pre-prepared or using a gauze swab with added 5% iodine solution) placed around the tube. ▶

QRG 5.5.3 *continued*

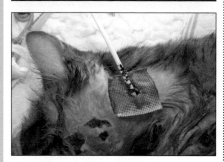

11 An adhesive dressing (e.g. Primapore) is placed over the iodinated swab; cutting a small V into the dressing will help facilitate easy placement. A soft, non-adhesive dressing (e.g. Soffban) is then placed around the neck, followed by a second light, conforming bandage layer (e.g. Vetwrap). At least one finger should be able to be placed underneath this dressing to ensure the dressing is not too tight. Padded collars are an alternative to keep the tubes in place (see Figure 1.13).

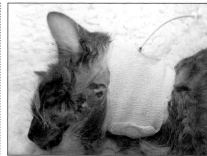

12 An Elizabethan collar prevents the cat displacing the tube. Cats prefer soft collars to rigid, plastic collars. Excess tubing can be coiled and placed underneath the conforming dressing or the taped inside the collar

13 Feeding can be commenced once the cat has recovered *completely* from anaesthesia. The tube should be flushed before and after feeding with at least 5 ml of warm water to help prevent tube blockage. This volume can be part of the daily maintenance fluid requirements. See QRG 5.5.1 for details of administering foods.

Stoma site care and tube removal

- The stoma site needs to be attended carefully to prevent cellulitis and infection. It should be inspected visually twice daily to assess for evidence of tube/suture migration and cellulitis. Cleaning the stoma site with iodinated solution (5%) or sterile saline should be performed at least once daily.

- Oesophagostomy tubes may be left in place for a number of weeks (e.g. 3–4 weeks). The tube is simply pulled out once the sutures are removed. Sedation is rarely required and the incision site can be left to heal by second intention (takes ~ 3 days). Early removal, if the cat starts eating voluntarily, or following self-removal, does not appear to pose a problem.

Ataxia

Laurent Garosi

Classification and clinical signs

> **Ataxia** is defined as an uncoordinated gait. It can arise from:
>
> - A sensory peripheral nerve lesion or a spinal cord lesion (general proprioceptive ataxia)
> - A vestibular lesion (vestibular ataxia)
> - A cerebellar lesion (cerebellar ataxia).
>
> Ataxia can be further divided into:
>
> - Hypometria (shorter protraction phase of gait)
> - Hypermetria (longer protraction phase of gait).

- General proprioceptive (GP) ataxia reflects the lack of information reaching the CNS responsible for the awareness of the movement and position of the neck, trunk and limbs in space. As a consequence, there may be a delay in the onset of protraction of the limb, which may cause a longer stride than normal. The cat may walk on the dorsal part of its foot or may drag its digits. These signs often overlap with those caused by upper motor neuron (UMN) paresis.
- Unilateral vestibular ataxia is characterized by leaning/rolling/falling to the affected side and a head tilt to the side of the lesion.
- Bilateral vestibular ataxia is characterized by a head sway from side to side, loss of balance to one side, and symmetrical ataxia with a crouched posture closer to the ground surface.
- Cerebellar ataxia is characterized by a strong, bouncy, uncoordinated gait with exaggerated movement of limbs and normal motor strength.
- Further, vestibular or cerebellar ataxias are accompanied by other signs of dysfunction of the vestibular apparatus or cerebellum, respectively (see below).

A thorough neurological assessment (see QRG 1.6) should first be performed to localize the lesion.

UMN paresis and GP ataxia
From a lesion localization point of view, UMN paresis and GP ataxia visible in the gait can occur as a consequence of a lesion affecting the brainstem or spinal cord. Compared to UMN paresis, disorders of the lower motor neurons (LMNs) only cause paresis and not ataxia. The pathways of the GP sensory system are anatomically adjacent to most of the UMN pathways necessary for gait generation. The change in the gait therefore generally reflects a combined dysfunction of both UMN paresis and GP ataxia, with delayed onset of protraction of the limb and lengthened stride.

Vestibular ataxia
Vestibular ataxia occurs with lesions affecting either the peripheral or central vestibular apparatus. In addition to ataxia, animals will often have concurrent neurological signs that reflect a vestibular disorder, such as head tilt (see Chapter 5.16) or head sway, pathological nystagmus, or positional strabismus. Cats with vestibular ataxia often have a broad-based gait (especially in the pelvic limbs) with leaning towards the side of decreased vestibular tone. Some animals may have substantial swaying when walking and will occasionally fall; recumbent animals may be seen to roll. Weakness or paresis is only seen with central vestibular disease and is not a feature of peripheral vestibular disease.

Cerebellar ataxia
Cerebellar ataxia can be seen in cats that have lesions within the cerebellar cortex. Other signs of cerebellar disease, such as intention tremors, are often present. Cerebellar ataxia is characterized by hypermetria and dysmetria. Hypermetria associated with cerebellar ataxia consists of overflexion during limb protraction and is therefore distinct from the over-reaching, long-strided gait noted in animals with combined GP ataxia/UMN paresis. Dysmetria is a component of cerebellar ataxia and manifests as a loss of synchronous limb movements.

Differential diagnoses

Differential diagnoses should be established based on the neuroanatomical origin of the ataxia (Figure 5.6.1).

Disease mechanisms (VITAMIND)	Cerebellar ataxia	Peripheral vestibular ataxia	Central vestibular ataxia	GP ataxia
Vascular	Brain infarct Brain haemorrhage	None	Brain infarct Brain haemorrhage	**Fibrocartilaginous embolic myelopathy (FCEM)** Vascular malformations Spinal cord haematoma or haemorrhage
Inflammatory/ Infectious	Infectious encephalitis (*Toxoplasma*, bacterial, **FIP**) Meningoencephalitis of unknown aetiology (presumed immune-mediated)	**Otitis media/interna** **Nasopharyngeal polyp**	Infectious encephalitis (*Toxoplasma*, bacterial, **FIP**) Meningoencephalitis of unknown aetiology (presumed immune-mediated)	Meningomyelitis/myelitis: infectious (*Toxoplasma*, FeLV, **FIP**, fungal); or of unknown aetiology Epidural abscess/empyema
Trauma	Head trauma	Head trauma	Head trauma	Spinal fracture/luxation Traumatic disc herniation
Toxic	Marijuana Fluorouracil Metronidazole	Aminoglycosides Topical otic iodophors (e.g. povidone–iodine) Loop diuretics (e.g. furosemide) Topical chlorhexidine	Metronidazole	N/A
Anomalous	Cerebellar hypoplasia Intracranial intra-arachnoid cyst, dermoid/epidermoid cyst	Congenital vestibular disease (infrequent but reported in Siamese, Burmese and Tonkinese cats)	Intracranial intra-arachnoid cyst, dermoid/epidermoid cyst	Spina bifida (esp. Manx) Myelodysplasia (spinal defect) Feline Chiari malformations
Metabolic	N/A	N/A	N/A	N/A
Idiopathic	N/A	Acute idiopathic peripheral vestibular disease	N/A	N/A
Neoplastic	**Primary or metastatic brain tumour**	**Middle and/or inner ear tumour**	**Primary or metastatic brain tumour**	**Primary or metastatic spinal or spinal cord tumour**
Nutritional	N/A	N/A	Thiamine deficiency	Vitamin B12 deficiency Hypervitaminosis A
Degenerative	Lysosomal storage diseases Cerebellar abiotrophy Other neurodegenerative disease	N/A	Lysosomal storage diseases Other neurodegenerative disease	Intervertebral disk disease (esp. caudal lumbar segments) Storage diseases

5.6.1 Differential diagnoses of ataxia by neuroanatomical localization. Common causes of ataxia in cats are highlighted in bold. NA = not applicable.

Diagnostic approach

The presence of ataxia should suggest a lesion of the spinal cord, brainstem, cerebellum or peripheral vestibular apparatus; multifocal disease with involvement of at least two of these regions should also be a consideration. Associated neurological signs are used to localize the lesion to one of these parts of the nervous system (Figure 5.6.2). Correct anatomical diagnosis is crucial in establishing a differential list as some causes of ataxia are specific to certain regions of the nervous system. Additionally, the choice of ancillary diagnostic tests is guided by lesion localization and the differential list.

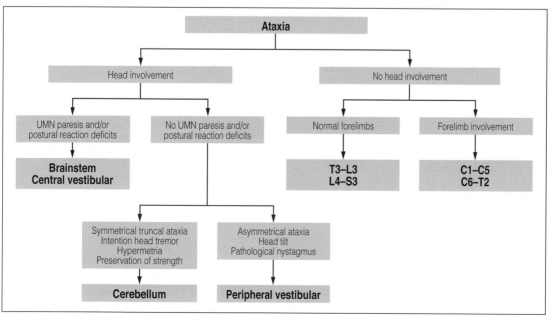

5.6.2 An approach to localizing the region of the nervous system from which ataxia may arise.

Diagnostic tests required

Appropriate diagnostic test selection is dependent upon the region of the nervous system affected.

Spinal cord disease:

- Vertebral column radiographs are a cost-effective screening test for identifying obvious vertebral fractures, luxation, osseous lytic tumours and discospondylitis
- Advanced imaging – preferably MRI rather than CT (Figures 5.6.3 and 5.6.4)
- Cerebrospinal fluid analysis.

Brainstem and cerebellar disease:

- Thorough history to investigate the possibility of toxic or nutritional causes
- Assessment for evidence of systemic disease (e.g. blood pressure assessment to exclude hypertension, routine haematology/biochemistry, FeLV/FIV/*Toxoplasma* serology, assessment for FIP)

- MRI of the brain (Figure 5.6.5) is suggested, as CT is less sensitive for detecting soft tissue changes within the caudal fossa due to beam-hardening artefacts
- Cerebrospinal fluid analysis.

Peripheral vestibular system disease:

- Otoscopy ± ear swabs (see Chapter 5.15)
- Pharyngeal examination (to rule out polyps)
- Bulla radiographs (ventrodorsal, laterolateral, rostrocaudal open-mouth, lateral oblique)
- MRI of the brain and peripheral vestibular apparatus is suggested as it may be challenging to discern central from peripheral vestibular disease based on physical examination; CT provides inferior imaging of the caudal fossa due to beam-hardening artefacts
- Myringotomy for cytology and culture of lesions extending into the middle ear (see QRG 5.15.2).
- Cerebrospinal fluid analysis if concurrent involvement of central structures is possible.

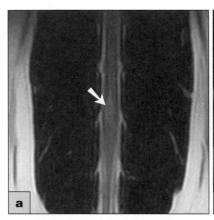
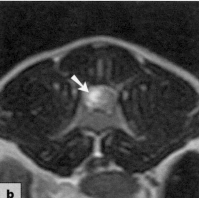

5.6.3 Dorsal **(a)** and transverse **(b)** T2-weighted MR images of the lumbar spinal cord in an ataxic cat with ischaemic myelopathy (suspected fibrocartilaginous embolic myelopathy). Note the focal ill-defined hyperintensity within the spinal cord (arrowed).

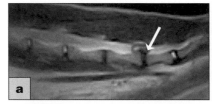
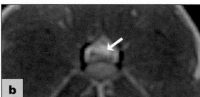

5.6.4 Sagittal **(a)** and transverse **(b)** T2-weighted MR images of the caudal lumbar spine in a cat with disc extrusion (arrowed) at L6/7 causing marked spinal cord compression.

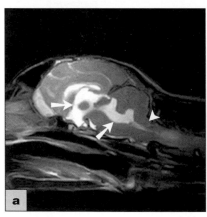
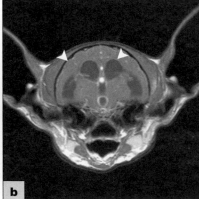

5.6.5 **(a)** Sagittal T2-weighted and **(b)** transverse T1-weighted contrast-enhanced MR image of a cat with the dry form of CNS FIP. On the transverse image, there is marked dilatation of the lateral and third ventricles, as well as enhancement of the ependymal lining and meninges (arrowheads). On the sagittal image, the third and fourth ventricles (arrows) are markedly dilated, causing compression and caudal foramen magnum herniation (arrowhead) of the cerebellum, as well as oedema within the cranial cervical spine.

Azotaemia

Kathleen Tennant

Azotaemia is defined as: an elevation in non-protein nitrogeous waste products in the blood.

Urea and creatinine are the products most frequently measured, and azotaemia refers to an elevation in blood concentration of one or both of these substances.

- Urea is a small molecule, freely filtered at the glomerulus and with some reabsorption occurring within the tubules and collecting ducts.
- Creatinine is freely filtered at the glomerulus and not reabsorbed.

Azotaemia may be caused by pre-renal, renal or post-renal disorders. Figure 5.7.1 demonstrates an approach to identifying which of these categories of disorder is the most likely cause.

> **PRACTICAL TIP**
>
> Urine specific gravity (USG) should always be measured using a refractometer, not with urine dipsticks.

Pre-renal azotaemia

Azotaemia dependent on rate of formation of urea/creatinine

> Urine SG variable, but cats should be able to concentrate urine (USG ≥1.035).

Increased concentrations of urea without elevations in creatinine may occur after a high-protein meal or

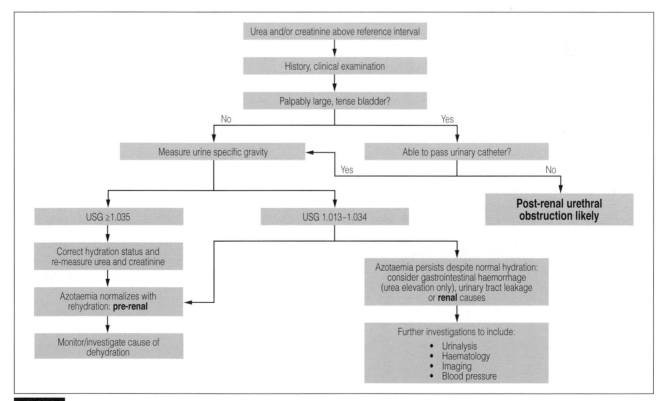

5.7.1 Diagnostic approach to differentiate pre-renal, renal and post-renal azotaemia

gastrointestinal haemorrhage, as the blood concentration of nitrogenous breakdown material temporarily increases. To reduce the effect of diet on urea values, blood samples taken after a 6-hour fast are preferred.

Other features of gastrointestinal haemorrhage might also be expected if this is the sole cause of persistently elevated urea without creatinine elevations: the presence of melaena, reductions in total protein, thrombocytosis and, in the longer term, the development of microcytic/hypochromic anaemia are all supportive. If suspicious, positive faecal occult blood testing after 3–5 days of a white meat diet may be used as further evidence to demonstrate gastrointestinal haemorrhage.

Small increases in urea may be noted with increased endogenous protein catabolism secondary to pyrexia or corticosteroid administration.

Creatinine is produced at a steady rate by non-enzymatic breakdown of creatine in skeletal muscle. The more muscle mass a cat has, the higher the usual creatinine concentration. An individual with significantly more or less muscle mass than the reference population may require a different interpretation of creatinine elevation (i.e. a high 'normal' value compared to a healthy adult cat reference interval may be clinically significant in a cachexic hyperthyroid cat with little muscle).

Azotaemia secondary to dehydration/ hypovolaemia

> With normal renal function, USG is usually ≥1.035 and signs of dehydration may be evident on clinical examination or other laboratory investigations (e.g elevated red cell mass, total protein).

Dehydration and hypovolaemia decrease renal perfusion and glomerular filtration rate, resulting in slower removal of urea and creatinine. Slower urine transit through the tubules and ducts also allows some urea to be reabsorbed into the blood. As creatinine is not reabsorbed, blood elevations occur more slowly than for urea.

The effect of decreased plasma volume directly increases the relative concentrations of both urea and creatinine. This should resolve quickly and completely with restoration of fluid volume and renal perfusion.

Renal azotaemia

> A decrease of 66–75% in renal function will result in accumulation of blood urea and then creatinine, with a USG that shows inadequate concentration.

- Azotaemia with USG 1.008–1.012 suggests loss of renal concentrating ability (kidney disease).
- Azotaemia with USG 1.013–1.034 suggests that some concentrating ability remains but is inadequate to compensate fully for losses. Cats with chronic kidney disease (CKD) retain urine-concentrating ability for longer than dogs with CKD; so USG is often higher than might be expected (USG >1.020) but is still inappropriate in the face of azotaemia.

Rarely, cats without kidney disease may present as azotaemic with non-concentrated urine (e.g. those with nephrogenic diabetes insipidus, diabetes mellitus or decreased medullary hypertonicity secondary to diuretic therapy).

Acute *versus* chronic kidney disease

- **Acute kidney injury** (AKI) is that in which a sudden onset and usually severe decline in glomerular filtration rate (GFR) occurs. In some cases, the changes are reversible.
- **Chronic kidney disease** is characterized by a progressive decline in GFR and renal function, which occurs slowly enough for compensatory mechanisms to engage.

Differences in clinical presentation and historical findings may help to distinguish between acute and chronic kidney disease (Figure 5.7.2; see also Chapter 13), although all features are not present in all cases.

Investigation	Acute kidney injury	Chronic kidney disease
History	Sudden onset. Possible cause noted (e.g. toxin, hypotension/NSAIDs concurrently). Urination volume may be normal or decreased, or urination may have ceased	Insidious onset. Uraemic signs (halitosis, mouth ulcers, gastrointestinal signs, dehydration). Polyuria, polydipsia. Poor appetite
Clinical examination	No weight loss. Other signs may relate to underlying cause (e.g. neurological dysfunction with ethylene glycol toxicity). Kidneys normal to enlarged on palpation and may be painful	Weight loss. Dehydration. Kidneys generally small and firm on palpation. Possible pale mucous membranes secondary to anaemia

5.7.2 Initial examination findings in acute and chronic kidney disease.

Acute kidney injury

Causes: **Nephrotoxins** may be endogenous (hypercalcaemia, myoglobin, free haemoglobin) or exogenous. Exogenous agents, including drugs, recognized to predispose to, or cause, AKI include:

- Non-steroidal anti-inflammatory drugs (NSAIDs)
- Aminoglycosides
- Ethylene glycol
- Ciclosporin
- Sulphonamides
- Heavy metals
- Iodine-based contrast agents
- Lilies.

Conditions leading to **poor renal perfusion** may cause kidney disease in isolation or may compound the effects of nephrotoxins or other renal injury. These would include:

- Hypotension or hypovolaemia (e.g. due to shock, haemorrhage, anaesthesia, decreased cardiac output)
- Thrombosis/infarct
- Hyperviscosity syndromes (e.g. polycythaemia).

Other diseases with the potential to induce AKI are those where the renal parenchyma is directly affected by pathogens (urinary tract infections including proximal urinary tract/pyelonephritis), degeneration/inflammation (glomerulonephritis) or mechanical damage (urinary tract obstruction). Hypokalaemia has also been reported to cause kidney disease.

Further investigations:

- Drug, supplement and environmental history should be obtained, and any suspicious agents removed.
- Urinalysis will help to eliminate urinary tract infections and is vital to check for crystals that may give a clue to the underlying cause (e.g. sulphonamide crystals associated with antibiotic treatment; calcium oxalate monohydrate crystals in ethylene glycol toxicity). Proteinuria, if present, may be a sign of kidney disease; and possible associated loss of antithrombin (most often measured as antithrombin III) in the urine may predispose to further damage from thrombotic disease.
- Haematology and full biochemistry will aid in the identification of more widespread disease and organ dysfunction. Clotting disorders likely to lead to thrombosis or infarct may be uncovered.
- Blood pressure monitoring will identify the dangerously hypotensive or hypovolaemic (along with clinical examination).
- Imaging will identify abnormal morphologies. Ultrasonography with an experienced operator may allow blood flow to be assessed in the renal arteries.
- Inorganic phosphate and potassium may accumulate in the blood if there is failure to excrete. Hyperkalaemia may lead to bradyarrhythmia, progressing to atrial standstill.

Chronic kidney disease

Azotaemia may result when cats lose 66–75% of renal function: their ability to minimally concentrate urine may remain with losses at the lower end of this range, but ability to tolerate further damage is reduced.

Causes: In many cases the underlying cause of CKD is never found: an initial insult gives rise to a limited number of pathological responses which may appear similar on histopathological and post-mortem examination. CKD may follow on from causes of AKI (see above) and the end-stage of CKD – with loss of a critical mass of nephrons – may result in an AKI picture ('acute on chronic').

- Urinary tract infections, transient hypovolaemia and NSAIDs may contribute.
- Successful treatment of hyperthyroidism and a return to 'normal' renal perfusion may unmask an underlying borderline CKD.
- Tubular and interstitial damage is often more prominent than glomerular abnormalities. Inability to concentrate urine and the accumulation of renally excreted analytes such as urea, creatinine and inorganic phosphate often outstrip renal protein loss. A urine protein:creatinine ratio of >0.4 is associated with poorer prognosis.
- Hypertension may result, and may worsen renal function, as well as causing cardiac, ocular and neurological pathology.
- Reduced renal mass may lead to reduced erythropoietin production, decreased erythrocyte production and survival, possible gastrointestinal haemorrhage and, thus, a non-regenerative anaemia, which can be severe.

Further investigations: These may include:

- Imaging to demonstrate often smaller, scarred kidneys
- Urinalysis including culture
- Blood pressure monitoring for hypertension
- Investigations as for AKI (see above).

Post-renal azotaemia

> Post-renal azotaemia is that in which (despite adequate renal filtration) excretory products do not exit the body in urine.

Elevations in urea and creatinine may be accompanied by significant hyperkalaemia; phosphate may also be elevated, depending on degree of tubular leakage and chronicity.

Causes

Causes of post-renal azotaemia include:

- Urethral obstruction
- Bladder leakage or rupture
- Ureteral (bilateral) obstruction, ligation or rupture
- Renal pathology or rupture (rare).

Investigations

These may include:

- Serum biochemistry: to detect azotaemia, hyperkalaemia, hyperphosphataemia and metabolic acidosis
- Physical examination: can detect a turgid or non-palpable bladder. Some cats with ruptured bladders may still be able to urinate
- Imaging: may show abdominal fluid (uroabdomen). Obstructions or gross anatomical disruptions may be detected
- Abdominal fluid analysis: fluid may have a higher creatinine value than peripheral blood and may smell of urine. Potassium concentrations may also be higher in the abdominal fluid compared to the blood, although potassium eliquilibrates rapidly between the two, meaning that the absence of a higher value in the abdominal fluid cannot rule out the presence of uroabdomen
- Urinalysis: may demonstrate the presence of crystals, mucous plugs and/or haemorrhage.

Cat bite abscesses

Martha Cannon

Cat bite abscesses are a very common presenting problem in veterinary practice. They arise following a bite from another cat, when the canine teeth penetrate the skin and effectively inject bacteria from the saliva into the soft tissues below.

Clinical presentation

Often there are minimal signs in the first 1–2 days following the cat fight but then, as the bacteria multiply, cellulitis develops, with local inflammation, heat and soft tissue swelling. Since the initiating entry wound is small it has usually sealed within hours of the bite occurring, so bacteria and inflammatory products are trapped within the soft tissues. If the focus of infection is not recognized and treated, the continued multiplication of bacteria and recruitment of leucocytes to counter the infection produce an accumulation of pus as the abscess forms. Thereafter, the typical signs will be recognized.

- **Focal swelling** at the site of the bite: often rapidly enlarging and initially firm but then fluctuant. Infected cat bites are initially very painful but as the abscess enlarges and the skin becomes separated from the underlying tissue the site may become less painful over time.
  - Common sites include the forelimbs, head and the base of the tail (Figure 5.8.1). Abscesses at the base of the tail may be very painful and can cause temporary flaccid paralysis of the tail, which must be distinguished from fractures and tail-pull injuries. Bites to the limbs may cause severe lameness.
- **Pyrexia** may develop, with associated signs of malaise and inappetence.
- There may be significant **enlargement of local lymph nodes**.
- On close examination a **puncture wound** or wounds will usually be found (Figure 5.8.2), but may only be apparent after clipping of the fur. If the abscess is painful this may need to be done under sedation or general anaesthesia.
  - As the abscess enlarges, the skin around the tooth entry sites becomes necrotic and the abscess may rupture, releasing an amount of

foul-smelling pus (Figure 5.8.3). In general, once the abscess has ruptured the site will be significantly less painful and any systemic signs, such as malaise and inappetence, will usually be markedly improved.

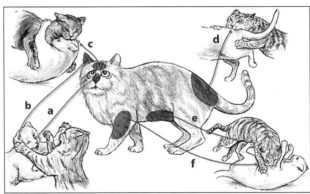

5.8.1 Target areas likely to be subjected to injury from cat bites. The head (a–c), antebrachium (f), tail base (d), axilla, and ventral abdomen (e) should be subjected to increased scrutiny during physical examination. (Reproduced with permission from Malik R, Norris J, White J and Jantulik B (2006) 'Wound cat'. *Journal of Feline Medicine and Surgery* **8**, 135–140.)

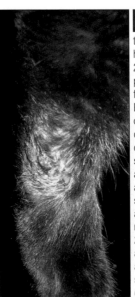

5.8.2 A wound on a cat's hock, showing the typical appearance of a bite that has occurred within the last 24–48 hours. One or more small puncture wounds can usually be found to confirm the diagnosis. Early intervention at this stage will often prevent an abscess from developing. Treatment involves clipping and cleaning the site, short-term (24–48 hours) use of an NSAID such as meloxicam, and a 5–7-day course of broad-spectrum antibiotic such as amoxicillin. There should be marked improvement within 24–48 hours; if this is not achieved, further investigation and more aggressive treatment should be recommended. (© Martha Cannon)

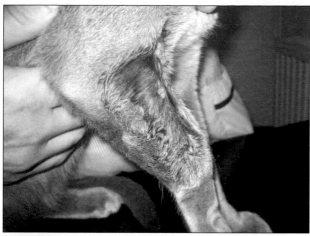

5.8.3 A bite wound on a cat's carpus: after 48–72 hours an accumulation of pus is developing. In this case the skin around the puncture sites is becoming necrotic and the pus is being released. In such cases there may be little to gain by incising the skin over the abscess, as drainage is already occurring. Treatment is as described for Figure 5.8.2 and the abscess should heal rapidly as long as the owner can bathe the site, massaging out any further small amounts of pus that may form. (© Martha Cannon)

Approach to treatment

Cat bite abscesses vary hugely: from small superficial abscesses, in an otherwise clinically well non-pyrexic cat; to extensive cellulitis or deep large abscesses, when the cat may be pyrexic with signs of malaise and inappetence; to rare cases of life-threatening septicaemia. Clinical judgement needs to be used to determine how aggressively each individual case should be managed, and a single treatment protocol for every case may not be appropriate. The key requirements of treatment are discussed below.

Release of trapped pus

Trapped pus should be released, if possible, and the dead space flushed with copious quantities of warm sterile saline.

If the abscess has already ruptured, is small and superficial, or the skin over the abscess is becoming necrotic and denervated it is often possible to lance and/or flush the abscess in the conscious cat. Application of topical local anaesthetic cream (EMLA) can be helpful. In cases where a more extensive area is involved, when the abscess has not already ruptured, when the abscess is in an awkward location or the cat is particularly sensitive over the affected area, then sedation or anaesthesia will be preferable and will allow more controlled lancing and more thorough flushing.

Choice of sedative combination or anaesthetic protocol will depend on the clinical condition of the individual case and any concurrent diseases. In young, otherwise healthy, cats a combination of ketamine, butorphanol and medetomidine provides good anaesthesia and short-term analgesia (see Chapter 3). Alternatively, sedation with midazolam and ketamine may be used.

When lancing an abscess, ensure that the incision is large enough to allow complete drainage. The incision should usually extend at least half to two-thirds of the width of the abscess cavity. Choose a dependent site for the incision, which will allow further pus to drain as it forms over the subsequent few days. In very severe cases it may be helpful to place a Penrose drain to encourage ongoing drainage but *this is rarely necessary* if adequate flushing can be achieved.

> **WARNING**
>
> **DO NOT** suture the incision closed as this will encourage further pus accumulation. It is wise to warn the owner ahead of time that the incision will not be stitched up.

Owners should bathe the incision site with sterile saline or 0.05% chlorhexidine solution at least twice daily over the subsequent few days to keep the wound open and encourage further drainage of pus. To produce a 0.05% solution of chlorhexidine from a 4% stock solution, mix 6.25 ml of stock solution with 500 ml of water.

Antibacterial treatment

The abscess usually contains a range of aerobic and anaerobic bacteria, including *Staphylococcus, Streptococcus, Pseudomonas, Pasteurella multocida* and *Escherichia coli*.

- A broad-spectrum antibiotic is appropriate (e.g. amoxicillin, amoxicillin/clavulanate); or an antibiotic with good spectrum against anaerobic bacteria may be chosen (e.g. clindamycin).
- Fluoroquinolones and third-generation cephalosporins (e.g. cefazolin) are **not** usually required and should **not** be used as a first-line treatment.

If the abscess has been adequately lanced and flushed a short course (5–7 days) of treatment should be sufficient. Bites to the top of the head can prove refractory to treatment and a more prolonged course (10–14 days) may be appropriate.

Supportive treatment

- If pyrexia and/or dehydration are present, consider the need for **fluid therapy**; this can be provided subcutaneously if only mild dehydration is present (see QRG 13.2), or intravenously if it is more severe (see QRG 4.1.3)
- **Provide analgesia** and **anti-pyretic** treatment as appropriate. In otherwise healthy cats a short course of treatment with an NSAID (e.g. meloxicam, robenacoxib) is usually appropriate. However, NSAIDs should not be used in any cat that is dehydrated, hypotensive or showing any renal compromise.

Prognosis

Uncomplicated cat bites usually respond very well and very rapidly to appropriate treatment. The cat should be re-examined within 2–3 days of initial treatment, by which time signs will usually be resolving.

If the abscess appears refractory to treatment consider the following:

- Is the owner able to dose the antibiotics as prescribed? If owners are unable to medicate their cat adequately despite appropriate advice (see QRG 3.1), it may be necessary to use an injectable antibiotic.
- Is there a foreign body within the wound (usually a piece of tooth or claw) that was not identified at the time of initial flushing?
- Does the abscess involve a joint space?

- Is the cat immunocompromised (e.g. due to FIV or FeLV infection)?
- Is there an unusual organism involved, e.g. *Nocardia, Mycobacterium,* L-form bacteria, poxvirus? Cytology, PCR tests and/or bacterial culture may be required. For bacterial culture and/or sensitivity testing, a swab taken from non-necrotic granulation tissue will be most likely to produce representative results.

Constipation

Albert E. Jergens

Constipation is a common clinical sign in cats of all ages, but is especially seen in older cats (>10 years). It is characterized by infrequent, incomplete or difficult defecation, with passage of hard or dry faeces. Constipation can develop with any disease that impairs the passage of faeces through the colon. Delayed faecal transit allows removal of additional salt and water, which produces drier faeces. Chronic faecal impaction with overt distension may result in diminished colonic motility, secondary to smooth muscle degeneration. Obstipation is intractable constipation caused by prolonged retention of hard, dry faeces.

Aetiology

The major causes of feline constipation are relatively few (Figure 5.9.1).

Key differential diagnoses include dyschezia and tenesmus caused by colitis. Cats with colitis show increased frequency of defecation with production of small amounts of faeces containing fresh blood and/or mucus. Stranguria (caused by cystitis/urethritis) may also mimic constipation but is associated with haematuria and abnormalities on urinalysis (e.g. pyuria, crystalluria, bacteriuria).

Clinical approach

A thorough history and physical examination should be carried out.

History
This may include the following:

- Straining to defecate with small or no faecal volume
- Presence of hard, dry faeces
- Infrequent defecation
- Elimination of liquid, mucoid stool – sometimes with blood present after prolonged tenesmus
- Occasional vomiting, inappetence and/or lethargy.

Physical examination
Abdominal palpation reveals a colon filled with hard faeces. Other findings depend on the cause of the problem. Rectal examination (if possible; usually needs to be performed under general anaesthesia)

Dietary
- Bones, hair, foreign material
- Decreased water intake

Environmental
- Changes in environment
- Hospitalization
- Dirty litter box

Drugs
- Opioids
- Diuretics
- Barium sulphate
- Anticholinergics

Painful defecation – due to
- Anorectal disease – anal sacculitis, rectal foreign body, rectal prolapse
- Pelvic trauma
- Perianal disease

Mechanical obstruction
- Extraluminal – narrowed pelvic canal, sublumbar lymphadenopathy
- Intraluminal – colonic/rectal neoplasia, rectal stricture, rectal prolapse

Neuromuscular disease
- CNS disease
- Peripheral nervous system disease (dysautonomia)
- Idiopathic megacolon

Metabolic/endocrine disease
- Hypokalaemia
- Hypocalcaemia

5.9.1 Causes of constipation in cats.

may reveal a mass or stricture, foreign material, perianal disease or a narrowed pelvic canal.

Risk factors
These include:

- Drug therapy, e.g. opioids, anticholinergics, barium sulphate
- Metabolic disease causing dehydration or electrolyte abnormalities, e.g. hypokalaemia
- Pica (ingestion of foreign material)
- Excessive grooming (hair ingestion)
- Pelvic fracture.

Diagnostic investigations

The diagnostic approach when trying to identify an underlying cause for constipation relies on excluding systemic disease (e.g. via routine blood work) and using diagnostic imaging.

- Complete blood count, biochemical profile and urinalysis are normal in the majority of constipated cats, but diseases associated with dehydration (e.g. renal disease) and electrolyte disorders need to be excluded. Elevated PCV and total protein may be observed in dehydrated cats, and pre-renal azotaemia with concentrated urine (USG ≥1.035) may also be present.
- Abdominal radiography will reveal colonic faecal impaction and may reveal underlying causes such as colonic/rectal foreign body, sublumbar lymphadenopathy, or a fractured or narrowed pelvis.
- Pneumocolon, which is usually present following effective faecal evacuation, may define an intraluminal mass or stricture; therefore radiographs taken post-evacuation can be useful.
- Ultrasonography can be valuable in detecting extraluminal masses. It is easier to perform once the colon has been emptied although the presence of air in the colon after faecal evacuation can also make ultrasonography difficult.
- Colonoscopy may be needed to identify colonic/ rectal mass or stricture.

Extraluminal masses and colonic/rectal strictures are less common than the other causes of constipation. If referral is required for procedures such as ultrasonography or colonoscopy, it is reasonable to attempt medical management first and only to seek referral in cases that are refractory to medical therapy.

Treatment

General treatment goals are directed at relieving colonic impaction, correcting any dehydration and electrolyte abnormalities, and preventing constipation from recurring (Figure 5.9.2). Clients should be counselled to discontinue medications that may cause constipation, to feed an appropriate diet and to encourage activity. General anaesthesia with manual removal of faeces may be required if enemas and medications are unsuccessful. In some cats with chronic obstipation or megacolon, subtotal colectomy may be the only and best long-term treatment option.

The therapeutic interventions used will be dependent on the individual case and severity and chronicity of the constipation. With cases of severe constipation and megacolon, a multimodal approach using manual evacuation followed by dietary therapy and a combination of laxatives (e.g. one from each category) ± a pro-motility agent may be most effective.

Enemas

Mild episodes of constipation may resolve with the use of a lubricant sodium citrate micro-enema (e.g. Micralax), without the need for anaesthesia. Other types of enemas, such as warm water enemas with or without lactulose, can also be used. These enemas

Therapy	Rationale and recommendations
Fluid therapy	
Intravenous or subcutaneous route may be used	Use i.v. route if significant dehydration. Add potassium supplement (KCl) if indicated to correct hypokalaemia (see QRG 4.4.1)
Enemas	
Sodium citrate micro-enema (e.g. Micralax)	One-off administration for very mild constipation. NB Avoid sodium phosphate enemas as these may cause severe hypocalcaemia
Warm water enema (± lactulose)	Use tepid water at 20 ml/kg administered q8–12h
Dietary modifications	
Supplement with fibre (e.g. bran, beet pulp, pumpkin, or psyllium ¼ teaspoon daily in divided doses)	Serves as a bulk-forming agent. Commercial high-fibre diets are available
Low-residue, easily digestible diets	Some cats do better on low-residue diets, also commercially available
Drug therapy	
Lubricant laxatives	Mineral oil/liquid paraffin per rectum. White petroleum oral paste (e.g. Katalax)
Osmotic (disaccharide) laxatives	Lactulose: 1 ml/4.5 kg orally; adjust dose to effect. Polyethylene glycol, PEG3350 (e.g. Colyte oral solution, Miralax): 1.9 g/meal or to effect in individual cats
Emollient laxatives	Docusate sodium: 50 mg/cat orally q12–24h
Stimulant laxatives	Bisacodyl: 5 mg/cat orally q12–24h. Dantron (e.g. in Normax 50 mg dantron is combined with 60 mg docusate sodium per 5 ml suspension or one capsule; dose 5 ml or one capsule orally q12–24h)
Pro-motility agent	Cisapride: 2.5–10 mg/cat orally q8–12h
Surgery	
Subtotal colectomy	Indicated in cats with obstipation or megacolon that is uncontrolled with medical management

5.9.2 Therapeutic interventions for constipation.

can be administered rectally using a well lubricated dog urinary catheter or soft feeding tube.

Manual evacuation

More severely affected cats or those unresponsive to enemas may require general anaesthesia for a warm water enema plus manual evacuation. Fluid therapy to correct dehydration and/or electrolyte disturbances should be performed prior to anaesthesia. An endotracheal tube should be placed to prevent aspiration if manipulation of the colon induces vomiting. The faecal mass is softened with the enema and manually reduced, 'milked' distally, and removed manually. With very severe cases this may have to be performed as separate procedures spread over a few days, to prevent prolonged anaesthesia and reduce the risk of colonic perforation. Other treatments should be instituted once the faeces have been removed.

Diet

Dietary management should be instigated once the colon has been emptied. Insoluble fibres act as a bulk-forming laxative and high-fibre diets can be useful in some cases, with the aim of promoting more frequent defecation. Alternatively, wheat bran or psyllium can be added to the normal diet to increase fibre intake. In other cases, however, this worsens the problem by significantly increasing faecal volume and a low-residue diet may be more appropriate.

Laxatives

All cats should be well hydrated before receiving laxatives, as they inhibit water absorption in the colon and so can result in dehydration. There are four different classes of laxative (see Figure 5.9.2).

Lubricant laxatives

Lubricant laxatives include liquid paraffin, mineral oil and white petroleum (e.g. Katalax). These laxatives lubricate the passage of faeces. They may be beneficial for mild constipation as a short-term treatment, but they can interfere with the absorption of nutrients if they are used long term. There is also a high risk of aspiration of mineral oil and liquid paraffin, and so their use should be limited to rectal administration.

Osmotic laxatives

Osmotic laxatives (e.g. lactulose, polyethylene glycol) are poorly absorbed and therefore result in osmotic retention of water in the colon. These are safe to use long term.

Emollient laxatives

Emollient laxatives (e.g. docusate sodium) work by promoting the retention of water within the faeces. They are often used in combination with another agent (e.g. combined with dantron (see below)). Docusate should not be used with mineral oil since it can promote its absorption.

Stimulant laxatives

Stimulant laxatives (e.g. dantron, bisacodyl) work by stimulating colonic smooth muscle contraction. They are usually reserved for use in cases of megacolon or other forms of constipation that are refractory to the other treatments.

- Dantron is combined with docusate sodium in co-danthrusate (e.g. Normax), which is particularly useful for intractable cases of constipation.
- Bisacodyl is a very effective stimulant but is only useful in the short term, as chronic use results in damage to myenteric neurons.

Pro-motility agent

Cisapride has been very useful in the past; however, it was withdrawn from the human market due to development of arrhythmias in some human patients and so it is now more difficult to obtain, although some compounding pharmacies still provide it in a formulation appropriate for dosing cats.

smoke, dust, aerosols, air fresheners, keep the cat out of the bedroom.

■ Steam therapy for 10–15 minutes twice daily, delivered either via a paediatric nebulizer or by placing the cat in a steamy environment (e.g. bathroom; or secure the cat within a carrier and place a bowl of steaming water outside the cage door, then cover the bowl and carrier with a towel) will moisten airways and encourage movement of airway secretions.

When to consider referral

In many cases of coughing, a diagnosis can be rapidly reached with tests widely available in first-opinion practice. Referral should be considered for patients requiring endoscopic or CT examination of the nasopharynx, trachea and lower respiratory tract, if intrathoracic tissue sampling is indicated and in patients refractory to treatment or where a definitive diagnosis remains elusive.

References and further reading

Corcoran B (2010) Clinical approach to coughing. In: *BSAVA Manual of Canine and Feline Cardiorespiratory Medicine*, pp. 11–14. BSAVA Publications, Gloucester
Foster S and Martin P (2011) Lower respiratory tract infections in cats – reaching beyond empirical therapy. *Journal of Feline Medicine and Surgery* **13**, 313–332
Padrid P (2010) Asthma. In: *Consultations in Feline Internal Medicine*, vol. 6, ed. J August, pp. 447–457. Elsevier Saunders, St. Louis
Venema C and Patterson C (2010) Feline asthma: what's new and where might clinical practice be heading? *Journal of Feline Medicine and Surgery* **12**, 681–692

QRG 5.10.1 Bronchoalveolar lavage (BAL)
by Angie Hibbert

Indications

■ To investigate coughing, bronchial or alveolar radiographic changes
■ To harvest samples of bronchial fluid/mucus and cells for diagnostic purposes (cytology and microbial culture)

Contraindications

■ Patient not stable enough to undergo anaesthesia (e.g. severe hypoxaemia)
■ Unstable asthma
■ Coagulopathy

Possible complications

■ Bronchospasm
■ Haemorrhage
■ Trauma leading to pneumothorax
■ Iatrogenic infection

Equipment

■ Sterile lavage catheter (6–8 Fr *soft* urinary catheter with an end hole)
■ 4 x 10 ml syringes with caps
■ Warmed sterile 0.9% saline
■ Sterile lubricating gel
■ Mouth gag
■ Collection pots (EDTA for cytology, sterile plain tubes or universal pots for microbial culture)
■ Microscope slides
■ 21 G hypodermic needle
■ Sterile ET tube of an appropriate size
■ Pulse oximeter
■ Elbow port: connects the endotracheal (ET) tube to a T-piece and allows simultaneous insertion of the lavage catheter whilst oxygen and the volatile agent are delivered continuously during lavage

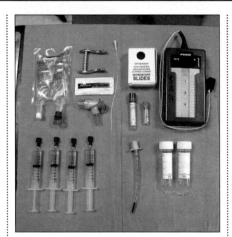

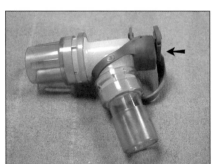

A 15 mm elbow port available from Veterinary Instrumentation. The arrow indicates the channel for passing the catheter.

Patient preparation

1 To reduce the risk of bronchospasm, terbutaline can be given pre-anaesthesia; 1–2 doses pre-lavage are recommended (e.g. 0.015 mg/kg s.c. or i.m. at 4-hourly intervals, with a dose given at the time of premedication). Onset of action may take 15–30 minutes when terbutaline is given subcutaneously or intramuscularly and is usually notable by an increase in heart rate. Terbutaline should also be available for giving during the procedure if bronchospasm still occurs.

2 Place an intravenous catheter, induce general anaesthesia and intubate using a sterile ET tube; an injectable induction agent should be available to deepen the plane of anaesthesia if required (e.g. propofol or alfaxalone).

3 Attach the elbow port to the breathing system and ET tube.

4 Apply a pulse oximeter to the patient's tongue.

5 Position the patient in lateral recumbency, with the most affected side ventral.

Procedure

1 When ready to start the procedure, prepare four lavage syringes; draw up 5 ml of *warm* sterile saline and 5 ml of air into each 10 ml syringe.

2 Gently introduce a soft urinary catheter aseptically via the elbow port into the ET tube until resistance is felt; at this point the catheter should be lodged within a distal airway.

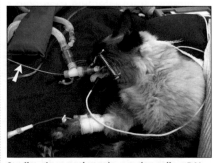

Sterile urinary catheter inserted to collect BAL (white arrow). Elbow port (black arrow). ▶

QRG 5.10.1 *continued*

3 Attach one of the lavage syringes to the end of the urinary catheter and instill the aliquot of warmed saline via the catheter, using the pre-drawn 5 ml of air to flush the fluid completely through the catheter.

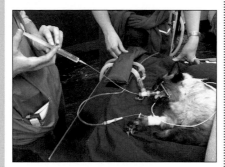

4 Immediately apply suction to the syringe to retrieve the fluid. Retrieval of 40–50% of the infused volume should be expected; elevating the caudal half of the cat may help. A good quality sample is indicated by a foamy 'cap' to the fluid (as shown below) as this indicates retrieval of surfactant from the distal airways; a single good quality sample is usually adequate for diagnostic purposes. Coupage is not performed when using this technique with the cat in lateral recumbency, as it may prevent retrieval of the lavage fluid, by redistributing fluid into other airways.

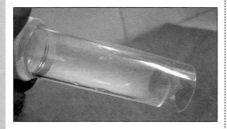

5 Collect fluid samples for cytology (EDTA tube), microbial culture (plain sterile collection pots for aerobic bacteria, *Mycoplasma* spp. ± fungal culture) and PCR for *Mycoplasma felis* ± *Bordetella bronchiseptica*.

6 Monitor respiratory rate, pattern and oxygen saturation closely throughout the procedure, aiming to maintain a steady respiratory rate and depth of breathing with S_pO_2 >95%.

7 Instillation can be performed 2–3 times if a good sample is not achieved initially, provided the patient does not develop any signs of hypoxia (shallow respiratory pattern, tachypnoea, S_pO_2 <95%).

8 Following completion of BAL, continue administration of 100% oxygen and volatile agent via the ET tube for 3–5 minutes, to allow time to detect any immediate complications of the procedure, e.g. bronchospasm. Continue oxygen supplementation via the ET tube until extubation.

9 For in-house cytology, centrifuge the collected EDTA sample, make a smear of the cellular pellet on a glass microscope slide and stain with Diff-Quik or similar. A differential cell count should be based on counting a minimum of 200 cells per slide. The presence of neutrophils (degenerate or not), bacteria and eosinophils are the most important features to evaluate, but the value of submitting samples to a clinical pathologist with expertise in evaluating feline airway cytology should not be underestimated.

Monitoring and aftercare

The cat's respiratory rate and pattern, and ideally pulse oximetry, should be monitored continuously during the procedure and in the recovery period following anaesthesia, due to the associated potential complications, which may induce dyspnoea and hypoxaemia. Oxygen supplementation (via a facemask) may need to be continued following extubation until the cat is able to maintain sternal recumbency and pulse oximetry shows adequate levels of oxygen saturation (S_pO_2 >95%). Respiratory pattern and rate should be monitored over the following 12 hours (in the hospital or by the owners if the cat recovers from the procedure without any immediate complications).

Potential complications associated with BAL include:

- **Bronchospasm:** This typically manifests as dyspnoea and hypoxaemia (S_pO_2 <95%), with wheezes and crackles audible on pulmonary auscultation. A dose of terbutaline (0.015 mg/kg i.v.) can be administered; if this does not stabilize the patient, consider administration of a short-acting steroid (e.g. dexamethasone sodium phosphate 0.1 mg/kg i.v. once). See Chapter 10 for further details of emergency management of bronchospasm as part of feline asthma syndrome
- **Upper airway obstruction by mucus and airway exudates:** This typically manifests as rattling inspiratory noise ± coughing and gagging with hypoxaemia following extubation. A suction unit (or 5 ml syringe attached to a sterile urinary catheter) should be kept nearby and can be used for clearing any secretions from the oropharynx. Try to maintain the cat in sternal recumbency. If the cat resents suctioning of the oropharynx, re-induction of anaesthesia may be required to clear the upper airway effectively.
- **Pneumothorax** is a rare complication, typically manifesting as dyspnoea and hypoxaemia, with a restrictive breathing pattern (i.e. shallow and rapid) with abdominal effort that progresses to a paradoxical pattern (loss of coordination between thoracic and abdominal wall movements). Lung sounds may be absent dorsally and there will be increased resonance on percussion of the thorax. Thoracocentesis should be performed as an emergency (see QRG 4.2.4). If there is continued air accumulation, a thoracic drain may need to be placed (see QRGs 4.2.5 and 4.2.6).

If complications occur in the recovery period and rapid reversal of hypoxaemia and dyspnoea cannot be achieved medically, re-induction of anaesthesia for intubation and ventilation may be required to increase oxygenation and enable investigations to determine the cause of dyspnoea.

Dehydration

Samantha Taylor

Dehydration is a loss of body water/solutes from the body and is a common finding in feline practice.

> **Body water**
>
> - Total body water makes up approximately 60% of the bodyweight of a normal cat.
> - This water is distributed between two body compartments: extracellular fluid (ECF) and intracellular fluid (ICF).
> - ECF can be further divided into plasma and interstitial fluid.

Dehydration is frequently encountered in cats because of their small size and the fact that the majority of a healthy cat's water intake comes from food, so any drop in food intake can result in fluid deficits. Dehydrated cats usually have an interstitial fluid deficit, and severe cases will also have lost plasma volume. Untreated dehydration results in electrolyte disturbances and further reduced food intake. Management of dehydration is vital for recovery from many different conditions.

Clinical assessment

Physical examination

Dehydration should ideally be checked for in a full physical examination of all patients, but especially in cats presenting with clinical signs that result in fluid losses or a reduced fluid intake, such as anorexia, depression, lethargy, vomiting/diarrhoea and polyuria. Subclinical dehydration (<5%) may be suspected in such patients even in the absence of physical examination findings consistent with dehydration.

It is important to estimate the level of dehydration:

- To gauge the severity and need for emergency treatment to prevent the cat's condition deteriorating
- To calculate fluid therapy accurately.

Physical examination findings associated with increasing levels of dehydration are shown in Figure 5.11.1.

Estimated level of dehydration	Physical examination finding
<5%	Not detectable
5–8%	Subtle loss of skin elasticity Slightly dry, tacky mucous membranes
8–10%	Definite loss of skin elasticity (visible skin tenting) Dry, tacky mucous membranes Eyes may appear slightly sunken
10–12%	Severe skin tenting Dry, tacky mucous membranes Eyes sunken in orbits Prolonged capillary refill time (CRT)
>12%	Severe skin tenting Dry, tacky mucous membranes Eyes sunken in orbits Signs of shock: tachycardia/bradycardia, hypotension, poor pulse quality, pale mucous membranes, prolonged CRT, weakness/collapse. This constitutes an emergency (see QRG 4.1.3 for treatment)

5.11.1 Physical examination findings in dehydrated cats.

Interstitial fluid volume deficits result in the common clinical signs of dehydration, including skin tenting (Figure 5.11.2) and dry mucous membranes. Findings such as sunken eyes are seen with moderate/severe dehydration (Figure 5.11.3). Skin turgor can be affected by factors other than dehydration, including body condition score and age. Using the skin over the axilla for assessment of tenting may be more useful than using skin in the 'scruff' region.

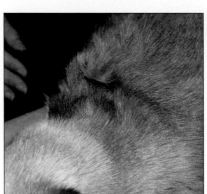

5.11.2

Skin tenting in the 'scruff' region of a dehydrated cat.

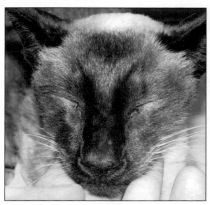

5.11.3
A slightly sunken-eyed appearance in a cat that had been receiving large doses of diuretic and was assessed as approximately 8% dehydrated.

Other parameters

Other objective parameters can be assessed if dehydration is suspected and can also be used to monitor the progress of fluid therapy. Such parameters include:

- Bodyweight – at presentation and then at least daily during hospitalization
- Elevated total solids (total protein)
- Elevated urea and creatinine
- Elevated packed cell volume (PCV)
- Elevated urine specific gravity (USG ≥1.035), although, depending on the cause of dehydration, polyuric patients with suboptimal concentrating ability may remain isosthenuric, hyposthenuric or mildly hypersthenuric despite fluid deficits.

Diagnostic approach

Dehydration can be caused by multiple disease processes, and a logical approach to diagnosis (Figure 5.11.4) and treatment (see later) is required. Acute fluid losses may result from vomiting and diarrhoea for example, but chronic conditions can also cause mild/moderate dehydration (e.g. chronic kidney disease, see Chapter 13) and are particularly seen in geriatric cats.

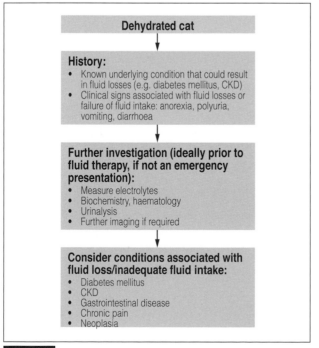

5.11.4 Clinical approach to the dehydrated cat.

Conditions that can result in chronic dehydration

- Chronic kidney disease (CKD)
- Diabetes mellitus
- Osteoarthritis (unwillingness to drink regularly)
- Chronic vomiting/diarrhoea.

Affected cats should be encouraged to increase their water intake at home (see QRG 13.1).

Management of dehydration

A plan for the correction of dehydration is given in Figure 5.11.5. Consideration should be given to obtaining samples prior to correction of dehydration, particularly for urinalysis with measurement of specific gravity.

The management of dehydration involves carefully considered fluid therapy, taking into account:

- Route of administration:
  - Subcutaneous fluid therapy (see QRG 13.2) – only indicated in cases of mild dehydration, often cats with CKD, and can be administered by owners at home in appropriate cases

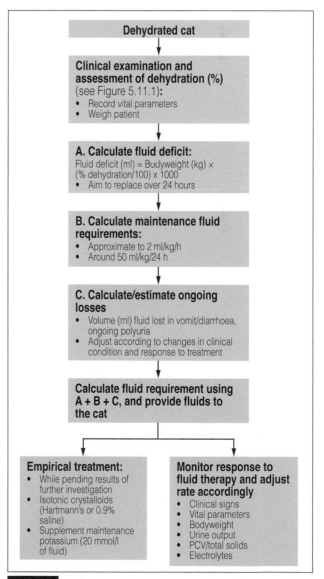

5.11.5 Management of the dehydrated cat.

- Intravenous fluid therapy (see QRG 4.1.3) – indicated in all moderate/severe cases and preferred in all dehydrated patients. Also allows administration of other medications intravenously
- Use of infusion pumps or syringe drivers (Figure 5.11.6) is desirable to ensure accurate fluid delivery rate: cats are sensitive to volume overload; also a simple change in limb position can result in a change in fluid rate
- Type of fluid:
  - Isotonic crystalloid solutions (0.9% saline, Hartmann's (lactated Ringer's) solution) are appropriate in the treatment of dehydration as they initially expand the intravascular space and fluid rapidly redistributes to the interstitial space. Such solutions are low in potassium and so supplementation is likely to be required (see QRG 4.6.1)
  - Dextrose saline is an isotonic solution but the dextrose is rapidly metabolized, leaving a hypotonic solution that can result in electrolyte abnormalities. Indications for use are limited
- Electrolyte abnormalities – ideally electrolytes are measured prior to the initiation of fluid therapy. Even in cats with normal electrolytes, consideration must be given to the effect of administration of an isotonic fluid, and potassium supplementation is recommended at maintenance dosage (see QRG 4.6.1)
- Monitoring response – fluid requirements change with time and correction of dehydration, so monitoring of clinical signs, urine output, bodyweight, PCV/total solids and vital parameters are important during fluid therapy to avoid overhydration and to assess the response to treatment.

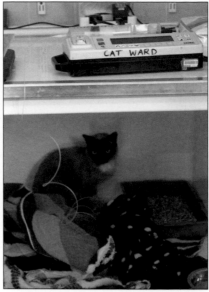

5.11.6

A cat receiving fluid therapy with a syringe driver to ensure an accurate administration rate.

PRACTICAL TIP

Remember electrolytes: balanced fluid therapy includes assessment and correction of electrolyte imbalances, particularly potassium.

WARNING

Cats are extremely sensitive to volume overload (see QRG 4.1.3 for signs of overhydration). Fluids must be administered incrementally with close monitoring.

A fixed fluid 'rate' is not appropriate, because fluid requirements will change as dehydration is corrected. 'Endpoints' should be used to adjust fluid therapy, including normalization of vital parameters and clinical signs of dehydration.

Diarrhoea

Albert E. Jergens

Diarrhoea is the most common clinical manifestation of intestinal disease in cats. It is caused by excess faecal water content, which results in increased frequency of defecation, stool fluidity and/or faecal volume.

- Disease of the small intestine may cause diarrhoea when intestinal contents exceed the absorptive capacity of the large intestine or cause colonic secretion of water.
- Disorders of the large intestine cause diarrhoea because there is no intestinal segment distal to this area to absorb water.
- The stool character and frequency of defecation is influenced by the anatomical site (small *versus* large intestine *versus* combination), patient activity, and/or presence of mucosal inflammation.
- Acute diarrhoea is of short duration (<2 weeks) while chronic diarrhoea persists for >2–3 weeks.

History and clinical examination

The clinical approach in establishing the cause for feline diarrhoea is aided by evaluation of the following factors:

- **Age/environment:**
  - Young animals are more prone to dietary, parasitic and infectious causes
  - Middle-aged cats are susceptible to metabolic/ systemic disease, hyperthyroidism, and infiltrative (inflammatory bowel disease, neoplasia) disorders
  - Environmental conditions, including overcrowding, poor sanitation and immune compromise, are well recognized risk factors due to the likely high infectious agent burden and the influence of stress
  - Free-roaming cats are at increased risk for diarrhoea due to parasites, infection (viral, bacterial, protozoal, fungal) and toxins.
- **Exposure to infectious agents:**
  - Bacterial pathogens: e.g. *Campylobacter jejuni*, *Escherichia coli*, clostridia, *Salmonella*
  - Systemic fungi: e.g. histoplasmosis,

blastomycosis in geographical areas where reported (not UK)
  - Protozoa: *Toxoplasma gondii*, *Giardia*, *Tritrichomonas foetus*, *Cryptosporidium* (rare), *Cystoisospora*
  - Viruses: feline leukaemia virus (FeLV), feline immunodeficiency virus (FIV), feline coronavirus (FCoV), feline parvovirus (FPV).
- **Clinical presentation:**
  - Diarrhoea is generally characterized as small intestinal (SI) or large intestinal (LI), or a combination (Figure 5.12.1)
  - Physical examination findings help to localize intestinal involvement, identify intercurrent disease in other organs, and confirm clinical disease severity (Figure 5.12.2).

Parameter	SI	LI
Faeces		
Mucus	Absent	Common
Fresh blood	Absent	Common
Melaena	Present/absent	Absent
Volume	Often increased	Normal to decreased
Quality	Variable – watery	Semi-solid to solid
Defecation		
Frequency	Normal to mild increase	Greatly increased
Dyschezia	Absent	Present/absent
Tenesmus	Absent	Present/absent
Urgency	Absent	Common
Associated signs		
Weight loss	Common	Uncommon
Vomiting	Present/absent	Uncommon
Appetite	Variable	Often normal
Activity of cat	Often decreased	Often normal
Borborygmus	Present/absent	Absent
Flatulence	Present/absent	Present/absent

5.12.1 General characteristics of small *versus* large intestinal diarrhoea in cats.

Parameter/ investigation	Findings
Observation	Mentation changes; weakness; lethargy
Posture	Arched back suggestive of abdominal pain
Hydration status	Skin tenting and/or tacky mucous membranes if dehydrated
Mucous membrane colour	Pallor: gastrointestinal blood loss, anaemia. Yellow: jaundice
Nutritional status	Malnutrition; emaciation
Thyroid gland palpation	Goitre
Abdominal palpation	Lymphadenopathy; distended bowel loops; abdominal pain; organomegaly; mass
Rectal palpation	Pain; mass/stricture; haematochezia

5.12.2 Potential abnormalities that may be observed on physical examination.

Causes

Acute non-specific gastroenteritis that is generally self-limiting is common: parasitic, dietary and infectious causes should be considered.

General causes for SI and LI diarrhoea include:

- Infections:
  - SI: *Cystoisospora* (formerly *Isospora*), nematodes, *Cryptosporidium*, *Giardia*, FPV
  - LI: *Tritrichomonas foetus*
  - SI and/or LI: *Campylobacter jejuni*, clostridia, *Salmonella*, *E. coli*, histoplasmosis, blastomycosis, toxoplasmosis, FeLV, FIV, FCoV, FPV
- Metabolic and systemic disorders:
  - Renal insufficiency
  - Hepatobiliary disease
  - Hyperthyroidism
- Dietary sensitivity and intolerance: predominantly mild LI diarrhoea but SI also
- Inflammatory bowel disease:
  - Lymphocytic–plasmacytic infiltrates predominate in both SI and LI disease
  - Eosinophilic and neutrophilic inflammation can also occur
- Neoplasia:
  - Lymphoma is most common, followed by adenocarcinoma and mast cell tumours
  - Tumours may occur in the small or large intestine or both
- Antibiotic-responsive enteropathy: prevalence in cats is unknown
- Maldigestion: exocrine pancreatic insufficiency (EPI) is the predominant cause.

Differential diagnoses

The list of potential causes for acute or chronic diarrhoea in cats is extensive (Figure 5.12.3).

Diagnostic approach

History, physical examination and selective diagnostic testing, including faecal examinations using fresh faeces, should always be performed. Components of the initial database include the following.

Cause	Acute diarrhoea	Chronic diarrhoea
Dietary causes	✓	✓
Parasites	✓	✓
Infections:		
■ Bacterial	✓	✓
■ Viral	✓	✓
■ Fungal	✓	✓
Intoxication	✓	✓
Obstruction:		
■ Intestinal foreign body	✓	✓
■ Intussusception	✓	✓
Infiltrative disease:		
■ Inflammatory bowel disease		✓
■ Neoplasia		✓
■ Histoplasmosis		✓
Dysbiosis (microbial inbalance)		✓
Maldigestion: EPI		✓
Hyperthyroidism		✓
Systemic disease:		
■ Hepatobiliary disease	✓	✓
■ Renal disease	✓	✓
■ Pancreatitis	✓	✓

5.12.3 Potential causes for acute or chronic diarrhoea in cats.

Faecal examinations and rectal cytology

Both faecal smears and rectal cytology are useful in defining potential causes for diarrhoea. Preparations are usually made in house and then analysed by a commercial laboratory but in-house analysis is possible.

Faecal smears

Smears are made by applying a small amount of faeces to a glass slide (best applied using the end of a cotton swab; the amount held on the end of a cotton swab is usually enough) and adding to it a few (1–3 usually adequate) droplets of saline and mixing with the cotton bud. For wet-mount preparations, a cover slip is applied and the slide examined with a microscope at X100 (oil immersion). For air-dried smears, the faecal emulsion is spread across a glass slide by application of another slide on top and using the surface tension between the two slides to make smears on both, which are air-dried and then submitted to a commercial laboratory.

Note that wet-mount slides (in-house analysis required within 30 minutes of faecal collection) are most useful to identify parasitic ova or protozoan parasites (*Giardia*, *Tritrichomonas foetus*; see www.ncsu.edu/project/cvm_gookin/Tfoetusvideo.mov for information on differentiating these parasites). Samples for wet-mount preparations in suspected cases of *T. foetus* infection can be collected using a colonic flush technique (see www.ncsu.edu/project/cvm_gookin/buttflush). Air-dried slides may detect bacterial spores (clostridia) and/or the presence of heterogeneous or homogeneous bacterial populations.

Rectal cytology

A gloved fingernail is used to abrade the rectal mucosa gently. The material collected is then dispersed across a glass slide. A thin smear is best for cytological review. Once dried, the smear can be stained with Diff-Quik, Wright's or Wright–Giemsa to facilitate examination.

Normal cytology comprises sheets of uniform columnar epithelium with some goblet cells and some faeces; squamous cell epithelial differentiation may be present on samples collected from around the anal opening, and bacteria should be a mixed population, with a predominance of rod-shaped bacteria. Abnormal cytology may reveal neutrophils (signifying acute active mucosal inflammation due to e.g. clostridial or *Campylobacter* infection, as neutrophils should be removed rapidly in the intestinal environment) or macrophages containing *Histoplasma* organisms, or lymphocytes in chronic colitis cases. Submission of the unstained smear for analysis by a commercial laboratory is always advised if one is not confident with in-house cytology.

Other faecal tests

These may include:

- Flotation for parasitic ova: can be done in house but usually submitted to a commercial laboratory
- Zinc sulphate centrifugation: more sensitive than flotation for parasitic ova and *Giardia* cysts; can be done in house but usually submitted to commercial laboratory
- ELISA/IFA for *Giardia* antigen: submit to commercial laboratory
- Faecal culture for enteropathogenic bacteria: submit to commercial laboratory.

Haematology and biochemistry

- A complete blood count should be performed:
  - Leucocytosis – suspect inflammation
  - Eosinophilia – caused by parasites, dietary sensitivity
  - Leucopenia – marked leucopenia may be seen during active FPV infection
  - Anaemia – diverse causes but includes anaemia of inflammatory disease or gastrointestinal blood loss; may see accompanying hypoproteinaemia, elevated urea and thrombocytosis with gastrointestinal blood loss
- Increased PCV and total serum protein may indicate dehydration
- Hypoproteinaemia (hypoalbuminaemia/ hypoglobulinaemia) may result from intestinal protein loss
- Hyperglobulinaemia may indicate antigen stimulation/inflammation
- Elevated urea may indicate pre-renal azotaemia or gastrointestinal blood loss. Increased liver enzymes may indicate primary hepatopathy or pancreatitis
- Serum thyroxine concentration should be measured in cats older than 6 years.

Urinalysis

This should be carried out to assess renal function, and to differentiate causes of azotaemia if present (see Chapter 5.7).

Tests for infectious agents

Viral enteropathy caused by FPV may cause acute haemorrhagic diarrhoea, vomiting, and depression. Diagnosis is made based on history (young cat, non-vaccinated, overcrowding) and exclusion of other causes for haemorrhagic gastroenteritis, as well as demonstration of the virus in faeces. In practice, test kits to detect FPV antigen in faeces have an acceptable sensitivity and specificity; tests marketed for the detection of *feline* parvovirus antigen, as well as those for detecting *canine* parvovirus antigen, may be used. Specialized laboratories offer PCR-based testing for FPV in whole blood or faeces. Testing of whole blood is recommended when no faecal samples are available. Serology for FPV is not useful, as tests do not differentiate between infection- and vaccination-induced antibodies.

Other tests:

- PCR for detection of FCoV and *Tritrichomonas foetus* in faeces
- FIV and FeLV tests, to screen for viral-induced inflammatory gut disease
- IgG and IgM antibody testing for *Toxoplasma gondii* infection.

Miscellaneous blood tests

The following are available from commercial diagnostic laboratories.

- **Folate** and **vitamin B12** (cobalamin) levels can reflect mucosal absorption in the proximal (folate) and/or distal (ileum) (vitamin B12) small intestine. Low levels indicate abnormalities in absorption and these assays serve to localize the extent of SI mucosal disease and act as biomarkers for treatment responses. It has been shown that chronic pancreatic and liver disease can also cause a deficiency in vitamin B12; absorption of this vitamin in the gastrointestinal tract relies on a pancreas-secreted intrinsic factor that may be reduced in pancreatic disease, and vitamin B12 has an enterohepatic recycling pattern that can be disrupted by liver disease. Reduced oral intake (e.g. in anorexia) may also contribute to reduced levels of vitamin B12.
- **Feline trypsin-like immunoreactivity** (fTLI); will be low if exocrine pancreatic insufficiency (EPI) is present.
- **Feline pancreatic lipase immunoreactivity** (fPLI); may be elevated if pancreatitis is present (see Chapter 12).

Intestinal biopsy

Mucosal biopsy specimens from the stomach and intestines are most commonly obtained via endoscopy. Referral is an option if this facility is not available in the practice.

An alternative is to obtain full-thickness gastrointestinal tissue specimens by laparotomy (see QRG 11.1) or laparoscopy (referral to a specialist usually required). As well as the stomach and small intestine (including the ileum), biopsy specimens from other organs (i.e. liver, pancreas, mesenteric lymph node) are recommended during laparotomy. LI specimens are not usually obtained at laparotomy.

An overview of treatment

Treatment of specific disorders causing diarrhoea can be found in Chapter 11; a general overview is given here.

Acute diarrhoea

Many causes of acute diarrhoea cause little morbidity and are self-limiting; often no treatment, or only palliative treatment, is required.

The diet should be modified and a highly digestible low-fat diet (e.g. Hill's d/d; Iams–Eukanuba low residue) should be fed, using small frequent feedings (3–6 meals/day) for 5–7 days. High-fibre diets can be useful in cats with colitis.

Empirical treatments with anthelmintics (pyrantel 5 mg/kg orally, repeat after 2 weeks; or fenbendazole at 50 mg/kg orally for 5 days), or a therapeutic trial using metronidazole (10–20 mg/kg orally q12h for 5–7 days) may also prove beneficial, even in cats negative for parasites and other infectious agents.

Selected patients with acute diarrhoea may require correction of fluid deficits (see QRGs 4.1.3 and 13.2). Symptomatic therapy with probiotics (e.g. Prostora max, Iams-Eukanuba; Fortiflora, Purina) each administered for 14 days may shorten the clinical course of acute diarrhoea. When infectious pathogens (bacteria, viruses) are the aetiological factors, established hospital protocols that inhibit disease transmission should be rigorously enforced (e.g. informing personnel, barrier nursing, use of isolation facilities).

Therapy for FPV includes: excellent nursing care; correction of hydration/electrolyte deficits with intravenous fluids (e.g. crystalloids such as lactated Ringer's solution); and parenteral antibiotics (e.g. penicillins) for haemorrhagic diarrhoea ± leucopenia.

Chronic diarrhoea

Treatment of chronic diarrhoea will be specific, depending on the underlying cause:

- Repeat anthelmintics: If giardiasis is suspected, treat with metronidazole (10–20 mg/kg orally for 7 days). Use pyrantel as a broad-spectrum de-wormer for treatment of other potential parasites. Toxoplasmosis is best treated with clindamycin (10–12.5 mg/kg orally or i.v. q12h) or trimethoprim/sulphonamide (15 mg/kg orally q12h) or azithromycin (10 mg/kg orally q24h) for a minimum of 4 weeks or for 2 weeks beyond clinical cure
- Prebiotics and probiotics: To modulate microbiota imbalances. Treat for a minimum of 4 weeks to optimize efficacy; longer treatment durations are likely to be needed to achieve benefits in host immunity
- Nutritional therapy: Using an intact protein or hydrolysate elimination diet to reduce dietary antigen load
- Antibiotics (e.g. metronidazole for clostridial infections, erythromycin for *Campylobacter jejuni*) if justified due to presence of a bacterial enteropathogen or evidence of an impaired mucosal barrier (bloody diarrhoea, sepsis)
- Immunosuppressive drugs (e.g. prednisolone) in biopsy-proven immune-mediated diseases, such as IBD. Metronidazole is advocated as an immunomodulating drug but its effects may be due to correction of intestinal microbial imbalances (dysbiosis)
- Adjunctive B12 vitamin therapy for hypocobalaminaemia. Treat cats with parenteral (subcutaneous) cyanocobalamin (250 μg/cat once weekly for 4 weeks) then recheck serum cobalamin
- Therapy for hyperthyroidism if confirmed by elevated thyroxine concentrations (see Chapter 14)
- Antifungal agents (e.g. itraconazole, 10 mg/kg orally q24h for 2–3 months or until active disease is gone) for gastrointestinal histoplasmosis or blastomycosis.

Haematuria

Danièlle Gunn-Moore

Haematuria (blood in the urine) is commonly seen in feline practice and can vary from very mild and only detectable on dipsticks (most common) to severe gross haematuria. It may be caused by blood leaking into any part of the urinary tract (kidneys, ureters, bladder, urethra) or the associated reproductive tract (e.g. prostate, prepuce, uterus, vagina), or it can result from a haemostatic defect, where the degree of haematuria may be very severe and grossly evident (Figure 5.13.1).

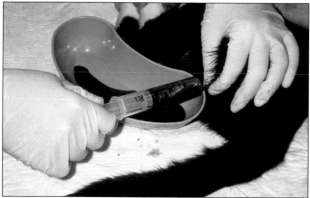

5.13.1 Severe haematuria; clots caused urinary obstruction.

Aetiology and differentials

Haematuria is most commonly caused by lower urinary tract (LUT) conditions such as feline idiopathic cystitis (FIC), and in these cases will often occur concurrently with other LUT signs such as dysuria, pollakiuria and inappropriate urination (see Chapters 5.21 and 13).

Causes of haematuria are listed in Figure 5.13.2. Only those that may occur without concurrent LUT signs will be further discussed in this chapter; disorders that may cause other LUT signs in addition to haematuria are discussed in Chapters 5.21 and 13.

Trauma

Haematuria can result from trauma to any part of the urinary tract. It can be accidental or iatrogenic. It is important to look for other signs of trauma (e.g.

- Feline idiopathic cystitis (FIC)
- Urolithiasis [a]
- Urinary tract infection (UTI) [a]
- Trauma [a]
- Renal cysts, e.g. polycystic kidney disease (PKD)
- Renal infarcts
- Neoplasia [a]
- Idiopathic renal haemorrhage
- Haemostatic defect: coagulopathy or thrombocytopenia

5.13.2 Causes of haematuria. [a] Disease can be within the kidneys, ureters, bladder or urethra.

shredded nails, lacerations, abdominal bruising, broken bones, shock) and to assess the integrity of the urinary tract (rupture may be suggested by unexplained azotaemia or uroabdomen (see Chapter 4.10); diagnosis is confirmed if creatinine concentration in the abdominal fluid is higher than that in plasma; see Chapter 5.1).

Renal cysts

These are most commonly associated with PKD in Persian cats (Figure 5.13.3). By damaging local blood vessels, haemorrhage can occur into the cysts, occasionally resulting in haematuria. Renal cysts can also be seen in any breed of cat with significant chronic kidney disease (CKD). In all cases the cats are likely

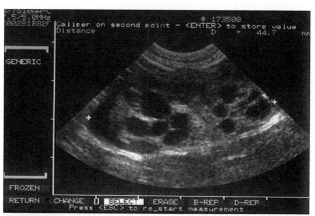

5.13.3 Ultrasound examination showing multiple anechoic renal cysts and a perirenal pseudocyst (visible as anechoic 'rim' on left-hand side of scan) in a 9-year-old Persian cat with hereditable PKD.

to have clinical signs associated with CKD (e.g. polyuria and polydipsia), but occasional cases may present with haematuria alone. Diagnosis is made by ultrasound examination. A genetic test is available for the diagnosis of hereditable PKD in Persian cats and related breeds (see Chapter 2).

Renal infarcts

These are most commonly seen in older cats with CKD and/or systemic hypertension (see Chapter 5.18). Clinical signs may be associated with CKD (e.g. polyuria and polydipsia) and/or systemic hypertension (e.g. intraocular haemorrhage, signs associated with cerebrovascular accidents), or congestive heart failure; occasional cases present with haematuria alone.

Neoplasia

Transitional cell carcinomas (TCCs), adenocarcinoma, leiomyoma, lymphoma and a number of other tumours may occur in feline bladders. TCCs are seen most frequently although they are still rare; they may occur as isolated tumours or multiple tumours arising more diffusely in the bladder wall, which may be secondary to chronic bladder inflammation. Clinical signs include haematuria, dysuria, pollakiuria and periuria (see Chapter 18), although haematuria may be the only sign. Diagnosis is made by identifying the mass (Figure 5.13.4) and then aspiration or biopsy. Neoplastic cells are rarely present in the urine.

The most common tumours in the kidneys are lymphoma (usually bilateral and causing diffuse hyperechogenicity; Figure 5.13.5) and adenocarcinoma (usually unilateral); haematuria may be the only sign.

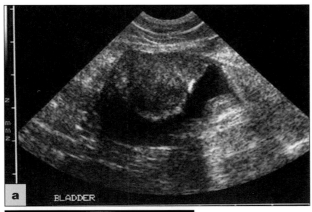

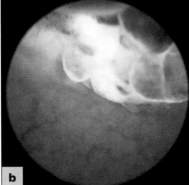

5.13.4 Bladder TCCs identified by **(a)** ultrasonography and **(b)** cystoscopy. Image (b) is from a dog. The gross appearance of a TCC is similar in both dogs and cats; however, in dogs TCCs tend to arise from the trigone region of the bladder whereas in cats they frequently occur in sites distant to the trigone. (b, courtesy of P Lhermette)

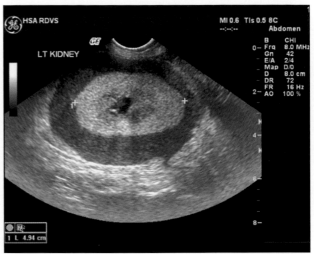

5.13.5 Ultrasound appearance of a kidney from a cat with renal lymphoma.

Idiopathic renal haemorrhage

This is a rare cause of haematuria, and haematuria is the only sign. Affected cats rarely lose enough blood to become anaemic. Diagnosis can be made after excluding all other causes and, if possible, visualizing a blood-stained urine jet in the bladder, via cystoscopy or at cystotomy. Severe cases that become anaemic may require unilateral nephrectomy; the blood loss therefore needs to be localized to the correct kidney if this is being considered.

Haemostatic defects: coagulopathy or thrombocytopenia

These are rare causes of haematuria. Coagulopathy can be associated with congenital (e.g. hereditary vitamin K-responsive coagulopathy in Devon Rex) or acquired clotting defects (e.g. warfarin poisoning, liver disease), whilst thrombocytopenia is most commonly associated with disseminated intravascular coagulation (DIC). Haematuria may be the only clinical sign of disease in cats with haemostatic defects if the blood loss does not cause anaemia and there is no associated systemic disease.

Diagnostic approach

Diagnosis entails finding out where in the urogenital tract the blood is coming from and determining the cause. The presence or absence of other LUT signs, and the severity of haematuria, will also help to indicate which causes are most likely.

Signalment

- PKD is seen mainly in Persian cats, and haemorrhage into the cysts is typically seen in older individuals.
- FIC is seen mainly in cats aged 4–7 years.
- UTIs are seen mostly in older cats, particularly those with CKD, diabetes mellitus (DM), hyperthyroidism, systemic immunosuppression, or following urethral catheterization.
- The most common cancer of the urogenital tract in cats is TCC and it usually affects older cats.
- Entire female cats may develop an open pyometra which may be mistaken for haematuria.

History

- Previous episodes of FIC, urolithiasis or UTI indicate that a cat may be predisposed to that condition.
- It is important to determine whether there has been recent trauma (e.g. urinary catheterization, road traffic accident, dog bite).
- Previous bleeding (e.g. at neutering) may indicate a congenital clotting problem.
- Possible exposure to toxins should be considered (e.g. ethylene glycol, lilies, NSAIDs, aminoglycoside antibiotics, warfarin).

Physical examination

- Non-painful renomegaly may be found with PKD, renal lymphoma or other forms of renal neoplasia, feline infectious peritonitis (FIP), chronic hydronephrosis, perirenal pseudocysts (which are usually associated with end-stage CKD), amyloidosis (typically seen in Abyssinian cats), functional renomegaly (due to acromegaly or, less commonly, portosystemic shunts), or congenitally defective kidneys (e.g. 'horseshoe' kidney).
- Painful renomegaly is more commonly associated with acute ureteral obstruction, multiple renal abscesses, renal haemorrhage associated with trauma, pyelonephritis, nephroliths, or poisoning (e.g. ethylene glycol).
- A painful bladder and signs of dysuria may be associated with any cause of cystitis (FIC, UTI, stones, neoplasia, or trauma).
- Fever is rarely associated with UTI, but is commonly associated with FIP.
- The cat may have signs of systemic disease (e.g. polyuria, polydipsia and dehydration with CKD, DM or hyperthyroidism; collapse with urinary obstruction; uveitis with FIP; or petechial haemorrhages with thrombocytopenia).

Observation of urination

- If haematuria is present only at the beginning of the urine stream the bleeding is distal to the bladder.
- If haematuria is present throughout the urine stream the area of bleeding is in the bladder or proximal to it.
- If there are signs of straining or discomfort when urinating, the area of inflammation is usually from the bladder or urethra. However, occasional cases of renal haemorrhage can result in clots in the bladder which cause dysuria when the cat tries to pass them, and so this may complicate the clinical picture.

Cystocentesis

Free-catch urine samples should be compared with those obtained by cystocentesis. If urine from cystocentesis is haematuric, the blood cannot be coming from distal to the bladder, unless iatrogenic haemorrhage has occurred during cystocentesis (usually microscopic or seen as a swirl of blood in the needle; see QRG 4.11.4).

Urinalysis

Red colouring of the urine (Figure 5.13.6) may be due to haematuria, haemoglobinuria or myoglobinuria.

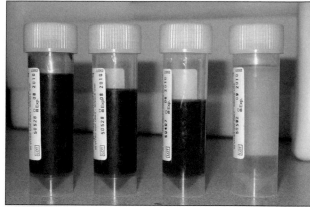

5.13.6 Urine samples: (left to right) haematuria, haemoglobinuria, bilirubinuria, normal urine.

Whole blood, haemoglobin and myoglobin all give a positive reaction on urine dipsticks. Sediment examination is needed to see whether erythrocytes (haematuria >10–20 erythrocytes/hpf) are present. With haematuria, sedimentation results in an erythrocyte pellet and clear supernatant; with haemoglobinuria (uncommon) and myoglobinuria (rare) the supernatant remains red-stained. With haemoglobinuria there should also be clinical and haematological evidence of intravascular haemolysis, while with myoglobinuria there should be evidence of muscle damage (e.g. elevated creatine kinase/AST).

Urinalysis and sediment examination (see QRG 4.11.3) are also necessary to look for:

- Evidence of UTI (e.g. increased leucocytes and erythrocytes)
- Large numbers of crystals that may predispose to urolithiasis
- Glucose or ketones that may indicate DM
- Reduced specific gravity (with DM, CKD, hyperthyroidism, corticosteroid administration).

Bacterial culture is needed to confirm a UTI; there will not always be an active sediment.

Haematology (including platelet count), serum biochemistry and clotting times

These are needed to assess the cat for systemic disease (e.g. DM, CKD, hyperthyroidism, FIP, clotting problems), particularly if there are other clinical signs or physical examination abnormalities, suspected UTI, or severe gross haematuria.

Imaging

Abdominal ultrasound examination

This is needed to assess the kidneys (shape, size, texture) and the presence of masses (neoplasia, FIP-associated granulomas), cysts, infarcts or hydronephrosis. In the hands of an experienced ultrasonographer it can be used to assess renal blood flow.

Ultrasonography is also useful to assess the ureters for distension, masses or stones, and the bladder for size, shape, wall changes, and the presence of stones, blood clots, etc. Only the proximal third of the urethra can be visualized by ultrasound examination. Retrograde urethrography (see QRG 5.21.1) and/or rectal examination are needed to evaluate the entire length of the urethra.

Abdominal radiography/CT

Routine radiography is useful for checking kidney and bladder size, shape and position, and to visualize radiopaque stones within the kidneys, ureters, bladder and urethra.

Intravenous urography (IVU) can assess renal perfusion (this technique is rarely required and therefore not described within this Manual, but see *BSAVA Manual of Canine and Feline Nephrology and Urology*; the reader should seek further advice if considering IVU). Single and double-contrast bladder studies (see QRG 5.21.1) can be useful in assessing bladder wall thickness, and to look for bladder masses and stones. CT, where available, can also be used to make many of these assessments. Retrograde urethrography is useful to assess the urethra for abnormalities such as stones, masses and strictures.

Cystoscopy

To confirm a diagnosis of renal haemorrhage it can be helpful to look at the ureteral urine jets to see which side is involved. This can be done at laparotomy, laparoscopy or using cystoscopy. The more common causes of haematuria should first be excluded, and then advice from a specialist sought to discuss whether further investigation is appropriate, with referral if necessary. The main reason for identifying which kidney is involved is if nephrectomy is being considered. This would be indicated if the degree of haematuria were so severe as to be causing significant anaemia.

Management

Appropriate treatment can be undertaken once the cause of the haematuria has been determined. Sometimes mild haematuria can be present, and the underlying cause can not be identified. The most important approach in these cases is to ensure that no other clinical or examination abnormalities are present, and to exclude a UTI. Monitoring is then prudent, and further investigation indicated if the haematuria persists.

Further reading

Archer J (2005) Urine analysis. In: *BSAVA Manual of Canine and Feline Clinical Pathology, 2nd edn*, ed. E Villiers and L Blackwood, pp. 149–168. BSAVA, Gloucester

Bartges JW (2000) The cat with discoloured urine. In: *Textbook of Small Animal Internal Medicine*, ed. EC Rand, pp. 96–99. WB Saunders, Philadelphia

Bartges JW (2006) Discoloured urine. In: *Problem-based Feline Medicine*, ed. SJ Ettinger and J Feldman, pp. 205–216. Elsevier Saunders, Philadelphia

Watson ADJ (2007) Dysuria and haematuria. In: *BSAVA Manual of Canine and Feline Nephrology and Urology, 2nd edn*, ed. J Elliott and GF Grauer, pp. 1–7. BSAVA, Gloucester

Hairballs

Margie Scherk

Hairballs typically present as a tubular wad of tightly or loosely packed ingested hair (Figure 5.14.1). The extreme is a true trichobezoar (Figure 5.14.2), a hard concretion consisting of hair, which is lodged in the stomach and is too large to vomit or pass through the pylorus and intestines.

Clients may, however, use the term hairballs to describe loose strands of hair in vomitus containing clear or coloured liquid, or even within regurgitated or vomited food. They may report that their cat extends his/her neck and appears to cough before dispelling the hairball ± liquid. It is therefore helpful to determine what exactly the client is referring to before determining what diagnostic and therapeutic approach to take.

Causes

Cats normally ingest small amounts of hair through grooming, and these pass normally in the faeces. This process can be disrupted either due to increased ingestion of hair (e.g. with skin or coat problems) or by abnormal passage of hair (e.g. changes in gastrointestinal motility). It is important to try to identify and treat the cause of the hairball rather than just its resulting effect; psychogenic or behavioural causes should also be considered (Figure 5.14.3). Many of the causes of hairballs will present with clinical signs associated with the underlying problem rather than just hairballs alone.

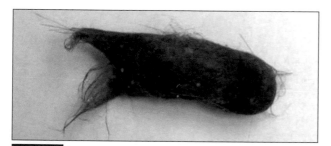

5.14.1 A typical hairball. (Courtesy of Susan Little.)

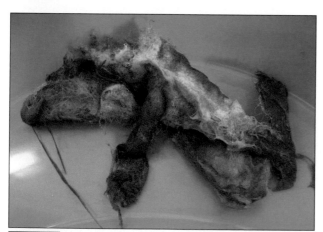

5.14.2 A large trichobezoar removed, at laparotomy, from the stomach of a middle-aged cat that was presented with a suspected gastric mass. The trichobezoar, which almost filled the stomach, has been cut open to show its contents. The cat had been grooming excessively and had gastrointestinal ileus of unknown origin. (Courtesy of The Feline Centre, Langford Veterinary Services, University of Bristol.)

Discomfort resulting in excessive grooming to soothe pain

■ Abdominal:
  – Cystitis (idiopathic, bacterial, urolithiasis), ureteronephrolithiasis, pyelonephritis
  – Gastroenteritis (IBD, infectious, parasitic)
  – Pancreatitis
  – Biliary tree disease (cholangitis, cholycystitis)
■ Degenerative skeletal disease

Digestive tract motility disorders
■ Oesophageal diseases (megaoesophagus, oesophagitis secondary to reflux or drug irritation, hiatal hernia) ■ Gastric diseases causing ileus (parasitic, neoplastic, infectious, inflammatory, post-surgical) ■ Intestinal diseases causing ileus (parasitic, neoplastic, infectious, inflammatory/IBD, intussusception, post-surgical) ■ Gastrointestinal foreign body ■ Hernia causing displaced viscera ■ Drug-induced dysmotility (e.g. opioids, atropine, loperamide)

Dermatological disorders resulting in excessive grooming due to irritation
■ Dermatophytosis ■ Allergic (atopy, food, contact, parasitic) ■ Ectoparasitic

Behavioural/psychogenic causes resulting in excessive grooming
■ Stress (environmental, social) ■ Temperament predisposing to compulsive/stereotypic behaviour

5.14.3 Causes of hairballs.

Empirical treatment pending results of investigations

While there are numerous therapeutic recommendations and commercial diets to reduce the frequency of vomiting hairballs, the underlying cause should always be addressed whenever possible. Below are considerations for cases in which an underlying cause is not easily apparent.

- **Hydration:**
  - Optimizing hydration by utilizing moist food, adding water to meals, and administering subcutaneous fluids will help to normalize cellular and neuromuscular function, thereby improving gastrointestinal motility
- **Hairball remedies:**
  - These consist of malt-flavoured petroleum jelly, with or without added vitamins. These products can be used copiously in the short term, and daily or intermittently at maintenance doses (2–5 cm/day) in the long term
  - Beet pulp and other fibres may help to increase motility; treats and diets containing these may be considered
- **Removal of excessive loose hair:**
  - Combing and brushing may help to reduce hairball formation. However, there is often a layer of loose hair left on the surface that the cat will swallow when completing grooming; a damp paper towel should be used to wipe these fine fibres away. Specialist combs/brushes such as the Furminator will reduce the quantity of loose hair, but must be used cautiously to avoid removing too much fur
- **Ensure that medications do not get stuck in the oesophagus:**
  - Drugs such as oral clindamycin and doxycycline pills/capsules can cause irritation and may result in oesophageal strictures, which may predispose to hairball formation.

Any oral medication that is not available in a liquid formulation should be flushed with a 3–6 ml water 'chaser'.

Diagnosis and treatment of underlying causes

A diagnostic approach to hairballs is summarized in Figure 5.14.4.

Oesophageal diseases

Diagnosis
Radiographs should be taken. Displaced viscera (suggesting a congenital problem or previous trauma) or megaoesophagus may be seen, both of which can be associated with hairballs.

A barium contrast imaging study can be used to identify oesophagitis (abnormal striations), a stricture or a foreign body within the oesophagus. Liquid barium (5 ml orally) may delineate a hairball (Figure 5.14.5). If a foreign body is not identified using liquid barium, further evaluation using barium paste mixed with canned food administered via a syringe may be required. Barium meals (canned food and, if necessary, barium pasted with dry food) are useful for evaluating strictures, as well as oesophageal motility through sequential exposures. Intravenous diazepam (0.2 mg/kg) can be given immediately before radiography to encourage feeding if the cat is reluctant to eat.

Referral may be indicated to look for a stricture, for biopsy of a mass, or to remove a foreign body. Fluoroscopy may be required to study a dynamic process such as a sliding hiatal hernia.

Treatment
Treatment will depend on the condition discovered. Correction or alleviation of the underlying problem will result in a reduction or cure of the hairball problem. If oesophagitis is diagnosed, oral medications should be given in a liquid format to avoid exacerbating oesophagitis.

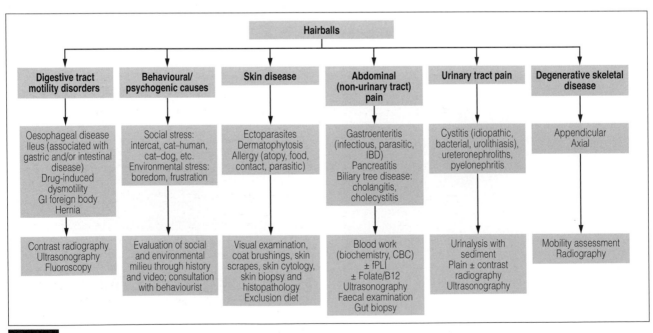

5.14.4 A diagnostic approach to the causes of hairballs.

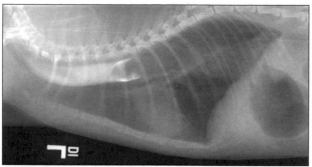

5.14.5 This cat was presented for inappetence and regurgitation with concurrent weight loss. On conscious plain radiography, aerophagia and a dilated oesophagus were suspected; so a follow-up image was taken immediately after oral administration of 5 ml of liquid barium. In this lateral view, the column of barium stops at the 4–5th rib, with a conical shape outlining the proximal portion of the hairball lodged in the oesophagus at this point. An orthogonal VD view is required for further localization. (Courtesy of John Graham.)

Gastric and intestinal disease

Radiography, ultrasonography and endoscopy may be performed non-invasively. Sometimes a hairball itself can be seen (Figure 5.14.6). Ultrasonography has the advantage of revealing motility. Biopsy may be required (laparotomy or endoscopy) to determine what is causing ileus or dysmotility. Faecal examination may be performed. Routine use of a broad-spectrum anthelmintic is recommended.

Gastric foreign bodies (including trichobezoars) will require surgical removal.

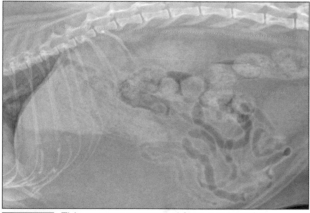

5.14.6 This cat was presented for a progressive decrease in appetite. The large falciform fat pad ventral to the liver occupies half the ventrodorsal dimension of the patient, indicating severe obesity. The obliquely longitudinal structure in the mid-cranial abdomen (the stomach) is filled with a radiodense object, representing some type of soft tissue foreign body. At laparotomy this was revealed to be a trichobezoar. (Courtesy of John Graham.)

Pancreatic disease

Ultrasonography in combination with a serum fPLI (feline pancreatic lipase immunoreactivity) test is the least invasive way to diagnose pancreatitis. General treatment of pancreatitis consists of analgesia, fluid therapy, and ensuring that the patient receives adequate amounts of a balanced diet (see Chapter 12).

Biliary tree disease

Radiography may reveal an opacity in the region of the gall bladder. Ultrasonography of the biliary tree will confirm choleliths and may also reveal any sludge and/or thickened biliary walls consistent with cholecystitis. Aspiration of bile for cytology (EDTA) and culture (plain) may be performed under ultrasound guidance (referral may be required for this). Bile cytology may show infection and/or inflammation.

Antibiotics should be chosen according to the results of sensitivity testing. Should finances be a concern, however, use of metronidazole for anaerobic bacteria, along with a fluoroquinolone for Gram-positive and Gram-negative aerobes should be considered.

Lower urinary tract disease

Urinalysis will be helpful by revealing whether infection, inflammation, idiopathic disease or crystals are present. Radiography and ultrasonography will also be useful.

Dermatological disease

Overgrooming may be generalized, rather than restricted to one region of the body, when dermatological disease is present. The cat should be evaluated for ectoparasites and dermatophytosis. If these are not found, treat for fleas (as these are difficult to confirm) and consider allergies (see Chapter 5.26).

Degenerative skeletal disease

Asking appropriate questions regarding mobility, jumping and climbing (both up and down), as well as overall energy levels, may suggest the presence of osteoarthritis or spondylosis deformans. Spondylosis deformans occurs secondary to the degeneration of intervertebral discs and is characterized by the formation of bony spurs or complete bony bridges around the diseased disc between affected vertebrae, to re-establish stability to the weakened joint. Radiographs may be taken to identify affected joints, although radiographic findings do not always correlate with clinical findings and normal radiographs cannot rule out the presence of either of these degenerative conditions.

Disease-modifying agents such as glucosamine/chondroitin sulphate (see Chapter 16), and therapeutic diets in conjunction with appropriately used NSAIDs and other analgesic agents (see Chapter 3), are warranted.

Behavioural and psychogenic causes

Cats may express overgrooming as a way to self-soothe when stressed. This stress may be: social (associated with other individuals (human, cat, dog, etc.) in the home); frustration (a change in, or loss of, routines); or environmental (no opportunity to express normal cat-appropriate behaviours). Individuals with temperaments predisposing to compulsive or stereotypic behaviour will start to overgroom and then be unable to stop. They may restrict excessive grooming to just one region (e.g. the forelimbs) or may generalize the behaviour. Consultation with a behaviourist is advised.

Head shaking and/or ear scratching

Natalie Barnard

Approximately 6–7% of feline patients presented at the veterinary surgery have ear disease, which can present as head shaking and/or ear scratching. The most common cause of head shaking and ear scratching in cats is otitis.

- **Otitis externa:** acute or chronic inflammation of the external auditory canal and tympanic membrane. Otitis externa (OE) is often a manifestation of an underlying skin disease.
- **Otitis media:** infection extends to involve the middle ear.

It is important to have a basic understanding of the anatomy of the cat's ear (Figure 5.15.1), as it is different from that of the dog.

Otitis can have many causes in cats:

- Ectoparasites: *Otodectes cynotis, Neotrombicula autumnalis, Demodex*
- Polyps (Figure 5.15.2)
- Infection: bacteria (Figure 5.15.3), yeast (Figure 5.15.4)
- Underlying allergic skin disease (cutaneous adverse food reaction, atopic dermatitis)
- Neoplasia
- Contact or irritant reaction to topical products.

In cases where the otitis is *unilateral*, this is more suggestive of polyps or neoplasia. *Bilateral* otitis is more commonly caused by parasitic infestation or allergic skin disease.

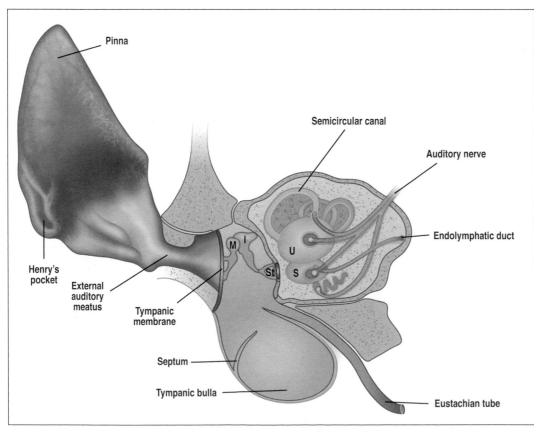

5.15.1

Anatomy of the feline ear, showing the presence of a septum in the bulla of the middle ear; this septum is not present in the dog.
I = incus;
M = malleus;
S = saccule;
St = stapes;
U = utricle.

Pinna

Semicircular canal

Auditory nerve

Endolymphatic duct

Henry's pocket

External auditory meatus

Tympanic membrane

Septum

Tympanic bulla

Eustachian tube

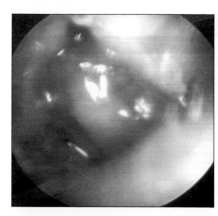

5.15.2 A polyp in the horizontal external ear canal of a young cat that presented with unilateral purulent otitis. The polyp was only visualized after flushing the ear canal with copious amounts of saline whilst the cat was anaesthetized.

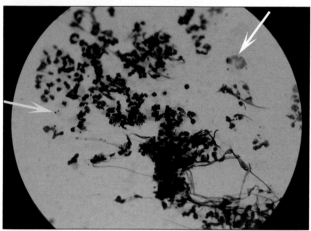

5.15.3 Coccoid bacteria (blue arrow) and degenerate neutrophils (white arrow) can be seen on this ear cytology smear from a cat with bacterial otitis. The coccoid bacteria are not often intracellular but their presence in large numbers indicates a problem. (Diff-Quik; original magnification X1000)

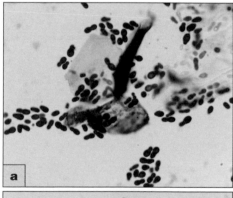
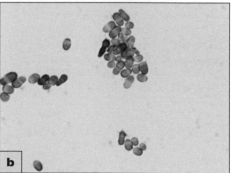

5.15.4 **(a)** These *Malassezia* organisms have a distinctive peanut or snowman shape. **(b)** Cats can also have different types of *Malassezia* from those found in dogs, with some having an oval or round appearance, as shown here. (Diff-Quik; original magnification X1000)

Skin diseases that affect the pinna can also present with head shaking and ear scratching; these include parasitic infestations, such as *Neotrombicula autumnalis*, and immune-mediated diseases, such as pemphigus foliaceus (which may cause pustules or crusting on the ear pinnae). Cats affected by immune-mediated diseases will often have other signs of skin disease in other areas of the body such as the face and feet (see *BSAVA Manual of Canine and Feline Dermatology*).

Diagnostic approach

A logical approach is required to determine the underlying cause (Figure 5.15.5).

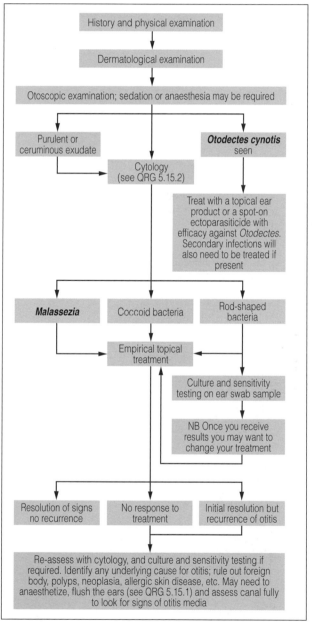

5.15.5 An approach to investigating otitis in cats that do not have neurological signs; for investigation of vestibular disease see Chapter 5.16.

History and general examination

Signalment can be helpful, as parasitic infestations such as *Otodectes* are more commonly seen in young cats. Purulent otitis in an older cat raises suspicion of an immune-mediated disease or a tumour in the external ear canal. If the cat has a chronic history of otitis, screening tests for retroviruses (see Chapter 19) should always be performed.

The cat should be examined for signs of neurological disease, such as head tilt (see Chapter 5.16), ataxia (see Chapter 5.6) or Horner's syndrome (miosis, enophthalmos, protrusion of the third eyelid, ptosis), which may be present with otitis media.

Dermatological examination

The skin should be examined over the whole of the cat, as this may give clues to the underlying cause, especially if allergic skin disease is suspected. The pinnae are examined carefully for signs of skin disease, such as crusting, ulcerations and alopecia. Sometimes harvest mites (*Neotrombicula autumnalis*) may be seen, especially in Henry's pocket (Figure 5.15.6).

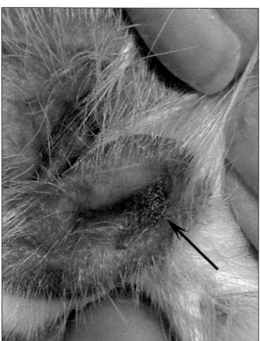

5.15.6 *Neotrombicula autumnalis* mites may be found in Henry's pocket at the base of the ear. The six-legged larvae cause a seasonal pruritic and papular dermatitis in cats. Mites can be seen from July to October in the UK. They are commonly found on the pinna, interdigital skin and face, and are easily seen with the naked eye as bright red-orange dots, which are tightly adherent to the skin, usually in clusters (black arrow). Treatment requires killing the mites and providing anti-inflammatory treatment if appropriate. Fipronil spray can be applied directly to affected areas and is usually effective at controlling the mites.

Otoscopy

Otoscopy must be performed carefully. If only one ear appears to be affected, the healthy ear should always be examined first. It may be necessary to sedate or anesthetize the cat if ear examination is too painful to be performed in the conscious patient.

The ear canal is assessed for patency or stenosis, proliferative changes, ulceration, exudate, foreign bodies, parasites, polyps (see Figure 5.15.2) and tumours. Tumours commonly seen in cats include ceruminal gland adenoma or adenocarcinoma and squamous cell carcinoma.

It is more common with otitis in cats to see a ceruminous otitis, with a black/brown discharge, than a purulent otitis. Flushing the ear (see QRG 5.15.1) may be appropriate in some cases if there is a concern about underlying tumours or polyps but the ear canal cannot be assessed fully due to the presence of purulent exudate. *Note, however, that samples for cytology should always be collected prior to flushing.*

Ear cytology and culture

This should be performed in all cases of otitis. (The technique is described in QRG 5.15.2.) Samples should be collected prior to using any form of ear treatment/flushing to give the most representative results. Cytology provides rapid results regarding the numbers and types of microorganisms and inflammatory cells that may be present. It also provides an accurate way to follow up cases of otitis and monitor response to treatment. Culture and sensitivity testing of swab samples should be performed when rods are seen on cytology, or when the cat is not responding to appropriate treatment and there are concerns regarding a resistant organism.

Treatment

Topical treatments can be chosen empirically, based on cytological findings, whilst awaiting sensitivity results (Figure 5.15.7). It is important to note that all authorized topical ear treatments are polypharmacy products containing an antibiotic, a steroid and an antifungal agent. It is also important to note that not all topical ear preparations are authorized for use in cats, and owners should be made aware of this.

Organisms seen on cytology	Organisms likely to be present	Topical treatment containing the following active ingredients is suggested
Coccoid-shaped bacteria	*Staphylococcus pseudintermedius, Streptococcus*	Fusidic acid, polymixin B, marbofloxacin [a], orbifloxacin [a], gentamicin [a] *Fluoroquinolones and gentamicin should be reserved for resistant infections as a second line treatment*
Rod-shaped bacteria	*Escherichia coli, Pseudomonas, Proteus*	Marbofloxacin [a], orbifloxacin [a], gentamicin [a], framycetin, polymixin B
Malassezia	*Malassezia pachydermatis*, lipid-dependent *Malassezia* species	Miconazole, clotrimazole [a], posaconazole [a], nystatin

5.15.7 Topical treatments for otitis externa in the cat. [a] There are no products authorized for use in cats containing these active ingredients.

If *Otodectes* infestation has been diagnosed, a topical treatment authorized specifically for killing *Otodectes* mites should be used. Topical ectoparasite treatments containing moxidectin and selamectin are used most frequently, as they are easier for clients to administer. It is important when using topical preparations in the ear that treatment is continued for long enough to kill *all* stages in the *Otodectes* life cycle; often this is a 3-week course of treatment.

Systemic treatment with prednisolone at an anti-inflammatory dose (1–2 mg/kg orally q24h) should be considered if the ear canal is very stenosed and inflamed.

WARNING

If the patient has neurological signs, or the tympanic membrane is known to be ruptured, do NOT use topical treatment but opt for systemic antibiotic treatment instead. If referral of the case is being considered, the referral centre should be contacted prior to starting such treatment.

When to refer

If patients have neurological signs and otitis media, referral should be considered as they may need advanced imaging and/or surgical intervention.

What to do if finances are limited

In-house cytology will enable the choice of appropriate treatment and monitoring without large financial outlays on submissions to external laboratories for culture. Topical treatment is generally more effective than systemic treatment, but should only be used if the patient does not have neurological signs or a ruptured tympanic membrane.

QRG 5.15.1 Ear flushing
by Natalie Barnard

If an ear canal is full of a purulent or ceruminous exudate, it is not possible to assess the integrity of the tympanic membrane. Flushing the ear canal can be beneficial to allow better visualization.
NOTE: Samples for cytology must be collected prior to flushing.

WARNING

- Ear flushing should only be performed under general anaesthesia.
- Clients must be warned that performing an ear flush could potentially cause temporary vestibular signs and temporary loss of hearing.

Equipment

- 500 ml bag of sterile saline
- Otoscope with two suitably sized heads
- Syringes: 2 ml, 5 ml
- Catheter of appropriate size depending on the patency of the ear canal; cat or dog urinary catheters can be used. The author prefers to use 6 Fr dog catheters if the ear canal is patent. If the ear canal is very narrow, a cat catheter may need to be used; the size will vary from patient to patient, depending on the severity of stenosis. The catheter should be cut to an appropriate length (around 4–5 cm) to make it more manageable.
- Two bowls: one 'clean' for the fresh saline; and one 'dirty' in which to place the fluid flushed from the affected ear

Technique

It is important that flushing of the ear is carried out whilst visualizing the ear canal, so that no damage is caused to any structures in the ear.

1 Examine the affected ear with an otoscope. Take a sample for ear cytology (see QRG 5.15.2) if not already done, and a sample for culture if required.

2 Take a clean 5 ml syringe and attach it to an appropriately sized urinary catheter cut to the right length for the patient. Draw up 1–2 ml of saline into the syringe.

3 Introduce the otoscope into the external ear canal. Once you are able to see as far as possible into the ear, move the lens on the otoscope out of the way to enable a catheter to be introduced through the otoscope head.

4 Whilst holding the otoscope and pinna in one hand, introduce the catheter into the affected ear and position the tip of the catheter as far as you can see it into the ear.

WARNING

- Be careful not to damage the tympanic membrane.
- Never stab blindly into the ear canal.

---

5 Introduce the saline slowly, whilst looking down the ear canal. You will see the saline fill the ear canal, and some of the saline will flood into the otoscope head and obscure your view. Before the saline reaches the top of the otoscope head, suck it back using the syringe and discard this in the 'dirty' bowl. This procedure is repeated many times until the fluid removed is clear.

PRACTICAL TIPS

- You will not be able to remove all the fluid introduced, but you should be able to remove most of it.
- Do not leave large quantities of saline in the affected ear.
- It generally takes 20–30 minutes to flush an ear.

---

6 You should now be able to visualize the external ear canal and hopefully the tympanic membrane.

- If the ear canal is clean and you can't see the tympanic membrane, but can see a black hole, it is likely that the tympanic membrane has ruptured and the cat has a middle ear infection. If the tympanic membrane is ruptured, choose appropriate systemic antibiotic treatment based on cytology findings, pending culture results if a sample has been sent.
- If you can see tissue at the base of the ear canal, a mass or polyp should be suspected (see Figure 5.15.2).

QRG 5.15.2 Ear cytology
by Natalie Barnard

Cytology should be performed in all cases of otitis and should be considered part of the minimum database required. **NOTE: Samples for cytology must be collected prior to flushing or applying any topical treatment.**

Equipment

- Glass slides
- Cotton buds/swabs
- Pencil
- Diff-Quik stain
- Microscope
- Immersion oil

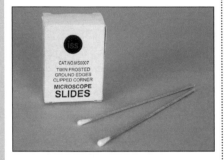

Sample collection

It is possible to collect a sample for cytology from most patients with ear disease. The process should be performed carefully to avoid damaging the patient's ear or causing further pain or discomfort. Samples should be collected prior to using any form of ear treatment/flushing to give the most representative results.

1 Place a cotton bud or swab into the affected ear to obtain a sample. In conscious patients aim for the junction of the vertical and horizontal canals. If the patient is uncomfortable, you may wish to take the sample using a swab that could then be sent on for culture if deemed necessary after looking at the cytology.

2 Remove the cotton bud/swab from the ear and gently roll it along the middle of a glass slide. Make a couple of rows to examine.

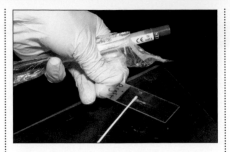

3 Stain with Diff-Quik once the sample is completely dry: 5 x 1-second dips in each of the three stains (blue, then red, then purple).

4 Rinse with water (tap water is fine), then gently blot the slide with a paper towel or leave it to air-dry.

PRACTICAL TIPS

- As the specimen has been fixed on to the slide, you will not remove the sample from the slide unless you rub the area hard.
- The slide might not look as if it has stained, but still examine it as material is likely to be present; most smears do not appear to be well stained to the naked eye, as they comprise waxy ear infections that only involve yeast.
- Generally slides will only look purple with heavy staining if there is a lot of pus on the slide.

5 Once dry, examine the slide using the microscope (see QRG 5.26.3). First find an area of interest using low-power (X4) objective; then progress through higher magnifications to using the oil immersion lens.

Examination

Look for bacteria, yeast and inflammatory cells, similar to looking at a tape strip sample.

- If you see coccoid bacteria, these are likely to be *Staphylococcus*. Such infections usually respond well to the antibiotics included in most ear treatments prescribed (e.g. fucidic acid in CanAural). If it is the first occurrence of an ear infection, there is no need to send a swab for culture and sensitivity testing. The exception to this is when the infection persists for >2 weeks or does not respond to treatment.
- If you see rod-shaped bacteria, a swab should always be submitted for culture and sensitivity testing because this may indicate a *Pseudomonas* infection and these can be more challenging to treat. They do not always respond well to routine prescribed treatment.
- When *Malassezia* is seen there is no need to send a swab for culture and sensitivity testing as it will not give you any additional information with regard to treatment.

Cerumen (wax) smear

A cerumen smear allows examination of waxy exudate for parasites such as *Otodectes*.

1 Use a cotton bud to collect some wax (enough to cover the head of a cotton bud) from the external ear canal and place this on a glass slide with some liquid paraffin.

2 Place a coverslip on top of the sample.

3 Examine using the low-power (X4) objective lens.

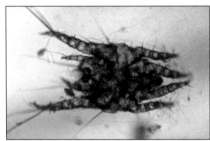

Otodectes mite from a cerumen smear. (Courtesy of University of Bristol Veterinary School)

Head tilt

Laurent Garosi

Head tilt is characterized by a rotation of the median plane of the head along the axis of the body, resulting in one ear being held lower than the other.

A head tilt often indicates a vestibular disorder (peripheral or central) and occurs as a result of the loss of antigravity muscle tone on one side of the neck. In addition to head tilt, other vestibular signs such as abnormal nystagmus, positional strabismus, falling, rolling, leaning, circling and ataxia are commonly associated. A head tilt alone may also be observed with otitis externa (Figure 5.16.1) or other causes of aural irritation.

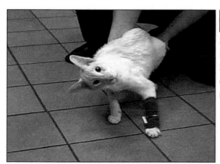

5.16.1
Severe right-sided head tilt in a Siamese cat caused by otitis media/interna.

Head tilt must be differentiated from a head turn:

- Compared to a head tilt, in a head turn the median plane of the head remains perpendicular to the ground but the nose is turned to one side
- A head turn is often associated with a body turn (pleurothotonus) and circling, and does not indicate a vestibular disorder but is indicative of a forebrain lesion, with the head turned towards the same side as the lesion.

Diagnostic approach

A cat presenting with a head tilt and other vestibular signs must have the lesion localized to either the peripheral (receptor organs in the inner ear or the vestibular portion of cranial nerve (CN) VIII) or the central (the brainstem vestibular nuclei or vestibular centres in the cerebellum) vestibular apparatus, before an appropriate differential diagnosis can be established and further testing conducted (Figure 5.16.2).

Disease mechanism	Peripheral vestibular disease	Central vestibular disease
Vascular	None	Brain infarct; brain haemorrhage
Inflammatory/ Infectious	**Otitis media/interna; nasopharyngeal polyps**	Infectious encephalitis (*Toxoplasma*, Bacterial, *Cryptococcus*, **FIP**); meningoencephalitis of unknown aetiology (presumed immune-mediated)
Trauma	**Head trauma**	**Head trauma**
Toxic	Aminoglycosides; topical otic chlorhexidine or iodophors (e.g. povidone–iodine); loop diuretics (e.g. furosemide)	Metronidazole
Anomalous	Congenital vestibular disease (infrequent but reported in Siamese, Burmese and Tonkinese)	Intracranial intra-arachnoid cyst; dermoid/epidermoid cyst
Metabolic	N/A	N/A
Idiopathic	**Acute idiopathic peripheral vestibular disease**	N/A
Neoplastic	**Middle and/or inner ear tumour**	**Primary or metastatic brain tumour**
Nutritional	N/A	Thiamine deficiency
Degenerative	N/A	Neurodegenerative disease

5.16.2 Causes of peripheral and central vestibular disease. FIP = feline infectious peritonitis; N/A = not applicable. Common causes of vestibular disease in cats are highlighted in bold.

Most lesions causing vestibular disorder affect a region, rather than a specific nerve or nucleus, so accompanying neurological abnormalities can often be used to localize the lesion to the peripheral or central vestibular system. Correctly identifying central vestibular disease requires identification of clinical signs that cannot be attributed to diseases of the peripheral vestibular system (see Figure 5.16.3 and Chapter 5.6); however, even if such signs are not present a central lesion cannot be excluded. Occasionally, intracranial vestibular lesions can result initially in signs indicative of a peripheral lesion. This is most commonly seen with extra-axial masses that compress CN VIII (vestibulocochlear) as it exits the brainstem or lesions that involve solely the vestibular nuclei.

Identification of ear disease, facial nerve paralysis (absent menace response, absent palpebral reflexes and/or asymmetry of facial muscles) and/or Horner's syndrome (miosis, enophthalmia, protrusion of the third eyelid, ptosis of the upper eyelid) is suggestive of peripheral vestibular disease due to the proximity of CN VII (facial nerve) and the ocular sympathetic nerve supply with CN VIII (vestibular nerve) in the region of the petrous temporal bone.

If in doubt about the localization of the lesion, the clinician should investigate the animal for central vestibular disease as well as peripheral vestibular disease (see also Chapter 5.6). Conversely, animals with acute severe peripheral vestibular disease may be so incapacitated that accurate interpretation of neurological examination findings may not be possible.

With both central and peripheral vestibular disease, the head tilt typically occurs ipsilateral to the side of the lesion. Less frequently, lesions affecting the caudal cerebellar peduncle, the fastigial nucleus and or the flocculonodular lobes of the cerebellum can cause central vestibular disease, resulting in a *paradoxical* head tilt, i.e. the head tilt occurs contralateral to the central lesion but the loss of balance and postural reaction deficits occur ipsilateral to the central lesion. There is usually also some evidence of a cerebellar disorder on neurological examination, such as a cerebellar ataxia (e.g. ipsilateral hypermetria) or a truncal sway.

The diagnostic approach is summarized in Figure 5.16.3.

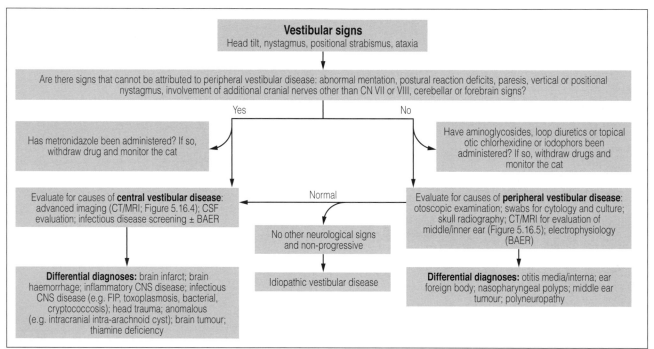

5.16.3 General diagnostic approach to head tilt and vestibular signs. BAER = brainstem auditory evoked response.

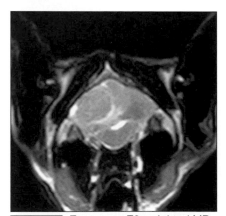

5.16.4 Transverse T2-weighted MR image of a cat with right-sided loss of balance and postural reaction deficit and left-sided paradoxical head tilt caused by a meningioma. Note the severe compression on the right side of the cerebellum and brainstem.

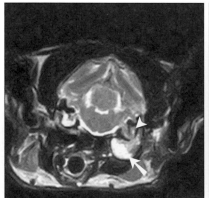 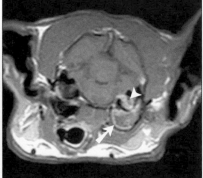

5.16.5 Transverse T2-weighted and T1-weighted contrast-enhanced MR images of a cat with left-sided otitis media/interna causing left-sided head tilt, facial nerve paralysis and Horner's syndrome. On T2-weighted images, the left bulla contains tissue that is mostly hyperintense to neural tissue (arrow). The signal from the perilymph in the left inner ear (arrowhead) is reduced compared to the normal right inner ear. The contrast-enhanced image shows marked enhancement of the periphery of the left bulla (arrow) and left inner ear (arrowhead).

Heart murmur

Kerry Simpson

> A heart murmur is caused by turbulent blood flow within the heart or the large vessels exiting the heart.

Heart murmurs are **graded** according to the criteria shown in Figure 5.17.1.

Murmur grade	Description
I	Audible in a localized area, only after prolonged listening with a stethoscope
II	Immediately audible; not as loud as the heart sounds
III	Immediately audible; of equal intensity to the heart sounds
IV	Immediately audible; louder than the heart sounds; no precordial thrill (palpable vibration evident over the heart)
V	Easily audible and associated with a precordial thrill; audible only when the stethoscope is held against the thoracic wall
VI	Easily audible with a precordial thrill; can be auscultated with the stethoscope lifted off the thoracic wall

5.17.1 Grading heart murmurs.

When assessing a murmur in a cat it is important to note whether it is **systolic or diastolic**. Diastolic murmurs are rare and are generally associated with severe or congenital heart disease. For example, the murmur associated with aortic regurgitation is diastolic, whereas the classic patent ductus arteriosus murmur has both a systolic and a diastolic component.

The **origin of the murmur** should also be noted. The majority of murmurs in cats are parasternal in origin, and therefore the clinician should be careful to include this area in their examination (see QRG 1.5).

Causes of heart murmurs

Many conditions can result in a heart murmur, including:

- Congenital heart disease (e.g. ventricular septal defect)
- Primary cardiomyopathy (e.g. hypertrophic cardiomyopathy (HCM))
- Secondary cardiomyopathies (e.g. thyrotoxic cardiomyopathy, hypertension)
- Anaemia
- Myocarditis/endomyocarditis – rare
- Infiltrative disease (e.g. lymphoma) – rare
- Heartworm disease.

Low-grade (I–II) systolic murmurs in clinically healthy cats are usually due to mild cardiac disease, most often HCM. As there is currently no evidence that early treatment of cardiac disease (i.e. prior to the onset of congestive heart failure (CHF)) is beneficial in such cases, the decision as to whether to investigate the cause of a murmur in a clinically healthy cat is problematical. Investigation is recommended if the cat: is very young, and congenital disease is suspected (e.g. noted at first presentation); is to be used for breeding; is to undergo anaesthesia; or needs high volumes of intravenous fluids. In other cases, or if the murmur is dynamic (i.e. present at high heart rates such as stress-induced tachycardia (heart rate >180 beats/min) but resolves when heart rate reduces), investigations may be of little benefit except in providing a baseline for that individual, thereby allowing disease progression to be monitored over time.

Clinical signs

If the cat is symptomatic, signs may include any of the following:

- Dyspnoea
- Lethargy
- Inappetence/anorexia
- Vomiting
- Ascites
- Oedema
- Cachexia
- Syncope
- Limb paralysis/paresis
- Collapse
- Cough (very rarely associated with cardiac disease)
- Cyanosis.

Assessing significance

The grade of a heart murmur does not necessarily correlate with the degree of severity of the heart problem, nor does the absence of a murmur rule out significant heart disease. Indeed, it has been demonstrated that 30–43% of cats presenting with aortic thromboembolism (ATE) do not have *any* auscultable cardiac abnormalities, and most of these cats show acute limb signs as the first indication of cardiac disease.

Cats with clinical signs that could be attributed to cardiac disease should ideally be assessed with echocardiography to rule out cardiac causes (see Chapter 9).

When a murmur is auscultated, the significance of that murmur needs to be considered. Between 15.5 and 44% of apparently healthy cats have murmurs on auscultation, either at rest or upon provocation (i.e. by raising the heart rate). However, when apparently healthy cats with murmurs are assessed, 22–88% have cardiomyopathy or congenital heart disease, and dynamic outflow tract obstruction (turbulence within either the right or left ventricular outflow tract, typically associated with a localized area of hypertrophy on the basal interventricular septum) is found in a proportion of the remaining cases. In studies there has always been a small proportion of cats with heart murmurs in which no underlying cause could be elucidated on echocardiography. With such a high incidence of murmurs in apparently healthy cats the relevance of a low-grade murmur can be hard to assess (see below).

Auscultation may reveal a gallop (audible S3 or S4) or arrhythmia in addition to the murmur; both of which are usually associated with significant cardiac disease, although non-cardiac causes exist, and it is recommended that these cases are investigated.

Diagnostic approach

In cats with clinical signs associated with cardiac disease, gallop sounds or arrhythmia, investigations are always recommended. Full evaluation should be performed when the cat is stable, i.e. pleural effusion has been drained, and/or diuretics administered. In cats with low-grade murmurs, the circumstances of the individual patient should be considered and options discussed with the owner; any breeding cat with a murmur should be assessed. Whilst echocardiography is required to assess chamber size, wall thickness and blood flow velocities, the clinician should also assess the cat for secondary causes, such as hypertension, hyperthyroidism, infection and arrhythmias (Figure 5.17.2). In addition, testing for pro-brain natriuretic peptide (pro-BNP) and troponin I (TnI) may be of use in cats with clinical signs suggestive of CHF, but where echocardiography is not available. Elevated values may be consistent with cardiac disease (especially arrhythmia or congestive heart failure), but as yet the effect of other diseases on these values has not been fully elucidated, and therefore, both false negative and false positive results can occur.

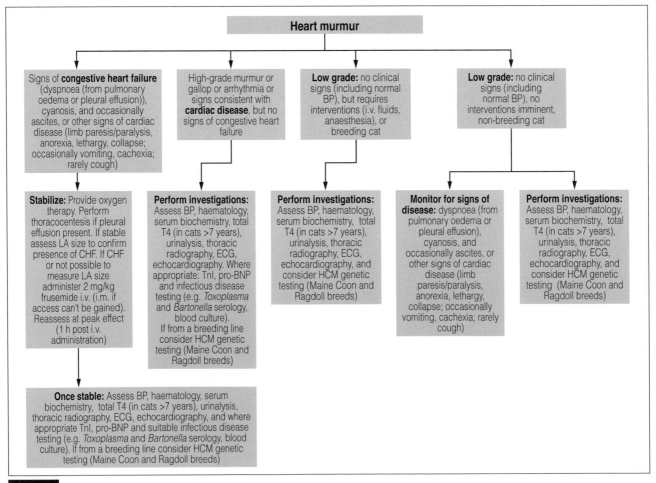

5.17.2 Diagnostic approach to heart murmur. BP = blood pressure; LA = left atrium.

Pedigree cats

HCM is known to result from genetic mutations in some breeds of cat. There is a familial incidence reported in many breeds, including:

- Maine Coon*
- Ragdoll*
- Turkish Van
- Cornish Rex
- British Shorthair
- Sphinx
- Siberian

- Persian
- Devon Rex
- Norwegian Forest Cat
- Scottish Fold
- Bengal
- American Shorthair

* Genetic mutation identified

Genetic tests are currently available for the known existing mutations in the Maine Coon and Ragdoll breeds. However, it is known that cats that are negative on genetic testing can still develop HCM, presumably due to further, as yet unidentified, mutations. Additionally cats that are positive on genetic testing may not necessarily develop HCM; a positive result is regarded as being a risk factor for HCM rather than an indication that disease will definitely occur. As it is recognized that cats with cardiac disease may not have any auscultable abnormalities, some recommend that all breeding cats from breeds with a familial predisposition to HCM are assessed regulary (annually if possible) by echocardiography.

Further reading

Drourr LT, Gordon SG, Roland RM and Boggess M (2010) Prevalence of heart murmurs and occult heart disease in apparently healthy adult cats. *Proceedings, American College of Veterinary Internal Medicine*, p.159

Nakamura RK, Rishniw M, King MK and Sammarco CD (2011) Prevalence of echocardiographic evidence of cardiac disease in apparently healthy cats with murmurs. *Journal of Feline Medicine and Surgery* **13**, 266–271

Wagner T, Luis Fuentes V, Payne JR, McDermott N and Brodbelt D (2010) Comparison of auscultatory and echocardiographic findings in healthy adult cats. *Journal of Veterinary Cardiology* **12**, 171–182

Hypertension

Sarah Caney

Systemic hypertension – a persistent increase in the systemic blood pressure – is now commonly recognized in feline practice. There are several reasons for this, including: an increased awareness of hypertension as a feline problem; increased access to diagnostic facilities; and, possibly, an increased prevalence of this condition related to the increasing average age of the cat population.

Idiopathic hypertension (also referred to as primary or essential hypertension) accounts for <20% of cases; most reported cases occur secondary to other medical problems. The most common secondary causes of hypertension are chronic kidney disease (CKD) and hyperthyroidism. Prevalence rates quoted have been highly variable: e.g. from 20% to 65% of CKD cats; from 9% to 23% of newly diagnosed hyperthyroid cats. Other diseases that have been associated with hypertension in cats include primary hyperaldosteronism (Conn's syndrome; see Chapter 4.6), chronic anaemia, phaeochromocytoma and erythropoietin therapy. A link between systemic hypertension and other feline endocrinopathies, such as diabetes mellitus, acromegaly and hyperadrenocorticism, has not yet been demonstrated. Most of the diseases commonly associated with hypertension are seen in older (senior and geriatric) cats; this explains why most hypertensive disease is seen in this group.

Clinical findings

Unfortunately, hypertension is often only suspected very late in the course of disease – typically once end organ damage (EOD) (also know as target organ damage) has occurred. The target organs most vulnerable to hypertensive damage are the brain, heart, kidneys and eyes; Figure 5.18.1 summarizes the typical changes seen.

Cats with systemic hypertension may be presented with signs referable to their underlying systemic disease, such as inappetence and weight loss in the CKD patient.

Organ affected	Pathology	Clinical findings	Reported approximate prevalence
Brain	Hyperplastic arteriosclerosis of cerebral vessels, oedema of the white matter, and microhaemorrhage development, resulting in hypertensive encephalopathy ± stroke	Many changes possible including behavioural (e.g. night vocalization, signs of dementia), ataxia, seizures, coma	15%
Heart	Left ventricular hypertrophy, cardiac failure (rare)	New murmur and/or gallop rhythm. Signs of congestive heart failure (rare)	50–80%
Kidneys	Glomerular hypertrophy and sclerosis, nephrosclerosis, tubular atrophy and interstitial nephritis, resulting in progression of CKD	Reduced urine specific gravity, increasing creatinine levels, proteinuria	Not known
Eyes	Hypertensive retinopathy/choroidopathy resulting in many changes, including intraocular haemorrhage (see Chapter 5.19), retinal oedema, retinal detachment (Figure 5.18.2), arterial tortuosity, variable diameter of retinal arterioles (Figure 5.18.3), papilloedema and glaucoma. Foci of retinal degeneration (hyper-reflectivity) may develop where damage has previously occurred	Visual deficits, blindness, mydriasis (Figure 5.18.4)	60–80%

5.18.1 End organ damage seen with systemic hypertension.

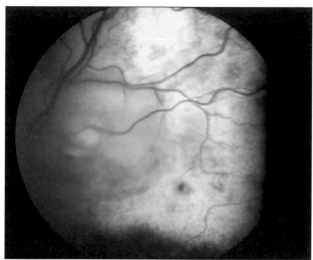

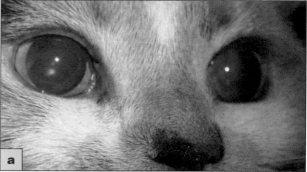

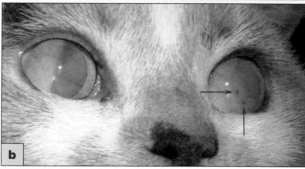

5.18.2 Fundus image showing early evidence of hypertensive damage. The main visible abnormality is a green circular area (from around 7 to 10 o'clock) representing a large serous bullous retinal detachment. Retinal vessels over this area can be clearly seen, although they are out of focus (indicating a serous effusion). Many smaller green/grey circular and oval areas indicative of retinal oedema and focal detachments are visible on the remainder of the retina. Oedema can be a prelude to retinal detachment. Both eyes had similar changes, and pupil size and pupillary light responses were normal. At this relatively early stage vision did not appear to be affected. (Courtesy of Sheila Crispin.)

5.18.4 Mydriasis. Dilation of the pupils is one potential indication of blindness associated with bilateral retinal detachment as a consequence of systemic hypertension. **(a)** Under normal consulting room light conditions, both pupils appear abnormally large. **(b)** When the room is darkened and a bright light is shone into the cat's eyes, there is a complete absence of both direct (constriction of the stimulated pupil) and consensual (constriction of the contralateral pupil) pupillary light response (PLR; see QRG 1.3) and both pupils remain the same size as before. Using a bright light source (a Finhoff transilluminator attached to an otoscope/ophthalmoscope handle in this case), the retina can be clearly seen in both eyes as a grey membrane containing blood vessels. Small retinal haemorrhages are visible billowing forwards within the vitreous in the left eye (red arrows). The retina usually remains attached around the optic nerve head and at the periphery, which is why it has the bulging appearance with folds as seen in the right eye. This retinal appearance is an abnormal finding, indicating bilateral serous retinal detachment. Unfortunately the blindness was permanent in this cat.

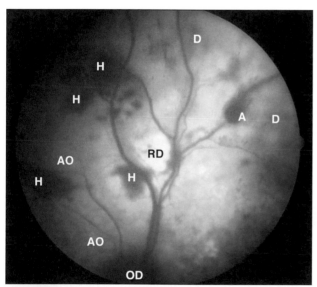

5.18.3 Fundus image showing significant evidence of hypertensive damage. Many abnormalities are present. There is widespread attenuation of the retinal arterioles, and arteriolar occlusion (AO) is apparent in a number of them. An aneurysm (A) is visible in a retinal arteriole. This swollen portion of arteriole is vulnerable to rupture, leading to intraocular haemorrhage. Multiple areas of retinal haemorrhage (H) are visible over the entire retina. In the centre of the image the retina appears bright and hyper-reflective, consistent with retinal degeneration (RD), which can occur as a consequence of any ocular pathology. Dorsal to this region there is retinal detachment (D) because of exudation (serous detachment). Part of the optic disc (OD) is visible at the bottom of the photograph; its definition is poor because of peripapillary and papillary oedema. Both eyes were similarly affected; the pupils were moderately dilated, the pupillary light response sluggish and incomplete, and vision was compromised. (Courtesy of Sheila Crispin.)

Diagnosis

Blood pressure should be evaluated as a routine part of check-ups of all cats of 7 years of age or older (see Chapter 2), and in younger cats if there is any reason to suspect they may be vulnerable to developing hypertension. Blood pressure should be assessed in cats presented with:

- Visual deficits
- Ocular disease – particularly where findings are consistent with hypertension
- Any disease reported to have an association with hypertension – particularly CKD and hyperthyroidism
  - 3- to 6-monthly blood pressure assessment is recommended in order to detect an increase in blood pressure prior to development of EOD
- Unexplained proteinuria
- Hypokalaemia (would increase suspicion for primary hyperaldosteronism)

- Auscultable cardiac abnormalities consistent with systemic hypertension (murmur, gallop; see QRG 1.5)
- Left ventricular hypertrophy
- Behavioural or neurological signs (especially older cats).

Ideally, diagnostic evaluation should include systolic (SBP) and diastolic (DBP) blood pressure measurement. As yet, however, there is little information on diastolic hypertension in cats and DBP is difficult to measure accurately. In humans diastolic hypertension is known to be an important cause of vascular damage. A detailed ophthalmic examination is essential in both the diagnosis and the assessment of the extent of ocular disease (see QRG 1.3).

Blood pressure measurement

This author recommends Doppler measurement of blood pressure (see QRG 5.18.1) since oscillometric techniques have been shown to be unreliable in conscious cats. Oscillometric machines fail to give a reading in a proportion of conscious cats and tend to overestimate low blood pressure and underestimate high blood pressure. High-definition oscillometry (HDO) machines are a newer version of the traditional oscillometric machines which allow real-time analysis of the oscillometric curve on a computer. Seeing the curve may allow artefacts to be identified but HDO devices have not yet been shown to be consistently accurate in determining SBP.

A number of different 'reference ranges' have been published for normal cats, citing normal SBP readings from 107 to 181 mmHg in healthy cats. When it is possible to measure it, the DBP of normal cats should be <95 mmHg. 'White coat' hypertension or stress-induced increases in the SBP are a significant issue when interpreting blood pressure results in cats. On average, the 'white coat' effect increases SBP by 15–20 mmHg. However, the effect is highly variable between cats and the increase can be as much as 75 mmHg.

Interpretation of SBP results

The American College of Veterinary Internal Medicine has published a classification system according to risk of target/end organ damage (Figure 5.18.5).

Risk category	Systolic BP (mmHg)	Diastolic BP (mmHg)	Risk of future EOD
I	<150	<95	Minimal
II	150–159	95–99	Mild
III	160–179	100–119	Moderate
IV	≥180	≥120	Severe

5.18.5 Classification of blood pressure in cats based on the risk of future EOD.

SBP ≥180 mmHg: severe risk of EOD

In general, cats with SBP ≥180 mmHg are genuinely hypertensive and therapy is justified. However, some healthy cats may *transiently* have SBP ≥180 mmHg. Hypertension should therefore *never* be treated solely on the basis of a single abnormal blood pressure reading. If evidence of EOD is present, the diagnosis of hypertension is confirmed and treatment can be

instituted. In the absence of EOD it is prudent to re-check the SBP on another occasion before pursuing treatment.

The author recommends the following steps are taken in cats with SBP readings ≥180 mmHg:

- Ensure that measurements are taken correctly (see QRG 5.18.1), allowing at least 5–10 minutes for acclimatization before readings are taken
- Perform a clinical and ocular examination: if there is evidence of EOD, the diagnosis of systemic hypertension has been confirmed
- If there is no evidence of EOD: repeat measurements on one or two separate occasions within 1–2 weeks (although if SBP is very high (230–250 mmHg) repeat SBP measurement and assessment for EOD should be performed within a day or two). If readings remain high, antihypertensive treatment is justified. Further investigations aimed at finding secondary causes of hypertension should be pursued.

SBP 160–179 mmHg: moderate risk of EOD

SBP readings that are persistently between 160 and 179 mmHg are believed to pose a moderate risk of EOD. Persistence is defined as being present on several occasions over a 2-month period. If there is evidence of EOD (e.g. hypertensive retinopathy) or if the cat is known to have CKD or any other condition known to be associated with hypertension, then antihypertensive therapy is justified. In the absence of either of these, it might not be possible to rule out 'white coat' hypertension, and further monitoring might therefore be more appropriate.

SBP 150–159 mmHg: mild risk of EOD

Cats in this group may have mild hypertension, but many normal cats will also give blood pressure readings in this range due to the 'white coat' effect. Treatment is not normally recommended unless there is evidence of EOD. For those cats with conditions known to predispose to hypertension, 1–3-monthly monitoring of blood pressure and evaluation for evidence of EOD is recommended once readings >150 mmHg are obtained.

SBP <150 mmHg

Most normal cats have SBP readings between 120 and 149 mmHg. This should be viewed as the ideal 'target range' following treatment for hypertension.

Management

The goals of management are to:

- Identify and treat potential underlying causes of the hypertension
- Identify EOD and characterize severity
- Reduce SBP to an 'ideal' reference range: 120–149 mmHg.

In any hypertensive cat, investigations for secondary causes should include serum thyroxine (T4), blood urea and creatinine, and urinalysis (including specific gravity, urine protein:creatinine ratio, and bacterial culture).

Additional diagnostic tests which may be considered include:

- More thorough laboratory evaluation, e.g. looking for hypokalaemia (common in cases of primary hyperaldosteronism, also present in around 20–25% cases of CKD)
- Abdominal ultrasonography, e.g. looking for an adrenal mass(es) (common in cases of primary hyperaldosteronism)
- Endocrine assays, e.g. serum aldosterone (elevated in cases of primary hyperaldosteronism), free T4 and cTSH. Elevated free T4 in combination with undetectable levels of canine TSH is consistent with hyperthyroidism, especially if the total T4 is ≥30 nmol/l.
- Where possible, echocardiography may be helpful. A degree of left ventricular hypertrophy is a common echocardiographic finding in hypertensive cats and generally does not require specific treatment.

Irrespective of the nature of the underlying disease, specific management with antihypertensive agents is required (see QRG 5.18.2), at least in the short term.

Prognosis

The long-term prognosis is very dependent on the presence, nature and extent of any underlying disease. In primary hypertensive cases it is usually possible to manage the hypertension and prevent future complications such as ocular haemorrhage.

Further reading

Brown S, Atkins C, Bagley R *et al.* (2007) Guidelines for the identification, evaluation and management of systemic hypertension in dogs and cats. *Journal of Veterinary Internal Medicine* **21**, 542–558

Caney SMA (2008) *Doppler Blood Pressure Measurement in Conscious Cats: A Guide for Veterinary Professionals.* [Available for download at www.catprofessional.com]

Caney SMA (2008) *Ocular Manifestations of Systemic Hypertension.* [Available for download at www.catprofessional.com]

QRG 5.18.1 Measuring blood pressure
by Sarah Caney

PRACTICAL TIPS

- Be patient; allow a minimum of 20 minutes for the procedure.
- Ask the owner, if appropriate, or a nurse to hold the cat gently with the minimum restraint possible (see QRG 1.2). The cat should feel comfortable.
- The animal should be positioned in such a way that the cuff is at the level of the right atrium.
- Use plenty of gel!
- Make sure that your equipment is well maintained: any cuffs that inflate unevenly or need securing with tape should be replaced.
- Record who performed the procedure, the equipment used, cuff size and location, and animal attitude and position, as well as the readings obtained. For continuity, the same person should repeat measurements using the same protocol.

Equipment

Choose a Doppler blood pressure monitor. The author recommends that headphones are always used to prevent the cat from hearing noise associated with the procedure.

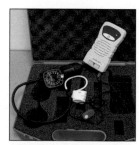

Patient preparation

Choose a suitable venue; a quiet place away from barking dogs, human traffic, telephones, etc., is preferred. The author prefers the owner to remain present and restrain the cat in order to reduce the stress associated with this procedure. Allow the cat to relax and settle for 5–10 minutes before starting the procedure; use this time to unpack your Doppler equipment and collect a history. If blood sampling or other procedures have been performed, allow at least 30 minutes for acclimatization – if at all possible, delay these procedures until after blood pressure measurements have been taken. Restrain the cat appropriately (see QRG 1.2).

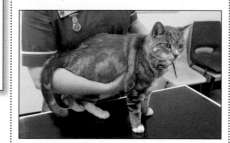

Technique

1 Select a cuff with a width approximating to 30–40% of the limb circumference between the elbow and the carpus. For most cats the ideal cuff width is 2.5 cm. (The tail can also be used for blood pressure readings; see QRG 1.2.) Secure the cuff in place and attach it to a handheld sphygmomanometer.

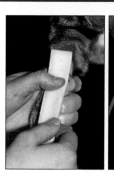

2 Prepare the common digital artery by wiping down the fur between the carpal and metacarpal pads with a surgical spirit-soaked cotton swab.

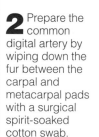
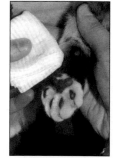

3 Apply a generous 'blob' of ultrasound gel to the prepared area between the carpal and metacarpal pads.

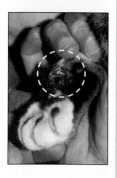

▶

QRG 5.18.1 *continued*

4 Apply gel to the Doppler probe. Make sure that the machine is switched off when this is done!

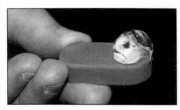

5 Gently place the probe over the prepared area, in line with the limb, and switch on the Doppler machine. Listen carefully for a pulse signal, moving the probe gently until a clear signal can be heard. If no pulse can be heard or if the signal is poor, turn off the machine, remove the probe and add more gel to the cat and the probe before repeating this step.

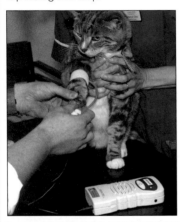

6 Gently inflate the cuff using the sphygmomanometer. Inflate the cuff an additional 10–20 mmHg beyond the point at which the pulse can no longer be heard.

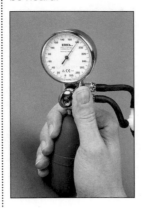

7 Slowly deflate the cuff and listen carefully for a return of the pulse signal. The systolic blood pressure (SBP) reading is the pressure at which the pulse can first be clearly heard.

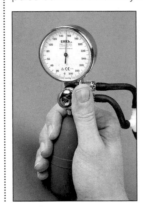

8 Continue deflating the cuff and listen for the diastolic blood pressure (DBP) – the pressure at which the audio signal of the pulse returns to pre-inflation sounds (although this may be hard to hear). Completely deflate the cuff once this reading has been collected.

9 Repeat steps 6–8 to obtain a series of three to seven blood pressure readings. Discard the first reading if it is very different from the others and continue to obtain more readings if a variability of >20% is seen in systolic readings obtained. Calculate the mean SBP and DBP; 120–149 mmHg is the ideal SBP for a cat.

Ocular assessment for hypertension should also be performed. Distant indirect ophthalmoscopy (see QRG 1.3) is an ideal way of visualizing large portions of the retina very quickly. Gross abnormalities can be seen, including retinal oedema and detachment, intraocular haemorrhage and vessel changes.

QRG 5.18.2 Treatment of hypertension
by Sarah Caney

Antihypertensive agents

There is no veterinary authorized treatment available for feline hypertension. A number of different agents have been used; most effective and extremely well tolerated is amlodipine, and this is considered the most appropriate first line treatment by most clinicians.

Response to therapy should ideally be assessed after 7–10 days of treatment by measuring SBP and monitoring end organ damage (EOD). In successfully treated cases, SBP should drop to 120–149 mmHg within 7–10 days of initiating therapy. Post-treatment SBP readings of 150–159 mmHg are acceptable, as long as there is no evidence of continued EOD. Once BP is stable, patients should be assessed every 1–2 months, reducing the frequency to a minimum of once every 3–4 months in very stable patients.

Class of agent	Agent(s) and oral dosage regime	Efficacy	Comments
Calcium channel blockers	Amlodipine 0.625–1.25 mg/cat q12–24h (maximum suggested dose 0.5 mg/kg/day)	High: typically reduces SBP by 30–55 mmHg	Often effective as sole therapy. Benazepril (or other agents) can be added if inadequate effect at the stated doses
ACE inhibitors	Benazepril 0.25–0.5 mg/kg q12–24h Enalapril 0.25–0.5 mg/kg q24h Ramipril 0.125–0.25 mg/kg q24h	Mild to moderate: typically reduce SBP by 10–20 mmHg	Reduce systemic and glomerular BP, hence of benefit in proteinuric cats. May provide additional benefits in cats with CKD (see Chapter 13). Benazepril often ineffective as a sole therapy, especially in marked hypertension (SBP >190 mmHg). In these cases, a combination of benazepril and amlodipine is usually very successful. Ramipril monotherapy has been reported to be successful in 69% of hypertensive cats (Van Israel *et al.*, 2009); there is currently no information on combining ramipril with amlodipine

Antihypertensive agents commonly used in cats.

▶

QRG 5.18.2 *continued*

Follow-up assessments should include:

- Measurement of blood pressure
- Assessment for evidence of EOD
- Periodic blood tests and urinalysis, including creatinine levels and assessment of proteinuria. Once stable, these assessments should be done every 6–12 months, according to the individual patient's needs.

Emergency treatment

Emergency treatment of hypertension may be indicated in some cases; e.g. in cats with very high blood pressure or where there is acute onset of EOD such as retinal detachment. In most of these cases, oral amlodipine is effective in safely but rapidly lowering blood pressure within 24 hours, but other options for emergency treatment are shown in the table below. Sodium restriction is not specifically recommended but high-salt diets should be avoided.

Reference

Van Israel N, Desmoulins PO, Huyghe B, Burgaud S and Horspool LJI (2009) Ramipril as a first line monotherapy for the control of feline hypertension and associated clinical signs. *Journal of Veterinary Internal Medicine* **23,**1331–1332 [abstract]

Agent	Dosage regime	Comments
Hydralazine	0.2 mg/kg i.v. or i.m., repeated q2h as needed	Blood pressure should be monitored frequently (e.g. every 20–30 min or using a continuous oscillometric monitor) and the drug dose and/or interval adjusted accordingly. Evidence of EOD should also be monitored at least daily
Enalapril	0.2 mg/kg i.v. or i.m., repeated q1–2h as needed	
Esmolol	50–75 µg/kg/min CRI	

Emergency treatment of hypertension.

Hyphaema

Natasha Mitchell

Hyphaema is the term used to describe the presence of blood in the anterior chamber. The entire chamber may be filled with blood (total hyphaema), or there may be a focal haemorrhage. Hyphaema can affect one eye (more likely an ocular disease) or both eyes (more likely a systemic disease). This condition presents a diagnostic challenge, as the presence of blood could prevent thorough inspection of the inside of the eye.

Causes

The blood–ocular barrier normally prevents free blood from entering the eye. This may be disrupted by the conditions outlined in Figure 5.19.1.

The most common cause of hyphaema in older cats is systemic hypertension (see Chapter 5.18).

When blood pressure is higher than normal, the eye attempts to autoregulate blood flow to maintain a steady perfusion. However, this results in precapillary arteriolar ischaemia and capillary permeability changes, leading to leakage of plasma proteins and blood. Retinal detachment can also tear retinal blood vessels resulting in bleeding.

Another common cause of hyphaema is due to formation of a pre-iridal fibrovascular membrane (PIFM). This pathological intraocular neovascularization is visible as a fine meshwork of blood vessels on the surface of the iris. It forms as a result of hypoxia caused by uveitis, neoplasia or retinal detachment. These new vessels are fragile and bleed easily. Non-clotting blood in the anterior chamber is likely to be due to a PIFM or a bleeding disorder.

- Systemic hypertension (Figure 5.19.2)
- Trauma:
  - Blunt trauma (e.g. RTA) (Figure 5.19.3a)
  - Penetrating trauma (e.g. cat claw corneal injury (Figure 5.19.3b))
- Following corneal or intraocular surgery
- Uveitis (Figure 5.19.4) due to bleeding of fragile blood vessels of induced pre-iridal fibrovascular membrane (PIFM)
- Uveal neoplasia (may also induce PIFM):
  - Lymphoma (Figure 5.19.5)
  - Melanoma
  - Adenocarcinoma
  - Haemangiosarcoma
- Glaucoma (Figure 5.19.6)
- Vasculitis:
  - Immune-mediated
  - Secondary to infectious disease
- Bleeding disorders:
  - Coagulation factor disorders (acquired, e.g. rodenticide poisoning (Figure 5.19.7) or liver disease; or inherited)
  - Platelet disorders (immune-mediated or sepsis)

5.19.1 Common causes of hyphaema.

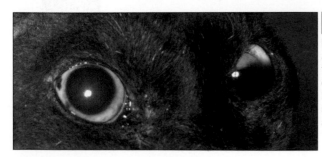

5.19.2 Bilateral intraocular haemorrhage in a hypertensive cat at initial presentation. In the left eye the hyphaema has settled ventrally with gravity, so that the dorsal half of the iris and pupil are visible. The fundus was examined through this and the retina was found to be detached. Haemorrhage in the vitreous of the right eye prevented fundus examination; the iris is visible because the haemorrhage is behind it, in the vitreous. There are some unrelated patches of pigment visible on the right iris, which are iris naevi or 'freckles'.

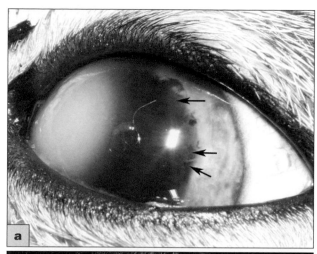

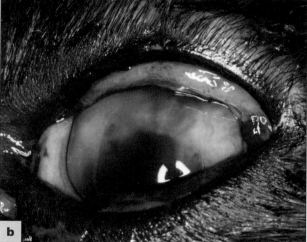

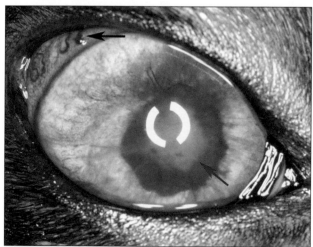

5.19.3 **(a)** Blunt trauma has caused corneal oedema (white area to the left of the picture) and hyphaema with an organizing blood clot, multifocally adhered to the yellow iris. There are small gaps visible between the blood clot and the iris (arrowed), which are important for the circulation of aqueous humour.
(b) Hyphaema from a cat claw injury on the upper eyelid. There is chemosis (bulging conjunctiva visible both dorsally and ventrally), conjunctival hyperaemia and mild corneal oedema, making the iris look dull.

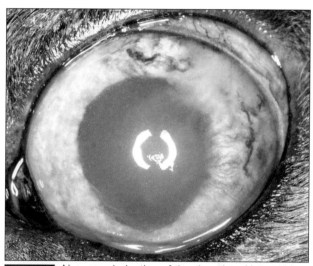

5.19.4 Uveitis with neovascularization of the iris (rubreosis iridis) due to PIFM formation. The fragile vessels are leaking protein (causing cloudy aqueous flare) and fibrin (forming a central cream-coloured clot (red arrow) in the anterior chamber), but not yet frank blood. Episcleral congestion is visible laterally (black arrow).

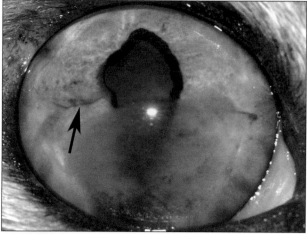

5.19.5 Fibrin and haemorrhage in the ventral aspect of the anterior chamber. The pupil is an abnormal shape (dyscoria) due to a pleated fold in the lateral iris (arrowed). The pigmented posterior surface of the iris is everted at the pupil margin (termed ectropion uveae). Lymphoma was subsequently diagnosed.

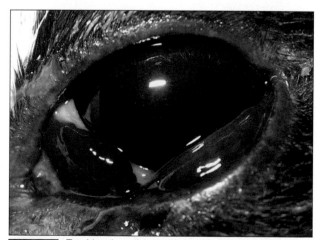

5.19.6 Neovascularization of the dorsal and lateral iris, due to a PIFM, along with corneal oedema. Conjunctivitis is visible dorsolaterally. There is mild corneal oedema throughout, obscuring a clear view of the iris, and the pupil is mid-dilated which was due to glaucoma. The PIFM can bleed, causing subsequent hyphaema (not present here).

5.19.7 Total hyphaema causing a dark red appearance to the eye. There are two areas of subconjunctival haemorrhage visible ventrally. This cat had rodenticide (flucoumafen) poisoning.

Clinical approach

The appropriate work-up depends on the presenting signs, and includes taking a full history, along with a thorough ocular (see QRG 1.3), neurological (see QRG 1.6) and physical examination. If the internal eye cannot be examined because of total hyphaema, examination of the contralateral eye may lead to a diagnosis, as it may show an earlier stage of the same disease if the underlying condition is systemic. Particular attention should be paid to fundus examination, which is much easier after pharmacological dilation with 0.5% tropicamide.

As systemic hypertension is the most common cause of hyphaema in older cats, blood pressure should be measured (see QRG 5.18.1). Estimation of intraocular pressure (IOP) is undertaken using tonometry when the equipment is available, as glaucoma can be a cause or a result of intraocular haemorrhage.

Laboratory tests may be indicated, such as haematology (including platelet count), biochemistry and urinalysis. If the cat is hypertensive, total T4 and aldosterone levels may need to be measured. In cases where uveitis is the main suspicion, tests for anti-FIV antibody, FeLV antigen, anti-*Toxoplasma* antibodies (IgG and IgM) and assessment for feline infectious peritonitis should be done (see Chapter 19). If a bleeding disorder is suspected, a clotting profile (prothrombin time (PT) and activated partial prothromboplastin time (APTT)) and buccal mucosal bleeding time (BMBT) measurement are indicated.

Ultrasonography of the globe is usually easy to perform in the conscious cat after application of topical anaesthetic (Figure 5.19.8). Normal findings are shown in Figure 5.19.9.

Ultrasonography is very useful for highlighting intraocular masses (Figure 5.19.10), retinal detachment, and ocular tunic disruption. Abdominal ultrasonography and thoracic radiography are also useful for diagnosing neoplasia or the presence of gunshot.

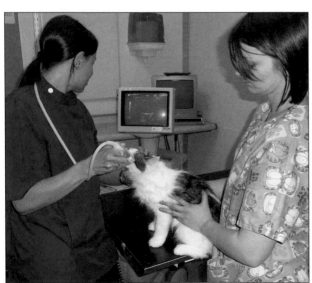

5.19.8 Ocular ultrasonography. The cat is gently restrained and a drop of topical anaesthetic is applied to the cornea. Coupling gel (e.g. K-Y jelly) is applied to the cornea, and the transducer is then gently applied directly to the cornea. Higher frequencies such as 7.5 or 10 MHz achieve the best resolution in the eye.

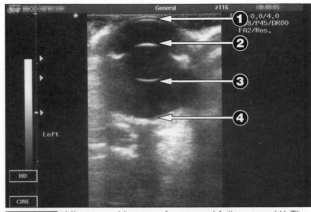

5.19.9 Ultrasound image of a normal feline eye. (1) The cornea – visible as a white line. The space between arrows 1 and 2 is the anterior chamber – it is black as it contains fluid. (2) The anterior lens capsule – visible as a white line. In the space between arrows 2 and 3 the lens appears black (it would be white if there were a cataract). (3) The posterior lens capsule – visible as a white line. In the space between arrows 3 and 4 the vitreous is liquid and appears black. (4) Posterior border of the globe – retina, choroid and sclera. (Courtesy of John Mould)

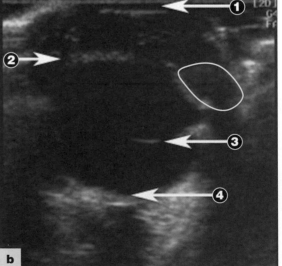

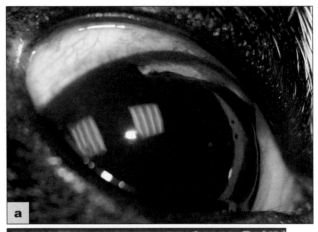

5.19.10 (a) The right eye of a 10-year-old cat with hyphaema almost filling the anterior chamber; a small section of the iris can be seen dorsally. (b) Ultrasound image, highlighting a mass within the iris. (1) The cornea. (2) The iris resting on the anterior lens capsule. (3) The posterior lens capsule. (4) The retina, choroid and sclera. The yellow outline delineates the mass. Continued rebleeding occurred due to PIFM, and the eye was later enucleated. Histology confirmed an iris melanoma.

Treatment plan

Hyphaema is a clinical sign rather than a disease. There is no specific treatment to eliminate the blood, but the outcome depends on correctly identifying and treating the underlying cause. In the absence of a specific diagnosis, the following treatment may be instigated.

- **Rest:** makes re-bleeding less likely. The blood will settle with time, allowing visualization of the internal eye.
- **Topical corticosteroids:** indicated for uveitis when corneal ulceration is not present. Prednisolone acetate 1% (Pred Forte, Allergan) has very good intraocular penetration and should be used initially q4–6h. If inflammation is under control in approximately one week, this may be reduced to q12h for a couple of weeks. Occasionally corticosteroids are required q24h long term, if signs of inflammation persist. NSAIDs are best avoided if possible as they may prolong clotting times.
- **Topical tropicamide:** to reduce synechiae formation by keeping the pupil dilated and therefore the posterior surface of the iris away from the lens. It is applied three times daily until the inflammation is under control, usually for one week. Topical atropine is not indicated unless there is a severe uveitis, and it may increase the risk of glaucoma.
- **Topical carbonic anhydrase inhibitors:** indicated if IOP is raised (e.g. Trusopt (dorzolamide) q8h). Continual monitoring is required, as the treatment may be stopped once the haemorrhage has resolved.
- **Surgical repair:** sharp or penetrating trauma (such as a cat claw injury) may need surgical repair; cases should be referred for assessment.
- **Enucleation** (see QRG 8.1): indicated in certain circumstances, e.g. if glaucoma is present and cannot be controlled medically.

> **WARNING**
>
> An attempt to aspirate the blood from the eye should NOT be made.

Prognosis

Prognosis depends on the underlying cause of the hyphaema. If the cause can be alleviated, then the blood is usually slowly absorbed and the hyphaema may resolve over one to several weeks without complications. Synechiae may develop due to blood- and fibrin-induced adhesions between the iris and intraocular structures, but these will often not impact upon vision or comfort (Figure 5.19.11).

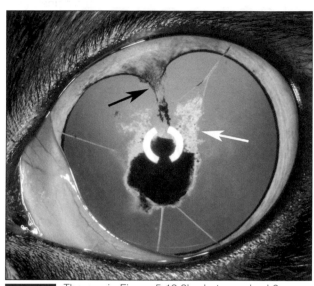

5.19.11 The eye in Figure 5.19.3b photographed 6 weeks later. There is a central resolving blood clot in the anterior chamber, with surrounding fibrin (white arrow) and synechiae to the iris (black arrow).

Uncommonly, glaucoma or cataracts may result, markedly affecting vision and, in the case of glaucoma, comfort of the eye. Following hypertension treatment it is possible for the cat with retinal detachment to regain some vision (Figure 5.19.12) but this depends on various factors, e.g. the length of time the retina has been detached.

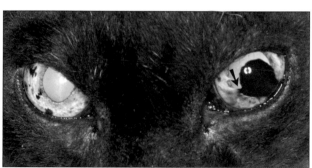

5.19.12 The cat in Figure 5.19.2 photographed 4 weeks after amlodipine treatment. There is restoration of vision, reabsorbed vitreal haemorrhage in the right eye, and a resolving blood clot in the left anterior chamber. There are anterior synechiae from the blood clot to the iris (arrowed). The iris freckles are obvious on the lateral aspect of the right iris; this is benign pigmentation but should be monitored in case melanoma develops.

Inappropriate urination, dysuria and pollakiuria

5.21

Samantha Taylor

Inappropriate urination, dysuria (difficult or painful urination) and pollakiuria (abnormally frequent urination) are distressing problems for owners.

- Behavioural house soiling must be distinguished from lower urinary tract disease, although there are often both medical and behavioural components (see Chapter 18).
- The term 'feline lower urinary tract disease' (FLUTD) is an umbrella term used to describe multiple conditions of the lower urinary tract with similar clinical signs such as dysuria, pollakiuria, haematuria or stranguria.
- 'Feline idiopathic cystitis' (FIC) is a specific diagnosis of bladder inflammation of unknown cause.

Further details of specific conditions and their management can be found in Chapter 13.

Clinical approach

History
With all cases of inappropriate urination, dysuria ± pollakiuria, thorough history taking is important. The following should be considered.

- Owners may mistake straining to defecate (dyschezia) for dysuria. Observation of urination and defecation can be helpful to distinguish these, e.g. observation of a urine stream or drips of urine, evaluating faecal consistency (normal *versus* dry and hard). Posture can be misleading, as cats with urethral inflammation can adopt a crouched or hunched posture similar to a defecation posture whilst straining to urinate.
- Due to the behavioural component of many urinary problems, the history should also include lifestyle information (indoor *versus* outdoor, other pets, family dynamics) and potential sources of stress (other cats, pets, etc.).
- Dietary history may also be important in case management (e.g. dry *versus* wet diet).
- Pattern of clinical signs: cats with FIC tend to

suffer multiple short episodes of dysuria, rather than continuous or progressive signs.
- Signalment:
  - Young to middle-aged cats are over-represented in the FLUTD patient group
  - Geriatric cats are unlikely to present with the first episode of FIC at an older age, but may have other diseases resulting in a predisposition to urinary tract infection (UTI), e.g. chronic kidney disease (CKD).
  - Urolithiasis is more frequently diagnosed in middle-aged cats, with female cats more likely to develop struvite urolithiasis, and male cats calcium oxalate urolithiasis. Certain breeds are predisposed to the development of urolithiasis.
- Other clinical signs: Urinary signs may prompt consultation but concurrent signs may suggest underlying systemic disease (e.g. PU/PD and/or inappetence in CKD).

Physical examination
A thorough physical examination should be performed.

- Bladder:
  - A large, painful bladder in a cat presenting with dysuria/pollakiuria may indicate urethral obstruction. This is an emergency and treatment should be started immediately (see Chapter 4.11)
  - Cats with non-obstructive FIC tend to have small, empty bladders due to the pollakiuria. Cats with FIC may have generalized bladder wall thickening. Rarely, a urolith or mass may be palpated within the bladder.
- Renal palpation:
  - Cats with CKD may present with dysuria due to a UTI and have small firm kidneys
  - Renomegaly may be detected in some cats with dysuria (Figure 5.21.1).
- Body condition score: Overweight or obese cats are predisposed to FLUTD, and weight management will form a part of the treatment.
- Examination for concurrent disease: Cats with conditions resulting in a reduced urine-concentrating ability may have a UTI.

- Neoplasia: lymphoma most common and usually bilateral (Figure 5.21.2); carcinomas less common and usually unilateral
- Hydronephrosis: ureterolithiasis, prolonged urethral obstruction, ureteral ligation following ovariohysterectomy; unilateral or bilateral depending on position or level of obstruction
- Feline infectious peritonitis (FIP): unilateral or bilateral
- Polycystic kidney disease: unilateral or bilateral
- Acute kidney injury: e.g. lily or ethylene glycol toxicity (see Chapter 4.9); often bilateral
- Amyloidosis: renal amyloidosis reported in Abyssinians; often bilateral
- Perinephric (perirenal) pseudocysts: unilateral or bilateral
- Acromegaly: bilateral
- Portosystemic vascular anomaly: renomegaly less common in cats than in dogs; bilateral

5.21.1 Differential diagnoses for renomegaly; note that not all conditions are associated with inappropriate urination, pollakiuria or dysuria.

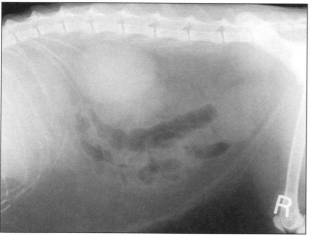

5.21.2 Lateral abdominal radiograph illustrating bilateral renomegaly in a cat with renal lymphoma.

Urinalysis

Urinalysis is vital in the investigation of cats with urinary signs. See QRG 4.11.3 for details on interpretation.

- Obtaining a sample via cystocentesis is preferred, to avoid contamination, and is vital for samples that are to be submitted for bacterial culture (see QRG 4.11.3). This may be difficult in cases with pollakiuria, due to small bladder size, although ultrasound guidance may be helpful.
- Alternatively, a free-catch sample may be obtained by the owner, using non-absorbable litter (Figure 5.21.3) and is suitable for basic urinalysis (e.g. dipstick, urine specific gravity (USG), sediment examination).
- Samples obtained by urethral catheterization from cats being anaesthetized (e.g. for urinary contrast studies or in cases of urethral obstruction) are suitable for most analyses, but iatrogenic haemorrhage may occur and placement should be as sterile as possible if the sample is to be used for bacterial culture.

Examination of urine sediment should be routine in the investigation of dysuria/pollakiuria or inappropriate urination. Pyuria and haematuria (see Chapter 5.13) are commonly found, and ideally bacterial culture is performed to exclude UTI. All samples should be examined as soon as possible to avoid artefactual crystalluria.

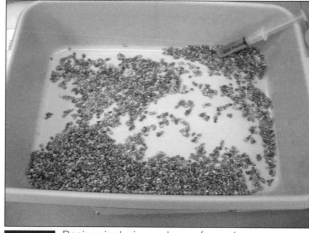

5.21.3 Basic urinalysis can be performed on a free-catch sample from non-absorbable cat litter.

Further investigations

Further clinical investigations may not be required in cases where a behavioural cause of inappropriate urination is suspected or when a there is strong clinical suspicion of FIC and the cat responds to treatment. However, cats with repeated episodes of clinical signs or abnormal findings on physical examination warrant further investigations. These include:

- Biochemistry and haematology
- FIV/FeLV testing
- Diagnostic imaging, including:
  - Plain abdominal radiography – check bladder size/shape and look for radiopaque uroliths (oxalate and struvite)
  - Contrast radiography (pneumocystogram and/or double-contrast cystogram, retrograde urethrography) – allows examination of bladder wall thickness, radiolucent uroliths (see QRG 5.21.1)
  - Ultrasonography – examination of bladder size, wall, renal structure and size
- Biopsy – if a mass or lesion has been identified, surgical biopsy may be obtained. The generalized bladder wall thickening seen in cases of FIC rarely warrants biopsy.

The clinical approach to inappropriate urination, dysuria and pollakiuria is summarized in Figure 5.21.4.

Inappropriate urination

Cats presented with inappropriate urination may not be dysuric. In such cases the owner may witness the inappropriate urination as spraying urine indoors or posturing to urinate outside the litter tray, but having no difficulty or pain passing **normal** volumes of urine.

Such cats may have a purely behavioural problem but an underlying medical problem must be excluded first. A full physical examination should reveal no abnormalities and urinalysis (preferably from a cystocentesis sample) should be unremarkable. Once medical conditions have been excluded a behavioural investigation and treatment plan can be considered. Consultation with a veterinary behaviourist may be required (see Chapter 18).

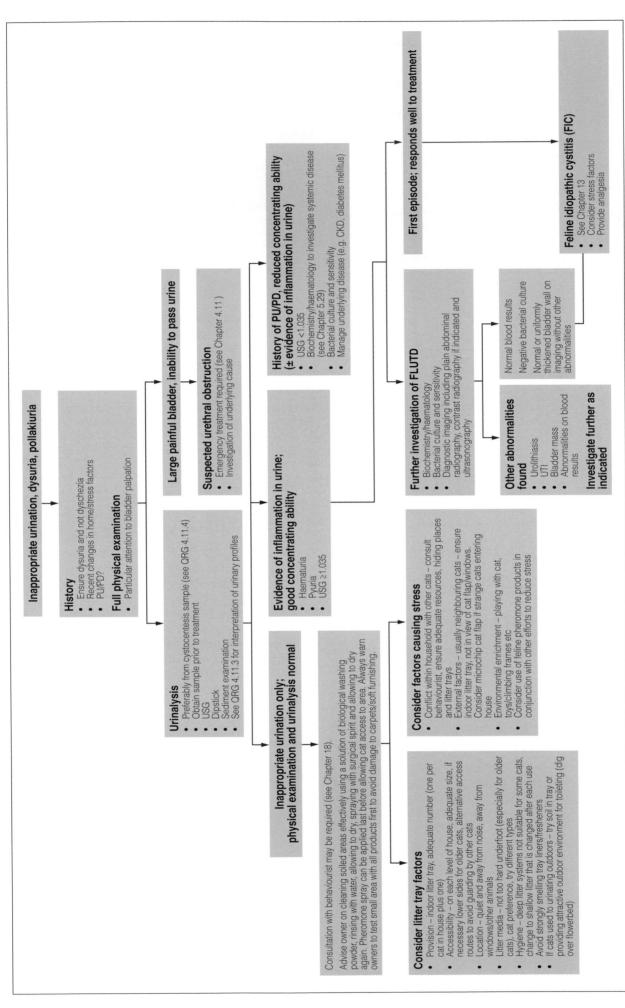

Inappropriate urination, dysuria, pollakiuria

History
- Ensure dysuria and not dyschezia
- Recent changes in home/stress factors
- PU/PD?

Full physical examination
- Particular attention to bladder palpation

Large painful bladder, inability to pass urine

Suspected urethral obstruction
- Emergency treatment required (see Chapter 4.11)
- Investigation of underlying cause

Urinalysis
- Preferably from cystocentesis sample (see QRG 4.11.4)
- Obtain sample prior to treatment
- USG
- Dipstick
- Sediment examination
- See QRG 4.11.3 for interpretation of urinary profiles

History of PU/PD, reduced concentrating ability (± evidence of inflammation in urine)
- USG <1.035
- Biochemistry/haematology to investigate systemic disease (see Chapter 5.29)
- Bacterial culture and sensitivity
- Manage underlying disease (e.g. CKD, diabetes mellitus)

Evidence of inflammation in urine; good concentrating ability
- Haematuria
- Pyuria
- USG ≥1.035

First episode; responds well to treatment

Further investigation of FLUTD
- Biochemistry/haematology
- Bacterial culture and sensitivity
- Diagnostic imaging including plain abdominal radiography, contrast radiography if indicated and ultrasonography

Normal blood results
Negative bacterial culture
Normal or uniformly thickened bladder wall on imaging without other abnormalities

Feline idiopathic cystitis (FIC)
- See Chapter 13
- Consider stress factors
- Provide analgesia

Other abnormalities found
- Urolithiasis
- UTI
- Bladder mass
- Abnormalities on blood results

Investigate further as indicated

Inappropriate urination only; physical examination and urinalysis normal

Consultation with behaviourist may be required (see Chapter 18).

Advise owner on cleaning soiled areas effectively using a solution of biological washing powder, rinsing with water, allowing to dry, spraying with surgical spirit and allowing to dry again. Pheromone spray can be applied last before allowing cat access to area. Always warn owners to test small area with all products first to avoid damage to carpets/soft furnishing.

Consider factors causing stress
- Conflict within household with other cats – consult behaviourist, ensure adequate resources, hiding places and litter trays
- External factors – usually neighbouring cats – ensure indoor litter tray, not in view of cat flap/windows. Consider microchip cat flap if strange cats entering house
- Environmental enrichment – playing with cat, toys/climbing frames etc
- Consider use of feline pheromone products in conjunction with other efforts to reduce stress

Consider litter tray factors
- Provision – indoor litter tray, adequate number (one per cat in house plus one)
- Accessibility – on each level of house, adequate size, if necessary lower sides for older cats, alternative access routes to avoid guarding by other cats
- Location – quiet and away from noise, away from windows/other animals
- Litter media – not too hard underfoot (especially for older cats), cat preference, try different types
- Hygiene – deep litter systems not suitable for some cats, change to shallow litter that is changed after each use
- Avoid strongly smelling tray liners/fresheners
- If cats used to urinating outdoors – try soil in tray or providing attractive outdoor environment for toileting (dig over flowerbed)

5.21.4 Clinical approach to inappropriate urination, dysuria and pollakiuria.

- **Age:** Geriatric cats, as well as being more likely to have conditions causing PU/PD and therefore a predisposition to UTIs, may have arthritis and an aversion to, or difficulty in, using the litter tray, resulting in house soiling. Such cats should have easy access to an indoor litter tray and be provided with soft litter media and a lower-sided tray.
- **Neurological problems:** Inappropriate urination may occur as a sign of cognitive dysfunction syndrome (see Chapter 17) or rarely with other central neurological pathologies but concurrent clinical signs would be expected
- **Litter tray:** The number, location, cleanliness and litter medium may affect the likelihood of cats using the litter tray.
- **Stress:** Many factors can result in stress and inappropriate urination, e.g. change in circumstances (house move, new baby), conflict with other cats inside/outside the home.

Differential diagnoses for dysuria and pollakiuria

Dysuria and pollakiuria often occur together. Affected cats often also develop inappropriate urination (see above) due to urgency and the association of pain and the litter tray.

Differential diagnoses for dysuria/pollakiuria include:

Common causes:

- FIC (most common cause)
  - Obstructive or non-obstructive
- Urolithiasis.

Less common causes:

- UTI (upper or lower), including pyelonephritis
- Trauma to bladder/urethra
- Neoplasia (bladder, urethra).

Urinary tract infection

Bacterial UTIs are uncommon in cats. Identification of infections should prompt investigation of an underlying cause, including:

- Conditions resulting in reduced urine-concentrating ability (diabetes mellitus, CKD, hyperthyroidism)
- Urethral catheterization
- Urinary diversion surgery (e.g. perineal urethrostomy)
- Immune system compromise (e.g. immunosuppressive treatment; retroviral infection; hyperadrenocorticism – rare in cats).

Empirical treatment

- Emergency treatment is required if urethral obstruction is suspected (see Chapter 4.11).
- If FIC (non-obstructive) is suspected:
  - Provide analgesia (e.g. buprenorphine 0.02 mg/kg i.v., i.m., s.c. or sublingually; NSAIDs such as meloxicam). Note that NSAIDs should only be used if renal function and hydration status are normal (see Chapter 3)
  - Identify stress factors and manage them if possible
  - Increase water intake (see QRG 13.1)
  - Antibiotics are rarely indicated and should only be used on the basis of a positive bacterial culture.

When to refer

Referral may be indicated in cases of recurrent FIC and should involve input from a veterinary behaviourist to manage stress factors. Cases of inappropriate urination (where medical causes have been excluded) may require referral to a veterinary behaviourist. Surgical treatment of cases of recurrent urethral obstruction may be required if a urethral stricture has developed (e.g. perineal urethrostomy).

If finances are limited

Urinalysis may be performed in-house inexpensively using a dipstick, USG and sediment examination to provide substantial amounts of information. If FIC is suspected, analgesia and advice to reduce stress and increase water intake may avoid further episodes without excessive expense.

QRG 5.21.1 Radiographic contrast studies of the lower urinary tract

by Myra Forster-Van Hijfte

Indications

When a cat shows recurrent and/or persistent lower urinary tract signs (stranguria, pollakiuria, haematuria), radiographic contrast studies may help identify the underlying cause, or at least rule out a number of causes. Radiographic contrast studies allow the assessment of the integrity of the bladder and urethra and the thickness of their walls, and will also document the presence of any foreign material (stones, plugs, blood clots). Contrast studies of the lower urinary tract may reveal abnormalities but will often not provide a definitive diagnosis. Further diagnostic tests are necessary, e.g. urine culture, cytology and sediment examination; stone analysis; histopathology and cytology of nodules or masses.

If the cat is older than 10 years when the first lower urinary tract signs occur, further imaging of the urinary tract is more likely to reveal abnormalities. In younger cats, feline idiopathic cystitis (FIC) is more common and further imaging is often unrewarding. In these cases the only abnormality detected on further imaging may be a thickening of the bladder wall. However, even in younger cats imaging is important to rule out other disease, before the diagnosis of FIC can be made.

Contraindications

The main contraindication is related to general anaesthesia. If the animal has urinary tract obstruction and consequential severe electrolyte and fluid imbalance, this needs to be corrected before anaesthesia is contemplated. In these cases it may be worth considering an ultrasound examination of the urinary tract. This does not require general anaesthesia, is less invasive, and allows good visualization of the bladder wall and any foreign material within the bladder. It does not, however, provide a good image of the urethra.

Patient preparation

Before the procedure the animal needs to be fasted for at least 12 hours (unless medically contraindicated).

It is important that any fluid and/or electrolyte imbalances are corrected prior to the general anaesthesia.

An enema may be necessary to prevent superimposition of a faeces-filled colon over the areas of interest.

The procedure is performed under general anaesthesia to allow for minimal discomfort of the cat and good positioning for radiography.

Equipment

- Urinary catheter: conventional cat catheter or a Jackson's cat catheter
- Sterile lubricating gel
- Surgical gloves
- 10 and 20 ml syringes
- Sample containers for the collection of urine
- Contrast medium: organic iodine-based water-soluble solutions, e.g. Urografin; Omnipaque (iohexol: 140 mg iodine per ml)

Technique

Plain ventrodorsal and lateral radiographs of the abdomen are initially taken. There may be obvious changes, such as radiopaque stones (struvite, calcium oxalate) within the urinary tract.

Positive contrast cystography

This is especially useful to document any damage of the bladder causing leakage of urine into the surrounding tissues. **NB The absence of obvious leakage of positive contrast medium into the abdomen does not fully rule out a bladder tear.**

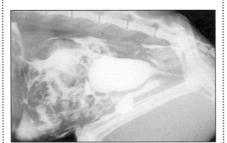

Lateral abdominal radiograph of a positive contrast bladder study, showing contrast medium leaking through the bladder wall indicating bladder rupture. (Courtesy of Danièlle Gunn-Moore)

- The procedure should be carried out as aseptically as possible: clean the external genitalia with dilute chlorhexidine and wear sterile gloves.
- The technique should be minimally traumatic.
- In the tom, a lubricated (using sterile lubricating gel) urinary catheter should be used and inserted into the urethra via the penis.
- The queen should be placed in ventral recumbency and the lubricated catheter guided over the mid-ventral part of the vagina into the urethra.
- The catheter should be inserted all the way into the bladder lumen and all of the urine removed using a syringe.

- Contrast medium should be injected via the catheter into the bladder (e.g. iohexol; approximately 5 ml/kg or until the bladder feels adequately distended on palpation) and radiographs taken after injection while the syringe is still attached to the catheter. Care needs to be taken that the weight of the syringe does not pull the catheter out of the bladder; it can be helpful to tape the catheter to the tail using micropore tape.

Double-contrast cystography

This is particularly helpful for assessing bladder wall thickness, any irregularities of the bladder wall, and any radiolucent bladder stones (e.g. cystine, urate).

If performed following a positive contrast cystogram:
1. Remove as much as possible of the initial positive contrast medium; a tiny amount will remain, lining the bladder wall.
2. Inject negative contrast medium (i.e. air) via the catheter into the bladder until the bladder is adequately distended.

If doing without an initial positive contrast cystogram:
1. Inject a small amount of positive iodine contrast medium (e.g. 1 ml iohexol) into the empty bladder.
2. Inject negative contrast medium (i.e. air) via the catheter into the bladder until the bladder is adequately distended.

Interpretation: Take care not to confuse air bubbles with radiolucent stones: air bubbles will be positioned at the periphery of the pooled positive contrast medium.

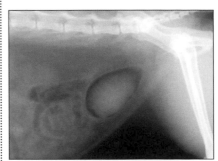

Lateral abdominal radiograph of a double-contrast bladder study, showing a thickened apical ventral bladder wall. This cat was diagnosed with feline idiopathic cystitis. (Courtesy of Danièlle Gunn-Moore)

▶

QRG 5.21.1 *continued*

Retrograde urethrography

Following the double-contrast cystography, positive urethrography allows for assessment of the urethra. Leakage of contrast medium suggests a urethral tear, whereas filling defects may be caused by neoplasia, urethral plugs or stones, and irregularities or strictures within the urethral mucosa.

Patient positioning for these radiographs is very important, as the urethra is very small and often not able to be visualized if the spine or pelvis is superimposed over it. Both lateral and ventrodorsal oblique views are often required to visualize the whole urethra.

1. Remove the air from the bladder via the urinary catheter.
2. Withdraw the catheter so that its tip is just within the end of the urethra. The tip of the prepuce or vulva should be clamped over the catheter (without occluding the catheter itself) using tissue forceps.
3. Radiographs are taken while the positive contrast medium (5–10 ml of iodine contrast medium, e.g. iohexol) is injected into the catheter. Care needs to be taken to adhere to radiation protection protocols.

Interpretation: Take care not to confuse a urethral stricture with a normal urethral contraction. If in doubt, the retrograde urethrogram should be repeated to see whether the narrowed urethra is a consistent finding.

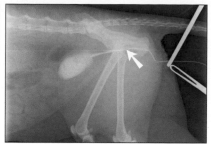

Positive retrograde urethrogram. There is a narrowing at the level of the pelvic obturator foramen (arrowed). This could be normal (urethral contraction) or abnormal. The contrast study needs to be repeated and a repeat radiograph taken to decide whether this is a consistent (and therefore abnormal) finding. (Courtesy of North Downs Specialist Referrals)

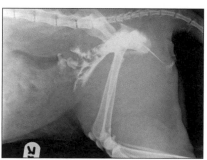

This 3-year-old neutered male DSH cat was involved in a road traffic accident. The retrograde urethrogram confirmed a ruptured urethra causing a uroabdomen, as shown by the leakage of contrast agent within the caudal abdomen and pelvic cavity. A prepubic urethrostomy was performed as a salvage procedure. (Courtesy of North Downs Specialist Referrals)

Intravenous urography

Contrast studies of the rest of the urinary tract (kidneys, ureters) require intravenous contrast medium. The contrast will be excreted via the kidneys and lower urinary tract, which will allow functional assessment (to a degree, provided the cat is well hydrated) as well as identifying anatomical lesions. See *BSAVA Manual of Canine and Feline Abdominal Imaging* for details of techniques.

Jaundice

Andrea Harvey

Clinical approach

Jaundice may be caused by pre-hepatic, hepatic and post-hepatic disorders. Figure 5.22.1 demonstrates an approach to identifying which of these groups of disorders is the most likely cause.

Once the most likely group of disorders has been identified, consideration needs to be given as to what the most common diseases are in each group (Figure 5.22.3).

Other basic clinical features need to be evaluated to direct the clinician to the most likely cause (Figure 5.22.4). These include:

- Cat's age and breed
- Other clinical signs present
- Duration of clinical signs
- Physical examination findings
- Other laboratory findings
- Other diagnostic imaging findings.

5.22.1 A diagnostic approach to differentiate pre-hepatic, hepatic and post-hepatic causes of jaundice.

[a] Tissue jaundice will only generally be evident when serum bilirubin exceeds approximately 50 µmol/l (reference range 0–15 µmol/l). The degree of hyperbilirubinaemia is also important in interpretation. There are no hard and fast rules but, generally, with pre-hepatic jaundice serum bilirubin is rarely above 50–100 µmol/l. FIP, pancreatitis, amyloidosis and sepsis also rarely result in serum bilirubin concentrations >100 µmol/l. When serum bilirubin is >200 µmol/l, this is most often caused by either hepatic lipidosis or post-hepatic obstruction, which may be a surgical emergency. Hepatic lipidosis may frequently result in serum bilirubin concentrations >200–300 µmol/l but, generally, the higher the serum bilirubin, the more likely that complete post-hepatic biliary obstruction is present.

[b] Haemolysis needs to be acute and severe (typically PCV<13%) to cause clinically evident jaundice, and caution should therefore be taken in over-interpreting a mild anaemia to be the cause. Cats will frequently have mild to moderate anaemia associated with chronic or inflammatory disease in hepatic and post-hepatic disorders. The degree of anaemia needs to be carefully interpreted with the degree of hyperbilirubinaemia, together with other clinicopathological features.

[c] If serum bilirubin is >100 µmol/l, abdominal ultrasonography is critical in identifying whether extrahepatic biliary duct obstruction is present. Where abdominal ultrasonography is not immediately available, if serum bilirubin is <100 µmol/l, other clinical features (see Figure 5.22.4) can be evaluated first to assist in identifying the most likely cause. Detecting early or partial extrahepatic biliary duct obstruction may require expertise in ultrasonography, and referral may need to be considered. For the practitioner, the priority is to know whether the case is a surgical emergency, and in this case the bilirubin is frequently >250 µmol/l and the gall bladder and common bile duct are grossly distended (see Figure 5.22.2).

Figure 5.22.1

```
                Presence of tissue jaundice
                          ↓
           Perform CBC and serum biochemistry
                          ↓
     Hyperbilirubinaemia confirmed and quantified[a]
                          ↓
          ┌───────────────┴───────────────┐
      PCV <15%                        PCV ≥15%
          ↓                               ↓
  Consider causes of            Abdominal ultrasonography[c]
  pre-hepatic jaundice[a,b]             ↓
  (see Figure 5.22.3)         ┌─────────┴─────────┐
          ↓                   │                   │
  Bile ducts and gall bladder    Bile ducts ± gall bladder
      not dilated                      dilated
          ↓                               ↓
  Hepatic jaundice most likely.   Post-hepatic jaundice
  Pancreatitis also not excluded.  (see Figure 5.22.2)
  Biliary rupture less common
  but can not be excluded and
  should be considered if
  presence of free abdominal
  fluid (see Chapter 5.1).
  Evaluate further for specific
  cause (see Figure 5.22.4 and
  Chapter 12).
          ↓                               ↓
  Evidence of acute pancreatitis.   No evidence of pancreatitis,
  Instigate medical treatment       or evidence of another
  accordingly (see Chapter 12)      post-hepatic disorder:
                                    refer for surgery
```

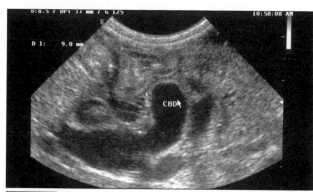

5.22.2 This ultrasound image of a 10-year-old male neutered DSH cat that had been presented with vomiting and acute-onset jaundice shows dilatation of the common bile duct (CBD) consistent with extrahepatic biliary tract obstruction. The normal diameter of the CBD in cats is <4 mm; in this case it measured up to 9 mm. On laparotomy the obstruction was found to be due to a cholelith in the CBD at the level of the duodenal papilla. Neutrophilic cholangitis was identified on hepatic histopathology, and this was thought to be the cause of the cholelithiasis.

Pre-hepatic disorders

- Haemolytic anaemia (see Chapter 5.4)

Hepatic disorders

- **Inflammatory hepatopathies** (neutrophilic cholangitis (acute or chronic); lymphocytic cholangitis)
- **Hepatic lipidosis**
- Feline infectious peritonitis
- Amyloidosis
- Sepsis
- Hepatotoxicity (e.g. paracetemol, diazepam, antithyroid medications)

Post-hepatic disorders

- **Pancreatitis**
- Cholecystitis
- Cholelithiasis (most commonly associated with neutrophilic cholangitis)
- Hepatobiliary mass
- Duodenal mass

5.22.3 Common causes of jaundice. The most common causes in cats are shown in bold.

Clinical features	Most common diagnoses
Age	
Young	FIP (typically 6 months to 3 years); lymphocytic cholangitis (typically 1–5 years)
Young to middle-aged (typically 2–8 years)	Pancreatitis; neutrophilic cholangitis; hepatic lipidosis
Middle-aged to older (typically >8 years)	Neutrophilic cholangitis; hepatic lipidosis; pancreatitis; neoplasia
Breed	
Siamese/Oriental	FIP; amyloidosis
Persian	FIP; lymphocytic cholangitis
Pedigree	FIP
History/Clinical signs	
Overweight with recent weight loss	Hepatic lipidosis
Weight loss despite a good appetite	Lymphocytic cholangitis
Any current medications	Consider possible hepatotoxicity (see Figure 5.22.3)
Abdominal pain	Pancreatitis; acute neutrophilic cholangitis; cholecystitis
Physical examination	
Pyrexia	FIP; neutrophilic cholangitis; sepsis
Hepatomegaly	Lymphocytic cholangitis; hepatic lipidosis; neoplasia
Ascites	Lymphocytic cholangitis; FIP; neoplasia; haemoabdomen associated with amyloidosis
Respiratory compromise	Could be associated with pleural effusion in FIP; neoplasia
Laboratory test results	
Neutrophilia	FIP; sepsis; neutrophilic cholangitis; pancreatitis
Left shift/toxic neutrophils	Acute neutrophilic cholangitis; sepsis
More marked increase in ALT compared to ALP	Hepatotoxicity; amyloidosis; hepatic neoplasia
Mild hyperbilirubinaemia with normal ALT and ALP	FIP; pancreatitis
More marked increase in ALP compared to ALT	Post-hepatic jaundice; cholangitis; hepatic lipidosis
Extremely elevated ALP with only mildly elevated GGT	Hepatic lipidosis
Marked hyperglobulinaemia	Lymphocytic cholangitis; FIP
Hypocalcaemia	Pancreatitis; sepsis

5.22.4 Most common diagnoses associated with specific clinical features. (continues) ▶

Clinical features	Most common diagnoses
Diagnostic imaging	
Radiopaque area in gall bladder	Cholelithiasis
Hepatomegaly	Lymphocytic cholangitis; hepatic lipidosis; neoplasia
Ascites	Lymphocytic cholangitis; FIP; neoplasia; haemoabdomen associated with amyloidosis; biliary tract rupture (uncommon)
Thickened gall bladder wall/sludge in gall bladder	Cholecystitis/acute neutrophilic cholangitis
Marked hyperechoic hepatic parenchyma	Hepatic lipidosis; lymphoma (less common)

5.22.4 (continued) Most common diagnoses associated with specific clinical features.

Empirical treatment pending investigations/results

- **Intravenous fluid therapy:**
  - 0.9% NaCl, usually supplemented with potassium chloride (KCl) depending on serum potassium concentration (see Chapter 4.6), but if potassium cannot be measured, supplement with 20 mmol/l KCl
  - 2–4 ml/kg/h is usually an appropriate fluid rate depending on degree of dehydration (see QRG 4.1.3).
- **Vitamin K:** If clotting times cannot be easily assessed, it is worth treating with vitamin K (1.0 mg/kg s.c. q12h) in case there is vitamin K-dependant coagulopathy, especially if there is the possibility of surgical intervention.
- **Assisted feeding:** If inappetent, and vomiting has been controlled, consider placing a naso-oesophageal feeding tube for short-term assisted feeding (see QRG 5.5.2).
- **Analgesia:** If abdominal pain is present, or if neutrophilic cholangitis or pancreatitis is suspected, administer buprenorphine (0.01 mg/kg sublingual or slow i.v. q8h).
- **Anti-emetics:** If vomiting/nausea is a feature, administer maropitant (1 mg/kg s.c. q24h for up to 5 consecutive days) and/or metoclopramide (CRI) (see Chapter 5.35).
- **Antibiotics:** If acute neutrophilic cholangitis or sepsis is suspected, based on clinical findings; broad-spectrum (e.g. amoxicillin/clavulanate, cefalexin) should be administered, initially parenterally.

When to refer

Given the large number of causes of jaundice, the difficulty in reaching a definitive diagnosis without accurate biliary ultrasonography and hepatic biopsy, and the intensive treatment required for many of these disorders, consideration should be given to referral of any jaundiced cat. In particular, referral is appropriate if post-hepatic obstruction is suspected, if liver biopsy is required, if the diagnosis is uncertain or if intensive treatment (e.g. for hepatic lipidosis) is required.

If finances are limited

Clinical judgement should be used, taking into consideration all of the above, in making a decision as to the most likely cause of the jaundice and this should be treated accordingly. See Chapter 12 for more details on management of specific disorders.

Lameness

Sorrel J. Langley-Hobbs

Cats have a tendency to roam, climb and jump; this means that they are prone to acquiring traumatic injuries such as fractures and dislocations (and also soft tissue ruptures; see Chapter 4.10). Fighting between cats as they defend their territory commonly results in bite injuries, which can lead to cellulitis, abscesses (see Chapter 5.8) and acute septic arthritis; these are important differential diagnoses for lameness in cats.

Developmental diseases are not common in cats. This probably reflects their relatively small size, agile nature and wider gene pool due to less frequent interbreeding and relatively few purebred animals compared to dogs. Some feline conditions are suspected of being hereditary or developmental; these include hip dysplasia (Figure 5.23.1) and patellar luxation (see Chapter 16).

Osteoarthritis (Figure 5.23.2) is being recognized more frequently in cats, due to increased awareness of its prevalence and also to the fact that cats are regularly reaching old age.

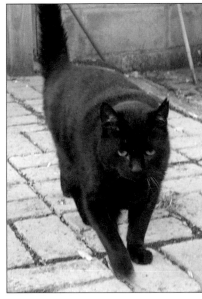

5.23.2
An 18-year-old male neutered DSH cat with severe bilateral stifle and hock arthritis and mild elbow arthritis. This cat was overweight and was dieted successfully to lose weight. Meloxicam was given (after blood screening to check that there were no contraindications to NSAID treatment) and the cat's lameness improved and his mobility increased.

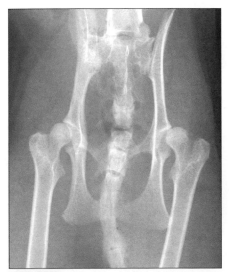

5.23.1 A 2-year-old female cat was presented with bilateral pelvic limb lameness and difficulty in jumping. On examination she exhibited signs of pain on hip extension. This ventrodorsal radiograph shows bilateral hip dysplasia with femoral head subluxation but minimal signs of degenerative joint disease. In such a case, conservative treatment should be tried initially; if unsuccessful, femoral head and neck excision could then be considered.

Initial investigation

Any cat with acute lameness that is suspected to have suffered trauma (e.g. from a road traffic accident (RTA)) should have a thoracic radiograph taken (see QRG 4.2.3) to check for injuries such as pulmonary contusions, pneumothorax, rib fractures or diaphragmatic rupture.

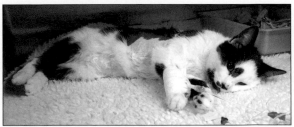

This 8-month-old female cat was presented with a pelvic fracture but was tachypnoeic. Radiography revealed a haemothorax. It is important to treat any life-threatening conditions before attending to fractures. The haemothorax was drained and the cat treated with cage rest for several days prior to treatment of the pelvic fractures.

Signalment

The first step in investigating lameness in cats is to take note of the signalment:

- Younger cats are more likely to have fractures than luxations
- Male entire cats are more likely to fight and therefore to have bacterial inflammatory causes of lameness
- Older animals are more likely to have osteoarthritis or neoplasia.

History

The history taken from the owners should include questions about:

- Whether the cat is an indoor or outdoor animal
- Whether it has gone missing for any length of time
- The duration and onset of lameness
- Progression and whether previous episodes have occurred.

Owners of cats may not necessarily report lameness but may be more concerned by a change in the cat's normal athletic behaviour, such as a refusal to jump on to a previously favoured piece of furniture, or an inability to climb the fence or go through the cat flap. These changes can severely influence the cat's normal behaviour. For example, its preferred sleeping place on the sunny windowsill may no longer be accessible, or it may no longer be able to escape the unwanted advances of the dog in the household. Food that was previously placed in a position easily accessible to the cat but out of the reach of the dog may have to be resituated so that it is still possible for the cat to eat the food but the dog is prevented from doing so.

Observation

A lame cat can present a challenge: walking and trotting a cat along a corridor to assess lameness is not usually possible and many cats do not have the patience to lie on their side and permit full orthopaedic examination. A cat that is shy may benefit from being removed from the cat carrier at the beginning of the consultation and being stroked and petted while obtaining the history from the owner. This can allow the cat to relax and become familiar with its surroundings. Observation of the cat standing and walking can then be carried out.

Observation of stance can help determine whether there is:

- Reduced weight-bearing on one limb (Figure 5.23.3)
- Abnormal angulation (Figure 5.23.4)
- Abnormal paw positioning
- Shifting of weight (Figure 5.23.5)
- A limb position that is suggestive of a muscular or neurological problem (Figures 5.23.6 and 5.23.7).

Observation of gait can confirm the presence of the reported lameness and will then make it easier to direct the subsequent majority of the orthopaedic examination.

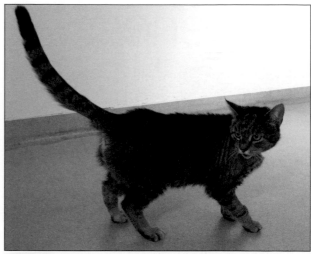

5.23.3 This 3-year-old male neutered 5 kg cat had a complete avulsion of his right triceps tendon, resulting in a dropped elbow. In the absence of a functional triceps muscle the elbow could not be extended. The cat had surgical repair of the avulsed tendon and postoperative external coaptation with a spica splint for 4 weeks to protect the repair during the initial phase of healing.

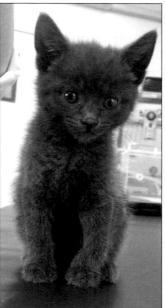

5.23.4

This 8-week-old kitten has premature closure of its left distal radial growth plate, resulting in carpal varus. This condition can be treated with ulnar and radial osteotomies and distraction osteogenesis to increase limb length, though in this case the owners opted not to treat.

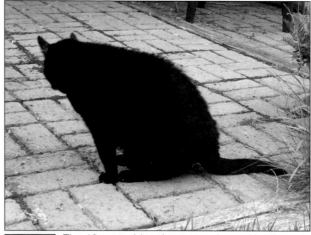

5.23.5 The 18-year-old male neutered cat with bilateral stifle arthritis shown in Figure 5.23.2 has a hunched stance as he shifts his weight on to his thoracic limbs while trying to rise.

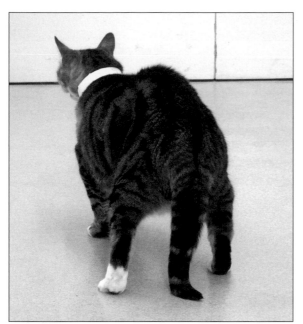

5.23.6 This 10-year-old male neutered cat with pelvic limb ataxia has a wide-based hindlimb stance. He was considered to have a neurological problem (diagnosis undetermined), although a bilateral stifle problem could also give a similarly abnormal stance.

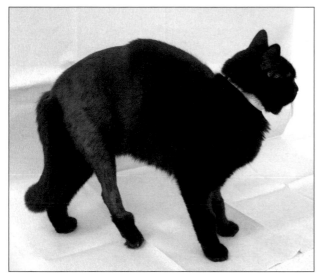

5.23.7 This cat has developed quadriceps contracture, leading to rigid extension of the right hindlimb subsequent to a femoral fracture of that leg. The cat had a mechanical lameness associated with the extended stifle but the leg was still considered functional. Treatment can be attempted in the early stages of quadriceps contracture; numerous different methods of treatment have been tried but the prognosis for recovery or reversal is guarded.

Orthopaedic examination

The orthopaedic examination should be done gently, with minimal restraint of the cat. A nervous cat will initially crouch in a sternal position. If the owner gently strokes the cat, the veterinary surgeon may be able to palpate and compare the thoracic and pelvic limbs for evidence of inflammation, swelling or muscle atrophy. A relaxed cat that will stand will enable a more thorough comparison. Some cats will tolerate lying on their side (on a warm non-slip surface, best tolerated on a comfortable bed placed on the table or floor) and will allow the individual examination of

each leg. This is performed from distal to proximal, assessing each joint for swelling, pain, instability and range of motion, and manipulation to detect crepitus. Each limb is also assessed for swelling, atrophy, pain, and for evidence of a change in shape or abnormal movement that may be indicative of a fracture. If it is not possible to perform the orthopaedic examination in a recumbent cat, then it is examined in a standing position using distraction techniques and, if necessary, gentle restraint of the head and neck. Some fractious cats and those in pain may require sedation/anaesthesia/analgesia in order to complete the orthopaedic examination.

Although the majority of the orthopaedic examination will concern the affected leg, all four legs should be examined if possible. At the very least, the contralateral limb should be checked, as developmental orthopaedic conditions can often be bilateral.

The examination of the cat should include a careful check for puncture wounds; these can be difficult to find but clues can include small areas of matted hair with some dried blood or inflammatory discharge that can indicate a tooth mark from a bite. Frayed nails in cats can indicate that they have suffered trauma – usually presumed to be an RTA (Figure 5.23.8). Pads should be evaluated carefully for conditions such as plasma cell pododermatitis (see Chapter 6).

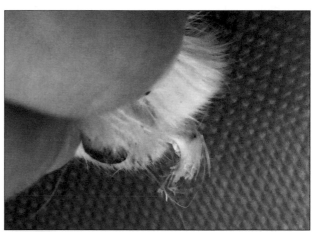

5.23.8 Scuffed nails are a common finding in cats after a road traffic accident.

PRACTICAL TIPS

- If cats really will not move or walk when presented to the surgery, owners can be asked to obtain video footage of the cat exhibiting its normal behaviour in its home environment.
- When there is a high suspicion of a cat bite injury (swollen painful hot area and a pyrexic cat) clipping the hair in order to look for bruising or puncture wounds can be helpful.
- Joints should be palpated carefully for ligament or tendon laxity and always compared with the contralateral limb; it is easy in cats to misinterpret normal joint laxity as a collateral ligament sprain.
- Cats are flexible and agile and their tendons and ligaments have a high degree of elasticity to permit the normal range of motion and athleticism.

Differential diagnoses

Some causes of feline thoracic and pelvic limb lameness are listed in Figures 5.23.9 and 5.23.10.

Cats that exhibit weakness or lameness of more than one limb may have systemic conditions (Figure 5.23.11) such as metastasis of a bronchial carcinoma to multiple digits (Figure 5.23.12), where the primary presenting complaint has been reported to be lameness (Gottfried *et al.*, 2000).

Area affected	Possible causes
Thoracic limb	Cat bite abscess, osteoarthritis, fracture, dislocation, soft tissue rupture, neoplasia
Scapula	Fracture, avulsion or disruption from body wall, neoplasia
Shoulder	Osteoarthritis, fracture, luxation, accessory centres of ossification, dysplasia, bicipital tenosynovitis, biceps tendon rupture, osteochondrosis
Humerus	Fractures, neoplasia, osteomyelitis
Elbow	Osteoarthritis, traumatic luxation, fracture, dysplasia, congenital or developmental luxation, elbow epicondylitis, synovial cysts, triceps tendon avulsion
Radius/ Ulna	Fracture, neoplasia, osteomyelitis, growth deformity
Carpus	Osteoarthritis, luxation, hyperextension
Foot	Fracture, luxation, plasma cell pododermatitis, digital carcinoma

5.23.9 Some localized causes of thoracic limb lameness in cats.

Area affected	Possible causes
Pelvic limb	Cat bite abscess, osteoarthritis, fracture, dislocation, soft tissue rupture, neoplasia
Pelvis	Fracture, sacroiliac luxation, neoplasia
Hip	Osteoarthritis, hip dysplasia, luxation, fracture, slipped capital femoral epiphyses
Femur	Fracture, neoplasia, osteomyelitis
Stifle	Osteoarthritis, mineralization of intra-articular structures, cranial or caudal cruciate ligament rupture, patellar luxation, patellar fracture, quadriceps rupture (patellar ligament rupture), stifle derangement (disruption or luxation), disruption of the proximal tibiofibular ligament, avulsion of the long digital extensor tendon, osteochondrosis
Tibia/ Fibula	Fracture, neoplasia, osteomyelitis
Tarsus	Osteoarthritis, luxation, malleolar fractures, rupture or avulsion of the Achilles tendon, luxation of the superficial digital flexor tendon, collateral ligament ruptures or sprains, tibiofibular ligament rupture, dorsal instability, talocalcaneal luxation
Foot	Fracture, luxation, plasma cell pododermatitis, digital carcinoma

5.23.10 Some localized causes of pelvic limb lameness in cats.

Hereditary and congenital musculoskeletal diseases

- Storage diseases: alpha-mannisodosis, mucopolysaccharidosis types I, II and VII, mucolipidosis type II
- Osteogenesis imperfecta
- Osteochondrodysplasia in the Scottish Fold cat
- Hypothyroidism
- Hereditary rickets
- Individual congenital disorders such as spinal dysraphism, syringomyelia, agenesis of bones

Diseases of bone

- Secondary hyperparathyroidism: renal, nutritional
- Vitamin D deficiency
- Hypervitaminosis A
- Osteomyelitis: bacterial, fungal
- Bone cysts
- Hypertrophic osteopathy
- Osteochondromas/osteochondromatosis

Diseases of joints

- Osteoarthritis
- Septic arthritis
- Erosive polyarthritis
- Non-erosive polyarthritis: immune-mediated, systemic lupus erythematosus, drug-induced, virus-associated e.g. calici virus, Lyme disease (borreliosis), osteochondrosis, synovial osteochondromatosis, synovial cysts

Diseases of soft tissues

- Muscle contracture and fibrosis: quadriceps, semitendinosus, biceps
- Myositis ossificans

Diseases of the feet

- Nails and nail beds:
  - Bacterial paronychia
  - Pemphigus foliaceus
  - Onychomycosis
  - Nail chewing
  - Idiopathic onychodystrophy
- Interdigital spaces:
  - Eosinophilic plaques
  - Trombiculosis
- Footpads:
  - Plasma cell pododermatitis
  - Metastatic calcinosis of the paws
  - Calicivirus infection
  - Contact irritant dermatitis

Diseases of the spine, nervous system and neuromuscular junction

- Intervertebral disc disease
- Spinal subarachnoid cysts
- Cord infarction
- FIP
- Discospondylitis
- Spinal empyema
- Congenital abnormalities
- Ischaemic neuromyopathy
- Myositis
- Diabetic neuropathy
- Hypokalaemic myopathy
- Myasthenia gravis
- Toxoplasmosis

5.23.11 Causes of generalized lameness and stiffness in cats. Osteoarthritis is the most common cause.

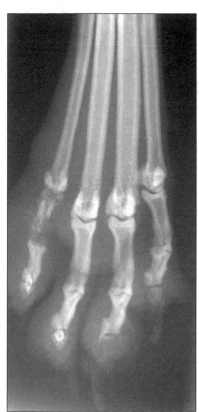

5.23.12

This 14-year-old cat was presented with a one-month history of lameness affecting several limbs. There was enlargement of multiple digits and radiographic evidence of bone lysis in the first phalanx of digit II and the third phalanx of digit IV. Thoracic radiography showed a pulmonary mass in the dorsocaudal lung fields and the presumptive diagnosis was bronchial carcinoma with metastasis to the digits.

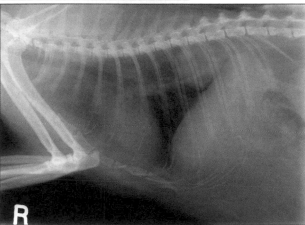

Further investigations

Following examination it may be possible to make a diagnosis. For example, medial displacement of the patella when the stifle is manipulated through its range of motion would be highly indicative of patellar luxation. The decision then needs to be made as to whether further investigation is necessary prior to treatment.

Further investigations of the affected limb, joint or bone to enable a diagnosis can include radiography, ultrasonography, MRI or CT, fine-needle aspirate cytology and/or arthrocentesis. Radiographs should be taken to evaluate fractures or other traumatic injuries to be able to classify the fracture and determine the appropriate treatment options. A whole 'catogram' can be useful to scan for thoracic and abdominal injuries (Zulauf *et al.*, 2008) although specific films focused on one area are preferred for a more complete examination of an area. If a systemic disorder is suspected, routine haematology, serum biochemistry or infectious disease testing may be indicated.

Management

Once the cause of the lameness has been determined, a plan for treatment is devised, taking into consideration the whole cat and prioritizing the treatment dependent on concurrent and perhaps more life-threatening injuries. Management of orthopaedic disorders is discussed in Chapter 16.

References and further reading

Cook JL, Innes JI, Houlton JEF and Langley-Hobbs SJ (2006) *BSAVA Manual of Canine and Feline Musculoskeletal Disorders*. BSAVA Publications, Gloucester

Gottfried SD, Popovitch CA, Goldschmidt MH and Schelling C (2000) Metastatic digital carcinoma in the cat: a retrospective study of 36 cats (1992–1998). *Journal of the American Animal Hospital Association* **36**, 501–509

Montavon PM, Voss K and Langley-Hobbs SJ (2009) *Feline Orthopedic Surgery and Musculoskeletal Disease*. Saunders Elsevier, Edinburgh

Zulauf D, Kaser Hotz B, Hassig M, Voss K and Montavon PM (2008) Radiographic examination and outcome in consecutive feline trauma patients. *Veterinary and Comparative Orthopaedics and Traumatology* **21**, 36–40

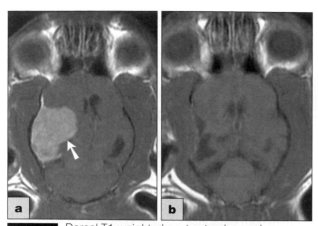

5.24.4 Dorsal T1-weighted contrast-enhanced magnetic resonance images of a cat with a large rostrotentorial meningioma (arrowed) **(a)** before and **(b)** after surgical resection via craniectomy.

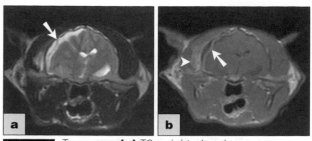

5.24.5 Transverse **(a)** T2-weighted and **(b)** T1-weighted contrast-enhanced magnetic resonance images of a cat with intracranial empyema secondary to a bite wound, that was presented with right forebrain signs. **(a)** There is fluid signal accumulation (arrowed) between the calvarium and brain on the right side. **(b)** Note the marked mass effect on the brain, contrast enhancement of the meninges (arrowed) and hyperintensity within the ventral part of the right temporalis muscles (arrowhead).

Ocular discharge

Natasha Mitchell

Ocular discharge is a common but non-specific clinical sign in cats, and may have numerous potential causes.

- A wet eye (serous discharge) may be caused by excessive tear production due to any form of ocular pain or irritation, poor distribution of the tear film, or impairment of normal tear drainage through the lacrimal system. Serous ocular discharge may become mucopurulent with chronicity.
- Ocular discharge as a result of inflammation is typically mucoid, mucopurulent or purulent, and is most often caused by bacterial infections, *Chlamydophila felis,* feline herpesvirus-1 (FHV), eyelid margin disease, or keratoconjunctivitis sicca (KCS).

Differential diagnoses

The most common causes of purulent ocular discharge in the cat are FHV infection and *C. felis*-associated conjunctivitis (Figure 5.25.1).

The most common conditions that cause an ocular discharge are:

- Eyelid abnormalities:
  - Entropion results in trichiasis, with resulting ocular discharge and blepharospasm (Figure 5.25.2a); this condition should be corrected surgically
  - Eyelid masses, e.g. tumours, lipogranulomas, hidrocystomas
  - Eyelid agenesis – usually the lateral upper eyelids are missing, resulting in poor blink and poor distribution of the tear film, and trichiasis can result in conjunctival and corneal irritation (Figure 5.25.2b). *Affected cats should be referred to assess whether they would benefit from corrective surgery.*
  - Lagophthalmos – an inability to blink completely (Figure 5.25.2c)
  - Misplaced cilia (distichiasis or ectopic cilia, both relatively uncommon in cats) – these cilia may cause increased tear production by stimulating conjunctival and corneal nerves, and they may lead to corneal ulcers or sequestra
- Lacrimal apparatus abnormalities:
  - Congenital aplasia of one or both lacrimal puncta (Figure 5.25.3)

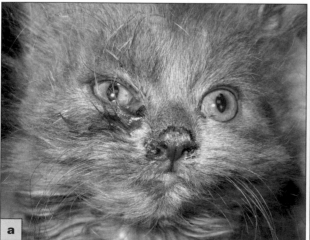
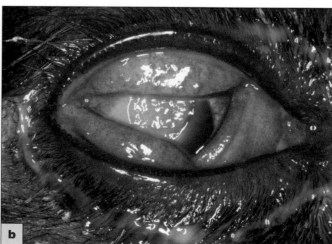

5.25.1 **(a)** Typical serous and mucoid discharge from the eye and nose of a kitten with FHV infection. **(b)** Purulent ocular discharge, chemosis dorsally and ventrally along with conjunctival hyperaemia of all visible conjunctival surfaces, and corneal opacity due to fibrovascular infiltration of a corneal ulcer. The cat was diagnosed with *Chlamydophila felis* infection.

- Misplaced lacrimal punctum
- Trauma
- Other acquired conditions, e.g. neoplasia, foreign body and dacryocystitis, are much less common
- Conjunctival disease:
  - Conjunctivitis – infectious (Figure 5.25.4a), allergic
  - Symblepharon (Figure 5.25.4b)
  - Trauma
- Corneal disease:
  - Ulceration (Figure 5.25.5a)
  - Sequestrum (Figure 5.25.5b)
  - Perforation
  - KCS
  - Foreign bodies
- Orbital disease:
  - Retrobulbar space-occupying lesions, e.g. abscess, tumour (Figure 5.25.6a) or sialocele (Figure 5.25.6b).

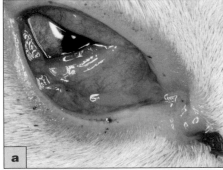
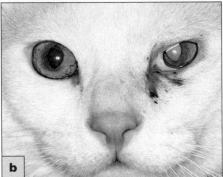

5.25.4 Conjunctival disease. **(a)** Mucoid to mucopurulent discharge typical of conjuctivitis in a cat with *C. felis* infection. Chemosis, conjunctival hyperaemia and third eyelid protrusion are also present. **(b)** Previous FHV infection has caused scarring over the lacrimal puncta, resulting in serous ocular discharge in the left eye. Third eyelid protrusion is present due to developing symblepharon along with typical signs of cat 'flu conjunctivitis, including chemosis, conjunctival hyperaemia and serous nasal discharge. The cornea was ulcerated behind the third eyelid, which is the cause of the symblepharon.

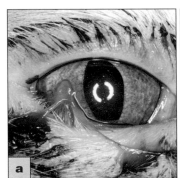
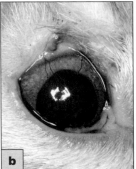
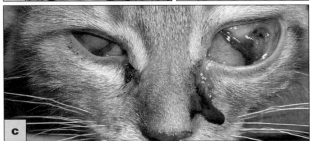

5.25.2 Eyelid abnormalities. **(a)** Mucopurulent ocular discharge with brown crusting caused by entropion of the lateral lower eyelid. **(b)** Purulent ocular discharge in a kitten with upper eyelid agenesis. The lateral half of the upper eyelid is missing. Poor blinking and the lack of meibomian glands to create tear film lipids have resulted in corneal neovascularization and a dull, dry appearance to the cornea. **(c)** Serous ocular discharge in a kitten with lagophthalmos due to left globe enlargement secondary to glaucoma, which also resulted in a ruptured corneal ulcer when it was not treated. The kitten was infected with FHV, and symblepharon (adherent conjunctiva) can also be seen on the right cornea. The left third eyelid is protruding due to ocular pain (as this can result in enophthalmos); the right third eyelid is partially protruded due to the conjunctival adhesions.

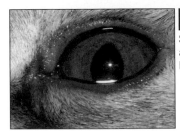

5.25.3 Serous ocular discharge in a cat with absence of the lower lacrimal punctum.

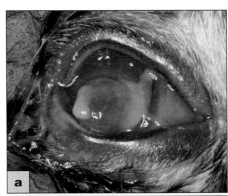
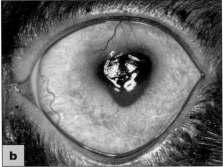

5.25.5 Corneal disease. **(a)** Purulent ocular discharge in a cat with a melting corneal ulcer due to *Pseudomonas aeruginosa* infection. **(b)** Corneal sequestrum inciting corneal neovascularization from the dorsal limbus, with some black crusty discharge on the lower eyelid.

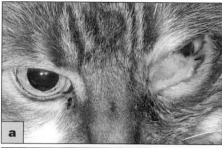

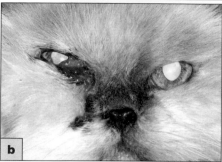

5.25.6 Orbital disease. **(a)** Purulent discharge with third eyelid protrusion due to exophthalmos caused by a retrobulbar tumour. Fluorescein dye has drained on to the face as the lacrimal puncta are closed due to conjunctival congestion. **(b)** Mucopurulent ocular discharge and third eyelid protrusion in the right eye of a Persian cat with a retrobulbar sialocele.

Imperforate lacrimal punctum(a) may occur unilaterally or bilaterally, and may affect the upper, lower or both lacrimal puncta. Affected cats present with chronic epiphora, and there is a negative Jones test (see below). Referral is recommended for surgery to recreate the lacrimal puncta.

Investigation

Investigation includes history-taking, clinical examination and careful ocular examination (see QRG 1.3). The following should be looked for particularly: eyelid conditions (upper eyelid agenesis, entropion, lagophthalmos); aplasia or misplaced lacrimal puncta; conjunctivitis; symblepharon; corneal conditions, such as ulcers, sequestra or foreign bodies; orbital disease; and dental disease.

The following procedures/tests may be indicated:

- It is useful to take a swab of the ocular discharge prior to examination as organisms may inadvertently be introduced later in the examination. The swab should be placed in culture medium and submitted for aerobic and anaerobic culture if no other cause for the ocular discharge can be found. Swab samples may also be taken for investigation of specific infectious causes (e.g. *Chlamydophila felis*, FHV)
- Next a Schirmer tear test (STT) should be carried out, which will help to distinguish between excessive tears, inadequate drainage, or KCS (less common than in the dog). It is appropriate to perform the STT at this point because stimulation of the eye during subsequent examination could produce extra reflex tears and lead to a falsely elevated result. KCS is diagnosed with a STT

reading of $\leq$10 mm/min, in conjunction with clinical signs of conjunctivitis and keratitis
- The presence of the lacrimal puncta should be observed with the aid of magnification, and they may be cannulated and flushed to confirm patency or blockage
- Fluorescein dye is applied and examined with a cobalt blue light: to check for the presence of a corneal ulcer (see Chapter 8); to investigate the patency of the nasolacrimal system (Jones test); and to check for a leaking corneal wound (Seidel's test). There is a blue light filter in most ophthalmoscopes, or a Wood's lamp can be used
  - Jones test: A drop of fluorescein is applied to the conjunctival sac; after 5–10 minutes the dye should be observable at the nares if the nasolacrimal system is patent (Figure 5.25.7). False negative results can be caused, however, by alternative drainage to the pharynx (especially in brachycephalic cats); therefore the mouth should also be checked for the presence of dye before deciding there is a blockage
  - Seidel's test: A positive Seidel's test occurs when the fluorescein dye beneath the wound is diluted by aqueous humour leaking from the wound; this appears as a black area within the green fluorescein beneath the wound (Figure 5.25.8).

Tear staining in Persian cats
Persian cats have multiple factors that lead to tear staining, which may be a cosmetic concern. These include: a shallow orbit; macropalpebral fissure; entropion of the medial aspect of the lower eyelid causing trichiasis, occluding the lower lacrimal punctum and wicking hairs on to the face; lagophthalmos; and poor corneal sensitivity centrally. Dark brown or black crusting at the medial canthus is not unusual, and the coloration is thought to be due to porphyrins in the tear film. Specific treatment is not usually required, apart from good eye hygiene by regularly wiping the discharge with previously boiled water soaked on cotton wool.

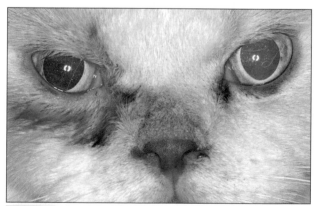

5.25.7 Jones test in a British Shorthaired cat. Fluorescein at the left naris (positive result) shows that the left nasolacrimal duct is patent. There is no fluorescein at the right naris, with fluorescein-stained tear overflow at the medial canthus (negative result), indicating an obstruction.

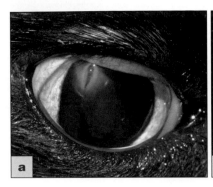

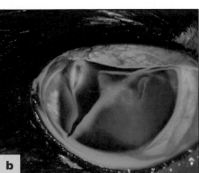

5.25.8 Seidel's test. **(a)** The right eye of a cat that had sustained a cat scratch injury. At the 11 o'clock position on the cornea, there is a dark linear opacity which is a wound, surrounded by a grey-whitish area of corneal oedema. Below this is a large pale brown area which is a fibrin clot in the anterior chamber. **(b)** Liberal fluorescein dye was applied and is a green colour. Beneath the corneal wound there is a dark triangular area which represents dilution of the dye with aqueous humour leaking from the wound. (Courtesy of John Mould.)

Overgrooming and pruritus

Natalie Barnard

The most common underlying cause for overgrooming in cats is pruritus, and this chapter discusses the approach to pruritic skin disease in cats. Diagnosing this is not always easy because there is a wide variation in clinical presentation and because owners often do not recognize that overgrooming is a problem (Figure 5.26.1); owners are often only aware their cat's behaviour is abnormal if they are able to compare the affected cat to another one in the household. It is for this reason that cats will often present with other clinical signs, such as a lesion from the eosinophilic granuloma complex or miliary dermatitis, and then it will also become apparent that the cat is actually overgrooming. To ascertain the cause of the overgrooming behaviour and pruritus, a thorough and logical diagnostic approach is required.

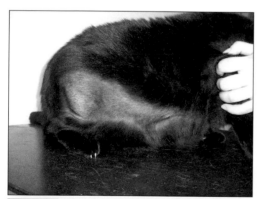

5.26.1 This 4-year-old DSH cat presented with a 6-month history of symmetrical flank alopecia. Hair pluck examination was used to confirm that this cat was overgrooming, and a diagnosis of atopic dermatitis was made by exclusion, as discussed later in the chapter.

History

Taking a history from the client will often highlight important information regarding the cat's signalment, lifestyle and management. The following points are particularly useful.

- **General health of the patient.** Are there any signs of systemic illness, such as asthma (which may fit with atopic dermatitis) or gastrointestinal signs (which may fit with cutaneous adverse food

reaction)? These may indicate the possibility of underlying allergic skin disease.
- **Lifestyle.** Cats that have free access to the garden and fields are more likely to encounter parasitic diseases and dermatophytosis.
- **Are any in-contact animals or humans affected?** If so, this narrows the differential diagnosis list considerably to particular infectious or parasitic agents. *Dermatophytosis may cause circular red skin lesions in the owner due to its zoonotic nature, and both cheyletiellosis and flea infestations can give rise to small papular lesions on owners, which are variably pruritic.*
- **Ectoparasite control regime.** Is there a strict regime in place? Always ask owners how frequently they treat their pets, including any in-contact animals in the house. Flea-allergic dermatitis (see Chapter 6) is a common cause of overgrooming and pruritus in cats (Figure 5.26.2).
- **Age of onset.** Parasitic causes of pruritus, such as *Otodectes* and *Cheyletiella* mites, are more likely to be seen in young animals less than 6 months of age or in animals that have recently been acquired

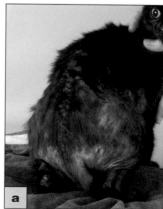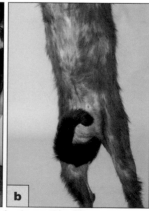

5.26.2 A cat with flea-allergic dermatitis. There are extensive signs of overgrooming on **(a)** the caudal dorsum and **(b)** the ventral abdomen and medial thighs. Flea dirt was found on a coat brushing sample, confirming the diagnosis. A strict flea control regime was instituted for all pets in the household and the environment was also treated. Prednisolone was used initially to control the patient's pruritus; this was then gradually tapered and discontinued.

from a rescue centre. In contrast, epitheliotropic lymphoma is usually a disease of older cats.

■ **Is there any seasonality to the problem?** If so, this could point more towards an underlying atopic dermatitis or a seasonal parasitic problem such as harvest mites.

■ **Does the patient respond to treatment with glucocorticoids?** Flea-allergic dermatitis and atopic dermatitis generally respond well to glucocorticoids.

Clinical examination

A general physical examination should be performed in all cases to look for signs of systemic disease and to check the patient's general health. Some causes of skin disease such as viruses (Figure 5.26.3) may have other systemic signs, e.g. cat 'flu in FHV infection.

Feline calicivirus and feline herpesvirus

■ FCV and FHV can both cause skin disease in cats that may be mistaken for other skin conditions in the early stages.
■ Both can be associated with pruritus.
■ In both cases the cats will usually also have signs of respiratory disease, which underlines the importance of taking a good general history and performing a general physical examination.
■ FHV dermatitis often presents as a facial dermatitis and can be severe in some cases. Lesions commonly seen include oral or skin ulcers on the face, trunk and footpads.
■ FCV dermatitis is typically a transient, self-limiting vesiculo-ulcerative disease. Oral ulcers are most commonly seen but in some cases ulcers occur on the lips and nasal philtrum or, rarely, elsewhere on the body.

Feline poxvirus

■ Feline poxvirus can also cause viral dermatitis. It is most commonly seen in rural hunting cats in the autumn (acquired via bites from rodents, etc.). *Poxvirus infection can be zoonotic.*
■ Primary skin lesions comprise a small scab on the face, neck or forelimbs; this may abscessate.
■ Secondary skin lesions develop a few weeks later and include papules, nodules, scabs, alopecia ± pruritus.
■ Systemic signs (more likely in immunosuppressed cats) can include pyrexia and pneumonia.
■ Diagnosis is by virus isolation from a scab, serology or skin biopsy.
■ Treatment is non-specific: supportive care, and broad-spectrum antibiotics if secondary bacterial infection is present. *Note that glucocorticoids can exacerbate disease.*
■ Prognosis is generally good.

5.26.3   Viral skin disease in cats.

The inside of the mouth should always be checked, as eosinophilic granulomas may be present on the tongue or soft palate (Figure 5.26.4) but general anaesthesia may be required for visualization of some of these lesions.

Dermatological examination

■ Examine the whole animal from nose to tail, including the ventral abdomen.
■ Signs of overgrooming are often apparent on the ventral abdomen in cats, often referred to as 'fur mowing' (Figure 5.26.5).
■ Signs of overgrooming may also be apparent on the limbs.
■ Examine the patient for any other signs of allergic skin disease such as miliary dermatitis or lesions from the eosinophilic granuloma complex.

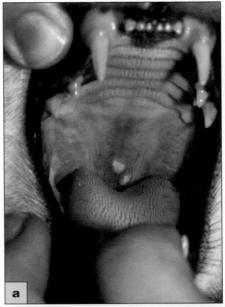

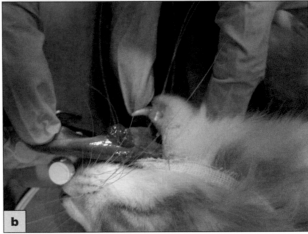

5.26.4   **(a)** Two small white plaques consistent with eosinophilic granulomas are evident on the roof of the mouth of this cat with atopic dermatitis. The cat presented with alopecia, due to overgrooming and pruritus, of the ventral abdomen. This cat was not showing any clinical signs related to the lesions in the oral cavity. **(b)** A large eosinophilic granuloma is present under the tongue of this cat with atopic dermatitis; initial presentation was of overgrooming and pruritus of the hindlegs only. However, upon further questioning regarding the cat's eating habits, it was found that some dysphagia was evident.

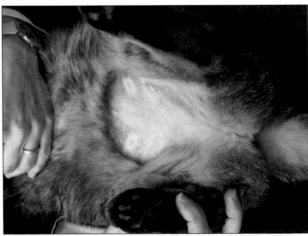

5.26.5   Alopecia on the ventral abdomen of a cat with flea-allergic dermatitis; this type of alopecia is sometimes referred to as 'fur mowing'.

Miliary dermatitis

Miliary dermatitis is a descriptive term used to describe a cutaneous reaction pattern of inflammation commonly seen in cats with a wide variety of skin diseases that cause pruritus and overgrooming. Cats with miliary dermatitis have a fine crusting papular dermatitis.

Differential diagnoses for miliary dermatitis include:

- Flea-allergy dermatitis
- Superficial pyoderma
- Dermatophytosis
- Cheyletiellosis
- Ear mites
- Allergic skin disease (cutaneous adverse food reaction, atopic dermatitis)
- Pemphigus foliaceus
- Cutaneous adverse drug reaction.

Eosinophilic granuloma complex

Eosinophilic granuloma complex (EGC) is a term used to describe a cutaneous reaction pattern in cats that involves several different syndromes, some of which can be pruritic. EGC syndromes comprise:

- Eosinophilic plaque
- Indolent ulcer (rodent ulcer, eosinophilic ulcer)
- Eosinophilic granuloma (linear granuloma).

EGC can arise from multiple different causes and should always highlight the need for a thorough investigation and logical diagnostic approach. Commonly an allergy investigation is required.

Clinical features

Eosinophilic plaque

- Single to multiple erythematous, well circumscribed, raised, eroded or ulcerated plaques.
- **INTENSELY PRURITIC**.
- Lesion distribution: anywhere on the body; commonly on the ventral abdomen and medial thighs.
- Regional lymphadenopathy may be present.

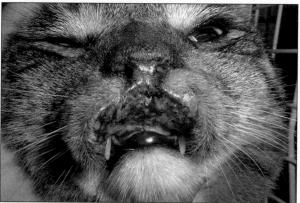

Severe rodent/indolent ulcer of the upper lip, a manifestation of the eosinophilic granuloma complex; this lesion had been present for 6 months. This is a very classical appearance, although not all lesions are this severe. If the lesion is very extensive and affecting the nasal planum, as here, skin biopsy is recommended to ensure that it is an indolent ulcer and not a neoplastic lesion such as a squamous cell carcinoma.

Eosinophilic granuloma

- Lesions usually occur singly.
- Can be variable in appearance: raised firm linear plaques; papular to nodular; oedematous or firm swellings; erythematous; ulcerated; alopecic and/or eroded.
- Usually not painful, nor pruritic.
- Lesion distribution: most common on the caudal aspect of the thigh (linear granuloma), chin or lip (swelling), or in the oral cavity.
- Regional lymphadenopathy may be present.
- Lesions in the oral cavity are characterized by papules, nodules, or well circumscribed plaques; usually on the tongue or palate (see Figure 5.26.4). Cats with oral lesions may be dysphagic.

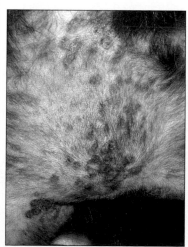

This cat had multiple small eosinophilic plaques on her distal ventral abdomen (the tail is at the bottom of the photo); these lesions were intensely pruritic. The surface of the lesions was moist, and an impression smear revealed large numbers of eosinophils with some coccoid bacteria. The bacteria indicated secondary infection, which is commonly seen in these cases.

Indolent ulcer

- Lesion distribution: commonly affects the upper lip; also reported in the oral cavity.
- Begins as a small crater-like ulcer with raised margin.
- Can be unilateral or bilateral.
- May enlarge progressively and become disfiguring.
- Not painful, nor pruritic.
- Regional lymphadenopathy may be present.

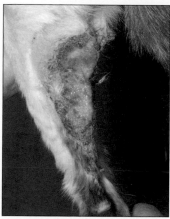

A linear granuloma on the caudal aspect of a cat's thigh; the cat was subsequently diagnosed with atopic dermatitis. An impression smear revealed large numbers of eosinophils and this, combined with the classical presentation which is pathognomonic, allowed a diagnosis of an eosinophilic granuloma to be made.

▶

Differential diagnoses for EGC

EGC arises most commonly due to allergic skin disease: flea allergy, cutaneous adverse food reaction or atopic dermatitis. The main differential diagnoses for EGC are:

- Infections: bacterial, viral or fungal (rarely dermatophytosis can present like an EGC, so a fungal culture should always be performed to exclude this differential)
- Trauma
- Neoplasia: squamous cell carcinoma, mast cell tumour or cutaneous lymphoma.

Diagnosis

Diagnosis is usually based on history, clinical findings and ruling out other differential diagnoses. An impression smear from a moist lesion may reveal large numbers of eosinophils, but neutrophils and bacteria may predominate if the lesion is secondarily infected. It is important when making an impression smear that the glass slide is placed directly on to the lesion and that the area is not aseptically prepared. Skin biopsy (see QRG 5.3.3) is also useful to characterize the lesion and will help rule out some of the differential diagnoses for EGC. The three types of EGC lesion have characteristic histological appearances. Cats with an eosinophilic granuloma or eosinophilic plaque may also have a peripheral eosinophilia.

Once an EGC lesion has been identified, investigation to find the underlying cause should be undertaken. This will usually include a full allergy investigation to rule in/out flea allergy, cutaneous adverse food reaction and atopic dermatitis (see Chapter 6).

Differential diagnoses in overgrooming and pruritus

- Ectoparasites, especially fleas
- Allergic skin disease (see Chapter 6):
  - Flea-allergic dermatitis
  - Cutaneous adverse food reaction
  - Atopic dermatitis
- Dermatophytosis (see Chapter 6).

Diagnostic approach

This is summarized in Figure 5.26.6.

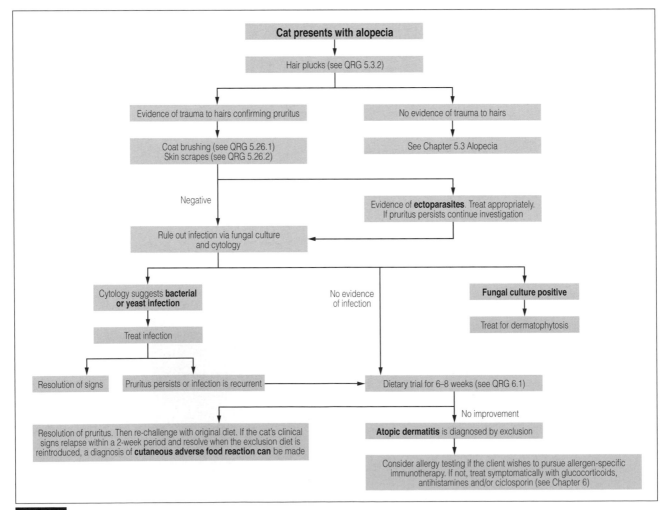

5.26.6 A diagnostic approach to a cat presenting with overgrooming and pruritus.

Diagnostic tests required

- A coat brushing (see QRG 5.26.1) will help determine whether fleas are present and may also detect *Cheyletiella* mites.
- Skin scrapes (see QRG 5.26.2) can also be used to detect mites.
- Hair plucks (see QRG 5.3.2): broken or chewed hairs confirm that the cat is overgrooming and thus likely to be pruritic.
- Cytology (see QRG 5.26.3): impression smears are especially useful when eosinophilic plaques are present, not only for identifying an eosinophilic lesion but also to identify secondary infection that may require treatment.
- Fungal culture (see Chapter 5.3).
- Dietary trial: to exclude a cutaneous adverse food reaction (see QRG 6.1).
- If a diagnosis of atopic dermatitis is made, allergen-specific IgE serology may be appropriate (see Chapter 6).

Treatment recommendations

- Institute a rigorous flea control regime for all animals in the house and the environment if not already in place (see Chapter 6).
- Treat any secondary infection; cefalexin 15 mg/kg orally q12h or clindamycin 5.5 mg/kg orally q12h are suitable choices. Treatment is usually for a minimum of 3 weeks or 1 week past resolution of clinical signs.
- Treatment with glucocorticoids (prednisolone 1 mg/kg orally q24h for 7 days and then on alternate days for seven doses) is useful in the initial stages of investigation to make the cat more comfortable. Glucocorticoid treatment is essential if the cat has EGC lesions; in these cases treatment with daily prednisolone should be continued until the lesions have resolved, and then gradually tapered (see Chapter 6).
- Once infections are controlled, consider starting a dietary trial (see QRG 6.1).

When to refer

Some cases of allergic skin disease are challenging to manage. If the cat is not responding to treatment it is worth considering referral.

What to do when finances are limited

Cats respond well to treatment with glucocorticoids, which are often very effective at controlling allergic skin disease. Ectoparasites are the most common cause of allergic skin disease in the cat, so strict flea control regime should never be compromised.

The cost of some veterinary diets can be prohibitive for clients. Some commercial diets are suitable if they have limited ingredients and are thought to be suitable for the patient based on their previous dietary history. In cases of allergic skin disease, dietary trials (see QRG 6.1) should be performed where possible.

Atopic dermatitis is a diagnosis of exclusion and is not made by blood testing, so making the diagnosis is not expensive. Allergy testing can be costly, however. It is performed to enable selection of allergens to formulate a course of allergen-specific immunotherapy and therefore should only be undertaken when clients want to pursue this course. If the client has limited funds, treatment of atopic dermatitis with glucocorticoids and antihistamines is inexpensive and effective (see Chapter 6).

QRG 5.26.1 Coat brushing
by Natalie Barnard

A recent study has shown that this method of looking for evidence of fleas is much more sensitive than a wet paper test.

1 Brush the cat's coat over a table top or piece of paper.

2 Collect together the brushed material using a glass slide; you should have a pile of hairs and scale.

3 Gently remove the excess hairs from your sample.

4 Mount the remaining scale on to a glass slide.

EITHER Place it on to a slide that has some liquid paraffin on it, placing a coverslip over the top of the sample.

OR Collect the scale on adhesive tape and stick this on to the slide.

5 Examine the sample using a low-power objective X4 or X10. You are looking for flea dirt and *Cheyletiella* mites and their eggs.

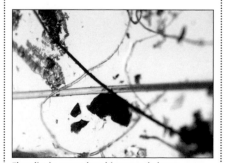

Flea dirt in a coat brushing sample has a characteristic red crystalline appearance.

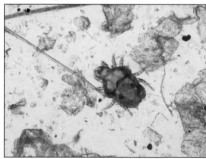

Cheyletiella mite, as seen under the X10 objective lens, in a coat brushing sample. Note the waisted appearance.

QRG 5.26.2 Skin scrapes
by Natalie Barnard

Indications

To identify skin parasites such as:

- *Demodex gatoi*
- *Demodex cati*
- *Notoedres cati*
- *Cheyletiella blakei.*

WARNING

Skin scraping should not be carried out on patients with conditions associated with fragile skin, e.g. hyperadrenocorticism.

Equipment

- No.10 scalpel blades
- Microscope slides
- Liquid paraffin
- Coverslips
- Pencil to label slides Scissors or clippers
- Cotton bud

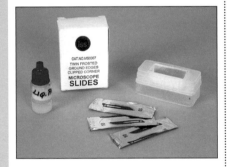

Technique

1 Choose an appropriate area to scrape, new fresh lesions are best. The area may need to be clipped if it is haired. This needs to be done carefully to avoid removing surface scale and crust that may contain important information that you want to scrape; use clippers gently, or scissors, but do not go too close to the skin.

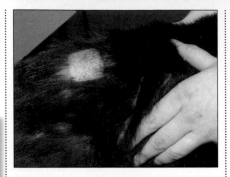

2 Apply liquid paraffin to the skin before scraping. This can be applied with a cotton bud or your finger. It is important to do this to enable you to collect the material you scrape.

3 Use a blade and start scraping the skin at an angle of ~45 degrees, in the direction of hair growth, for a minute or so (length of time depends on factors such as skin thickness, crusting present, etc.), covering the same area of skin until you have capillary ooze, which basically means a small ooze of blood will be present at the end of scraping. You do not need to scrape until you have lots of blood present, as this will affect your sample and make it difficult to examine.

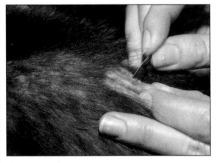

4 Collect the scraped material on the blade and place it on a slide containing liquid paraffin; you may need to transfer your material several times to the slide until you get capillary ooze.

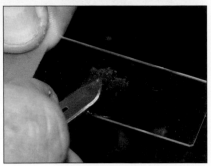

5 Once you have transferred all the material to the slide, cover it with a coverslip. Examine with the microscope using the low-power objective lens X4 or X10.

Results

The most common parasite you are likely to find from a cat skin scrape is *Cheyletiella. Notoedres* and *Demodex* mites (see Figure 19.19) are rarely seen in cats in the UK.

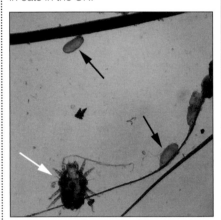

Cheyletiella mite (white arrow) viewed under the X4 objective lens. Note the characteristic waisted body shape. Two *Cheyletiella* eggs are visible (black arrows). (Total original magnification X40.)

QRG 5.26.3 Skin cytology using tape strips and impression smears

by Natalie Barnard

Indications

- To identify whether there is evidence of bacterial or yeast infection of the skin.
- To look for the presence of inflammatory cells.
- Can be used in cases with ulcerative lesions, crusting lesions and/or moist inflamed skin.

Equipment

- Clear adhesive tape: Scotch tape is good as this does not dissolve in the stains. Avoid any 'magic' tapes which are cloudy. You may need to experiment with several different tapes to find which is best
- Microscope slides
- Pencil to label slides
- Diff-Quik stain, water for rinsing slides and paper towel for drying
- Immersion oil

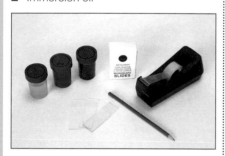

Making a tape strip preparation

1 Find a suitable area to sample (e.g. moist, ulcerated and/or inflamed). Take a piece of adhesive tape approximately 10 cm in length. Hold it at both ends but do not touch the middle of the tape as you do not want to examine your fingerprints at the end of the procedure! Gently press the tape three or four times against the piece of skin you wish to sample, pressing the same piece of tape to the same area of skin each time; the sample will then be several layers of cells thick.

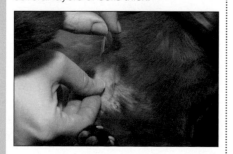

2 Attach one end of the piece of tape to the labelled slide and then fold it back on itself to form a loop so that the sticky side of the tape containing the sample is uppermost. Fix the free end of the tape to the slide.

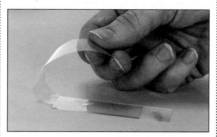

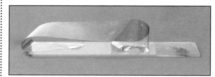

3 Stain the sample. If using Diff-Quik:

- Dip the slide in the first stain (light blue, fixative) for 1–2 seconds only otherwise the tape may become cloudy.

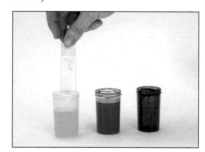

- Then make 5 x 1-second dips in each of the other stains (red followed by dark purple). There is no need to rinse the tape between each stain.

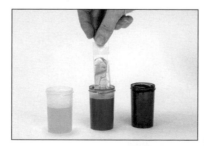

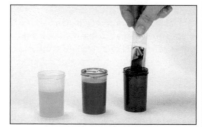

NOTE: If staining an impression smear (see later) the slide requires 5 x 1-second dips in each stain, including the light blue fixative.

4 Rinse the stain off the slide with water (tap water is fine); rinse until the water runs clear.

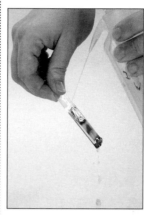

5 Unwrap the loop of tape and stick it on the opposite side of the glass slide, i.e. your label will be on the opposite side of the slide to your sample. The tape will not stick – as it is wet – but the previously sticky side of the tape should now be in contact with the glass slide.

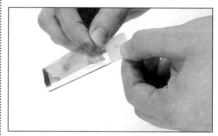

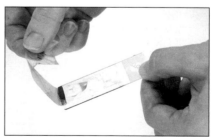

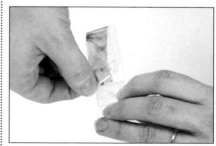

QRG 5.26.3 *continued*

6 Blot the sample dry with a piece of paper towel. Do not be concerned if there is water underneath the tape.

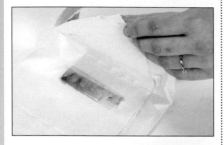

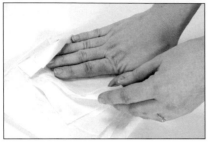

Making a direct impression smear

Moist exudate can be collected from pustules, erosions, ulcers and draining lesions to make an impression smear. Gently press a glass microscope slide against the moist surface of the skin to collect a sample. Alternatively, material may be collected using a swab and gently smeared on to the microscope slide. Allow the sample to dry and then stain (e.g. with Diff-Quik as shown above).

Examination

The slide is now ready to be examined. For a tape sample, keep the tape uppermost.

First examine under low power using the X4 objective, to find an area of interest, and then gradually increase the magnification, finally to use the oil immersion X100 objective. You will only be able to see microorganisms and cells using the oil immersion lens (total magnification will be X1000 due to X10 eyepiece).

Using the oil immersion lens

1. Ensure the lowest objective (usually X4) is in place.
2. Place the slide you wish to examine on to the microscope stage; ensure the stage is fully racked up, i.e. as high as it will go. It is always safer to move the stage *away from* the objective lens rather than towards it, to ensure that the specimen and lens are not damaged.
3. Set the light on a low to medium intensity.
4. Look down the eyepiece(s) and then slowly lower the stage until the sample comes into focus.
5. Scan the slide systematically in parallel rows. Start at one corner and work in either a horizontal or a vertical pattern.
6. When you identify an area of interest under low power, gradually move up through the low power lenses to the X40 lens, racking the stage up and down as needed to ensure that the lens does not make contact with the slide. Once in focus using the X40 lens, move your eyes away from the eyepiece, turn up the light intensity and raise the condenser, so that you can see a bright spot of light under the slide.
7. Lower the stage slightly and place a drop of immersion oil on the slide over the spot of light.
8. Move the oil objective lens into place, taking care not to let the objective crash into the slide.
9. Gradually raise the stage up to the lens very slowly. Watch closely from the side and you will see the drop of oil sucked up onto the lens. When this happens, look down the eyepieces and use the fine focus to bring the image into focus.
10. Once you have examined your sample under oil, remove the slide and clean the oil from the immersion lens.

Examples of results

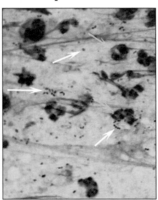

Coccoid bacteria (white arrows) and neutrophils (blue arrows) under oil immersion lens (X1000 total magnification).

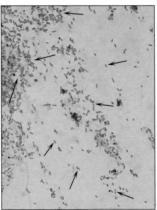

Very large numbers of rod-shaped bacteria (black arrows indicate a few of these) under oil immersion (X1000 total magnification).

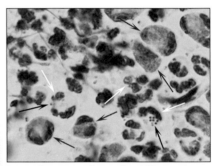

Impression smear of an eosinophilic granuloma, viewed under oil immersion (X1000 total magnification). Neutrophils can be seen (white arrows) together with intracellular coccoid bacteria (black arrows), and eosinophils (red arrows) containing pink granules within their cytoplasm. The cat was treated with antibacterials to treat the secondary infection and prednisolone to control pruritus and treat the eosinophilic granuloma.

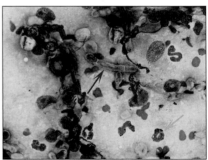

Impression smear of a fungal granuloma caused by *Alternaria*, viewed under oil immersion (X1000 total magnification). Fungal hyphae (red arrow) and neutrophils (blue arrows) can be seen.

Pica

Samantha Taylor

Pica is the abnormal appetite for non-food material, e.g. wool and other fabrics, cat litter, houseplants or licking concrete or stones. It can arise as a behavioural problem or can be the result of an underlying medical problem such as anaemia. Thorough history-taking may suggest whether the pica is due to a behavioural or a medical condition.

Behavioural pica

Behavioural pica is often a chronic problem, with affected cats being otherwise healthy. However, cats may be presented for complications as a result of behavioural pica such as ingestion of linear foreign bodies or toxic substances. Behavioural pica may increase during times of stress (e.g. house move, new pet).

Fabric eating

Siamese and related breeds are particularly prone to fabric eating and this is often a chronic problem starting at a young age. It has also been reported in Burmese cats. It is presumed that there is a genetic component to this habit and, although incompletely understood, it is thought that the endorphin release the cat experiences makes the habit addictive. Some cases are very difficult to manage and consultation with a veterinary behaviourist is highly recommended. Treatment via a behaviourist includes avoidance of the desired materials, using play and environmental enrichment to occupy and distract the cat, and, occasionally, medication.

Cats kept exclusively indoors may be more likely to develop pica. Houseplant ingestion (particularly dangerous if toxic plants such as those from the *Lilium* family are ingested (see Chapter 4.9) and chewing electric wires are seen in this group.

Pica secondary to a medical condition

Pica may also be a clinical sign of chronic anaemia (of various underlying causes). Affected cats may be presented for ingestion of cat litter for example (Figure 5.27.1), or licking concrete surfaces. Owners may not have noticed other clinical signs of anaemia (pallor, lethargy, inappetence). Melaena may be noted in cats with gastrointestinal blood loss.

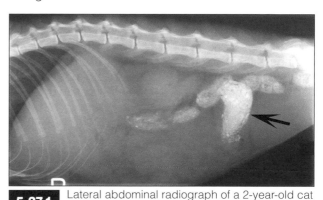

5.27.1 Lateral abdominal radiograph of a 2-year-old cat presented with severe anaemia and related pica, which comprised ingestion of cat litter. The pica had resulted in small intestinal obstruction that necessitated surgery. There is mineralized material in both the small and large intestine. Dilation of the small intestine (arrowed) indicated obstruction (small intestinal diameter in the cat should not exceed 12 mm and it was >12 mm in this case). This loop of bowel was identified as small intestine as it is not in the position or orientation of the ascending, transverse or descending colon; a ventrodorsal view would help confirm this. (Courtesy of Andrea Harvey)

Pica is also occasionally seen in association with gastrointestinal disease. Affected cats consume excessive grass or plant material and present with a concurrent history of vomiting, diarrhoea, weight loss or inappetence. Investigation for underlying gastrointestinal disease is appropriate in such cases.

Grass/outdoor plant ingestion in cats

Grass ingestion is common in cats. The reason for this is not fully understood but it is suspected that grass has some beneficial effects on the gastrointestinal tract, including easing nausea. Grass eating is not problematic unless the cat also exhibits clinical signs of gastrointestinal disease, such as vomiting (besides vomiting the ingested ▶

Polyphagia

Darren Foster

Polyphagia is defined as an excessive intake of food. In animals this presents as an increased appetite. Polyphagia can be either physiological (e.g. from increased energy demands such as with exercise, cold, pregnancy or lactation) or pathological (e.g. from malassimilation/malabsorption of nutrients, increased metabolic rate, an inability to use nutrients). Polyphagia may also occur with highly palatable diets or for behavioural reasons (e.g. boredom, following neutering) or with certain medications (e.g. corticosteroids and some anticonvulsants). Polyphagia may therefore be accompanied by weight gain or weight loss.

Aetiology

Common causes of polyphagia are shown in Figure 5.28.1. If apparent polyphagia is present without any change in bodyweight, this may represent the early stages of the condition associated with any of the causes listed.

Clinical approach

Signalment and a thorough history (including, in particular, specifics regarding diet and calculation of caloric intake, changes in lifestyle, presence of vomiting/diarrhoea, polyuria/polydipsia) and physical examination (in particular, palpation for abdominal masses, intestinal abnormalities, palpation for goitre, cardiac auscultation) are vitally important in narrowing the list of differential diagnoses.

Polyphagia with weight gain

The causes of polyphagia with weight gain (Figure 5.28.1) should be easily elucidated from history-taking. Overfeeding, extremely palatable foods and boredom are common causes. Iatrogenic polyphagia is common with administration of certain drugs such as corticosteroids, anticonvulsants, progestogens and benzodiazepines.

Polyphagia with weight loss

In the majority of cases, further investigations such as a complete blood count and biochemistry panel are

Polyphagia with weight gain

- Overfeeding
- Boredom
- Palatable food
- Iatrogenic (glucocorticoids, anticonvulsants)
- Hyperadrenocorticism

Polyphagia with weight loss

Physiological causes

- Pregnancy
- Lactation
- Exercise
- Cold environment

Pathological causes

- Malassimilation/malabsorption
  - Infiltrative gastrointestinal disease, e.g. **inflammatory bowel disease**, neoplasia (e.g. **lymphoma**, mast cell tumour, adenocarcinoma)
  - Exocrine pancreatic insufficiency
  - Right-sided heart failure
  - Lymphocytic cholangitis
- Inability to utilize nutrients
  - **Diabetes mellitus**
  - Gastrointestinal parasitism, e.g. ascarids, *Giardia*
  - Acromegaly, hyperadrenocorticism
- Increased metabolic rate
  - Hyperthyroidism

5.28.1 Causes of polyphagia; common pathological causes are highlighted in bold.

indicated, along with urinalysis (specific gravity and dipstick). Depending on the history and physical examination findings, additional investigations may also be required to reach a diagnosis. Causes such as pregnancy, lactation, cold environment and exercise can be excluded/identified with a thorough history.

Inability to use nutrients

Diabetes mellitus can be diagnosed by detecting significant hyperglycaemia with concurrent glycosuria (± ketonuria). Stress-related causes of hyperglycaemia and glycosuria can be excluded by measuring serum fructosamine concentrations (which should only be elevated in cats with diabetes mellitus (DM)) and/or assessing for glycosuria in a home-collected urine sample (see Chapter 14).

Diseases that result in secondary DM (usually insulin-resistant DM, i.e. unstable whilst on >2 IU/kg per dose of insulin), such as acromegaly and hyperadrenocorticism, require more specific testing. Hyperadrenocorticism may be diagnosed with a combination of imaging (abdominal ultrasonography; brain and/or abdominal CT or brain MRI) and endocrine function testing (ACTH stimulation and low-dose dexamethasone suppression test). However, other clinical signs will often be present (e.g. skin fragility, thin skin, pot belly) that increase suspicion of these more unusual endocrinopathies (see *BSAVA Manual of Canine and Feline Endocrinology*).

Parasitism can be confirmed by faecal analysis or a therapeutic trial with worming medications such as fenbendazole.

Malassimilation/malabsorption

Gastrointestinal signs such as vomiting and diarrhoea often accompany diseases that lead to malassimilation or malabsorption, but owners may not observe these signs (especially with outdoor toileting). Cats have a great capacity to absorb water from the colon, making diarrhoea less common than in other species.

Diffuse infiltrative small intestinal disease can lead to polyphagia with weight loss. In early or mild disease, maintenance of bodyweight may be possible if sufficient polyphagia compensates for the degree of malabsorption. Clinical findings may include diffuse intestinal thickening and mesenteric lymph node enlargement. Infiltrative disease may be inflammatory or neoplastic (low- or high-grade intestinal lymphosarcoma, mast cell tumours). Rarer causes include lymphangiectasia. Diagnosis involves imaging of the gastrointestinal tract (ultrasonography) and, ultimately, histopathology of biopsy specimens taken via endoscopy or exploratory laparotomy. Lowered serum concentrations of folate and/or vitamin B12 (cobalamin) may also indicate the presence of malabsorption in the proximal and/or distal (ileum) small intestine, respectively (see Chapter 5.12).

Exocrine pancreatic insufficiency is a rare disease in cats. Suspicion is raised with a combination of weight loss, polyphagia and steatorrhoea. Demonstrating a sub-normal fasting serum trypsin-like immunoreactivity (TLI) confirms the diagnosis.

Increased metabolic rate

Hyperthyroidism (see Chapter 14) is usually easily diagnosed by demonstrating an elevated serum thyroxine (T4) concentration in combination with compatible history (polyphagia, polydipsia, polyuria, vomiting, diarrhoea, hyperactivity) and clinical findings (poor body condition, palpable goitre, tachycardia ± a heart murmur and hypertension).

Neoplasia

Some cats with neoplasms may maintain or have an increased appetite. An abdominal mass (see Chapter 5.2) or thickened loops of intestine may be palpable. Occult neoplasia may be detected by: thoracic radiography (to look for lung metastases); abdominal ultrasonography (presence of masses, infiltration of gastrointestinal walls); evaluation of abdominal lymph nodes; sampling of any masses or enlarged lymph nodes (e.g. by fine-needle aspiration if possible); or whole body CT examination.

Further reading

Behrend EN (2010) Polyphagia. In: *Textbook of Veterinary Internal Medicine*, ed. SJ Ettinger and EC Feldman, pp. 175–179. Saunders Elsevier, St. Louis
Tilley LP and Smith FWK Jr (2007) Polyphagia. In: *Blackwell's Five-minute Veterinary Consult*, p. 1109. Blackwell, Ames, Iowa

Polyuria and polydipsia

Sarah Caney

Polydipsia is a reasonably common clinical sign reported by owners of older cats. Most commonly polydipsia occurs as a compensatory response to polyuria, and therefore polyuria and polydipsia (PU/PD) are usually grouped together when considering differential diagnoses and the diagnostic approach. In indoor cats that use a litter tray, polyuria may be noticed by owners as an increase in the volume of 'wet clumps' of litter in the litter tray. In cats that toilet outside, however, polyuria almost always will go unnoticed. Regardless of the cat's lifestyle, polydipsia is more frequently the clinical sign noticed by owners and will therefore be the focus in this chapter.

Whilst the list of differential diagnoses for polydipsia is relatively long (Figure 5.29.1), in most cats the diagnosis is usually one or more of the following:

- Diabetes mellitus
- Chronic kidney disease (CKD)
- Hyperthyroidism.

Classification	Causative condition or factor
Physiological	For example: change in diet (wet to dry; offering 'tasty' liquids)
Endocrine	**Hyperthyroidism.** *Polydipsia often mild in these cases*
	Diabetes mellitus (including secondary to hyperadrenocorticism, acromegaly or hyperprogesteronism). *Marked polydipsia (>100 ml/kg/day) often present*
	Hyperadrenocorticism
	Central diabetes insipidus (CDI). *Absolute deficiency in amount of circulating ADH. Primary (congenital) or secondary (e.g. head trauma, CNS neoplasia) causes. Complete CDI associated with hyposthenuria (USG 1.004–1.008) and profound polydipsia (often >200 ml/kg/day)*
	Hypoadrenocorticism. *Rare*
	Primary hyperaldosteronism. *Uncommon*
	Phaeochromocytoma. *Rare*
	Hypertestosteronism. *Rare*

5.29.1 Causes of polydipsia. The common causes are in bold. ADH = antidiuretic hormone (vasopressin); USG = urine specific gravity. (continues) ▶

Classification	Causative condition or factor
Renal	Acute kidney injury (AKI)
	Chronic kidney disease (CKD). *Variable polydipsia reported according to severity of renal disease*
	Pyelonephritis
	Nephrogenic diabetes insipidus (NDI). *Failure of the renal tubule to respond to ADH. Primary and secondary (e.g. pyelonephritis, hyperthyroidism, pyometra) causes. May be complete or partial. Complete NDI associated with hyposthenuria (USG 1.004–1.008) and profound polydipsia (often >200 ml/kg/day)*
	Primary renal glycosuria
	Post-obstructive diuresis
Electrolyte disturbances	Hypercalcaemia
	Hypokalaemia
	Hyponatraemia
Compensatory polydipsia	Gastrointestinal water loss (e.g. vomiting, diarrhoea)
	Respiratory water loss (e.g. open-mouth breathing)
	Water loss through the skin (e.g. severe exudation or severe pruritus resulting in overgrooming and salivary loss)
	Accumulation of fluid in body cavities
Hepatic disease	
Pyometra	
Haematological	Polycythaemia and hyperviscosity syndrome
Behavioural/neurological	For example: brain tumour; possibly cognitive dysfunction
Psychogenic polydipsia	Not well described in cats
Iatrogenic	For example: diuretic therapy; phenobarbital; salt supplementation (some urinary diets include added salt to increase thirst and reduce USG)

5.29.1 (continued) Causes of polydipsia. The common causes are marked in bold. ADH = antidiuretic hormone (vasopressin); USG = urine specific gravity.

Water intake

Quantification of water intake is usually recommended to confirm suspected polydipsia. However, clear guidelines regarding what constitutes normal and abnormal water intake are lacking:

- Many clinicians estimate that normal cats drink 20–50 ml/kg/day
- Textbooks define polydipsia as water consumption >100 ml/kg/day.

Many factors need to be taken into consideration when assessing a cat's water consumption.

- **Diet:** Cats eating a dry diet will drink more than cats eating a wet diet. Cats offered appetizing liquids such as milk may choose to drink more.
- **Grooming behaviour:** Grooming results in water loss via saliva on the coat. Grooming is used as one mechanism to reduce body temperature and so is increased in cats living in warm climates. Meticulous groomers, and cats with skin disease, are likely to have greater water consumption than other cats. This category may also include cats staying at a boarding cattery, where there may be little to do other than eat, sleep and groom.
- **Activity:** Increased activity may be associated with an increase in water requirements.
- **Play:** Some cats enjoy playing with water (e.g. a dripping tap) and tend to have a greater water intake. Providing water fountains for cats often increases drinking.
- **Other factors:** The amount of water consumed by a cat may be influenced by factors including the type, size and location of the water bowl, e.g. cats prefer to drink from large-diameter bowls filled to the brim.

Most owners of healthy cats do not see them drinking unless they are indoor-only and fed a dry diet. Many cats prefer puddles and ponds to the water offered by owners and, particularly in cats allowed free access outdoors, it can be difficult for owners to know how much their cat is drinking. Given these considerations, and the lack of clear guidelines for water consumption, a better definition of polydipsia may be: 'drinking more than is considered normal for that cat'. Many cats reported as polydipsic by their owners will still have a water consumption of <50 ml/kg/day.

While measurement of water intake is helpful in diagnosis (the magnitude of the polydipsia helps to narrow down the diagnostic list) it is not always easy for owners to do this. Water intake should be monitored with the cat in its home environment, since hospitalized patients often drink less. In multi-animal households, knowledge of total household water consumption is useful in monitoring progression of illnesses such as CKD and diabetes mellitus. Water intake is usually an excellent indicator of diabetic control (Figure 5.29.2).

If hospitalized, urine output can be measured using non-absorbent cat litter or clean aquarium gravel. Measuring the urine specific gravity can also be helpful; if USG is >1.040 it is unlikely that the cat's thirst is pathological. Exceptions to this would include those cats with increased loss of fluids (e.g. from diarrhoea or exudative skin disease), where a compensatory thirst is required to prevent dehydration.

Approach to diagnosis

An approach to a cat with polydipsia is illustrated in Figure 5.29.3 (overleaf).

A thorough history and physical examination may reveal clues as to the cause of the polydipsia, even if this is the sole/major clinical sign reported by the owner. Quantification of water intake to confirm the polydipsia and define the severity is helpful, if possible (see above).

Urinalysis

Urinalysis comprising urine specific gravity (USG) and dipstick testing is a quick and cost-effective way of confirming significant polydipsia (USG will be ≤1.040) and of identifying diabetes mellitus (glucose positive on dipstick).

If USG is ≤1.040, haematology, serum biochemistry (including calcium, potassium, sodium and total serum thyroxine) and more detailed urinalysis (including sediment examination (see QRG 4.11.3), urine protein-to-creatinine ratio (UPC), bacterial culture) should be performed. A cystocentesis sample (see QRG 4.11.4) is required for culture. Older cats with USG ≤1.040 are more vulnerable to bacterial urinary tract infections but, unfortunately, many of these are clinically 'silent' in terms of urinary signs. Vague systemic clinical signs such as malaise, lethargy and dementia may be present in some of these cats.

In those cats with a compensatory polydipsia due to excessive fluid loss, concentrated urine (USG >1.040) should be produced.

> **PRACTICAL TIP**
>
> Remember that dipstick estimates of USG are very inaccurate and refractometers should always be used for USG measurement.

Further tests

If urinalysis fails to identify a cause of polydipsia, further investigations may be indicated.

Time point	24-hour water consumption	Comments
Diabetes mellitus just diagnosed	370–510 ml (92.5–127.5 ml/kg/day)	Toots is severely and persistently polydipsic
Diabetes well controlled	120–180 ml (30–45 ml/kg/day)	Toots's water intake has dropped dramatically. Serum fructosamine results confirm that the diabetes is now well controlled. Although fed a totally wet diet, Toots's water intake is still noticeable due to IRIS Stage 2 chronic kidney disease in addition to her diabetes mellitus
Urinary tract infection	260–290 ml (65–72.5 ml/kg/day)	Toots's increase in water intake prompted veterinary assessment, at which point a urinary tract infection was diagnosed by culture of a cystocentesis urine sample. Once treated, Toots's diabetes mellitus once again came under control

5.29.2 An example of the usefulness of water consumption measurement in cats. (Data extracted from records relating to Toots: a 13-year-old female neutered DSH cat with diabetes mellitus and CKD.)

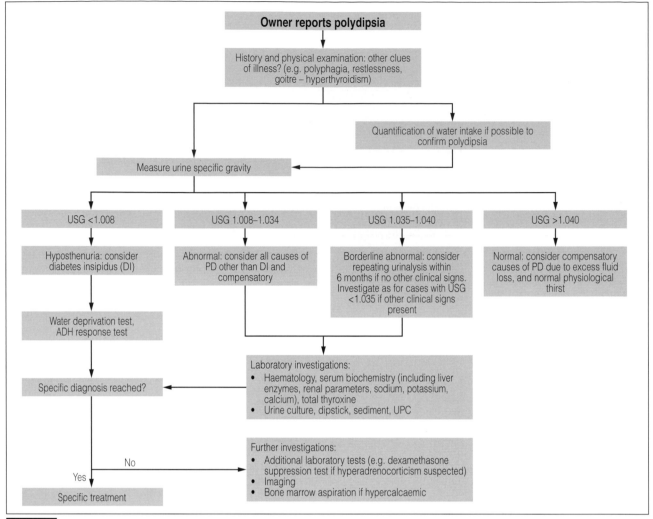

Owner reports polydipsia

History and physical examination: other clues of illness? (e.g. polyphagia, restlessness, goitre – hyperthyroidism)

Quantification of water intake if possible to confirm polydipsia

Measure urine specific gravity

| USG <1.008 | USG 1.008–1.034 | USG 1.035–1.040 | USG >1.040 |

Hyposthenuria: consider diabetes insipidus (DI)

Abnormal: consider all causes of PD other than DI and compensatory

Borderline abnormal: consider repeating urinalysis within 6 months if no other clinical signs. Investigate as for cases with USG <1.035 if other clinical signs present

Normal: consider compensatory causes of PD due to excess fluid loss, and normal physiological thirst

Water deprivation test, ADH response test

Specific diagnosis reached?

Laboratory investigations:
* Haematology, serum biochemistry (including liver enzymes, renal parameters, sodium, potassium, calcium), total thyroxine
* Urine culture, dipstick, sediment, UPC

Further investigations:
* Additional laboratory tests (e.g. dexamethasone suppression test if hyperadrenocorticism suspected)
* Imaging
* Bone marrow aspiration if hypercalcaemic

No Yes

Specific treatment

5.29.3 An approach to a cat with polydipsia.

* Laboratory tests:
  * Pre- and postprandial bile acids (to detect hepatopathies)
  * ACTH stimulation test (hyperadrenocorticism, hypoadrenocorticism, hyperprogesteronism)
  * Dexamethasone suppression test (hyperadrenocorticism)
  * Endogenous adrenocorticotropic hormone (ACTH) (hyperadrenocorticism)
  * Insulin-like growth factor 1 (acromegaly)
  * Plasma aldosterone and renin (hyperaldosteronism)
  * Plasma parathyroid hormone levels (primary hyperparathyroidism)

Most of these tests are not often performed in first-opinion practice, and the advice of a specialist should be sought regarding their performance and interpretation.

* Imaging:
  * Thoracic and abdominal radiography (may detect, for example, cardiomegaly with

hyperthyroidism, acromegaly; hepatomegaly with diabetes mellitus)
  * More advanced imaging may necessitate referral depending on experience available but may include:
    – Echocardiography (e.g. left ventricular hypertrophy with acromegaly)
    – Abdominal ultrasonography (e.g. adrenomegaly with hyperadrenocorticism and acromegaly)
    – Cervical ultrasonography (parathyroid tumour)
    – MRI or CT (e.g. pituitary macro tumour with hyperadrenocorticism, acromegaly).
* Bone marrow biopsy (see QRG 5.4.3) (for investigation of unsolved hypercalcaemia).
* Water deprivation test/modified water deprivation test (for diabetes insipidus (DI)) and ADH response test (for central DI, e.g. following head trauma or resulting from a neoplasm) are rarely indicated, as DI is so rare in cats; it may be wise to seek the advice of a specialist when considering these tests.

Pyrexia and hyperthermia

Mike Lappin

Elevated body temperature in cats (>39.2°C) can arise due to hyperthermia or pyrexia (fever).

- **Hyperthermia** results from increased muscle activity, increased environmental temperature, or increased metabolic rate. Stress-associated hyperthermia appears to occur in many cats, sometimes during transport to the veterinary clinic. Opioids and ketamine have been associated with a mild to moderate, self-limiting (a few hours) perioperative hyperthermia in cats.
- **Pyrexia** occurs when the thermoregulatory set point in the hypothalamus is raised, resulting in increased body temperature from physiological mechanisms, inducing endogenous heat production or heat conservation. The alteration in thermoregulatory set point is induced by soluble factors, such as cytokines, released by leucocytes activated due to, for example, bacterial (such as following a cat bite), viral, fungal and parasitic agents, neoplasia, tissue necrosis, vaccination or primary immune-mediated diseases. The thermoregulatory set point can also be altered by intracranial disease (e.g. trauma, neoplasia) and some drugs (e.g. tetracyclines). Shivering and vasoconstriction are important physiological responses to a thermoregulatory set point change, and result, respectively, in generation or conservation of heat.

Hyperthermia should be differentiated from pyrexia by determining whether the cat has been exposed recently to increased environmental temperature, or has increased muscle activity due to excitement, physical exertion or seizures. Apparently normal cats with elevated body temperature should be encouraged to lie quietly in a cool examination room accompanied by the client for 15–20 minutes, and body temperature should then be measured again. However, if elevation is only mild (≤39.6°C) and stress is also evident, repeat measurement may not be required.

If hyperthermia has been ruled out and no obvious cause of pyrexia is apparent (clinical signs and clinical examination are unrewarding and a short course of an antibacterial such as amoxicillin has failed to resolve the pyrexia), where high body temperature persists for >2 weeks the case can be classified as **pyrexia of unknown origin** (PUO).

Causes

Overall, infectious causes of pyrexia are more common than primary immune-mediated diseases or neoplasia in cats (see Figure 5.30.1). Many causes of fever in cats have clinical findings that can be used to rank the primary differential diagnoses prior to performing diagnostic investigations or instituting a therapeutic plan.

Signalment

The age, breed and sex of the cat can help narrow the differential list; e.g. young cats often have infectious diseases whilst older cats often develop neoplasia. Feline infectious peritonitis is most common in purebred cats. Male cats are more likely to fight, partly explaining the increased incidence, compared to females, of FIV and haemoplasma infections, as well as common presenting problems like cat bite abscesses.

History

It is necessary to determine whether the cat is being administered any medicines, since some drugs (e.g. tetracyclines) can induce pyrexia. Vaccination can also induce pyrexia; usually within 7 days (Moore *et al.*, 2007). Which vaccines have been administered and the interval used may help rank the differentials for pyrexia, as vaccine-induced immune responses can wane with time, making cats more susceptible to some infections (e.g. FHV, feline calicivirus).

The owner should be questioned as to whether the cat fights or hunts, as these activities may be associated with some of the differential diagnoses for pyrexia (e.g. cat bite abscess or cellulitis, FIV or FeLV infection, haemoplasma infection, toxoplasmosis, poxvirus). Determining the prey species for outdoor cats may be helpful, as they can transmit infectious diseases associated with pyrexia: e.g. songbirds (salmonellosis), rabbits (tularaemia), rodents (*Toxoplasma gondii*).

Since many causes of pyrexia are transmissible, the environment of the cat should be assessed with regard to recent exposure to other cats (potential FHV, FeLV, feline coronavirus), excrement (potential *Campylobacter*), ectoparasites (e.g. *Ctenocephalides felis* may transmit *Bartonella*) or bite wounds (e.g. cat bite abscess, potential FIV, FeLV or haemoplasmas). Some infectious agents have limited geographical distribution and so the travel history of the cat is important (e.g. *Ixodes* ticks may transmit *Anaplasma phagocytophilum* in parts of Europe). It should also be determined whether family members have similar clinical signs of disease, as some agents are zoonotic (e.g. *Salmonella*).

Owners should also be questioned concerning any clinical signs involving organ systems commonly associated with pyrexia (e.g. oral cavity, central nervous system, cardiopulmonary system, urogenital system, subcutaneous tissues, limbs, peritoneal cavity, gastrointestinal tract, liver and pancreas).

Physical examination

Anorexia, depression, hyperpnoea, reluctance to move, and stiffness from muscle, joint or meningeal discomfort are common non-specific manifestations of pyrexia in cats. Clinical signs or physical examination findings associated with the primary organ systems involved with the primary infection, or with tissue necrosis, neoplasia or immune-mediated disease may be evident. In some cases, the only significant finding on physical examination is pyrexia.

- Some oral cavity diseases (e.g. FCV infection) are associated with pyrexia. The oral cavity should be examined carefully for: dental disease; infiltrative diseases; increased mucus; red, pale or icteric mucous membranes; petechiae; or tonsillar enlargement.
- The nares should be examined for evidence of discharges. Mucopurulent discharges generally indicate primary or secondary bacterial (e.g. *Bordetella bronchiseptica*; *Pasteurella*) or fungal infection (e.g. *Cryptococcus neoformans*).
- The body should be examined carefully for any evidence of cat bite abscesses or cellulitis, focusing on regions commonly affected by bites (see Chapter 5.8).
- The chest should be auscultated carefully for: cardiac murmurs (see QRG 1.5) (e.g. from bacterial endocarditis); muffled heart or lung sounds (e.g. from pyothorax or FIP); or pulmonary

crackles or wheezes (e.g. from bacterial pneumonia or bronchitis). *Bartonella* infection has recently been associated with bacterial endocarditis and myocarditis in cats. The anterior chest should be gently compressed to check for mediastinal masses (e.g. lymphoma or thymoma).

- The external lymph nodes and spleen should be palpated; enlargement may indicate immune stimulation or neoplasia.
- Cats showing clinical signs of stiffness should have their muscles, long bones and spinal column palpated to assess for conditions such as myositis (potentially infectious (e.g. *Toxoplasma gondii*) or immune-mediated), bacterial osteomyelitis or discospondylitis. The joints should be palpated separately, and gently extended and flexed while evaluating for swelling, pain or redness (potential immune-mediated or infectious causes of polyarthritis).
- The abdomen should be palpated for evidence of organomegaly (e.g. neoplasia), peritoneal effusion (e.g. peritonitis), or pain (e.g. peritonitis or pancreatitis).
- A thorough ophthalmic examination (see QRG 1.3) should be performed to evaluate for evidence of anterior or posterior segment inflammation. Uveitis occurs with several infectious agents associated with pyrexia in cats, including *Toxoplasma gondii*, FeLV, FIV, FHV, *Bartonella henselae*, *Ehrlichia* and fungi (see Chapter 8). However, the lack of uveitis does not exclude these differentials.

Diagnostic plan

Obvious causes of pyrexia (e.g. subcutaneous abscessation, bite wounds, upper respiratory infections) are treated appropriately, or a further diagnostic plan is formulated. Readers are referred to relevant sections of Chapters 4 and 5 for details on diagnostic evaluation for cats with clinical signs of respiratory, gastrointestinal, liver, urinary, cardiac and dermatological disease.

For cats with pyrexia without a readily apparent cause, a complete blood cell count, serum biochemistry panel, urinalysis, FeLV antigen assay and anti-FIV antibody assay are indicated as a minimum. The results of these assays are usually used to make a further diagnostic plan or to direct the therapeutic plan.

Figure 5.30.1 lists some of the more common causes of apparent PUO that may not have other clinical examination findings that direct the diagnostic investigations or therapeutic plan.

Syndrome/agent	Other findings	Diagnostic plan	Therapeutic plan
Infectious			
* *Anaplasma phagocytophilum*	*Ixodes* exposure, polyarthritis	PCR, serology	Doxycycline
Bartonella	*Ctenocephalides felis* (flea) exposure, uveitis, cardiac murmur, hyperglobulinaemia	PCR, serology	Doxycycline
* *Ehrlichia*	Tick exposure, cytopenias, proteinuria	PCR, serology	Doxycycline

5.30.1 Diagnostic and therapeutic plans for some causes of pyrexia of unknown origin in cats. Worldwide geographical variation in the prevalence of some of the infectious diseases listed exists; those reported in the area in which the cat lives should be considered. Asterisks indicate those regarded as being **less common** causes of PUO. See Chapter 19 for more detail on diagnosis and treatment of infectious diseases. (continues) ▶

Syndrome/agent	Other findings	Diagnostic plan	Therapeutic plan
Infectious (continued)			
Feline infectious peritonitis	Lymphopenia, hyperglobulinaemia, uveitis, effusions, organomegaly	Combination of diagnostics	Treatment not effective; palliative steroids, interferon could be tried
* *Francisella tularensis*	Lagomorph exposure	Serology	Doxycycline
Haemoplasmas	History of fighting, haemolytic anaemia	PCR	Doxycycline
* *Rickettsia felis*	*Ctenocephalides felis* exposure	Serology	Doxycycline
Salmonella (songbird fever)	History of hunting, gastrointestinal signs in 50%	Blood culture	Based on susceptibility
Toxoplasma gondii	History of hunting, uveitis, muscle pain, CNS disease, dyspnoea, hepatic disease	Serology	Clindamycin
* *Yersinia pestis* (plague)	Travel history, lymphadenopathy, pneumonia	Culture, fluorescent antibody test, serology	Doxycycline
Neoplasia			
	Varies by organ system involvement	Thoracic and abdominal radiography, biopsy	Treat specific disease; control non-specific pyrexia
Primary immune-mediated diseases			
Haemolytic anaemia		Spherocytes, agglutination, Coombs' test; exclude drugs and haemoplasmas	Prednisolone
* Thrombocytopenia		Exclude infectious causes	Prednisolone
* Polyarthritis		Exclude *Anaplasma* and mycoplasmas	Prednisolone

5.30.1 (continued) Diagnostic and therapeutic plans for some causes of pyrexia of unknown origin in cats. Worldwide geographical variation in the prevalence of some of the infectious diseases listed exists; those reported in the area in which the cat lives should be considered. Asterisks indicate those regarded as being **less common** causes of PUO. See Chapter 19 for more detail on diagnosis and treatment of infectious diseases.

Treatment plan

Hyperthermia

Cats with hyperthermia from stress do not need primary treatment, as their temperature will decrease while in a cool examination room.

Cats with hyperthermia from increased muscle activity or increased metabolic rate should be treated for the primary disease causing these, e.g. myopathy, hyperthyroidism. Whilst awaiting management of such disorders, treatment of marked hyperthermia (>41°C) comprises cooling the cat with intravenous fluids at room temperature (gastric, bladder or peritoneal lavage with room temperature fluids have also been reported for treatment of severe hyperthermia but are very rarely required). This cools the animal's core without causing peripheral vasoconstriction, which would limit further cooling. Fans can also be used.

Pyrexia

In cats with suspected infectious, neoplastic, or primary immune-mediated causes of pyrexia, multiple specific and non-specific therapeutic options are available.

Intravenous administration of fluids at room temperature (see QRG 4.1.3) may help maintain body temperature at safe levels (<39.2°C). Using a cool cage, or directing a fan towards the cat may also be effective. *However, it should be remembered that, since pyrexia in general is biologically helpful, artificial lowering of body temperature with fans, drugs (e.g. NSAIDs) or by other means is usually not indicated.*

Treatment of the primary disease should result in resolution of pyrexia in 2–3 days. However, if chronic pyrexia is present that results in morbidity (depression, inappetence), multiple NSAIDs are available (see Chapter 3) that can be used to decrease body temperature transiently, if indicated and if risks for toxicity are minimized. Prednisolone (1 mg/kg orally q24h) can be used to lessen pyrexia while waiting for response to the primary therapy if absolutely necessary, or if immune-mediated disease is suspected; ideally, prednisolone should be avoided if immune-mediated disease is not suspected, and consideration should be given to referral of the cat to a specialist.

It can be difficult to differentiate primary immune-mediated from infectious causes of pyrexia in some cats. This is particularly true for the flea- and tick-associated blood-borne infections. Oral doxycycline (10 mg/kg q24h or 5 mg/kg q12h) is effective for most of these infections (but see Chapter 3 for possible side effects). Administration of prednisolone (2 mg/kg orally q24h) is unlikely to exacerbate vector-borne diseases in cats, and will help control pyrexia and other clinical manifestations of disease. Thus, use of doxycycline and prednisolone concurrently is considered for cats with primary immune-mediated and vector-borne diseases on the same differential list.

Reference

Moore GE, DeSantis-Kerr AC, Guptill LF *et al.* (2007) Adverse events after vaccine administration in cats: 2,560 cases (2002–2005). *Journal of the American Veterinary Medical Association* **231**, 94–100

Raised liver parameters

Kathleen Tennant

Aminotransferase enzymes

Aminotranferase enzymes commonly measured are alanine aminotransferase (ALT) and aspartate aminotransferase (AST). Increases in the concentrations of these enzymes indicate injury or insult to the hepatocellular elements of the liver, giving rise to hepatocellular death and rupture, or leakage in less severe injury.

Alanine aminotransferase

ALT is present free in the cytoplasm of hepatocytes, in concentrations markedly higher than in blood. Release into the blood occurs where there is any loss of integrity of the cell membrane, making this a relatively sensitive marker of hepatocellular damage, whether mechanical, toxic or hypoxic in origin. The half-life of the enzyme in the circulation is approximately 60 hours.

Elevations are generally considered as mild (2–3 times the upper reference interval), moderate (4–9 times) or severe (10 times or more). Although the number of hepatocytes affected relates to the magnitude of increase, there is no direct correlation between the magnitude of the elevation and the severity or reversibility of the hepatocellular changes. An acute widespread disease is likely to cause greater elevations than a low-grade chronic one, but the degree of eventual hepatic compromise may be the same.

Increases may be caused by primary liver disease, or may occur when there is primary pathology distant from the liver (e.g. gastrointestinal or pancreatic disease) and the liver undergoes secondary changes (Figure 5.31.1). That is not to say that the liver is histopathologically or functionally normal in these 'secondary' elevations, but the likelihood is that the changes may resolve if the primary distant pathology is resolved. One of the most common causes for mild elevations of ALT is hyperthyroidism, where increased metabolic rate and altered perfusion lead to tissue hypoxia. Very severe muscle damage can result in ALT elevations, but such muscle disease is extremely uncommon in cats.

Aspartate aminotransferase

AST is present in the cytosol of hepatocytes but is also bound to mitochondria; thus more damage may be required to bring about an elevation of AST than of ALT.

- Hypoxia (e.g. in anaemia)
- Trauma
- Primary neoplasms (e.g. hepatocellular or bile duct carcinoma)
- Metastatic neoplasms
- Inflammatory liver disease (e.g. neutrophilic cholangitis/lymphocytic cholangitis)
- Hepatic lipidosis
- Toxins (e.g. paracetamol, oral diazepam)
- Response to extrahepatic disease (e.g. hyperthyroidism, inflammatory bowel disease, pancreatitis)
- Drugs (e.g. phenobarbital, corticosteroids)

5.31.1 Some causes of increased ALT concentrations. The elevations seen in response to corticosteroid therapy are due to structural changes in the liver and not to induction of enzyme expression by the drug.

This and a shorter half-life in the circulation (1 hour) makes AST a less sensitive, though more specific, marker for hepatocellular damage than ALT, and persistent elevations in AST are more concerning. Serial measurement of ALT and AST together can give a much clearer picture of whether a single insult has occurred or there is ongoing hepatocellular damage.

AST is also present in muscle, and thus the source of the AST elevation must be defined. Release of AST due to muscle damage is likely to be accompanied by an elevation in creatine kinase (CK) concentrations (and possibly a rise in ALT if damage is very severe).

Cholestatic/biliary tract markers

Alkaline phosphatase

Alkaline phosphatase (ALP) is present on the canalicular and microsomal membranes of hepatocytes and biliary epithelium. In healthy cats it is secreted into the biliary tract. Cholestasis (blockage of the biliary tract) results in increased formation of ALP via induction of enzyme expression and accumulation on the sinusoidal hepatocyte membranes, thus increasing serum levels. This induction takes approximately 8 hours and so ALP elevations may not be noted in the very acute stages of a cholestatic event. ALP is a somewhat insensitive marker for cholestasis in cats; bilirubin (see below) tends to rise more swiftly. The half-life of ALP in the circulation in cats is a relatively short 6 hours, making elevations more significant than in dogs. Other cholestatic markers can be used in addition (gamma-glutamyl transferase (GGT), bilirubin) to increase sensitivity and specificity. Cholestasis may be caused by direct occlusion of the biliary system by a physical obstruction, as occurs with some post-hepatic causes, but disruption of architecture and cell swelling with hepatic parenchymal disease and inflammation in the biliary system itself can also give rise to cholestatic effects.

Causes of increased liver ALP activity are listed in Figure 5.31.2.

Hepatic causes
■ Inflammatory liver disease (e.g. neutrophilic cholangitis/lymphocytic cholangitis)
■ FIP
■ Hepatotoxicity (e.g. paracetamol, oral diazepam)
■ Hepatic lipidosis (ALP elevation usually more marked than GGT elevation)
■ Sepsis
■ Intrahepatic neoplasms (e.g. hepatic or biliary carcinoma, lymphoma)
Post-hepatic causes
■ Pancreatitis
■ Cholecystitis
■ Cholelithiasis
■ Neoplasms (e.g. biliary, pancreatic or duodenal adenocarcinoma)

5.31.2 Some causes of increased liver ALP activity.

ALP isoenzymes

In addition to the liver isoenzyme of ALP, distinct bone, renal and gut isoenzymes occur. The renal isoenzyme is secreted into urine, not impacting significantly on serum levels. The gut isoenzyme has a very short half-life such that elevations are not generally noted. The bone isoenzyme increases in situations where there is increased osteoblastic activity and bone turnover. ALP elevations in hyperthyroid cats come from this source as well as from liver ALP, and elevations might be expected in rapidly growing individuals. Note that there is no steroid-induced ALP isoenzyme in the cat.

Gamma-glutamyl transferase

GGT is found on the biliary epithelium; concentrations rise in cholestasis, with increases related to biliary hyperplasia and possible induction secondary to bile acid accumulation. Elevations generally mirror those of liver ALP in cholestatic disease (see above), the exception being in hepatic lipidosis, where approximately 80% of cats have a proportionately greater ALP than GGT elevation. GGT is also present on pancreatic, intestinal and renal tubular membranes and is therefore not entirely liver-specific; however, it remains a more sensitive marker for hepatic disease than ALP in all but hepatic lipidosis. The half-life of GGT in the circulation in cats has not been established definitively but is believed to be similar to that of ALP.

Liver function markers

Bilirubin

Bilirubin is formed by the uptake and destruction of haem by macrophages in the liver and spleen, and to a lesser extent in bone marrow. The major source in healthy cats is from the normal destruction of senescent erythrocytes, with minor contributions from other haem-containing substances such as myoglobin. Bilirubin is released from the macrophage and is attached to albumin for transport to the liver. In the hepatocyte, conjugation with glucuronide occurs and the resulting conjugate is moved actively into the bile canaliculi; this is the slowest part of the process. Excretion into bile and movement from the gall bladder into the gut results in direct excretion in faeces, or transformation into urobilinogen which is reabsorbed and excreted renally. Any conjugated bilirubin which escapes back into circulation becomes attached to albumin and has a half-life in the circulation of approximately 10–14 days. This gives rise to the phenomenon of persistent icterus after correction of a cholestatic event.

> Cats are dependent on hepatocyte conjugation, with none occurring in the kidneys as is the case for many other species. Bilirubin in feline urine is therefore always abnormal.

There are some important considerations for bilirubin assays and their interpretation:

■ Bilirubin in blood samples is exquisitely sensitive to degradation by ultraviolet light, to the point that very significant decreases can occur in samples left in daylight for 1 hour.

■ Methods for total bilirubin concentration can be variably affected by interference from sample haemolysis.

■ Although reference intervals and methodologies are validated for the different fractions of bilirubin, these are not the most commonly available: the majority of methods are for total bilirubin concentrations.

■ In some stages of disease, relative increases in unconjugated over conjugated bilirubin suggest an increase in formation due to accelerated haem breakdown; disproportionate increases in conjugated bilirubin suggest an accumulation beyond the rate-limiting step in the liver and are more associated with hepatic cholestasis or post-hepatic obstruction. However, with time, competition between the unconjugated and conjugated forms for reuptake by hepatocytes can lead to variable proportions, and interpretation becomes difficult. In these circumstances, the use of other laboratory and imaging results may be of more use than overinterpretation of bilirubin fractions.

Pathological increases in bilirubin can be caused by an increase in formation by macrophages where there is increased red cell destruction (e.g. in haemolytic anaemia). Increases caused by reduced ability to take up and/or conjugate bilirubin may be seen in a variety of diseases causing overall reduced hepatic function. Overspill back into circulation increases with hepatic cholestasis and post-hepatic obstruction.

Hyperbilirubinaemia may also be a feature of FIP (approximately 25% of cases) and septicaemia: in both of these situations other features are required for diagnosis (see Chapter 19); feline sepsis-associated hyperbilirubinaemia is often accompanied by lethargy, pallor, tachypnoea, bradycardia and hypothermia.

Serum bile acids

Bile acids are formed by the liver and after conjugation are excreted via the biliary system. Contractions in response to fatty meals, or occasional 'housekeeping' contractions of the gall bladder, empty the bile acids along with the other components of bile into the duodenum. In the gut they are important in the absorption of fats, and are taken back into the entero-hepatic circulation. If the portal venous system is intact, the bile acids are delivered back to the hepatic parenchyma, where hepatic function is required to reclaim the bile acids from the blood to be recycled and re-excreted in bile.

Bile acids are measured either in fasting samples (fasted serum bile acids, FSBA) or 2 hours after a meal (postprandial bile acids, PPBA) to provoke gall bladder contraction and provide a maximal challenge of bile acids to the system. Approximately 20% of paired FSBA and PPBA samples will have a preprandial value higher than the post, possibly due to the 'housekeeping' contractions of the gall bladder; this is of no clinical consequence. In the fasted state, with bile acids accumulated in the gall bladder, there may be little challenge to the functional ability of the liver or to the integrity of the portosystemic circulation in the recycling of bile acids. Time may allow even a pathologically inefficient system to reclaim bile acids from portal and/or systemic circulation and return blood levels to normal. Therefore, a single normal FSBA result is not enough to rule out poor liver function: the challenge of capturing and recycling a mass release following feeding (PPBA assay) gives a more accurate view.

Causes of elevated bile acids include the following:

- Portosystemic shunts: Bile acids will increase in concentration where portosystemic shunting blood vessels allow them to spill unreclaimed into the systemic circulation. FSBA values may be normal, slightly or markedly elevated, but very high levels (>100 μmol/l) can be more reliably seen in a PPBA sample
- Cholestatic disorders: These impair the enterohepatic circulation and may result in

elevation in either FSBA or PPBA concentrations, often before there is an increase in bilirubin
- Hepatic disease: Any hepatic disease that results in impaired hepatic function or decreased hepatic mass leads to decreased reclamation and variable amounts delivered into systemic circulation. Values for PPBA of >25 μmol/l have been shown to correlate with histopathological changes in the liver
- Extrahepatic diseases (e.g. pancreatitis, gastrointestinal disease): These may give rise to modest elevations in FSBA or PPBA concentrations (usually <40 μmol/l, although occasionally higher values may be obtained).

PRACTICAL TIP

In cats that are hyperbilirubinaemic due to cholestatic or post-hepatic causes, FSBA and PPBA concentrations are inevitably elevated and there is no extra information to be derived from their measurement.

Bile acid levels are naturally dynamic, and serial measurements are influenced by so many factors that serial measurement cannot be easily used as a marker of improvement or worsening of hepatic function. While values in the high hundreds decreasing to reference interval or just above following surgery for portosystemic shunts are noted in some cases, amelioration of clinical signs and the improvement of serum albumin concentration and clotting function are often more significant.

Ammonia

Serum concentrations of ammonia may increase in either hepatic dysfunction or portosystemic shunting, and this is a major contributor to hepatic encephalopathy. Ammonia is extremely labile: haemolysis or storage of the sample for more than a few minutes will cause elevations. Samples should be collected into a cold syringe and EDTA container to be separated immediately from the red cells, preferably in a chilled centrifuge. Ammonia may then be measured immediately in house or sent frozen to an external laboratory. There are few advantages over paired serum bile acid testing.

Regurgitation

Myra Forster-van Hijfte

Regurgitation is the retrograde passive expulsion of undigested food, water and/or saliva without any obvious effort. There should be no forceful contraction of abdominal muscles, as this would indicate vomiting (see Chapter 5.35) rather than regurgitation. In the cat it is important to remember that, unlike in the dog, the caudal third of the oesophagus contains smooth muscle (giving a herringbone appearance to the oesophageal mucosa in that area).

Causes

Regurgitation is caused by abnormalities within the oesophagus, anywhere from the proximal oesophageal sphincter to the cardia. Causes of regurgitation in the cat are:

- Oesophagitis: secondary to reflux of gastric acid into the oesophagus, e.g. during general anaesthesia or secondary to drugs when incompletely swallowed (some formulations of doxycycline and clindamycin have been implicated; Figure 5.32.1)
- Foreign body: these can be lodged in the oesophagus (fish hook or needle being the classical examples)
- Acquired oesophageal stricture: mainly due to non-treated, severe oesophagitis
- External compression causing narrowing of the oesophageal lumen: for instance caused by a vascular ring anomaly or a cranial mediastinal mass
- Oesophageal mass lesion, such as a squamous cell carcinoma, lymphoma, abscess or granuloma.
- Oesophageal motility problems (including megaoesophagus) caused by myasthenia gravis, feline dysautonomia, lead toxicity, general neuromuscular disease, or oesophageal dysmotility in the Siamese and Oriental breeds with concurrent delayed pyloric outflow. Megaoesophagus can also be idiopathic.

Clinical presentation

It is important to obtain a good history, as owners often have difficulty differentiating regurgitation from vomiting. It can be helpful if the owners record a

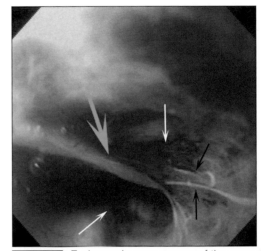

5.32.1 Endoscopic appearance of the oesophagus of a cat with severe oesophagitis following ingestion, and incomplete swallowing into the stomach, of a doxycycline tablet. In addition to the ulceration and bleeding (white arrows), fibrinous strands (black arrows) are seen crossing the oesophageal lumen, and a free flap of mucosa (green arrow) is seen draping into the lumen. These fibrinous strands and flap of mucosa indicate that this cat is at risk of developing an oesophageal stricture. (Courtesy of The Feline Centre, Langford Veterinary Services, University of Bristol)

video of an episode. It is very important to make this differentiation (Figure 5.32.2), as the further diagnostic approach differs markedly between vomiting (see Chapter 5.35) and regurgitation. Additional questions to consider are: the age of onset of the clinical signs; whether there has been any ingestion of toxins, drugs or foreign bodies; or whether the cat has had a recent general anaesthetic.

Cats with regurgitation usually have marked weight loss. Their appetite can be good and they usually remain bright, unless there are further complications. Signs of pain during swallowing or excessive gulping can be seen, especially in cases with oesophagitis or luminal foreign bodies. Assessment of the cranial rib spring is important, since this can be reduced with anterior mediastinal lymphoma (more common in young cats, especially Siamese and Oriental breeds) or thymoma (more common in older cats), which can cause compression of the oesophagus. The clinician

Clinical sign	Regurgitation	Vomiting
Change in appetite	Varies according to cause but appetite often good	Varies according to cause
Pain on swallowing	Possible	No
Nausea and/or other prodromal signs (e.g. swallowing or gulping)	No	Possible
Hypersalivation	May be present	Usually only seen immediately before vomiting, if present
Retching/abdominal effort during episode	No	Yes
Timing with respect to feeding	May occur immediately after feeding (proximal oesophageal disease) or have longer lag time (distal or generalized oesophageal disease)	Variable
Character of food returned	May be tubular in appearance and may appear partially digested; cat may re-eat it	May be partially digested

5.32.2 Comparison of clinical signs in regurgitation and vomiting.

needs to be aware that the cranial rib spring does reduce in the normal older cat.

Additional clinical signs depend on the underlying cause of the regurgitation. For example, if the cause is generalized neuromuscular disease there will be generalized weakness as well as a functional abnormality of the oesophagus; if dysautonomia is present there may be concurrent mydriasis, megacolon, protruding third eyelids, etc.

If aspiration pneumonia has developed secondary to regurgitation, the cat will develop coughing, dyspnoea and a fever.

Diagnostic approach

Blood and urine tests

Full biochemical and haematology profiles and urinalysis are used to determine the health status of the cat. Blood tests are generally not useful to determine the underlying cause of an oesophageal problem, although they might identify associated complications such as electrolyte imbalances or anaemia of inflammatory disease. Electrolyte imbalances are best identified and corrected prior to further diagnostic investigations to avoid any complications. The FeLV/FIV status of the cat should also be determined (though these diseases have a low prevalence within the UK).

Diagnostic imaging

Survey radiography of the thorax (lateral and dorsoventral views) can be helpful. The normal oesophagus cannot be seen on survey thoracic radiography; if the oesophagus is visible, its shape and size should be assessed and also whether there are any other abnormal opacities in or around it. The lungs should be examined to determine whether there is any evidence of aspiration pneumonia (alveolar pattern particularly in the cranioventral lung fields).

PRACTICAL TIPS

- Ideally radiography should be done on a conscious animal, as sedation (and especially general anaesthesia) can cause the appearance of a dilated oesophagus on radiography. It is then unclear whether this dilation is true or caused by the sedation or anaesthesia.
- If conscious radiography is not possible, minimal sedation (using acepromazine 0.01–0.1 mg/kg i.m. or s.c.) can be used.
- Minimal rather than heavy sedation or anaesthesia will also minimize the risk of aspiration pneumonia.

Survey radiography can be very helpful in the diagnosis of the following:

- Megaoesophagus: focal (e.g. secondary to vascular ring anomaly, or other obstruction) or generalized
- Anterior mediastinal mass (e.g. lymphoma, thymoma)
- Oesophageal or perioesophageal masses
- Radiopaque foreign bodies.

Contrast studies

Contrast radiography can be used to assess the oesophageal lumen and mucosa, although this is not often performed. Although administration of barium paste may help identification of lesions and/or confirm the presence of megaoesophagus, it is contraindicated if there is any possibility of oesophageal perforation (because barium causes marked mediastinitis) or aspiration, or if endoscopy is going to be performed within the next 24–48 hours. If endoscopy is contemplated, iodine-based soluble contrast medium can be used as an alternative. However, both barium and iodine-based contrast media have serious consequences when aspirated: barium will cause severe inflammation; and iodine-based contrast media are hypertonic, causing an osmotic draw of fluid and subsequent pulmonary oedema. For this reason contrast studies are often avoided in cases with oesophageal disease. Generally, a combination of plain radiography and/or endoscopy is preferred for diagnosing most conditions. Referral should be considered for endoscopy if required.

Endoscopy

Endoscopy is a very useful tool for identifying structural abnormalities within the oesophagus. It is less useful for diagnosing functional abnormalities, but as they are usually a diagnosis by exclusion it is necessary to examine the oesophagus endoscopically.

Endoscopy of the oesophagus can be performed at referral centres, or in practice if there is appropriate experience. A 7.8–10 mm diameter 4-way tip deflection, flexible gastroscope is ideal and can be used to identify strictures, foreign bodies and oesophageal masses. A smaller diameter endoscope (3–6 mm diameter) may be required to visualize the oesophagus beyond a stricture or mass, and to allow assessment of the extent of a mass or stricture. Referral for endoscopy is to be encouraged in view of the potential risks of aspiration in many of these patients during anaesthesia and the possible need for further intensive treatment of some of the possible lesions (e.g.

strictures). Although endoscopy can be used to diagnose oesophagitis, trial treatment for this in suspected cases may be rewarding in causing an improvement in the cat's clinical signs and then preclude the need for referral. It is difficult to obtain endoscopic biopsy specimens of a relatively healthy oesophagus due to its tough nature.

Fluoroscopy

Fluoroscopy is required to document functional motility disorders of the oesophagus definitively (including swallowing abnormalities) and will generally require referral.

Further tests for neurological or muscular disease

If all of the above tests are inconclusive, or a motility disorder is found, further diagnostic investigations of the neurological system should be considered, especially if abnormalities are detected on a standard neurological examination (see QRG 1.6). Central neurological disease involving the brainstem, or a peri-pheral neuropathy, can cause megaoesophagus. In cases where a neurological disorder is suspected, referral for further investigations (e.g. MRI, nerve conduction velocity measurement, nerve biopsy) should be considered.

If a primary muscle disease is suspected, changes in the muscular system, such as muscle wastage or muscle swelling, may be noticed. Creatine kinase may be increased on serum biochemistry. The electrical activity within the peripheral muscles can be assessed using electromyography (EMG), but it is difficult to assess the muscle of the oesophagus, and referral is indicated for such investigations.

Other diseases associated with regurgitation in the cat include lead poisoning (possible exposure from old paint or batteries), myasthenia gravis, acetylcholinesterase toxicity and feline dysautonomia. Further details on these conditions can be found in the *BSAVA Manual of Canine and Feline Neurology*.

Treatment

Oesophagitis

The signs of oesophagitis can be very subtle and this is a disease that is probably underdiagnosed. Early recognition of (the potential development of) oesophagitis is paramount so that treatment can be started and the development of oesophageal strictures as a consequence of oesophagitis prevented. If oesophagitis is suspected based on the history and clinical signs, trial treatment can be instigated without necessarily obtaining a definitive diagnosis to see whether there is an improvement.

Intravenous fluid therapy may be necessary to treat and/or prevent dehydration secondary to anorexia and adipsia.

Other treatment options include:

- Sucralfate suspension: (2 ml orally q8h) to provide cytoprotection and promote mucosal healing. Sucralfate needs an acidic environment to be active, so give at least 1–2 hours before any acid secretion inhibitors
- Gastric acid secretory inhibitory therapy (to reduce the acidity of any (further) gastric reflux): e.g.

omeprazole (0.75–1 mg/kg orally q24h), cimetidine (5–10 mg/kg orally q6–8h), famotidine (0.5–1 mg/kg orally q12–24h) or ranitidine (2 mg/kg slow i.v. over 5 min or orally q12h or s.c. q12h). Ranitidine will also promote gastric emptying, which may reduce the likelihood of reflux.

If the cat is also vomiting, food should be withheld and an anti-emetic given. The anti-emetic metoclopramide promotes gastric emptying too, and can be particularly effective when given via a constant rate infusion (1–2 mg/kg i.v. over 24 hours in crystalloid fluids using an infusion pump); an alternative non-prokinetic anti-emetic is maropitant (see Chapter 5.35 for further details on anti-emetics).

Oesophagitis can be painful, so provision of analgesia can be important in treatment; an opioid such as buprenorphine is usually effective in acute cases.

Nutritional support is important. Food is usually withheld for 24 hours whilst medications are initiated. Thereafter, a low-fat diet of a soft consistency (such as a wet intestinal support diet; *NB low-fat diets promote more rapid gastric emptying*) is usually best handled by an inflamed oesophagus, although this can be variable. Some cats do better with a 'sloppier' food, others with dry kibble, so it is worth trying foods of different consistency if regurgitation and/or signs of oesophagitis persist. Placement of a gastrostomy feeding tube can be considered while the oesophagus heals if the cat is not vomiting and severe oesophagitis is present. Referral for this procedure is recommended if the practice does not have experience of placing gastrostomy feeding tubes under endoscopy; placement using endoscopy will also allow endoscopic examination of the oesophagus, to ensure that more serious disease such as a stricture is not present.

If the oesophagitis is very severe, anti-inflammatory medication with prednisolone (0.5–1 mg/kg orally q24h) has been advocated by some to try and prevent stricture formation; advice should be sought from a specialist before giving prednisolone treatment in these circumstances.

Oesophageal strictures

A stricture may develop if oesophagitis is severe or left untreated (Figure 5.32.3). Usually strictures occur within 3 weeks of the initial insult.

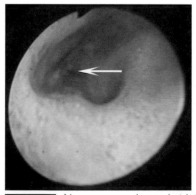

5.32.3 Narrow oesophageal stricture in a cat following severe oesophagitis; the small lumen is just visible (arrowed). The cause of the stricture was not known but it was believed to be secondary to severe untreated oesophagitis due to gastro-oesophageal reflux during general anaesthesia. (Courtesy of The Feline Centre, Langford Veterinary Services, University of Bristol)

Bougienage or balloon dilation under endoscopic inspection can rectify the problem but referral is required due to the specialist equipment and expertise required to dilate the stricture and deal with any potential complications. It should be noted that the procedure often needs to be repeated several times. Although the complication rate for stricture dilation is low, there is always the potential of causing rupture of the stricture with usually fatal consequences (pneumothorax, mediastinitis). If these complications occur, surgery can be contemplated (once the pneumothorax has been dealt with) but a very poor prognosis has to be given. It is essential to provide therapy after dilation to reduce the recurrence of the stricture using anti-inflammatory medication (prednisolone at 0.5–1 mg/kg orally q24h), liquid sucralfate and possibly some added gastric acid secretory inhibitors (see above). Recently the use of a biodegradable polydioxanone self-expanding stent at the level of the stricture site after dilation has been described that was successful in preventing recurrence of the stricture; again referral to a specialist for this procedure is necessary.

Oesophageal foreign body

Cats may ingest foreign bodies (e.g. needles, fish-hooks) and these can be retrieved endoscopically under certain circumstances; referral for endoscopic removal should be considered. Endoscopic removal depends on the size and shape of the foreign body and the duration of the problem. The longer the foreign body has been within the oesophagus, the more likely complications will occur because of mucosal inflammation and ischaemia, secondary to the pressure of the foreign body *in situ*.

Oesophageal surgery to remove a foreign body is fraught with complications, especially dehiscence of the oesophageal wound and secondary infections. It is not possible to remove a significant amount of oesophageal tissue as this would result in traction on the wound. It is sometimes possible to push an oesophageal foreign body further into the stomach, so that it can be removed surgically via a gastrotomy.

Removal of an oesophageal foreign body should be followed by treatment for oesophagitis (see above).

Oesophageal masses

These are rare in the cat. Squamous cell carcinoma is the most common neoplasm of the oesophagus, followed by lymphoma. Biopsy samples can be obtained at endoscopy; sampling oesophageal tissue can be difficult with endoscopic biopsy forceps due to the tough nature of normal oesophageal tissue, but abnormal tissue is usually easier to acquire. Surgical removal of the mass has similar complications to surgical foreign body removal from the oesophagus. Lymphoma can be treated with chemotherapy (see Chapter 21).

Neuromuscular disease

Treatment of neuromuscular disease of the oesophagus depends on the underlying cause. Cats with megaoesophagus will require supportive care and additional medication to treat the underlying disease. It is worth trying food of different consistencies to see which is best tolerated by the patient; usually a wet low-fat food is preferable but some cats do better on dry food. Small frequent meals and postural feeding (holding the cat's forelimbs up, with the head higher than the trunk during feeding (Figure 5.32.4) and afterwards for 15 minutes if possible) are recommended to facilitate passage of food down the abnormal oesophagus and into the stomach. If postural feeding is not possible, the owner can try just holding the cat up for 15 minutes after feeding. However, some cases will require placement of a gastrostomy feeding tube.

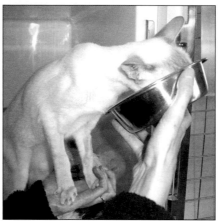

5.32.4 Postural feeding in a 17-week-old Siamese kitten with pyloric dyssynergia (also known as pyloric stenosis) with associated megaoesophagus. Pyloric dyssynergia is a condition seen most commonly in young Siamese cats and is often associated with concurrent megaoesophagus; the dyssynergia is due to abnormal pyloric function rather than a mechanical stenosis. Medical treatment with prokinetic agents (e.g. metoclopramide or ranitidine) can be tried, or surgical pyloroplasty. The cause of the megaoesophagus is not known, but it can resolve following effective treatment of the pyloric dyssynergia. This kitten was fed a low-fat high-protein diet – to encourage weight gain – alongside medical management with metoclopramide. (Courtesy of The Feline Centre, Langford Veterinary Services, University of Bristol)

References and further reading

Frowde PE, Battersby IA, Whitley NT and Elwood CM (2011) Oesophageal disease in 33 cats. *Journal of Feline Medicine and Surgery* **13**, 564–569

Harai BH, Johnson SE and Sherding RG (1995) Endoscopically guided balloon dilatation of benign esophageal strictures in 6 cats and 7 dogs. *Journal of Veterinary Internal Medicine* **9**, 332–335

Leib MS, Dinnel H, Ward DL *et al.* (2001) Endoscopic balloon dilation of benign esophageal strictures in dogs and cats. *Journal of Veterinary Internal Medicine* **15**, 547–552

Skin masses, nodules and swellings

Natalie Barnard

Skin masses, nodules and swellings are a common presentation as they are visible to owners and often worry them. Solid, cystic or oedematous elevations of the skin may be epidermal or dermal, or may extend into the subcutaneous fat and panniculus. All masses and nodules are composed of accumulations of cells, which can be neoplastic, inflammatory, or a mixture of the two.

History

It is important to ascertain whether there are any signs of the cat being systemically unwell. Information about the lifestyle of the cat may also be helpful; for example, if the cat is a hunter or a fighter then this may pre-dispose to injuries that provide an opportunity for the entry of unusual organisms such as mycobacteria and fungi. Neoplasia may be more likely in an older cat, although a cat of any age that has a white nose and ears and sunbathes regularly has an increased risk of developing squamous cell carcinoma.

Clinical examination

A general physical examination should always be per-formed to look for signs of systemic disease such as enlarged lymph nodes, pyrexia and weight loss.

Dermatological examination

The whole cat should be examined for other signs of skin disease, to avoid missing smaller additional lesions. It is important not to focus only on the lesion the cat is presented for.

Sometimes lesion distribution can give important clues to the diagnosis (Figure 5.33.1).

Differential diagnoses

Nodules, swellings and masses can be classified as follows:

- Inflammatory lesions (Figure 5.33.3):
  - Infectious inflammatory
  - Non-infectious inflammatory
  - Miscellaneous – plasma cell pododermatitis

Location	Possible diagnoses
Nose	Fungal granuloma (see Figure 5.33.2); squamous cell carcinoma, especially if the cat is white
Face and neck	Cat bite abscess; mycobacterial infections
Ventral abdomen	Panniculitis caused by mycobacterial infections; cat bite abscess
Forelimb	Cat bite abscess; mycobacterial infections
Tail base	Cat bite abscess

5.33.1 Location of skin mass, nodule or swelling and possible diagnoses. Mycobacterial infections include feline leprosy and tuberculosis. See Chapter 5.8 for more details on cat bite abscess.

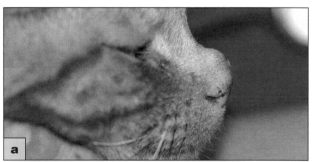

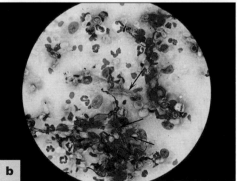

5.33.2 **(a)** DSH cat presented with a swelling on the dorsal aspect of its nose. **(b)** Fine-needle aspirate smear from the swelling (Diff-Quik; original magnification X1000). Fungal elements can be seen (examples are arrowed) plus large numbers of inflammatory cells, confirming the lesion to be a fungal granuloma. It is not possible to identify the species on cytology alone but the causative fungus was identified by culture as *Alternaria*. Treatment with systemic itraconazole for 3 months led to a complete resolution of the lesion.

- Neoplastic lesions:
  - Common skin tumours are: squamous cell carcinoma; basal cell tumours; fibrosarcoma; and mast cell tumours (Figure 5.33.4). It is important to note that malignant neoplasms form a greater proportion of skin tumours in cats than in dogs.

Plasma cell pododermatitis

Plasma cell pododermatitis is a unique condition of the cat that affects only its footpads. It is uncommon and its aetiology and pathogenesis are unknown, although it can be associated with FIV infection. No age, sex or breed predilection has been identified.

Clinical signs

- Soft painless swelling of multiple footpads on multiple paws; usually the central metacarpal and metatarsal pads are affected.
- Occasionally: pain, lameness, ulceration and secondary infection can occur.

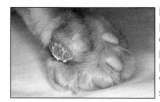

Plasma cell pododermatitis of the central metacarpal pad of a forelimb. The pad surface is slightly white/mauve and scaly.

Differential diagnoses

- Eosinophilic granuloma complex
- Bacterial or fungal granulomas
- Neoplasia
- Autoimmune conditions

Diagnosis

Usually confirmed on skin aspirate or biopsy samples, but the clinical appearance is suggestive.

Treatment

Plasma cell pododermatitis will sometimes regress spontaneously without treatment. Prednisolone can be used (1–2 mg/kg orally q24h; occasionally up to 4 mg/kg q24h) until remission is achieved. It can take several weeks for there to be an improvement. Once in remission, treatment is then tapered and either discontinued or maintained at the lowest effective alternate-day dose. Treatment with doxycycline (10 mg/kg orally q24h) may be used if prednisolone treatment is contraindicated, but doxycycline treatment is not always effective and clinical improvement is slower than with prednisolone. Ciclosporin has also been used successfully in some cases.

Infectious – bacterial

- Abscesses secondary to cat bites (see Chapter 5.8)
- Cutaneous mycobacterial infections (especially feline leprosy)
- *Actinomyces/Nocardia*: these organisms are soil saprophytes and the most common route of infection is through a contaminated wound

Infectious – fungal

- Dermatophyte granulomas
- Opportunistic saprophytic fungal infections; phaeohyphomycosis infections due to *Alternaria* are commonly seen in the UK
- *Cryptococcus*

Non-infectious

- Urticaria
- Eosinophilic granuloma complex (see Chapter 5.26)
- Panniculitis (excluding that caused by mycobacteria)

5.33.3 The most common infectious and non-infectious causes of nodular skin lesions in the cat. Mycobacterial skin disease is discussed in detail in Chapter 6.

Tumour	Origin	Location	Clinical features
Basal cell tumour	Epithelial origin	Head, neck, thorax	Older adult cats affected. Well circumscribed solitary lesions that can be pigmented and ulcerated. Slow growing. Treatment is wide surgical excision. Do not routinely metastasize. Siamese, Himalayan and Persian cats over-represented
Squamous cell carcinoma	Epithelial origin	Pinna, nasal planum, eyelids	Older animals affected. Strong association with non-pigmented lightly haired skin in white cats. Solitary lesions that can be proliferative and erosive. Often ulcerated. Wide surgical excision/ radiotherapy/photodynamic therapy required
Mast cell tumour	Round cell origin	Head, neck	Two distinct forms recognized in cats: • Mastocytic mast cell tumour (most common): usually seen in older cats; Siamese predisposed. Often a solitary lesion which is firm and well circumscribed. Most behave in benign manner. Surgery is the treatment of choice • Histiocytic mast cell tumour (less common): seen in younger cats and can regress spontaneously
Fibrosarcoma	Mesenchymal origin	Trunk, distal limbs, pinna	Can be spontaneous, or induced by feline sarcoma virus (FSV), or may be vaccine-associated (see Chapter 21). FSV-induced lesions occur in cats <5 years old. Older cats can have fibrosarcomas that are not associated with vaccines or sarcoma virus. Rapidly infiltrating dermal or subcutaneous masses that are poorly defined.

5.33.4 Common skin tumours found in cats.

Diagnostic approach

Specimens that may be required include:

- Hair plucks for a trichogram (see QRG 5.3.2)
- Fine-needle aspirates for cytology (see QRG 5.33.1). Sedation or anaesthesia may be required for sensitive or painful lesions, e.g. on the face or feet; butorphanol or medetomidine are possibilities for sedation
- Impression smears for cytology
- Swab samples from the surface of the lesion for microbial culture and sensitivity (if cytology suggests a bacterial infection, i.e. degenerative neutrophils, intra/extracellular bacteria)
- Skin biopsy samples (see QRG 5.3.4) for histopathology and culture. Tissue culture will give more reliable results than a surface swab and is essential if a mycobacterial or fungal infection is suspected.

Impression smears are useful if the lesion is exudative with a moist, eroded or ulcerated surface. It is not necessary to prepare or clean the surface of the lesion. Take a glass microscope slide and gently press this on to the area to be sampled. Label the slide and allow it to air dry. Once dry, stain with Diff-Quik (see QRG 5.26.3) and examine using a microscope. You will need to use oil immersion to see cells and microorganisms.

Interpretation of fine-needle aspirate cytology is summarized in Figure 5.33.5.

Other potentially useful diagnostic tests include:

- Blood biochemistry and haematology to assess the cat's general health, and/or if sedation or anaesthesia will be required
- Retrovirus testing (FeLV/FIV), especially in cats with fungal granulomas or mycobacterial infection
- In cases with mycobacterial skin infection: imaging (radiography and ultrasonography) of the chest and abdomen to investigate whether there is systemic involvement (e.g. calcified lung masses, lymphadenopathy).

Empirical treatment whilst awaiting results

Treatment given will depend on the underlying cause of the lesion. When fungal elements are seen it is reasonable to excise solitary lesions, if possible, and start treatment with itraconazole (see Chapter 6). If a mycobacterial infection is suspected, pending a definitive diagnosis, interim treatment with a fluoroquinolone may be recommended in cases with localized lesions. If, however, there are signs of systemic involvement, double or triple therapy for mycobacterial infection (see Chapter 6) should be instituted, pending diagnosis, as this will decrease the chance of the mycobacterial agent developing resistance. If cytology of ulcerated masses (e.g. a squamous cell

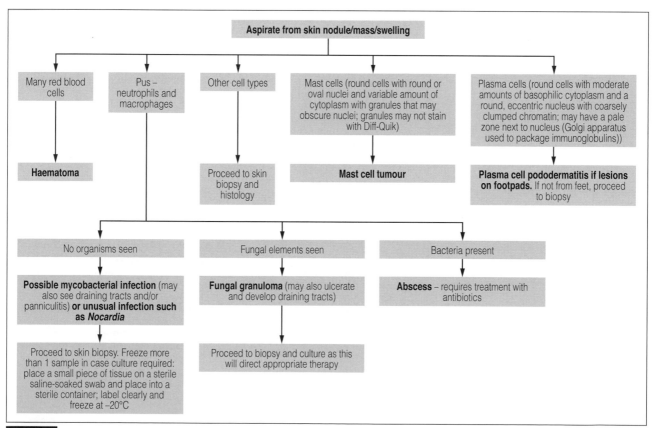

5.33.5 Interpretation of fine-needle aspirate cytology.

carcinoma) indicates secondary bacterial infection, this should be treated appropriately with antibacterials (e.g. cefalexin 15 mg/kg orally q12h) pending skin biopsy results. Treatment with antibacterials should be continued until 1 week past resolution of infection, monitoring using cytology and clinical signs.

When to refer

Referral should be considered if the mass is neoplastic and not easily resectable, or in cases where chemotherapy or radiation may be required as an adjunct to surgery. Referral should also be considered for cases of mycobacterial infection.

What to do if finances are limited

This will depend on the cause of the skin mass. Cases of mycobacterial infection require prolonged treatment and monitoring, which may not be affordable for some clients, so this needs to be discussed in detail before embarking on therapy.

QRG 5.33.1 Fine-needle aspiration
by Kathleen Tennant

Indications

Cytology of samples obtained by fine-needle aspiration (FNA) should be regarded as a useful screening test. Definitive diagnosis is sometimes possible, but in many cases cytology may serve better to rule out differential diagnoses or narrow them to a category (e.g. inflammatory *versus* neoplastic). Some tissues or lesions give much better cell yields and/or a greater chance of a definitive diagnosis than others.

Lesions for which it is always worth attempting FNA

Dermal or intradermal lesions

There are many inflammatory and neoplastic changes that can be diagnosed definitively using FNA. Caution is needed with mammary masses, as cytologically benign areas can be very close to malignant areas; histopathology is better for a more complete assessment up to the surgical margins, but an aspirate yielding malignant cells still has value in confirming malignancy.

Enlarged lymph nodes

FNA can be very useful in the diagnosis of large cell lymphoma (see Chapter 21), though histopathology may be required where the results are equivocal or a small cell lymphoma is involved, as these may have an appearance identical to that of aspirates from a normal lymph node. As well as confirming that such a malignancy exists, prognosis and behaviour for large *versus* small cell lymphomas, and even subtypes within these categories, varies enough for this information to be useful when planning treatment and advice to the owner. Evidence of immune stimulation or inflammation (lymphadenitis) can be seen on cytology, occasionally with causative organisms. FNA cytology is more specific than it is sensitive for finding evidence of metastatic disease in a lymph node; histopathology is more sensitive, due to the larger sample volume.

Intra-abdominal masses

Many masses arising from abdominal organs (see Chapter 5.2) have a reasonable cell yield. It is very important to examine the mass and the surrounding tissues ultrasonographically and to have a clear idea of the area being aspirated, as some tumours/organs are extremely vascular. Experience with abdominal ultrasonography is required to perform FNA on abdominal masses.

> **WARNING**
>
> Clotting times (prothrombin time (PT) and activated partial thromboplastin time (APTT)) should ideally be checked before aspirating masses associated with the liver, spleen or kidney or other well vascularized organs, although in practice this may not always be possible due to financial or time constraints.

Aspirates from many lesions in the abdomen have a tendency to yield delicate cells that are easy to rupture, so a light hand is required when making smears.

Masses within the thoracic cavity

Ideally, FNA should only be attempted under ultrasound guidance, as the risks of accidently puncturing vascular structures are high; in some circumstances it may be possible to perform 'blind' aspiration of solid masses or areas of lung if they are directly against the body wall.

Lesions for which it is sometimes worth attempting FNA

Some tissues or organs may show only limited changes despite the presence of important pathology, or generally do not yield many cells from which a diagnosis can be attempted. FNA may still be worth a try, but the limitations should be explained to the owners. In many cases histopathology may be preferable, or necessary to make a definitive diagnosis.

Liver lesions

FNA of the liver has variable reliability in diagnosing different conditions.

- **Good reliability: hepatic lipidosis/ widespread lymphoma.** Where FNA cytology demonstrates hepatic lipidosis or lymphoma, it agrees well (good specificity) with the gold standard of histopathology. However, due to the smaller area being sampled there is still a chance that FNA may miss a focal change or an underlying cause for lipidosis.
- **Limited reliability: neutrophilic or mixed inflammation/cholestasis.** FNA has good specificity, but a poorer sensitivity becomes evident when neutrophilic inflammation and cholestasis (appearance of pigment in casts outside the hepatocytes) are being looked for. If they are obviously present on FNA they are almost certainly present on histopathology, but many cats without these changes in small aspirates are shown to have them on histopathology of liver sections.
- **Poor reliability: lymphocytic and/ or plasmacytic inflammation:** FNA has a poor detection rate for lymphocytic/plasmacytic inflammation (poor sensitivity).
- **Very poor reliability: hyperplasia/ benign neoplasia/well differentiated neoplasia of hepatocytes.** FNA gives few or no hints as to structure and is poor at distinguishing between the causes of some hepatic masses in which the individual hepatocytes appear very similar, i.e. hepatic nodules (hyperplasia), hepatoma (benign neoplasia), and well differentiated hepatic carcinoma (malignant ▶

QRG 5.33.1 *continued*

neoplasia). Histopathology reveals the behaviour and arrangement of these hepatocytes and is far superior in these cases.

Thyroid masses

Thyroid mass cells are very delicate and easy to rupture. FNA samples from the thyroid gland may also appear the same cytologically whether they are from an adenoma or a carcinoma, so FNA samples cannot distinguish benign from malignant masses.

Masses of connective tissue origin

Some masses of connective tissue origin (e.g. sarcomas) may not give a good cell yield on FNA as the matrix they produce 'glues' the cells in place, making them hard to aspirate. Sometimes a mixture of needle sizes and using both the passive needle redirection technique and the active aspiration technique (see below) may increase the chance of obtaining a diagnostic sample.

Procedure
Patient preparation

- Superficial lesions may sometimes be sampled in conscious cats, but sedation or anaesthesia may be required for deeper aspirates and/or where there is the possibility of critical structures being damaged if the cat moves during sampling.
- Identify the area to be aspirated. This may be done visually, by palpation, or using imaging (usually ultrasonography).

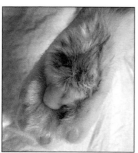

A mass above the metacarpal pad of a young cat's foot.

- Consider whether the area to be aspirated is uniform in appearance so that aspirates from any area of the mass are likely to be representative. If there is a varied appearance to the mass visually, by palpation or via ultrasonography (e.g. fluid contents and capsule in a cystic type lesion) there may be an advantage to aspirating several areas within the mass. The gross appearance of the mass, including factors such as size, location, firmness and the presence of haemorrhage/ulceration, should be noted before surgical preparation is undertaken. Clipping the area may allow better visualization of superficial lesions and may uncover important features such as

ulceration, pigmentation, bruising or wounds, which may alter the differential diagnosis.

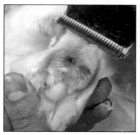

Clipping has revealed puncture wounds on the mass.

- Surgical preparation of the site to be aspirated lessens the chance of introducing infection. For masses in a subcutaneous or body cavity location surgical scrubbing is essential. However, it may not be appropriate for delicate superficial lesions, such as vesicles, which would be destroyed by the scrubbing involved.

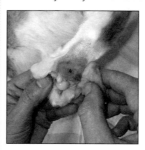

Active aspiration technique

1 The needle is introduced into the lesion with a 5 or 10 ml syringe attached. A 23–25 G ¾-inch needle is usually adequate for superficial masses. Smaller gauge needles may give a smaller cell yield than larger needles but are less likely to lead to excessive haemorrhage. Longer or spinal needles may be needed for deeper or intracavitary masses, e.g. up to 3.5 inches for gall bladder aspiration.

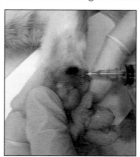

2 A small amount of negative pressure (2–3 ml is usually adequate) is then applied to obtain the aspirate. Material becoming visible within the hub of the needle is a good indication that aspiration has been successful, but is not always seen.

PRACTICAL TIP

Slight redirection of the needle within the mass during suction may ensure a better cell yield.

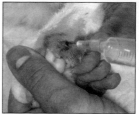

The needle is redirected within the lesion with slight suction from the syringe.

3 The pressure/suction is released before the needle is withdrawn to ensure that the material is not evacuated into the barrel of the syringe. Occasionally more solid, unyielding masses may require more negative pressure to obtain a sample, but there is more risk of cell rupture.

Needle redirection technique

1 The needle is introduced with a syringe attached but without the application of any suction.

2 The needle is then gently redirected within the mass to gather a core of cells in the barrel of the needle as it is pushed through the tissue.

3 The needle is then withdrawn.

This technique is particularly helpful when aspirates are collected under ultrasound guidance, leaving one hand free to direct the probe.

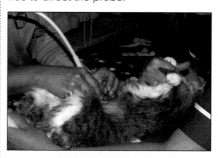

PRACTICAL TIPS

- If using ultrasound guidance, care should be taken to remove excess ultrasound gel from the area of skin through which the needle is introduced, as gel can obscure cellular detail and alter the staining characteristics of the sample.
- The needle should be introduced close to the ultrasound probe to make visualization and tracking of the needle point easier.
- Although a one-handed active aspiration technique with a syringe attached is possible, in many cases introducing the needle alone and redirecting its path within the area of interest is not only adequate but easier to achieve one-handed.
- A spinal needle of appropriate length may be used to access more deeply located lesions.

►

QRG 5.33.1 *continued*

Sample preparation

1 For both the active aspiration and needle redirection techniques, once the needle is withdrawn from the lesion it is quickly detached from the syringe. Air (5 ml) is then drawn into the syringe and it is reattached to the needle.

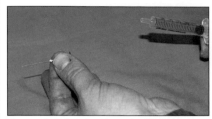

The needle is detached from the filled hub.

2 The collected material is propelled on to the slide using a sharp compression of the syringe plunger. Where a great deal of material has been obtained, it is split between several slides to make multiple smears.

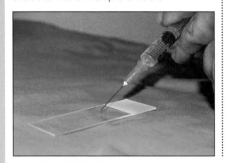

PRACTICAL TIPS

- Ideally, the sample on each slide should be the size of a single drop of blood; if more than this is used, the resulting smear may be too thick to allow visualization of the internal detail within individual cells.
- Locating the material close to the centre of the slide makes staining and microscopy considerably easier than for material at the very margins of a slide.

3 A second clean microscope slide ('spreader') is placed over the original slide containing the sample, and the material is allowed to spread between the two slides. Both the original slide and the spreader slide become coated in material from a single aspirate.

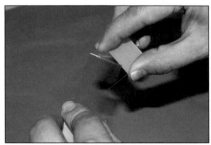

WARNING

Use the surface tension between the two slides only. No downward pressure should be exerted, as this may rupture the cells.

4 Using a smooth movement, the slides should be drawn apart, spreading the material as evenly as possible across the surface of both.

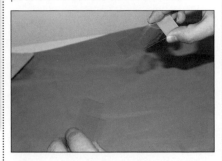

5 Both smears should then be placed aside to air dry before staining.

PRACTICAL TIP

Thick or viscous samples can be encouraged to dry by using a hairdryer on a low setting or by vigorous slide waving.

Further reading

Dunn JK and Gerber K (2005) Diagnostic cytology. In: *BSAVA Manual of Clinical Pathology, 2nd edn*, ed. E Villiers and L Blackwood, pp. 305–339. BSAVA Publications, Gloucester

Sneezing and nasal discharge

Andrea Harvey and Richard Malik

Sneezing and nasal discharge are common present-ing clinical signs in cats, indicating disease within the nasal cavity or nasopharynx. Unlike many other pre-senting clinical signs, the differential diagnoses for these signs are relatively limited, and diagnostics are also limited to a number of key procedures.

Differential diagnoses

- Feline upper respiratory tract (URT) infection caused by feline herpesvirus (FHV) or feline calicivirus (FCV), possibly with secondary bacterial infection (*Bordetella bronchiseptica*, mycoplasmas and/or normal flora – especially obligate anaerobes) (see Chapter 19)
- Dental disease with oronasal fistula/tooth root abscess
- Developmental or trauma-induced anomalies (e.g. cystic bone lesions, choanal atresia)
- Foreign body (e.g. blade of grass)
- Neoplasia (lymphoma most common, carcinoma also seen)
- Nasopharyngeal polyp
- Nasopharyngeal stenosis
- Fungal infection (*Cryptococcus* most common; prevalence very dependent on geographical location, e.g. rare in UK, common in Australia)
- Chronic rhinitis: usually a diagnosis after other conditions have been ruled out, but cats that have suffered previously from cat 'flu (see Chapter 19) are predisposed to chronic rhinitis.

Diagnostic approach

When taking the history and performing the physical examination, the clinician should particularly focus on the characteristic features of the potential disease pro-cesses that can cause sneezing and nasal discharge.

- URT infection is typically acute in onset, resulting in bilateral serous or purulent nasal discharge with or without an ocular discharge. It is most common in young cats, but can occur at any age. Vaccinated cats can also be affected. The cat may also be systemically unwell and may have other

signs of URT viral infection such as lingual ulcers (e.g. with FCV) or corneal ulcers (e.g. with FHV).
- Foreign bodies are typically associated with acute-onset severe sneezing/gagging, often accompanied by pawing at or rubbing the face due to facial discomfort. The nasal discharge usually starts a day or two later and is typically very purulent, pungent smelling and most often unilateral, though it can be bilateral.
- Neoplasia occurs most commonly in older animals and is more likely to be associated with dyspnoea and a haemorrhagic and/or unilateral nasal discharge than with chronic rhinitis, which often presents as sneezing and bilateral nasal discharge.
- Nasopharyngeal polyps, nasopharyngeal stenosis and neoplasia, in particular, are likely to be associated with easily audible stertor. Cats with nasopharyngeal polyps are usually young cats and they may also have signs of middle ear disease.

History
Important historical features that allow the differential diagnoses to be prioritized include:

- Age (e.g. nasopharyngeal polyps in younger cats, neoplasia in older cats)
- Speed of onset (e.g. very sudden onset seen with foreign bodies)
- Duration of clinical signs (e.g. neoplastic causes may be associated with more chronic histories)
- Progression: Is the condition improving (e.g. with acute rhinitis or, occasionally, a dislodged foreign body), waxing and waning (e.g. with chronic rhinitis) or becoming progressively worse (e.g. with neoplasia or fungal disease)?
- Any temporal relation to, for example, a visit to a cattery, show or boarding facility, which could have reactivated FHV through stress?
- Nature of the discharge (serous, purulent, haemorrhagic) and whether unilateral or bilateral (Figure 5.34.1). Epistaxis is especially seen with neoplastic lesions.
- Presence of additional clinical signs (e.g. conjunctivitis with some infectious agents, Figure 5.34.2)

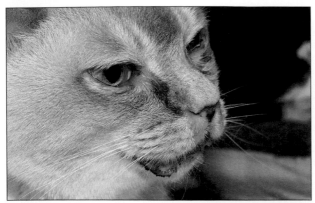

5.34.1 A 7-year-old male neutered Burmese cat from a multi-cat household, where another cat had also been sneezing. He was presented with severe bilateral purulent nasal discharge with no other clinical signs. Disease was thought most likely to be due to FHV infection and the cat was treated empirically with doxycycline and famciclovir. The nasal discharge resolved fully within a week. (Courtesy of Samantha Taylor)

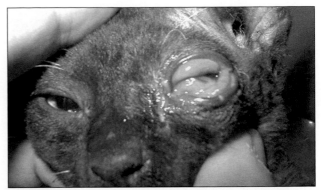

5.34.2 This kitten was presented with nasal discharge and concurrent conjunctivitis and keratitis, the latter strongly suggesting nasal disease was referable to FHV infection. Concurrent chlamydophilosis would also be a possible cause for the ocular signs but *Chlamydophila* is not usually associated with corneal ulceration and was not identified by PCR on plain conjunctival swabs. Treatment with amoxicillin/clavulanate and famciclovir were successful in resolving clinical signs within several days.

It is also important to find out whether any in-contact animals have had similar clinical signs (e.g. infectious causes), and whether the cat has been vaccinated. If similar clinical signs have been present in the past, do signs recrudesce with stress? Has there been a favourable response to any therapy provided in the past?

Physical examination

- Listen carefully for snoring or stertorous breathing (most commonly caused by a nasopharyngeal polyp, nasopharyngeal neoplasia or stenosis).
- Look for nasal discharge, focusing on assessing the nature of any discharge (serous, purulent, haemorrhagic), determining whether it is worse or predominantly on one side.
- If there is also ocular discharge, is conjunctivitis or keratitis evident?
- Are there any ulcers in the oral cavity, or skin ulcers in the vicinity of the naso-ocular region (suggestive of FHV dermatitis)?
- Is there any distortion of the nasal planum or the bones overlying the nasal cavity or frontal sinus, or pain on sinus percussion? Facial asymmetry can be a feature of neoplasia or fungal granulomas
- Is epiphora present – on one side, or both?
- Look inside the nares – does the mucosa look normal? Are any proliferative lesions evident within either naris, e.g. a neoplastic lesion or fungal granuloma?

Usually, once a good history has been taken and a physical examination has been performed, a list of the most likely differential diagnoses can be formulated based on these features plus signalment, clinical experience and intuition.

Deciding on empirical treatment *versus* further investigations

The next step is deciding whether to treat on the basis of a presumptive diagnosis (e.g. a trial of famciclovir 30–40 mg/kg orally q12h plus antibiotics such as doxycycline or amoxicillin/clavulanate for suspected FHV-associated rhinitis; Figure 5.34.2) or whether to proceed to further diagnostic investigations, which may require general anaesthesia and be associated with significant expense and some morbidity. Trial treatment is quite a reasonable first step, as many cases of FHV-associated disease will improve markedly with therapy, whereas cancers, fungal infections and foreign bodies will generally not improve. Further investigation should be performed particularly in recurrent or severe cases, or if the signalment, history and clinical findings are suggestive of conditions that will require physical intervention, such as foreign body, polyp or neoplasia.

Further diagnostic investigations

If further diagnostic investigations are required, the choice will be dependent on the cat's signalment and presenting signs. Possible tests are outlined below. In most cases of sneezing and nasal discharge it is possible to make a definitive diagnosis using one plain intra-oral radiograph (to rule out metallic foreign bodies), nasopharyngeal assessment including retro-flexed endoscopy (if available) or a vigorous nasal flush, combined with nasal biopsy.

Infectious disease testing

Oropharyngeal swabs may be taken for FCV isolation (swab placed in viral transport medium) and/or FCV and FHV PCR (plain swab). This is helpful in identifying an aetiological agent in URT infections; results are unlikely to influence therapy in the individual cat but may be useful for knowing viral status for management of multi-cat or breeding households. If ocular signs are present, ocular swabs may also be submitted for infectious disease testing (see Chapter 5.25).

Antigen tests for *Cryptococcus* (latex polysaccharide antigen test) or filamentous fungi (galactomannan or beta-glucan assays) are quite sensitive and specific for these agents, although the latter are not yet widely utilized. It is advisable to contact the laboratory for further information on sampling requirements prior to taking samples. Some antibiotics can result in false positive results in some of these assays.

FeLV and FIV testing should particularly be considered for cats with recurrent URT infections (see Chapter 19).

Haematology and serum biochemistry

Haematology and serum biochemistry usually provide little or no useful information concerning diseases of the nose and/or nasopharynx but may be advisable in clinically unwell or older patients in order to assess general systemic health, particularly prior to performing procedures that require general anaesthesia. If epistaxis alone is present, platelets, coagulation times and blood pressure should be assessed to look for systemic causes of epistaxis. It is not necessary to assess coagulation times in cases of a localized haemorrhagic nasal discharge, since this will be a result of local disease (e.g. neoplasia, fungal infection).

Diagnostic imaging

Radiography: Plain radiographs are of very limited benefit when evaluating cats with nasal discharge and sneezing, although they will identify radiopaque foreign bodies (uncommon but do occasionally occur) and some nasopharyngeal masses. A full series of nasal radiographs can be very time-consuming to obtain and are likely to fail to provide a definitive diagnosis. Intra-oral dorsoventral views of the nasal cavity are most useful. Radiographs of the lateral pharynx and bullae can sometimes be helpful in looking for a nasopharyngeal polyp, which may have middle ear involvement. Dental radiography can be used to evaluate disease of the tooth roots, and thoracic radiographs are indicated if pulmonary complications are suspected (e.g. bronchopneumonia with FHV infection, metastases with neoplasia).

CT and MRI: The best overall delineation of the nasal disease process is afforded by advanced imaging – either CT or MRI. Although it is said that MRI produces superior soft tissue detail, the speed, lower expense and exquisite bony detail obtained with CT (especially fast helical CT) make this the imaging modality of choice for nasal disease. However, imaging still does not usually provide a definitive diagnosis, and advanced imaging is expensive and usually requires referral; its use should be discussed first with a specialist to determine whether or not it is likely to be of value.

Evaluation of the nasopharynx

QRG 5.34.1 describes how the nasopharynx can be evaluated in both conscious and anaesthetized cats.

Rhinoscopy

If a fine rigid endoscope is available, anterior rhinoscopy can be of help in visualizing the nasal cavities, although visibility may be poor due to excessive mucus or bleeding. Fungal mycelium (whitish plaques) and tumours (mass lesions) can sometimes be seen, but since many nasal diseases extend to the nasopharynx, retroflexed retrograde rhinoscopy (see QRG 5.34.1) is usually more helpful if the equipment is available.

Nasal flush and biopsy

A vigorous nasal flush (see QRG 5.34.2) is helpful in identifying fungal disease and neoplasia through cytology of the resulting nasal flush fluid, and also for flushing out a nasopharyngeal foreign body. It is a cheap procedure to perform and can be used without advanced imaging and rhinoscopy if these are unavailable or unable to be performed for financial reasons.

Nasal biopsy (see QRG 5.34.2) can also be performed, particularly to confirm or exclude neoplasia. Bacterial culture of nasal discharges is rarely helpful, but culture of nasal biopsy specimens may be helpful in assessing antibiotic sensitivity in persistent infections.

QRG 5.34.1 Evaluating the nasopharynx

by Andrea Harvey and Richard Malik

Indications

- Evaluation of stertor (most commonly caused by nasopharyngeal polyp, neoplasia or stenosis)
- Suspected nasopharyngeal foreign body (e.g. acute-onset sneezing/gagging, facial discomfort, and/or nasal discharge)
- Suspected nasopharyngeal neoplasia, polyp, fungal granuloma (nasal discharge, epistaxis, nasal asymmetry, stertor)

Examination in the conscious cat

Some cats are amenable to a thorough oral examination without being anaesthetized. It may then be possible to get a view of the nasopharynx by grasping the cat's tongue with your fingers and extending it rostrally, using the projecting lingual papillae to help obtain a firm grip. If this is done successfully, the soft palate develops a V-shape, and a momentary glimpse of the nasopharynx can be obtained, which may be sufficient to allow you to see a grass blade or a polyp in the caudal nasopharynx. If there is a large mass lesion in the nasopharynx, it is also sometimes possible to see a 'bulging' of the soft palate. However, general anaesthesia will almost always be required to investigate further or remove a grass blade or polyp if present.

PRACTICAL TIP

Polyps are usually situated more caudally than nasopharyngeal lymphoma or fungal granulomas.

Examination in the anaesthetized cat

Considerations for anaesthesia in a cat with nasopharyngeal disease

Before a cat is anaesthetized for assessment of the nasopharynx, the clinician should be aware that these cases can be at high risk of upper airway obstruction. This is usually due to the presence of associated discharge, and stimulation of the nasopharynx will also often result in excessive mucus and saliva secretion, in addition to tissue oedema/inflammation. It is prudent to ensure that necessary equipment is ready prior to anaesthesia, including the following:

▶

QRG 5.34.1 *continued*

- Suction equipment
- Swabs and cotton buds to help remove secretions
- A laryngoscope
- Various sizes of endotracheal (ET) tubes
- A dog urinary catheter in case of difficulty intubating (see Chapter 3).

The cat should be pre-oxygenated and intubated with an ET tube that is as large as possible. Pulse oximetry monitoring should be used throughout, and suction equipment kept to hand throughout induction, the procedure and recovery.

Palpation

Once anaesthetized, the nasopharyngeal region should be palpated through the soft palate. Normally, the soft palate 'gives' on palpation, but if a polyp, granuloma or neoplasm is present it is generally possible to appreciate the presence of a mass lesion by palpation. Such a mass lesion may be sampled by fine-needle aspiration (see QRG 5.33.1) of the mass through the soft palate.

Retraction of the soft palate

This is best done with the cat in dorsal recumbency, and is a useful technique for visualizing foreign bodies such as blades of grass and soft tissue masses within the nasopharynx. The nasopharynx can be further evaluated using simple adjunct tools such as a laryngoscope, spay hook or forceps, and/or a dental mirror to facilitate observation of the area of interest. The authors' preference is to apply a few drops of lidocaine to the free edge of the soft palate via a cannula and to use Allis tissue forceps to pull the soft palate rostrally while a laryngoscope is used to highlight the nasopharynx.

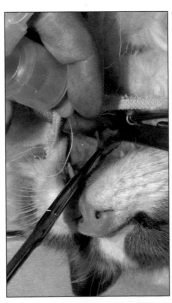

This 6-year-old male neutered DSH cat was presented with an acute history of sneezing and pawing at his face after having been outside in the owner's garden. The cat had no nasal discharge or stertor. These signs, with their acute onset, are the typical presentation for a nasopharyngeal foreign body. Retraction of the soft palate using Allis tissue forceps and the use of a laryngoscope allowed a blade of grass to be seen in the nasopharynx. Grass blades appear to get lodged while a cat is chewing on long grass, or if grass is ingested and then vomited up. This grass blade was removed intact using a pair of forceps; retrograde rhinoscopy was not required.

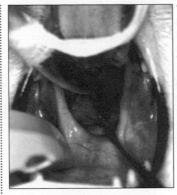

This 1-year-old female neutered DSH cat was presented with a history of several weeks of progressively worsening stertor. There was no nasal discharge or sneezing. Under anaesthesia, a firm 'bulging' of the soft palate was palpable. With the cat in dorsal recumbency the soft palate was retracted rostrally using a spay hook, and a nasopharyngeal polyp (the red lesion just caudal to the tip of the spay hook) was seen. This was successfully removed by traction using grasping forceps.

Diagnostic imaging

Plain radiography, CT and MRI can all provide a measure of the extent of the lesion, its precise anatomical location and presence of a foreign body but imaging does not negate the need for direct visualization of the nasopharynx (see above). Plain radiographs are the most practical modality to use in general practice, with the most helpful views being an intraoral dorsoventral view of the nasal cavity and a lateral view of the skull and pharynx, with the patient extubated in order to be able to assess the nasopharynx. In the majority of cases, however, these are of limited value in reaching a diagnosis, and extubating the patient may not be desirable. Advanced imaging is not usually required, but may be considered in some cases where a diagnosis has not been possible using other methods; this should be discussed first with a specialist to determine whether or not it is likely to be of value before proceeding

Retrograde rhinoscopy

If a flexible endoscope is available (either a small gastroscope or a bronchoscope) then a very good view of the nasopharyngeal region can be obtained by fully retroflexing the endoscope into a U-shape and inserting this into the mouth, hooking the free end over the top of the soft palate, rotating it to be in a midline position (look for the endoscopic light pointing rostrally through the soft palate to show that you are in the correct position), and then pulling the endoscope rostrally. Retrograde rhinoscopy will be of particular value when foreign body, nasopharyngeal mass (tumours or polyp) or nasopharyngeal stenosis (where the nasopharyngeal opening is reduced in size) is suspected but cannot be seen using the techniques described above. Referral may be required for this procedure.

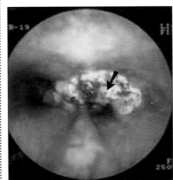

View of the nasopharynx obtained by retrograde rhinoscopy. This 5-year-old male neutered DSH cat was presented with a chronic mucopurulent nasal discharge and progressively worsening stertor. A fungal (cryptococcal) granuloma can be seen (arrow) occluding the posterior nares. Orientation of the image can be determined by pushing a finger against the soft palate; the resultant indentation can be seen at the bottom of the image here.

QRG 5.34.2 Nasal flushing and biopsy
by Andrea Harvey and Richard Malik

Indications

Nasal flush only:

- Where a foreign body is suspected or has been identified and flushing is required to attempt to dislodge it
- Where a mass has been identified or is suspected, and nasal flushing is successful in dislodging enough tissue for histopathology (this can occur with fungal granulomas and nasal lymphoma)
- In chronic rhinitis, to flush out tenacious secretions (this can be therapeutic).

Nasal flush and biopsy:

- Where a soft tissue mass has been identified or is suspected, and has not been dislodged with vigorous nasal flushing
- Where a cause (e.g. foreign body or polyp) of the clinical signs has not yet been identified; flushing can be used to collect samples for cytology, and nasal biopsy samples obtained for histopathology.

Equipment

- Suitably sized mouth gag
- Gauze swabs
- Gauze bandage
- Throat packs: these can be made by rolling up a small piece of gauze swab and tying a gauze bandage around it; the swab can be packed into the throat, whilst the bandage remains outside the mouth to allow easy retrieval. Alternatively, a small sponge with a tie attached can be used

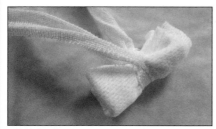

Throat pack

- Laryngoscope
- Suction equipment
- Lidocaine
- Allis tissue forceps and/or spay hook
- Dental mirror
- 3–5 mm diameter tip (or smaller) endoscope
- Cotton buds
- Small bowl of tap water
- 2 formalin pots
- 1 plain collection tube
- 1 or 2 EDTA collection tubes
- 0.9% saline (warmed)
- 2–4 x 10 ml syringes and needle for drawing up saline

- Suitable nasal biopsy forceps – e.g. alligator forceps with sharp cupped tips, otoscope biopsy forceps or endoscopic GI biopsy forceps. The bigger the forceps that can be inserted, the larger the samples that can be retrieved.

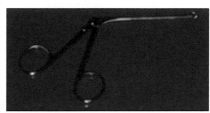

Alligator forceps

Patient preparation

- The nasopharynx should be evaluated prior to performing nasal flush or biopsy (see QRG 5.34.1).
- Since nasal biopsy can cause significant haemorrhage, haematological parameters (PCV and platelets) should be checked and found to be normal prior to taking biopsies. The authors do not routinely assess coagulation times unless the cat has any other systemic abnormalities (e.g. liver disease).
- General anaesthesia is required and anaesthetic considerations are important (see QRG 5.34.1). With nasal flush ± biopsy, there is the additional concern of even more risk of upper airway obstruction and aspiration, because of the nasal flush fluid and haemorrhage from biopsy. In addition to having suction equipment and gauze swabs and cotton buds to hand, the pharynx should be packed (see below) and consideration given to using a cuffed ET tube.

Performing a nasal flush

1 With the cat anaesthetized and with an ET tube in place, the pharynx is packed with gauze swabs or small pieces of sponge attached to a tie.

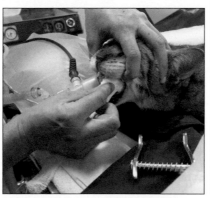

2 One of the authors (AH) prefers to have the cat positioned in sternal recumbency, with the head and neck facing ventrally over the edge of the table, to encourage fluid to drain out rostrally after flushing.

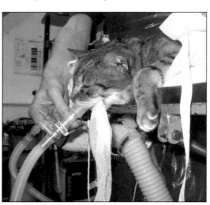

The other author (RM) prefers cats to be positioned in dorsal recumbency. Firm tape can be used to hold the cat's head in position against the table top using the maxillary canine teeth as points of anchorage (not shown here). Gauze tape can be hooked around the mandibular canine teeth to open the jaws (not show here) or, if a third person is available, it is ideal if they can hold the tongue (as shown here) and ET tube 'up' and away from the palate.

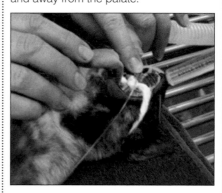

3
- Two to four 10 ml syringes are filled with sterile 0.9% NaCl that has been warmed to 38°C. The end of the syringe is wedged into one nostril.
- One hand is used to hold the syringe in place and to occlude the contralateral nostril, while injecting 10 ml saline as quickly as possible using the other hand.
- A collection dish is held underneath the cat's head to collect any material that drains from the nose or pharynx.
- Unless a foreign body has been dislodged and thus the cause already identified, fluid is then transferred to an EDTA tube for cytological assessment.
- The procedure is repeated for the other side of the nose. ▶

QRG 5.34.2 *continued*

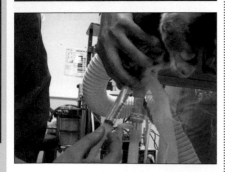

4 After flushing, the throat packs can be removed and examined for any foreign material, or dislodged tissue. Usually foreign bodies and many mass lesions will be dislodged with two or three attempts.

Portions of dislodged tissue can be:

- Used to make impression smears for cytological assessment
- Placed in formalin for histopathology
- Retained for fungal culture if fungal infection is suspected on the basis of gross appearance, or suggested by cytology or histopathology.

Routine bacterial culture of flush fluid is rarely helpful, but in cases of chronic rhinitis culture can sometimes be useful in directing antibiotic therapy if a resistant infection is identified (culture of tissue collected by biopsy is more helpful).

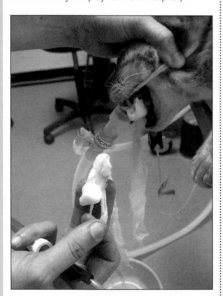

5 Following the procedure the pharynx should be examined, and any remaining secretions or fluid suctioned out.

Performing nasal biopsy

1 The anaesthetized cat, with ET tube in place, is positioned in sternal recumbency with new throat packs placed (so that any blood resulting from biopsy is not aspirated). Care must be taken not to risk penetrating the cribriform plate: forceps can be pre-measured from the nares to the medial canthus of the eye and a piece of tape used to mark the forceps at this point. The forceps must not be inserted beyond this.

WARNING

The tape must not be allowed to get wet and slip during the procedure.

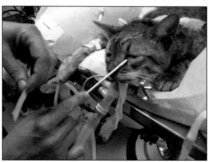

Pre-measuring the forceps. This cat has a mouth gag in place because retrograde rhinoscopy had just been performed; a gag is not necessary for nasal biopsy

2 0.1–0.2 ml of 1% lidocaine is instilled into the nares via a cannula and a few minutes allowed for this to take effect.

3 The forceps are inserted anterograde into the ventral meatus. The forceps are opened and then lodged up against any area of resistance, before closing and retracting them. The head should be directed slightly ventrally, to encourage any blood to flow cranially to the nostrils rather than caudally into the pharynx. Gauze swabs and cotton buds should be on hand to help stop any haemorrhage, which inevitably occurs.

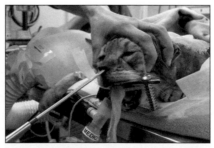

4
- Tissue collected is placed in formalin pots (labelled with the side collected from). A small amount of tissue is also reserved in a plain pot on a moistened sterile gauze swab, for bacterial and fungal culture.
- Both sides of the nose should be sampled, with at least six samples collected from each.
- Note: It is important to remember to wash the forceps in water after each sample has been placed in formalin (using the forceps), prior to inserting them into the nose again to avoid formalin entering the nose.

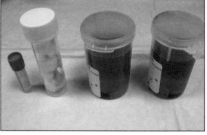

Typical samples collected from nasal investigations. From left to right: nasal flush fluid in EDTA tube for cytology; secretions from nasal flush on a gauze swab for bacterial and fungal culture; tissue samples from the left and right sides of the nose in formalin for histopathology

5 Following the procedure, the throat packs should be removed once haemorrhage appears to have ceased.

The pharynx should then be carefully examined and any remaining blood or blood clots removed with swabs or cotton buds, and any secretions suctioned, prior to recovering the cat from anaesthesia.

The pharynx should be evaluated continually for any ongoing haemorrhage prior to extubation, and anaesthesia should be maintained until any haemorrhage has ceased.

The cat should be monitored very closely in the recovery period, ensuring that suction equipment, laryngoscope, ET tubes and intravenous anaesthetic agent are kept close to hand until the cat is fully recovered.

Analgesia should be provided for at least 24 hours following biopsy.

Vomiting

Albert E. Jergens

Vomiting is a common clinical sign in feline practice and involves retching with active expulsion of gastric and/or duodenal contents that may be bile-stained. It is important to differentiate vomiting from dysphagia and regurgitation (see Chapter 5.32), which reflect primary disorders involving the oral cavity and oesophagus, respectively. Vomiting may be acute or chronic and have either an intermittent or a persistent clinical course.

Causes

Vomiting may be caused by a variety of gastrointestinal and non-gastrointestinal disorders (Figure 5.35.1).

Gastrointestinal causes	5.35.1
■ Food intolerance/food allergy ■ Gastritis (lymphocytic–plasmacytic, eosinophilic) ■ Foreign body ■ Neoplasia ■ Inflammatory bowel disease ■ Infectious disease (viral, bacterial) ■ Motility disorders	General causes of vomiting in cats.
Non-gastrointestinal causes	

■ ***Extra-abdominal disorders:***
  – Azotaemia/uraemia
  – Hyperthyroidism
  – Heartworm disease
  – Drugs/other intoxicants
  – Vestibular disease
■ ***Intra-abdominal disorders:***
  – Hepatobiliary disease
  – Pancreatitis
  – Peritonitis	

Clinical approach

The clinical approach to establishing a cause for vomiting is guided by evaluating the following parameters:

- **Age:**
  - Young animals are more likely to ingest foreign bodies and acquire infectious agents (e.g. parvovirus, ascarids)
  - Older animals develop metabolic/systemic disease (e.g. neutrophilic cholangitis) and neoplasia (e.g. lymphoma)

- **Vomiting duration:**
  - Acute vomiting (duration ≤7 days) should prompt consideration of dietary indiscretion, foreign bodies or intoxicants (e.g. paracetamol, ethylene glycol; see Chapter 4.9).
  - Chronic vomiting (duration >7 days) may be caused by numerous metabolic/systemic disorders (e.g. pancreatitis) and primary gastrointestinal disease (e.g. inflammatory bowel disease (IBD))
- **Haematemesis:**
  - Denotes blood in the vomitus due to erosive or ulcerogenic gastroduodenal disease. While uncommon in the cat, it can be caused by numerous disorders, including infiltrative mucosal disease (e.g. IBD, neoplasia such as lymphoma or mast cell tumours), NSAIDs or metabolic/systemic disorders (e.g. renal disease, hepatobiliary disease)
  - Investigate potential causes with thorough history, routine laboratory work-up (e.g. complete blood cell count, biochemistry profile, urinalysis) and advanced diagnostics, possibly to include imaging and endoscopic examination
- **Risk factors:**
  - Use of drugs, including chemotherapy (e.g. cyclophosphamide), antibacterials (e.g. amoxicillin/clavulanate, erythromycin, tetracycline hydrochloride), and NSAIDs (e.g. meloxicam)
  - Presence of systemic diseases secondarily affecting the gastrointestinal tract (e.g. renal disease, hyperthyroidism)
  - Dietary history – dietary changes and potential association of diet ingestion with vomiting
- **Geography:**
  - Infectious diseases are more prevalent in specific geographical regions (e.g. gastrointestinal histoplasmosis in midwest USA).
- **Clinical presentation:**
  - Cats with a normal physical examination and without signs of serious disease (see below) are considered to have 'non-serious disease'
  - Cats whose vomiting is associated with serious or systemic signs (e.g. lethargy, dehydration, fever, abdominal pain, icterus, anorexia) are considered to have 'serious disease'.

Diagnostic strategies

The diagnostic approach to vomiting is dictated by the presence or absence of serious gastrointestinal disease based on the history and physical examination findings. Benign, self-limiting disease should prompt minimal investigation. Further laboratory tests are warranted in cats with chronic vomiting and those with systemic signs of illness. Figure 5.35.2 summarizes the diagnostic approach to vomiting.

Treatment goals

General treatment strategic aims are to:

- Stop vomiting episodes
- Rehydrate the patient
- Correct any concurrent electrolyte abnormalities.

Cats with non-serious disease are generally treated as outpatients. Cats with serious clinical disease should be hospitalized and undergo diagnostic testing as shown in Figure 5.35.2.

Anti-emetics

Indications include patients that cannot rest and/or require correction of dehydration, electrolytes and acid–base imbalances. *Routine empirical use of anti-emetics is discouraged, since therapy may mask more serious disease, such as intestinal obstruction.* Anti-emetic options are:

- Maropitant:
  - 0.5–1 mg/kg orally or s.c. q24h
  - Acts as a selective neurokinin 1 antagonist.
- Metoclopramide:
  - 0.2–0.5 mg/kg i.m. or s.c. q8h
  - Consider CRI (0.01–0.02 mg/kg/h in crystalloid fluids such as saline or lactated Ringer's) if infusion pumps are available and/or the cat is unresponsive to intramuscular or subcutaneous dosing
  - Light-sensitive: wrapping the fluid bag/syringe and intravenous catheter in bandage is advisable if the prepared metoclopramide/crystalloid fluid mixture is to be used for ≥24 hours; if used within 24 hours, wrapping of the solution is unlikely to be needed
  - Dopamine antagonist and also provides central and peripheral (promotility) anti-emetic actions.
- Chlorpromazine:
  - 0.1–0.5 mg/kg i.m. or s.c. q8–24 h
  - Phenothiazines are potent centrally acting anti-emetics. Their alpha-antagonist actions

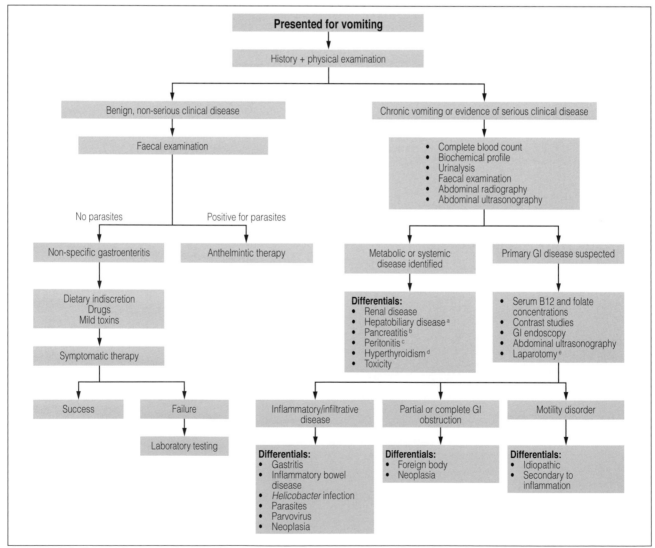

5.35.2 A diagnostic approach to vomiting in the cat. [a] Use bile acids and liver biopsy; [b] use abdominal ultrasonography and fPLI; [c] use abdominocentesis ± culture; [d] use total T4; [e] biopsy of multiple organs (liver, gut, pancreas).

may cause hypotension; avoid using this drug in epileptic animals since it may exacerbate seizures.
- Mirtazapine: 1.88–3.75 mg per cat orally q1–3d
  - In addition to having anti-emetic properties, this is an appetite stimulant and so may be desirable if anorexia is present and stimulation of eating is desired once vomiting has ceased.

Rehydration and feeding
Once vomiting ceases, small amounts of water should be introduced slowly. Food should be withheld for 12–24 hours then feeding begun with small, frequent meals of a highly digestible, low-fat diet (e.g. Hill's d/d, Iams-Eukanuba low-residue) for several days. A slow transition back to the cat's regular maintenance food should take place, by giving increasing amounts of its normal diet.

Fluid therapy
In cats with serious disease, subcutaneous or intravenous fluid therapy using crystalloids (saline or lactated Ringer's solution) should be given (see QRGs 4.1.3 and 13.2). Electrolyte imbalances (e.g. hypokalaemia, see QRG 4.6.1) should be treated specifically.

Other therapies
Symptomatic therapies for haematemesis may include:

- Cytoprotectants: e.g. sucralfate (250 mg/cat orally q8–12h) to provide cytoprotection and promote mucosal healing; needs an acidic environment to be active, so give at least 1–2 hours before any acid secretion inhibitors
- Antisecretory drugs to block acid production (e.g. famotidine, omeprazole).

Analgesia may be required for pain associated with gastrointestinal ulceration; an opioid such as buprenorphine is usually effective in acute cases (see Chapter 3).

Cats with chronic vomiting are treated according to their specific disease process, for example:

- Appropriate drug or dietary therapy for metabolic/systemic disease (e.g. chronic kidney disease)
- Foreign body removal at surgery
- Drug therapy for infiltrative mucosal disease (see Chapter 11)
- Antiparasitic medications (e.g. pyrantel, fenbendazole).

When to refer

Some cases of weight loss can be difficult to diagnose and manage, and referral may be indicated for further investigations (e.g. endoscopy for the investigation of gastrointestinal disease; hepatic biopsy; advanced imaging such as MRI). Cats with severe weight loss and cachexia may require intensive treatment and prolonged assisted feeding, which may warrant referral to a specialist centre.

What to do if finances are limited

The underlying cause of the weight loss may be indicated by initial investigations, for example in the case of hyperthyroidism; in such cases the cost of treatment and prognosis can be discussed. If investigations are limited by financial constraints, clinical judgement based on signalment and clinical signs must be used.

Managing skin disorders

Natalie Barnard

This chapter will focus on the management of the most important skin disorders encountered in feline practice, notably infectious and allergic skin diseases. Other sections of the Manual contain more information on the approach to specific skin problems, such as alopecia (Chapter 5.3), overgrooming/pruritus (Chapter 5.26), head shaking/ear scratching (Chapter 5.15) and skin masses (Chapter 5.33), including practical QRGs on Wood's lamp examination (QRG 5.3.1), hair plucks (QRG 5.3.2), skin biopsy (QRG 5.3.3), coat brushing (QRG 5.26.1), skin scrapes (QRG 5.26.2), skin cytology using tape strips and impression smears (QRG 5.26.3), ear flushing (QRG 5.15.1), ear cytology (QRG 5.15.2) and fine-needle aspiration (QRG 5.33.1).

Infectious skin disease

Dermatophytosis

Aetiology
Dermatophytosis in cats is usually caused by the fungus *Microsporum canis*. Cats become infected by coming into contact with either an infected animal or an infected environment.

Clinical features
Dermatophytosis can be seen in cats of any age, but those that are very young, very old or immunosuppressed are most at risk. Clinical signs vary greatly and so dermatophytosis should be considered a differential diagnosis for *all* feline skin conditions. Common clinical signs include:

- Variable pruritus
- Alopecia with crusting and scaling (Figure 6.1), often in a circular or irregular shape
- Focal, multifocal or diffuse lesions
- Variable erythema
- Broken or frayed hairs
- Fungal granuloma (Persians over-represented).

Diagnosis
History and dermatological examination may raise the index of suspicion for dermatophytosis, especially if other animals in the household are affected or if the owners have lesions ('ringworm'). Affected cats may give positive results with a Wood's lamp (see QRG

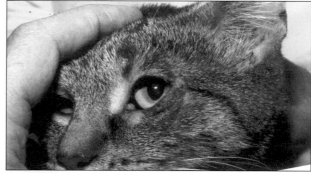

6.1 Periorbital alopecia, crusting and erythema due to *Microsporum canis* infection in a young cat.

5.3.1), although only 50% of *Microsporum canis* isolates fluoresce. Hair plucks may reveal spores on the hair shaft, though these are often hard to recognize without experience. If spores are seen on a hair pluck or if the cat has a positive Wood's lamp examination, empirical treatment with itraconazole (see later) may be started, as it can take up to 2 weeks to obtain fungal culture results.

A positive fungal culture confirms the diagnosis. Hair and scales from focal affected areas should be sent to an external laboratory for fungal culture. If lesions are diffuse, the Mackenzie toothbrush technique should be used to gather specimens (see Chapter 5.3). In-house fungal culture is possible but kits do not detect all species and false positives are common, so culture by an external laboratory is always recommended.

Management
Dermatophytosis will resolve spontaneously within a few months in healthy cats but, because of the zoonotic nature of this disease, infected individuals should be treated. When treating large multi-cat households/catteries, advice must be sought from a specialist early in the course of treatment as it can be very challenging and expensive for the client. Further discussion is provided in the *BSAVA Manual of Canine and Feline Dermatology*.

Antifungal treatment: Systemic treatment is the treatment of choice for dermatophytosis. Itraconazole is the only authorized systemic treatment for feline dermatophytosis and is very effective. It is used at 5 mg/kg orally q24h for 7 days; treatment is then stopped for 7 days and the cycle repeated. At least three 7-day periods of treatment are required as a minimum. In some cases, if a rapid clinical response is not seen, longer courses of treatment may be required. Itraconazole can be hepatotoxic to cats and it is therefore advisable to monitor liver enzymes (ALT and ALP) before and during treatment. If the cat becomes anorexic or loses weight, treatment should be discontinued while liver enzymes and liver function are evaluated.

Some texts advise clipping longhaired cats; this is a controversial practice but may help to reduce environmental contamination. Clipping must be performed in a place that can be easily cleaned and disinfected and should not take place in the veterinary surgery. Clients must be warned that clipping an affected cat may lead to a temporary worsening of its clinical signs.

A 2% miconazole + 2% chlorhexidine shampoo (Malaseb) is authorized as an aid in the control of dermatophytosis, as it helps to reduce environmental contamination. However, in the author's experience, bathing cats is generally very challenging for clients, especially as it needs to be performed twice weekly.

Treating in-contact animals: Specimens for fungal culture should be obtained from all in-contact cats. In some cases it may also be necessary to sample dogs and small mammals; these animals are often treated alongside the presenting cat, pending fungal culture results, as this is a highly contagious disease.

Treating large multi-cat households is challenging, especially if finances are limited. In this situation, affected animals with clinical signs should be kept separate from unaffected animals while receiving treatment. Fungal culture should be carried out on all cats, however, to determine whether any cat without clinical signs is an asymptomatic carrier that needs treatment. If previously unaffected animals start to show lesions, they should be added to the group being treated.

Decontaminating the environment: This is very challenging. The most important method is the physical removal of hair by vacuuming. Surfaces should also be disinfected, and contaminated bedding must be destroyed. Surfaces should be cleaned using a product that contains bleach.

Monitoring treatment: Fungal cultures should be performed every 4 weeks, taking hairs and scales from lesional areas or using the Mackenzie toothbrush technique if the lesions are no longer visible. Treatment should be continued for at least another 2 weeks after negative culture. Clinical resolution will always occur before mycological cure.

Feline acne

Aetiology
A primary keratinization problem leads to secondary bacterial infection of the skin.

Clinical features
Lesions are usually seen on the chin and occasionally the upper lips, and can include:

- Comedones
- Follicular casts
- Papules, pustules and crusts
- Swelling and oedema of the chin.

Diagnosis
This is based on history, physical examination and clinical signs. Other conditions such as demodicosis and dermatophytosis need to be excluded by skin scrape examination (see QRG 5.26.2) and fungal culture. Cytology (see QRG 5.26.3) of samples from the affected skin will reveal coccoid bacteria, degenerate neutrophils and macrophages. If the surface of the lesion is highly crusted it is often necessary to remove a small amount of the crust and take a sample from below to obtain meaningful cytology results. It is also possible to make an impression smear from the underside of the removed crust.

Management
Some cats may only have mild clinical signs (e.g. comedones) and will not require treatment.

Systemic antibiotic treatment is usually required in cats that are displaying signs of infection (i.e. large numbers of inflammatory cells and bacteria seen on cytology). Cefalexin, clindamycin and amoxicillin/clavulanate are appropriate choices. Treatment often takes several weeks (typically a minimum of 4 weeks) and should be continued for at least another 2 weeks after resolution of the papules and pustules.

Topical therapies are beneficial in all cases and have the aim of dislodging debris and dissolving the comedones. The use of antiseborrhoeic or antibacterial shampoos daily can be useful. In cats that have recurrent episodes of acne, long-term twice-weekly use of such shampoos may be a useful preventive measure. Topical antimicrobials can be used in some cases; mupirocin ointment can be applied twice daily if the cat will allow.

WARNING

Although benzoyl peroxide shampoo can be used in dogs, it should not be used in cats as it is too irritating and can be toxic.

Systemic prednisolone (1–2 mg/kg orally q24h for 7–10 days then gradually tapering over 2–3 weeks) may be useful in cases with marked swelling and to help to reduce scarring. It is important that any bacterial infection is treated **before** giving prednisolone treatment. In cases with marked swelling it is important that eosinophilic granuloma is also considered as a differential.

Malassezia dermatitis

Aetiology
Until recently *Malassezia* dermatitis was considered rare to uncommon in cats, but it is now recognized frequently in cats with all forms of allergic skin disease (including flea-associated disease, food allergies and atopic dermatitis) and in certain breeds such as the Devon Rex and Sphynx. It is also seen in cats with paraneoplastic alopecia, and may be the cause of the pruritus seen in these cases.

Clinical features

Clinical signs may include:

- Pruritus
- Greasy exudates
- Erythema
- Scaling
- Seborrhoea.

In Devon Rex and Sphynx cats with *Malassezia* dermatitis, the skin is greasy, and often a brown waxy discharge may be present around the nail beds, but there is often no pruritus.

Diagnosis

The most reliable way to diagnose *Malassezia* infection (see Figure 5.15.4) is through cytology of a tape strip sample (see QRG 5.26.3). The only time that culture is indicated is when a cat is not responding to appropriate treatment despite owner compliance. In addition to *Malassezia pachydermatis* (the yeast commonly found on dogs), cats also have several different types of lipid-dependent *Malassezia,* which do not grow on the routine culture media used at most commercial laboratories; a specific request for attempted culture of these species must be made when submitting samples. If there is concern that a cat has a resistant *Malassezia* infection that warrants sensitivity testing, the laboratory should also be contacted prior to sending the sample; it should be noted that fungal sensitivity testing is often very expensive.

Management

There are no authorized treatments for *Malassezia* dermatitis in cats but treatment with itraconazole at 5 mg/kg orally q24h for at least 3 weeks, or a 2% miconazole + 2% chlorhexidine shampoo (Malaseb, Dechra) used twice weekly, is effective. Monitoring during itraconazole treatment is as described for dermatophytosis.

Mycobacterial infections

It is recommended that a specialist is consulted to discuss the diagnosis (and management) of mycobacterial cases.

Aetiology and clinical features

Mycobacteria are aerobic, non-spore-forming bacteria, capable of causing the following diseases in cats.

Tuberculosis: Tuberculosis is quite rare but may be caused by *Mycobacterium bovis* or the vole variant *M. microti.* These species exist in a variety of small mammals, with cats infected via bite wounds when hunting. The cutaneous form is most commonly seen in cats, and causes non-healing wounds and nodules with draining sinus tracts on the face and limbs. Occasionally systemic gastrointestinal or respiratory signs are seen. Local or generalized lymph node enlargement is common, occasionally in the absence of other clinical signs. These organisms pose a zoonotic risk, although there are no reported cases of cats passing tuberculosis to people; human infection is usually acquired from other humans or from cattle. In the UK *M. bovis* infection is a notifiable disease and must be reported to the Animal Health Veterinary Laboratories Agency upon confirmation. Tuberculosis

lesions typically contain acid-fast bacilli but culture is slow, taking 2–3 months, or may be impossible.

Feline leprosy: Caused by *Mycobacterium lepraemurium,* this usually affects young adult cats. An alternative form is reported in Australia, caused by a novel undefined mycobacterium. Infection is thought to occur via bite wounds or soil contamination of a wound. There is no known zoonotic potential for these organisms. Feline leprosy is a cutaneous disease, with single or multiple mobile, non-painful nodules, which can be alopecic, ulcerated or haired, found primarily on the head and limbs. Acid-fast bacilli are variably present but culture is usually not possible.

Opportunistic (non-tuberculous) mycobacterial infections: Non-tubercular mycobacterial infections can be caused by saprophytic, usually non-pathogenic, organisms found in soil, water and decaying vegetation, which gain entry into the host via bites, scratches and other wounds. Although infections are caused by many different organisms (e.g. *Mycobacterium smegmatis, M. phlei, M. chelonae*), the clinical syndrome is similar. There is no known zoonotic potential. These organisms can sometimes be easy to grow in culture. Clinical signs comprise panniculitis with multiple small, draining, sinus tracts ('salt and pepper shaker' appearance), which may progress to form large, ulcerated, non-healing skin wounds. The subcutaneous fat of the inguinal fat pads and flanks are commonly affected. Systemic disease is rare but cats may be pyrexic and anorexic.

Diagnosis

A screen for systemic disease should take place if there is a compatible history and clinical signs.

Mycobacterial infections can be diagnosed using histopathology and/or tissue culture and/or PCR. Multiple (three to four) tissue specimens are obtained from affected regions and submitted in formalin for histopathology (nodular dermatitis or deep pyogranulomatous panniculitis) and Ziehl–Neelsen staining (mycobacterial organisms seen as acid-fast bacilli). Additionally, small (e.g. 0.4 cm^3) samples of these tissues should be preserved for culture, with one unfixed for submission for routine bacterial culture and two frozen in sterile containers without any preservative. One of the latter two samples can be sent for further specialist mycobacterial investigations (e.g. culture, PCR) should this be required. The other one is a reserve for further investigation. PCR can also be performed on fixed paraffin embedded tissue if this is all that is available. The organisms can be successfully cultured to a variable degree (see above).

> **WARNING**
>
> Until organisms are identified definitively, biopsy samples should be considered as having zoonotic potential.

Management

Small localized cutaneous nodules, caused by feline leprosy, may be surgically removed; adjunct antibiotic treatment with a fluoroquinolone (e.g. marbofloxacin at 2 mg/kg orally q24h) is also usually given. A fluoroquinolone can be prescribed when awaiting results in a cat with only cutaneous manifestations of myco-bacterial disease. However, since cases of mycobac-terial infection often require lengthy (6–9 months), intensive (up to three drugs at a time) and expensive treatment, it is advised that a specialist is consulted for advice on treatment. The prognosis for feline leprosy is good, but is guarded for tuberculosis and poor to guarded for opportunistic (non-tuberculous) mycobacterial infections.

Pyoderma

Aetiology
Pyoderma usually occurs secondary to an underlying skin disease (most commonly allergic skin disease).

Clinical features
Papules and pustules are most common, though pyoderma may sometimes present in the same way as miliary dermatitis or lesions of the eosinophilic granuloma complex. Lesions can be seen anywhere on the body.

Diagnosis
Diagnosis can be made through cytology (see QRG 5.26.3) or culture of samples from affected skin. For skin culture, a swab and transport medium should be used; the sample should be taken gently from the affected area, which can be defined based on finding bacteria on cytology.

Management
The underlying cause (e.g. ectoparasites, cutaneous adverse food reaction, atopic dermatitis) should be identified and treated.

Antibiotic therapy: Choice of antibiotic(s) will depend on the organisms seen on cytology:

- Cocci are most commonly *Staphylococcus* spp., which are Gram-positive and usually have a predictable sensitivity pattern. Cefalexin (15 mg/kg orally q12h), clindamycin (5.5 mg/kg orally q12h) or amoxicillin/clavulanate (12.2 mg/kg orally q12h) can all be used. At least a 3-week course is usually required and treatment should continue for at least 7 days past resolution of clinical signs.
- Rods may indicate a Gram-negative infection, such as with *Escherichia coli, Proteus* or *Pseudomonas* spp. A swab sample should always be submitted for culture and sensitivity testing. Treatment must be continued for at least 7 days past resolution of infection, as judged by improvement in clinical signs and cytology findings.

If there is a deep infection (furunculosis, draining tracts) treatment should be continued for at least another 2 weeks after resolution of clinical signs and negative cytology findings. For a resistant infection, treatment should be continued for 7–14 days after a negative culture result.

Viral dermatitis
Calicivirus, herpesvirus and poxvirus can all cause viral dermatitis (see Chapter 5.26).

Allergic skin disease

Atopic dermatitis
Atopic dermatitis is a pruritic skin disease that is commonly seen in cats.

Aetiology
Unlike in dogs, a genetic basis has not been proven in cats. The disease has a complex pathogenesis and is mainly caused by a type 1 hypersensitivity reaction to environmental allergens such as house dust mites and pollens. It gives rise to a number of cutaneous reaction patterns.

Clinical features
A variety of clinical signs can be suggestive of feline atopic dermatitis but none is pathognomonic. Signs include:

- Pruritus (may be seasonal; skin lesions are not always seen)
- Lesions of the eosinophilic granuloma complex (Figure 6.2)
- Alopecia
- Miliary dermatitis (see Chapter 5.26)
- Ceruminous otitis externa
- Secondary pyoderma or *Malassezia* dermatitis (see earlier)
- Erythematous macules, papules, excoriations or ulcerative lesions – usually located around the head, neck, ears, ventral abdomen and caudal thighs
- Allergic asthma (an uncommon concurrent clinical manifestation).

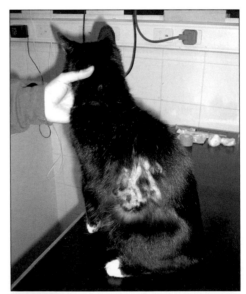

6.2 Eosinophilic plaques in a cat with eosinophilic granuloma complex (see Chapter 5.26); this can be a manifestation of atopic dermatitis or cutaneous adverse food reaction.

Diagnosis
Atopic dermatitis is a diagnosis of exclusion that can only be made: if the cat has compatible history and clinical signs; and when all other causes of pruritus (e.g. infection, ectoparasites, cutaneous adverse food reactions) have been ruled out. This is because all of these diseases can have similar, if not identical, clinical presentations.

Allergy testing:

> Allergy testing should only be performed when a diagnosis of atopic dermatitis has been made. The purpose of allergy testing is to identify allergens so as to enable avoidance or formulation of a course of allergen-specific immunotherapy; it is *not* to make a diagnosis of atopic dermatitis.

Allergy testing in cats is controversial. It can be performed by using either allergen-specific IgE serology or intradermal testing. It is important to realize that these tests assess different things:

- The intradermal test measures the skin's reactivity to an allergen that has been injected intradermally
- Serological tests measure the reactivity of antibodies present in the blood to a particular antigen.

Intradermal testing is still recognized as the gold standard in dogs, but the tests can be difficult to interpret in cats. Cats may only have very subtle reactions and there is a high incidence of false negatives. Technically the test may be difficult to perform because feline skin is much thinner than canine. An increased incidence of anaphylaxis with intradermal testing has also been reported in cats compared to dogs. It is important that cats sedated for intradermal tests are under minimal stress, as the stress response could also cause a false negative result. For the above reasons, many dermatologists will perform only serology in cats.

Serology detects allergen-reactive IgE in the cat's serum. It is important to use a laboratory where the test has been validated for cats. FcεRIα is a high affinity receptor of IgE and is used to detect allergen-specific IgE in serum samples; other antibodies such as IgM, IgA or IgG, whether allergen-reactive or not, do not bind to this receptor. It must be remembered that some normal cats can have positive reactions on this test; it is therefore important that the test is performed only once a diagnosis of atopic dermatitis has been made, and that the results are interpreted in light of the patient's clinical signs. For example, if a cat has clinical signs all year round and grass pollens are the only positive reaction, this is unlikely to be significant. It should also be borne in mind that a high value result does not necessarily indicate that this allergen is clinically more important compared with an allergen that has a lower value.

Management

Secondary infections: It is vital to manage any secondary infections that may be present, including *Malassezia* overgrowth and pyoderma (see above) as these can increase the cat's level of pruritus.

Avoidance: Reducing exposure to the offending allergens, if these have been identified by allergy testing, is beneficial but is often difficult to achieve, especially as house dust mites are the most commonly identified allergen. Spraying the house with an acaricide to reduce mite numbers may benefit some patients; permethrin agents are available that kill mites and are safe to use environmentally as long as there is good ventilation.

Allergen-specific immunotherapy: This is a safe and effective treatment for feline atopic dermatitis, in which gradually increasing quantities of an allergen extract are administered to a patient by subcutaneous injection, the purpose of which is to reduce or eliminate the symptoms associated with subsequent exposure to the causative allergen. Treatment should be trialled for between 9 and 12 months, as it can take this long for the benefits to be seen. Generally most patients will require additional treatment to control their clinical signs in the interim. A satisfactory response is generally regarded as a 50% reduction in pruritus and dermatitis; this is seen in 60–78% of cats treated with ASIT.

Corticosteroids: Corticosteroids (see Chapter 3) comprise the mainstay of treatment for cats with atopic dermatitis. Prednisolone at a dose of 1–2 mg/kg orally q24h for 7–10 days is used and then tapered to the lowest possible alternate-day dose that controls the cat's clinical signs. Methylprednisolone is an alternative (0.8 mg/kg orally q24h), which is also tapered to the lowest possible alternate-day dose. Some cats may respond differently to different types of corticosteroid, although the reason for this is not completely understood. Methylprednisolone acetate (4 mg/kg s.c. or i.m.) should only be used if the cat cannot be medicated orally, as this formulation has a long duration of effect and also possible associated side effects.

Ciclosporin: Ciclosporin has been used to treat feline atopic dermatitis and is authorized at a dose of 7.5 mg/kg orally q24h. Reported side effects seen when using ciclosporin in cats can include:

- Vomiting
- Weight loss
- Anorexia and subsequent hepatic lipidosis
- Diarrhoea and loose stools.

It is important to realize that ciclosporin causes immunosuppression and may induce serious infectious problems such as systemic toxoplasmosis or herpesvirus-associated disease, especially if given concurrently with steroids. Exposure to novel *Toxoplasma* infection via hunting or eating raw meat should be avoided if possible, but recrudescence of existing infection (see Chapter 19) is also possible on ciclosporin therapy. Diagnostic testing and prophylactic treatment for such conditions, e.g. clindamycin for toxoplasmosis or famciclovir for herpetic disease, may be considered.

Antihistamines: There are no antihistamines authorized for use in the cat but they can be useful in reducing clinical symptoms in 40–70% of atopic cats. They can be used alone, or in combination with glucocorticoids and essential fatty acids, and may have a steroid-sparing effect. Benefits are seen within 1–2 weeks of starting treatment. Sedation is a common side effect. Commonly used antihistamines include chlorphenamine (0.25 mg/kg q12h) and cetirizine (5 mg/cat orally q24h).

Essential fatty acids: These help control pruritus in 20–50% of cats but it can take up to 3 months before benefits are seen. A synergistic effect between

every other day for 2–4 weeks) due to its short duration of action; spinosad is a longer lasting (up to a month) oral preparation that is expected to be authorized in the UK soon for use in cats. Lufenuron is another longer lasting oral treatment, which can also be given by injection; it is an insect development inhibitor that should be used with an adulticide if a large population of fleas is present.

The treatment chosen needs to take into consideration patient factors such as: the level of flea control required; whether the cat can be medicated easily; the age of the cat (e.g. fipronil spray can be used in young kittens); and client factors (e.g. cost, ease of application).

Environmental control

As adult fleas represent only a small proportion of the life cycle in the cat's environment, **environmental control is vital**. The pupae are the most resistant stage of the life cycle and can persist in the environment for several months; no currently available products kill pupae. Many products are available for spraying the environment, and most combine an adulticide (e.g. permethrin) with an insect growth regulator (e.g. methoprene). These take time to apply but can be used safely in a well ventilated environment, applied according to the manufacturer's instructions. Several on-animal preparations (e.g. selamectin, methoprene) also have some action in the environment, but these do not replace the need for environmental control.

Cheyletiellosis

This is typically a very mild but highly contagious skin condition caused by surface-living *Cheyletiella* mites. These can affect many species and are not thought to be host-specific, readily transferring between dogs, cats, rabbits and humans. They are fairly large mites with four sets of legs and are easily recognized by their waisted body and accessory mouthparts that terminate in hooks (see QRG 5.26.2).

Clinical features
These include:

- Excessive scaling, often on the trunk and dorsum
- Variable pruritus
- Some animals can be asymptomatic carriers and

may act as a source of infestation for other animals.

Diagnosis
A diagnosis can be made by finding the mites on a coat brushing sample (see QRG 5.26.1) or skin scrape (see QRG 5.26.2).

Management
There are currently no authorized treatments for dealing with this ectoparasite in the UK. Fipronil spray may aid in control (affected cats need to be treated every 2 weeks). An imidacloprid 10% + moxidectin 2.5% spot-on treatment (Advocate) is reported to be safe and efficacious when treating canine cheyletiellosis, when two applications are used at 4-weekly intervals, but no studies are available in cats.

All in-contact animals need to be treated, and bedding and grooming equipment should be disinfected.

References and further reading

Guaguère E and Prelaud P (1999) *A Practical Guide to Feline Dermatology*. Mérial Animal Health

Gunn-Moore D, Dean R and Shaw S (2010) Mycobacterial infections in cats and dogs. *In Practice* **32**, 444–452

Heinrich NA, McKeever PJ and Eisenschenk MC (2011) Adverse events in 50 cats with allergic dermatitis receiving ciclosporin. *Veterinary Dermatology* **22**, 511–520

Jackson H and Marsella R (2012) *BSAVA Manual of Canine and Feline Dermatology, 3rd edn*. BSAVA Publications, Gloucester

Loewenstein C and Mueller R (2009) A review of allergen specific immunotherapy in human and veterinary medicine. *Veterinary Dermatology* **20**, 84–98

Mecklenburg L, Linek M and Tobin DJ (2009) *Hair Loss Disorders in Domestic Animals*. Wiley Blackwell, Oxford

Medleau L and Hnilica KA (2006) *Small Animal Dermatology: A Colour Atlas and Therapeutic Guide, 2nd edn*. WB Saunders, Philadelphia

Miller WH, Griffin CE and Campbell KL (2012) *Muller and Kirk's Small Animal Dermatology, 7th edn*. WB Saunders, Philadelphia

Noli C and Scaranpella F (2006) Prospective open pilot study on the use of ciclosporin for feline allergic skin disease. *Journal of Small Animal Practice* **47**, 434–438

Ordeix L, Galeotti F, Scarampella F *et al.* (2007) *Malassezia* spp. overgrowth in allergic cats. *Veterinary Dermatology* **18**, 316–323

Peterson ME, Kintzer PP and Hurvitz AI (1988) Methimazole treatment of 262 cats with hyperthyroidism. *Journal of Veterinary Internal Medicine* **2**, 150–157

Rhodes KH and Werner AH (2011) *Blackwell's Five Minute Veterinary Consult Clinical Companion: Small Animal Dermatology, 2nd edn*. Wiley-Blackwell, Oxford

Trimmer AM, Griffin CE and Rosenkratz WS (2006) Feline immunotherapy. *Clinical Techniques in Small Animal Practice* **21**, 157–161

Wassom and Grieve (2002) In vitro measurement of canine and feline IgE: a review of FcεR1α- based assays detection of allergen-reactive IgE. *Veterinary Dermatology* **9**, 173–178

Wisselik MA and Willemse T (2009) The efficacy of ciclosporin A in cats with presumed atopic dermatitis: a double blind, randomised prednisolone controlled study. *The Veterinary Journal* **180**, 55–59

QRG 6.1 Dietary trial for cutaneous adverse food reaction

by Natalie Barnard

NOTE: The description below is specifically for cats with *cutaneous* signs. Measures for a cat with gastrointestinal signs of food hypersensitivity are described in Chapter 11.

A cutaneous adverse food reaction can only be diagnosed by performing a dietary trial with a novel diet for 6–8 weeks (6 weeks minimum). It is vital that any infections/infestations are treated first because otherwise it is not possible to assess the benefit of the dietary trial.

Diet selection

A diet should be carefully selected based on the patient's history, avoiding proteins that the cat has been exposed to previously. The most common allergens are chicken, beef, fish and dairy products, which are commonly included in many commercial petfoods. Most commercial petfoods contain multiple ingredients; the owner should understand that a food labelled as 'tuna-flavoured', for example, will not just contain tuna. It is therefore necessary to feed a good quality diet with limited ingredients. Prescription diets are commonly used.

Several types of diet are possible:

- **Hydrolysed diets** (e.g. Purina HA, Hill's z/d ultra, RCW hypoallergenic). These diets have undergone enzymatic hydrolysis to disrupt the protein structure and reduce the antigenicity of the protein. These diets may not always use a novel protein. They are easily fed and palatable for most cats, in the author's experience. These diets are generally more expensive compared to the limited-antigen diets
- **Limited-antigen diets**. These are composed of a novel protein and carbohydrate source. They need to be selected carefully, based on the patient's dietary history. For example, if a cat has had a diet mainly consisting of chicken and fish, a suitable limited antigen diet with a novel protein would be, for example, Hill's d/d venison and green pea
- **Home-cooked diets**. The advantage of a home-cooked diet is that the protein and carbohydrate source can be carefully selected and it is known exactly what is in the food (e.g. rabbit and potato). However, cats will often not eat many of the novel carbohydrate sources. The main disadvantages of home-cooked diets are that they are labour-intensive in terms of preparation for the owner, and they are not nutritionally complete. Thus, they are generally not recommended in cats for long-term use, although they can be useful in the short term for identifying an appropriate carbohydrate and protein source.

PRACTICAL TIPS

- It is important to find a diet that the cat will eat, e.g. if the cat is used to eating a wet diet, a suitable wet diet for the food trial should be sought.
- To find a diet that the cat will actually eat, several diets may need to be tried.
- The diet needs to be fed strictly and so in a multi-cat household it may be helpful to have all the cats on the same diet.
- Some dermatologists advise keeping the cat indoors to avoid it feeding elsewhere; this is ideal if it is possible for the owner, but it is often very difficult to keep the cat confined. The author still recommends attempting a dietary trial, even if the cat continues to go outdoors; the owner can be advised to obtain a collar which states 'do not feed me I am on a special diet' for their cat, and/or they can provide any neighbour known to feed their cat with some of the exclusion diet.

Results

At the end of the dietary trial:

- **If there is no improvement** (the patient remains pruritic): In the absence of infection, ectoparasites or lack of compliance, this confirms that cutaneous adverse food reaction is not the cause of the cat's clinical signs
- **If there is improvement:** The patient now needs to be re-challenged with all aspects of its original diet over a 2-week period. *The dietary re-challenge is a vital part of the dietary trial. As allergic skin disease can wax and wane, deterioration must be seen with dietary re-challenge to confirm the improvement is not attributable to antimicrobial treatment, or a coincidence.* In some cases, an increase in pruritus can be noted within 24 hours of ingestion of the allergenic food, and in other animals it can take up to 2 weeks. When a reaction is seen the patient should be placed immediately back on to the exclusion diet and the clinical signs should resolve again, thereby confirming the diagnosis of a cutaneous adverse food reaction. If the owner wishes to identify the specific component the cat is allergic to, then each item needs to be added to the diet for a 2-week period without a reaction being observed, before concluding whether or not the item is acceptable.

Radiographic features of FORLs

- Loss of integrity of the periodontal ligament space (see white arrows on Figures 7.3b, 7.4b and 7.5b)
- Loss of the lamina dura
- Irregularities on the root surface
- Diffuse decrease in radiodensity of the entire root compared with adjacent roots (see black arrows on Figures 7.3b, 7.4b and 7.5b)

- Radiolucent areas within the root dentine, often extending into the crown dentine (see red arrows on Figures 7.3ab, 7.4ab and 7.5ab)
- Replacement of root substance by bone-like tissue (see blue arrows on Figures 7.3b, 7.4b and 7.5b)
- Resorbing roots present with clinically missing crown (see green arrow on Figure 7.4b).

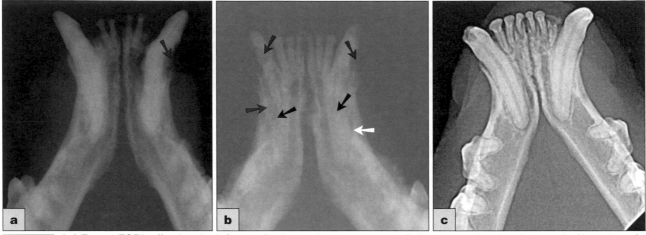

7.3 (a) Type 1 FORL affecting the left mandibular canine, seen as a radiolucency at the alveolar margin (the edge of the portion of bone that contains the tooth). The root and the periodontal ligament can still be distinguished from the surrounding bone. **(b)** Type 2 FORLs affecting both mandibular canine teeth. There are radiolucent areas in the crown as well as loss of the structure of the root and periodontal ligament. **(c)** Normal radiograph for comparison. (See box above for explanation of arrows.)

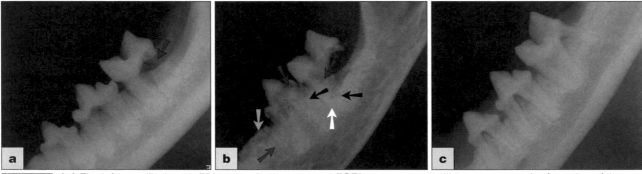

7.4 (a) The left mandibular 4th PM and molar have type 1 FORLs, seen as a radiolucent area at the furcation of the tooth. The roots of the 4th PM remain relatively unaffected, whilst the lesion has resorbed most of the coronal part of the distal root of the molar, with the apical two-thirds remaining unaffected. **(b)** The left mandibular 4th PM and molar on this radiograph are affected by type 2 FORLs. The left mandibular 3rd PM is missing clinically but ghost roots are visible radiographically. Although the outline of both roots of the 4th PM can be seen, only its most mesial root is visible. There is no periodontal ligament space around the roots, the lamina dura has been lost and the density of the dentine resembles bone. **(c)** Normal radiograph for comparison. (See box above for explanation of arrows.)

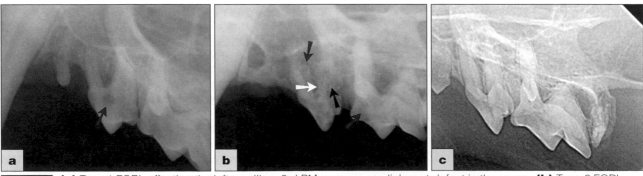

7.5 (a) Type 1 FORL affecting the left maxillary 3rd PM seen as a radiolucent defect in the crown. **(b)** Type 2 FORL affecting the left maxillary 3rd PM and 4th PM. The roots of the 3rd PM appear less dense and have lost the periodontal ligament and lamina dura. The mesiopalatal root of the 4th PM is most affected, with the mesiobuccal and distal roots retaining their periodontal ligament and the surrounding lamina dura. **(c)** Normal radiograph for comparison. (See box above for explanation of arrows.)

Treatment

Many FORLs were previously restored using glass-ionomer products, but the long-term success rate was poor. The current recommendation is that all affected teeth should be extracted, as the lesions will almost invariably progress and become more painful. Feline tooth extraction is usually difficult but becomes even more so when the integrity of the tooth is damaged by the destructive resorption process. There may be areas of ankylosis between the root and alveolar bone, which may or may not be visible on radiographs.

Type 1 FORLs

The whole root and remaining tooth substance must be removed. Often a surgical extraction technique is required to remove the teeth as the roots are prone to fracture (see QRG 7.2).

Type 2 FORLs

Crown amputation with intentional root retention has been proposed as an alternative to whole-tooth extraction. Studies have shown that the resorbing root continues to be resorbed. This technique is acceptable, provided preoperative radiographic assessment has been performed to establish that the lesion is of type 2. However, this technique is only appropriate for teeth that do not have any radiographic evidence of endodontic disease (disease of the pulp tissue (blood vessels, nerves, connective tissue) such as periapical inflammation) or periodontitis. In cats with gingivostomatitis the whole tooth should be removed.

Feline chronic gingivostomatitis

Feline chronic gingivostomatitis (FCGS) is a condition affecting many cats seen in general practice. The actual incidence of the disease is about 3% of all feline dental conditions. The term FCGS is a descriptive term rather than a diagnosis. It has also been termed plasmacytic–lymphocytic stomatitis, based on histopathological findings. The condition is characterized by severe inflammation – either locally or diffusely – affecting the gingiva and oral mucosa, often extending past the glossopalatine folds and into the fauces. The inflammation is usually of chronic duration and may have been present for months to years at the time of presentation. FCGS is often refractory to medical treatment (Figure 7.6).

Aetiology and pathogenesis

The aetiology of the syndrome is unknown but studies suggest that there may be an infectious and immune response component associated with the disease. An aberrant reaction to plaque accumulation in the mouth is believed to play a part in FCGS. This aberrant reaction may be due to the host's immune response either not being able to deal with the oral pathogens or showing an excessive reaction to oral pathogens. Cats with FCGS have been shown to have elevated serum immunoglobulins but low levels of salivary IgA, which forms part of the oral defence mechanism. Salivary IgA interferes with bacterial adherence and neutralizes pathogens and toxins produced by bacteria in the oral cavity.

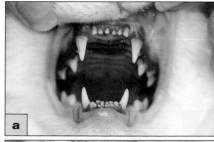
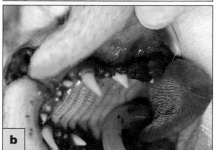

7.6 Feline chronic gingivostomatitis. **(a)** The canines and incisors of a 2-year-old male neutered DSH cat. The inflammation had been persistent despite medical treatment for the past 9 months. The inflammation present extends the whole width of the attached gingiva to the level of the mucogingival junction. **(b)** The same cat, showing severe gingivitis and inflammation of the premolars and molars extending beyond the mucogingival junction. The inflammation can be seen in the oral mucosa on the left side (top of photo) and also extends on to the palatal mucosa on the right side of the mouth (base of photo). The gingival tissue is also hyperplastic.

Role of feline calicivirus

FCV is detected in up to 100% of chronically affected cats (oropharyngeal swab) but no direct aetiological link has been shown in experimental studies. One study found that palatoglossitis, but not buccostomatitis, was linked with FCV infection.

Role of diet

In humans, chronic gingivostomatitis can be linked to intolerance to certain food ingredients, but there are as yet no studies in veterinary medicine; however, anecdotal reports have described that changing a cat's diet has helped improve FCGS.

Clinical features

Unlike many dental conditions affecting cats, FCGS may cause anorexia, dysphagia and weight loss. Affected cats often present with halitosis and ptyalism and sometimes bleeding from the mouth. They will often have poorly kept coats as the mouth has become too sore and uncomfortable to use for grooming. Oral examination reveals the extent of the inflammation; it usually extends beyond the gingiva to the oral mucosa lining the cheeks (buccal mucosa) and lips (labial mucosa), and caudally to the glossopalatine mucosa of the oropharynx. The palatal and lingual mucosae are usually not involved. The inflammation may be ulcerated or proliferative and will often bleed during gentle manipulation of the mouth (Figure 7.7). The inflammation is usually more intense at the level of the carnassial teeth (maxillary 4th PM and mandibular molar) (Figure 7.8). Some cats may have few or no teeth in the mouth but still show severe FCGS. A more thorough examination and full dental assessment should be performed under general anaesthesia (see QRG 7.1).

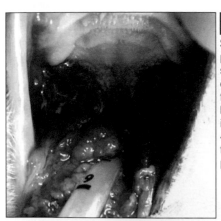

7.7 Severe proliferative stomatitis extending into the fauces. This cat had persistent inflammation for 4 years (despite treatment) prior to presentation.

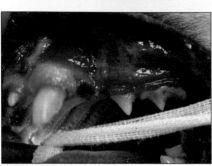

7.8 Inflammation is more severe caudally at the level of the left maxillary 4th PM and left mandibular molar, extending almost to the mucocutaneous junction at the commissure. Bleeding of the gingiva of the left mandibular molar is just visible in the bottom corner of the photo. Inflammation of the oral mucosa can be seen above the maxillary canine tooth (which is fractured) and the maxillary 2nd, 3rd and 4th PMs.

Diagnosis

Initial investigations should rule out any underlying systemic (e.g. kidney disease causing uraemic ulceration, hepatopathies or diabetes) or infectious causes (FIV, FeLV) for the stomatitis. This requires routine haematology and biochemistry, and virology (FIV and FeLV testing, and FCV virus isolation or PCR from oropharyngeal swabs). The choice of certain medications may vary depending on the results; for example, interferon may be used more frequently in cats that have tested positive for FCV.

A thorough dental examination should be performed (see QRG 7.1). All teeth should be evaluated for gingivitis and periodontal disease, and examined for FORLs (see above). Full-mouth radiographs should be taken whether teeth are present or not (Figure 7.9).

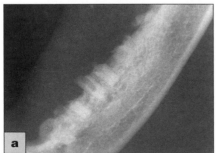

7.9 Intraoral radiography of the cat in Figure 7.7. **(a)** Intraoral radiograph of the left mandible, showing root remnants from all previously 'extracted' teeth. (continues)

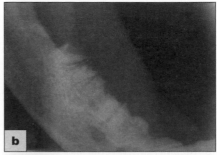

7.9 (continued) Intraoral radiography of the cat in Figure 7.7. **(b)** Intraoral radiograph of the right mandible, showing six root remnants. The root remnants have intact periodontal ligaments and show no signs of resorption. The root fragments also extend above the alveolar bone margin. This is the reason for the poor response to previous treatment; the root remnants remain a focus of infection, pain and inflammation.

Biopsy of the lesions should ideally be carried out, and biopsy should *always* be done if lesions are asymmetrical or if there is no response to initial treatment. There are reported cases where cats with chronic oral disease have developed squamous cell carcinoma (see Chapter 21).

Treatment

Different treatment protocols have been described for FCGS (Figure 7.10). Owners should be made aware that these cases are difficult to manage and some cats will require repeated treatments or, in very severe cases, lifelong management. Treatment protocols are based on reducing plaque accumulation in the mouth, treating existing dental disease and controlling inflammation. Ideally, plaque should be removed daily by brushing using a chlorhexidine-based product, as this also inhibits new plaque formation. However, this may not be possible initially due to the pain associated with FCGS.

- **Extraction of teeth:** (see QRG 7.2) The premolars and molars should be extracted, as well as any other teeth (incisors or canines) affected by gingivitis, periodontitis, endodontic disease or a FORL (Figure 7.11). Studies have shown that this sort of radical extraction results in up to 80% resolution of the gingivostomatitis and, based on this, it is now the treatment of choice.
- **Antimicrobial treatment:** Drugs effective against both Gram-positive aerobes and Gram-negative anaerobes (e.g. amoxicillin/clavulanate) should be used. Good concentrations are required in both bone and soft tissue. Ideally the antimicrobial should be used prior to dental treatment (for a minimum of 1 week prior to surgery) and continued for 4–6 weeks following surgery.
- **NSAIDs:** Meloxicam at 0.1 mg/kg orally q24h, provided renal parameters are within normal limits and no renal compromise is anticipated or present.
- **Opioid pain relief:** Buprenorphine at 0.02 mg/kg orally q8h.
- **Chlorhexidine-based mouthwashes or gel (0.12%):** Should be used as an adjunct to help control plaque accumulation on the oral mucosa and remaining teeth, e.g. canines. If using a mouthwash, 1 ml should be syringed into the mouth by gently placing the tip of the syringe behind the maxillary canines. Cotton buds soaked in the mouthwash can also be used to wipe the canine teeth. The gel can be applied with a cotton bud or finger to the canine teeth and wiped along the gingival margin if the cat allows.

7.10 Treatment protocols for FCGS. Combinations of these elements may need to be considered. (continues)

- **Interferon:** Interferons are cytokines that have antiviral, antiproliferative and immunomodulatory effects. Virbagen omega is a recombinant omega interferon of feline origin (rFeIFN-ω); the current recommended protocol for FCGS is a combination of subcutaneous injections (1 million IU/kg q48h for five injections), followed by an oral dose daily (a 10 million IU vial of interferon is diluted in 200 ml of saline to give a concentration of 50,000 IU/ml, and 1 ml is given orally q24h). The diluted solution is stable under refrigeration for 21 days, but can also be frozen in 20 ml aliquots and thawed as required. The duration of oral treatment is 1–3 months, depending on the clinical response. The inflammation improves gradually and will often take 3–6 months to subside completely. Interferon is used primarily in FCV-positive cats or in cases where inflammation persists following extraction of teeth. The author never recommends using interferon when plaque control is not optimal or where complete extractions have not been carried out.

- **Corticosteroids:** Can be used as a last resort but never as first-line treatment. Prednisolone at 2 mg/kg orally q12h can be given until resolution of clinical signs, and the dose can then be tapered accordingly. The dose can usually start to be tapered within a month of starting treatment, but some cats will need to remain on a low dose every other day to control inflammation. Do not use in conjunction with NSAIDs.

7.10 (continued) Treatment protocols for FCGS. Combinations of these elements may need to be considered.

WARNING

It is essential that all root remnants are removed during tooth extraction for FCGS. Inflammation will persist in the mouth as long as roots are present, even if they are being resorbed. Full-mouth radiographs should be taken following extraction to ensure that all roots and root fragments have been extracted.

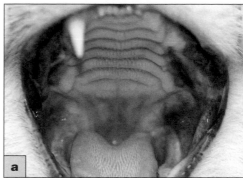
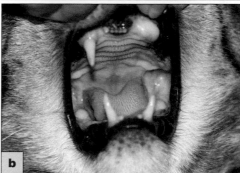

7.11 **(a)** This 6-year-old DSH cat had been treated for chronic gingivostomatitis 3 months previously by extraction of the PMs and molars, as well as the left maxillary canine. There is mild inflammation caudally, although all the extraction sites appear to have healed well. **(b)** The same cat at a recheck 6 months later. There appears to be resolution of the inflammation.

Further reading

Tutt C, Deeprose J and Crossley D (2007) *BSAVA Manual of Canine and Feline Dentistry, 3rd edn*. BSAVA Publications, Gloucester

QRG 7.1 Dental examination, scaling and polishing
by Lisa Milella

Examination of the mouth in a conscious cat is described in QRG 1.4; for an in-depth dental examination, general anaesthesia is always required. Sometimes pathology can only be identified once calculus has been removed from the teeth. Professional scaling and polishing is carried out to deal with plaque-retentive surfaces and reduce areas of plaque stagnation, ensuring that the mouth is then in the best condition to enable the client to provide ongoing plaque control.

Patient preparation

General anaesthesia is always required in order to perform a scale and polish because:

- Areas in the mouth may be painful
- The cat may resist examination of the mouth
- A secure watertight airway is needed to prevent aspiration of water (used for cooling equipment), debris or blood. The author recommends using a low-pressure high-volume cuffed endotracheal tube with care, to ensure a secure airway (see Chapter 3). Care must always be taken to ensure that the tube is fastened securely, to minimize any movement when manipulating the head during dentistry treatment.

The dental chart

Dental charts are available to aid reporting of dental records in patients. These should be completed and filed following any dental examination and/or treatment. The feline dental chart shown uses the modified Triadan tooth-numbering system, where individual numbers are assigned to individual teeth to enable accurate recording. The numbers correspond to the 30 teeth found in the permanent dentition of cats:

	Incisors	Canines	Premolars	Molars	TOTAL
Maxilla	3	1	3 (2nd, 3rd & 4th PM)	1	X 2 = 30
Mandible	3	1	2 (3rd & 4th PM)	1	

The maxillary 4th PMs and mandibular molars are the carnassial teeth.

▶

QRG 7.1 continued

Feline Dental Chart

Date	
Animal's name	Age
Owner's name	Sex
Breed	Client ref.

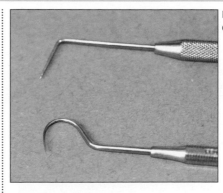

Differently shaped dental explorer probes.

Other hand instruments

- Hand curette – has a blunt, rounded toe with a sharp working edge. A Gracey curette pattern 5/6 is a useful size to clean below the gingival margin in cats
- Extraction forceps (e.g. 76N, with small narrow beaks)

Scaler

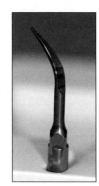

An ultrasonic scaler with a sickle-shaped tip is recommended.

The water setting should be set so that it produces a fine mist when in motion and a fine droplet off the point. The water reduces the heat generated by the tip, but also aids calculus removal through a process known as cavitation. The power setting of the scaler should be set according to the manufacturer's recommendations, but ideally at the lowest possible setting to avoid excessive heat generation.

Procedure

1 Examine the mouth using the periodontal probe and explorer probe and record findings on the dental chart.

Use the **periodontal probe** to check for bleeding of the gingival tissues, periodontal probing depths around all teeth, tooth mobility and furcation exposure. Insert the periodontal probe into the gingival sulcus, and *gently* advance the probe vertically. *Stop* when light pressure is resisted by attachment tissues. Guide the probe around the whole tooth circumference feeling for this 'stop'. Cats normally have probing depths <0.5 mm.

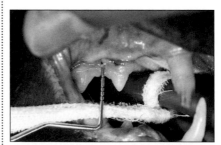

Using a periodontal probe to measure gingival sulcus depth around the distal root of the right maxillary 3rd PM. The probe has advanced 3 mm into the gingival sulcus, whereas the normal pocket depth in a cat should be <0.5 mm, indicating periodontal disease (the periodontal pocket depth should be recorded on the dental chart). Note also the fractured tip of the right maxillary canine.

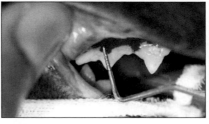

The gingiva starts to bleed when probed. This should be graded for every tooth in the mouth (see Gingivitis index on dental chart).

Full-size downloadable chart available to BSAVA members at www.bsava.com.

Equipment

Periodontal probe

The periodontal probe is a rounded, narrow, flat, blunt-ended, graduated instrument. The blunt end allows the probe to be inserted into the gingival sulcus without causing trauma. The periodontal probe is used to:

- Measure periodontal probing depth
- Assess the degree of gingival inflammation
- Evaluate furcation (area between the roots, generally lying below the main cusp) lesions
- Evaluate the extent of tooth mobility.

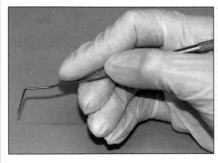

The periodontal probe is held in a modified pen grip, as with all dental instruments except elevators and luxators. Graduations (millimetres) are marked on the end of a periodontal probe to enable measurements of the gingival sulcus.

Explorer probe

The dental explorer probe is a sharp-ended instrument. It is used to explore enamel and dentine defects, such as fractures and FORLs. Explorer probes come in various patterns and it is personal preference as to which shape is used. The author's preference is the pattern number 6, a right-angled probe.

QRG 7.1 continued

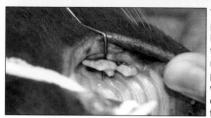

The periodontal probe is passed horizontally between the distal and the mesial roots of the maxillary 4th PM. The probe passes the whole way through, indicating complete exposure of the furcation of this tooth.

Use the **explorer probe** to check for defects of the crown, such as tooth resorption or pulp exposure in fractured teeth. The explorer is also useful for tactile examination of the subgingival tooth surfaces, and subgingival calculus and FORLs may be identified in this way. The explorer probe is only ever used on hard tissues.

WARNING

NEVER use an explorer probe in a conscious animal with suspected pulp exposure. This could be extremely painful for the patient and potentially dangerous for the operator. Thus dental examination should always be performed in an anaesthetized patient.

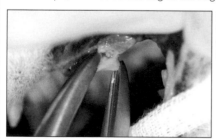

Using an explorer probe to check for defects in the crown in a different cat. A FORL is visible on the right mandibular 4th PM.

2 Rinse the mouth with a chlorhexidine mouthwash (e.g. Hexarinse). This reduces the bacterial aerosol created by ultrasonic scaling.

3 Remove any large pieces of calculus using extraction forceps, without contacting or damaging the gingiva.

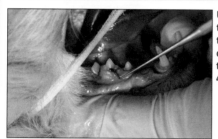

Using forceps to crack off a large piece of calculus from the left maxillary 4th PM tooth.

4 Scaling can now begin. Start descaling the crowns of the teeth above the gingival margin (supragingival scaling). Always use the side of the scaler tip and never the point, as that would damage the tooth enamel. Make sure that the tip is water-cooled. Clean all the buccal surfaces of the mandibular and maxillary dental arcades that are uppermost, and then all the lingual and palatal surfaces of the opposite mandibular and maxillary dental arcades.

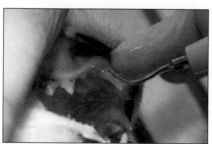

Ultrasonic scaler in use. The side of the tip is used against the tooth surface and the fine water spray can be seen. Here the buccal surface of the uppermost maxillary canine is undergoing descaling.

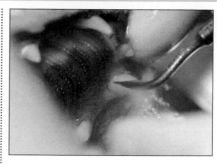

Scaling the palatal surface of the opposite maxillary canine.

5 If calculus is present below the gingival margin, use a hand curette to remove the calculus and any diseased cementum. The instrument is positioned below the gum margin with the working edge against the tooth surface to be cleaned, and then pulled towards the crown. Use an explorer probe to check that all calculus has been removed, or gently puff some air under the gingival margin using the air water syringe from the dental unit.

6 The teeth are then polished to remove any remaining plaque and small bits of calculus.

PRACTICAL TIPS

- Immense iatrogenic damage can be caused by polishing: always use a fine grit polishing paste with a soft rubber cup.
- Use plenty of polishing paste to reduce friction between the rotating cup and the tooth surface.
- Use enough pressure to flare the cup gently against the tooth surface. The cup can gently be flared below the gingival margin to clean any subgingival plaque.
- Set the speed of rotation so that the cup just slows down when it contacts the tooth surface. Too much pressure, too much friction or too high a speed rotation will result in excess heat being produced that can ultimately cause pulpitis (inflammation of the pulp – usually irreversible and leading to pulp necrosis).

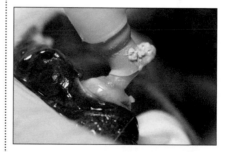

7 Rinse the mouth with water followed by a chlorhexidine mouthwash. Any further treatment such as extraction (see QRG 7.2) can then be carried out.

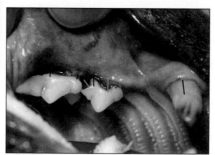

Following the scale and polish, FORLs (green lines) can now be seen on the distal root and crown of the right maxillary 3rd PM as well as at the furcation. Gingival recession (black lines) can also be seen, e.g. on the right maxillary 4th PM.

QRG 7.2 Tooth extraction
by Lisa Milella

Indications

- Severe periodontal disease (mobility, furcation exposure, periodontal probing depths)
- Tooth resorption (FORL)
- Chronic gingivostomatitis
- Complicated crown fracture, i.e. the pulp is exposed
- A tooth where the fracture extends subgingivally to involve the root, whether the pulp is exposed or not
- Teeth involved in a jaw fracture
- Unerupted teeth causing pathology
- Teeth causing malocclusions
- Supernumerary teeth

Equipment

- Luxator 3 mm straight and curved (not essential)
- Elevators – Couplands 1 (3 mm) and Super Slim (1.3 mm)
- Periosteal elevator
- Scalpel handle and blades
- Extraction forceps – pattern 76 N
- Selection of burs for bone removal and sectioning the teeth. The author recommends having a friction-grip round 1 and 2 available to remove bone, a 701 tapered fissure friction-grip bur to section teeth, and a large round diamond bur to smooth bone edges following the extractions
- High-speed turbine water-cooled handpiece
- Soft tissue protector, such as a plastic spatula
- Surgical kit for closure of oral flaps and monofilament absorbable suture material

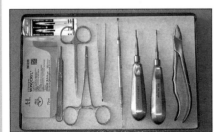

An example of a tray of instruments. Not all instruments listed are shown in the photograph. From the right hand side: extraction forceps; Super Slim and Couplands elevators; periosteal elevator.

Patient preparation

- The cat should always be anaesthetized using a cuffed endotracheal tube (see QRG 7.1 and Chapter 3) that is securely fastened to minimize any movement when manipulating the head during dentistry treatment.
- Pre-extraction radiographs should be taken to assess the tooth, its roots and pathology present.

- Appropriate pain relief should be given (preoperatively, intraoperatively and postoperatively). Ideally, an opioid should be given preoperatively, local anaesthesia should be used intraoperatively, and continued opioids should be given in the postoperative period. NSAIDs should also be used in otherwise healthy cats.
- The teeth should be scaled and polished (see QRG 7.1) prior to extraction, to ensure that the oral surgery is performed in a clean mouth.

Procedures

Non-surgical or closed technique

This technique is used for single-rooted teeth, except mandibular canine teeth, and multi-rooted teeth that have previously been cut into sections according to individual roots.

1 The gingival attachment is cut around the whole circumference of the tooth using a No.11 scalpel blade, as shown here, or a sharp luxator.

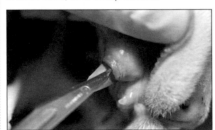

Before proceeding further, multi-rooted teeth (dental charts such as that in QRG 7.1 indicate position of roots in multi-rooted teeth) are sectioned into individual roots using a tapered fissure friction-grip bur (701) on a high-speed handpiece with water cooling. The furcation (area between the roots, generally lying below the main cusp) is identified by raising some of the gingival tissue away from the bone. Sectioning of the tooth starts from the furcation, working towards the cusp from the buccal to lingual/palatal aspect of the tooth. Care is taken not to damage the gingival attachment at the furcation.

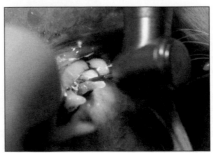

Sectioning the right mandibular 4th PM with a bur

To check that a multi-rooted tooth has been adequately sectioned, an elevator is placed between the two sections of the tooth and gently rotated – both sections of the crown should move independently.

2 Either a luxator or elevator of appropriate size (Couplands 1 for canines, Super Slim for all other teeth) is then inserted into the periodontal ligament space to cut the periodontal ligament fibres.

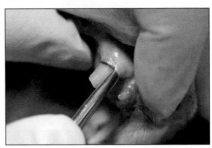

A Couplands 1 elevator being used on the right maxillary canine.

3 The elevator is used to work circumferentially around the tooth applying some apical and rotational pressure at an acute angle to the tooth root. The rotational pressure should be applied for 10 seconds at a time to break down the periodontal ligament fibres.

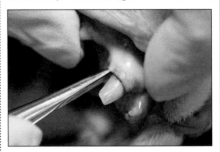

4 Once the tooth or section is mobile, it can be delivered from the socket using either fingers or extraction forceps. The forceps are applied as low down the root as possible. They are initially used in a rotational manner to break down any remaining periodontal ligament fibres prior to the tooth or section being lifted out of the socket to complete the extraction.

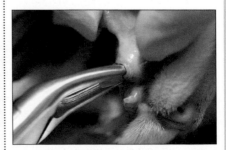

QRG 7.2 *continued*

Surgical or open technique

This technique should always be used for extraction of mandibular canine teeth, for retrieval of root remnants and if any abnormal tooth morphology exists (e.g. FORL). The surgeon may also prefer to use a surgical technique if multiple adjacent teeth need to be extracted.

1 Vertical releasing incisions of a few mm in length are made using a scalpel mesial and distal to the tooth/teeth to be extracted. The releasing incisions extend through the attached gingiva, into the free alveolar mucosa, just beyond the mucogingival junction.

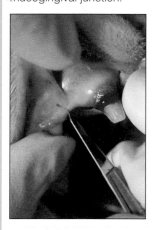

2 A mucoperiosteal flap is raised using a periosteal elevator.

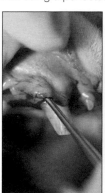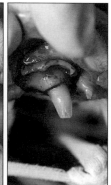

3 The buccal bone overlying the tooth is removed using a friction-grip round bur on a high-speed handpiece with water cooling; if a multi-rooted tooth is being removed, the tooth is sectioned at this stage as described earlier for the closed technique.

For a canine tooth, as an alternative to removing the overlying buccal bone, grooves can be made along the mesial, and distal aspects of the root, using a friction-grip round bur, to create space for placement of a dental elevator. Each groove is connected so that a window of bone overlying the root is removed together with the root.

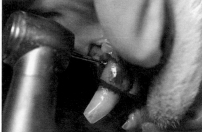

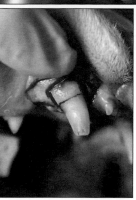

4 An elevator of an appropriate size is placed in the groove and periodontal ligament space and gently rotated to tear the periodontal ligament fibres as described earlier.

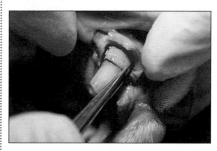

5 The tooth is extracted using forceps or fingers once movement has been created; when using forceps, they are once again used to twist the tooth gently without levering the root, to break down any remaining fibres and lift the tooth from its socket.

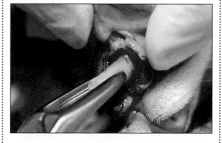

6 The edges of the socket are then smoothed using a large round diamond bur.

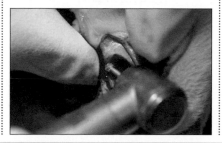

7 The mucoperiosteal flap is then replaced and sutured, with no tension, using a fine (1 metric; 5/0 USP) monofilament absorbable suture material. Simple interrupted sutures are placed (see Appendix).

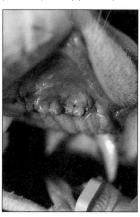

Crown amputation for type 2 FORLs

This technique is used when a tooth is undergoing resorption and there is no normal root structure remaining. This technique can only be used after a diagnosis of type 2 FORL has been made radiographically, as shown below (see main chapter text).

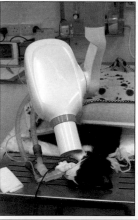

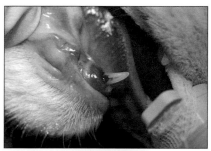

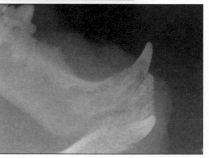

▶

QRG 7.2 *continued*

1 A No.11 scalpel blade is used to make releasing incisions and a periosteal elevator used to raise a small mucoperiosteal flap.

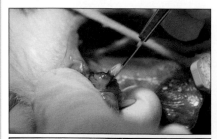

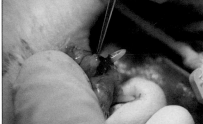

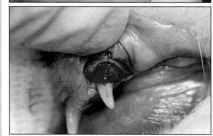

2 A small friction-grip round bur is used to remove the crown of the tooth, sectioning the tooth just below the level of the alveolar bone, taking care not to damage the soft tissue on the lingual/palatal aspect of the tooth.

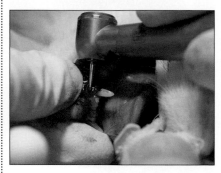

3 The loose fragment can then be removed using an elevator to cut the gingival attachment on the lingual aspect of the fragment.

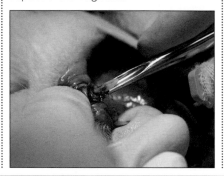

4 The alveolar bone margin is smoothed using a large round diamond bur.

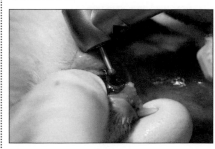

5 The flap is sutured closed using a fine (1 metric; 5/0 USP) monofilament absorbable suture material with simple interrupted sutures (see Appendix), ensuring that there is no tension on the sutures.

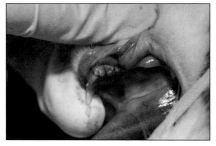

Management of eye disease

Natasha Mitchell

This chapter will focus on the management of some of the more common feline eye diseases encountered in first-opinion practice, notably conjunctivitis, corneal ulceration and uveitis. It also includes a practical QRG on enucleation. Further discussion of some of the aetiological agents associated with infectious ocular diseases can be found in Chapter 19.

Ocular and neurological examinations are described in QRGs 1.3 and 1.6. The diagnostic approach to commonly encountered problems can be found in relevant chapters, e.g. sudden-onset blindness (Chapter 4.8), hyphaema (Chapter 5.19) and ocular discharge (Chapter 5.25). Ophthalmic manifestations of hypertension are covered in Chapter 5.18. The *BSAVA Manual of Canine and Feline Ophthalmology* should be consulted for further discussion of feline ocular problems and diseases.

Conjunctivitis

Conjunctivitis is a common condition, particularly in younger cats, and may affect one or both eyes. Signs of conjunctivitis include ocular discharge (serous, mucoid or purulent; see Chapter 5.25), conjunctival hyperaemia and chemosis.

Aetiology

There are many possible causes of conjunctivitis but infectious causes are most common in cats. Other potential causes include eosinophilic keratoconjunctivitis (see below), allergic conjunctivitis (e.g. sensitivity to topical medication), foreign bodies, chemical injury, or secondary to ocular and adnexal conditions such as keratoconjunctivitis sicca (KCS) or entropion. FCV rarely causes conjunctivitis, despite being a major pathogen of the upper respiratory tract.

FHV

FHV is a common cause of conjunctivitis, particularly in younger cats (Figure 8.1). Primary infection is associated with upper respiratory tract (URT) infection (see Chapter 19). Ocular signs include those listed above and there may also be pathognomonic dendritic superficial corneal ulceration visible with fluorescein staining (Figure 8.2). Other potential ocular signs include blepharitis, symblepharon, keratitis, eosino-

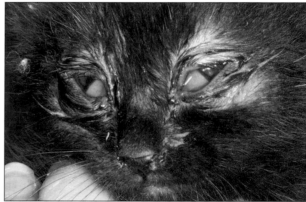

8.1 Bilateral serous ocular discharge, third eyelid protrusion with conjunctival hyperaemia and a corneal opacity in the left eye due to corneal ulceration in a kitten with FHV infection.

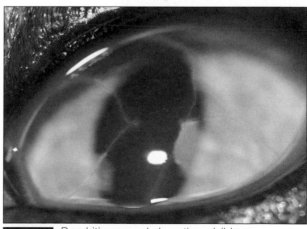

8.2 Dendritic corneal ulceration, visible as branching fluorescein-positive green lines. This is pathognomonic for FHV infection of the eye but is not always present.

philic keratoconjunctivitis (see below), corneal sequestrum (see below) and uveitis (see below).

Treatment of FHV conjunctivitis involves appropriate management of the URT infection (see Chapter 13), cleansing of ocular discharge, and topical broad-spectrum antibiotics such as fusidic acid to prevent secondary bacterial infections. While oral antibiotics may be given for the respiratory infection, it is still important to prescribe topical antibiotics. This is because corneal and conjunctival ulceration usually occurs and topical antibiotics may reduce adhesions that would lead to permanent symblepharon.

Topical antiviral treatment is also indicated and can be very effective, e.g. trifluorothymidine (1% solution available in the UK from Moorfields Eye Hospital, London – or contact your local human eye hospital) five times daily; however, it may be difficult to obtain, is expensive, and is not well tolerated by cats. Oral famciclovir has shown some very promising results in clinical cases but recommended dose ranges vary greatly, the latest pharmacological study suggesting a dose of 30–40 mg/kg q12h. Oral lysine has been advocated at a dose rate of 500 mg/cat q12h and is available as a paste, powder or gel. Lysine is safe, although reports of efficacy in the field and clinical cases are not consistent; it does inhibit replication of FHV *in vitro* but only in the absence of arginine, which may not be an achievable situation in clinical cases.

Chlamydophila felis

C. felis is a common pathogen in cats and typically causes bilateral pronounced chemosis and a mucopurulent or purulent ocular discharge (Figure 8.3). Treatment includes eye hygiene (gently bathing the eyes to remove ocular discharge daily, using cotton wool soaked with previously boiled and cooled water) and oral doxycycline at 10 mg/kg q24h for at least 4 weeks (treat 2 weeks beyond clinical cure) (see Chapter 3 re potential adverse effects of doxycycline). In multi-cat households it is also recommended that in-contact cats are treated to try to remove potential carriers. Follow-up vaccination can be considered in multi-cat households.

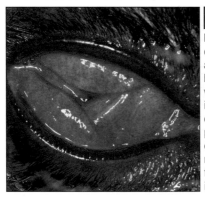

8.3 Purulent ocular discharge, chemosis and conjunctival hyperaemia in a cat with *C. felis* infection. A deep corneal ulcer is also present, although corneal ulceration is not typically a feature of *C. felis* infection.

Mycoplasma felis

M. felis has been reported to cause conjunctivitis, chemosis, and follicle and pseudomembrane formation, but has also been isolated from clinically normal cats. Therefore a positive culture or PCR result from a cat that does not have signs of conjunctivitis does not necessarily warrant antibiotic treatment. If there is a positive culture or PCR result from a cat *with* conjunctivitis, treatment should be given if the conjunctivitis has not cleared by the time the test results come back (the condition can also be self-limiting). Treatment consists of oral doxycycline at 10 mg/kg q24h for 3 weeks (see Chapter 3 re potential adverse effects).

Diagnosis

Diagnosis of conjunctivitis is straightforward, but consideration must be given to the underlying cause. As well as a thorough history, and ocular and physical examinations, useful diagnostic tests may include the Schirmer tear test (STT; see QRG 1.3), fluorescein staining, cytology, bacteriological culture (including specific request for *Mycoplasma*) and sensitivity testing, and PCR for FHV, *C. felis* and *M. felis*.

Corneal ulcers

Corneal ulceration is interruption of the corneal epithelium. It may be superficial, involving the epithelium only, or may involve the loss of corneal stroma, leading to a deeper ulcer (Figure 8.4). Chronic indolent

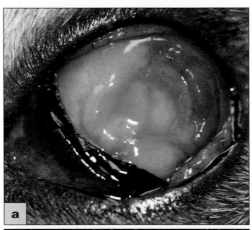

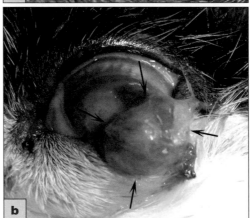

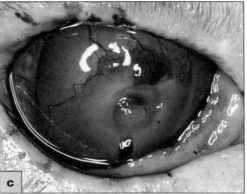

8.4 Corneal ulcers. **(a)** Very deep stromal ulcer. Medially there is corneal oedema, making the cornea appear white, while laterally there is stromal infiltration with blood vessels – a fibrovascular healing response. **(b)** Large deep corneal ulcer with rupture. A large clot of aqueous humour is present ventrally (arrowed), plugging the defect. **(c)** Deep central corneal ulcer, which had previously ruptured and then self-sealed, with corneal oedema and neovascularization visible around it.

ulcers are superficial corneal ulcers that have been present for >3 weeks, with a flap of non-adherent epithelium at the periphery. This flap allows fluorescein to be run beneath this loose epithelium. When the ulcer reaches the depth of Descemet's membrane, it is termed a descemetocele. The ulcer may be complicated by the persistence of the underlying cause, by the presence of infection, or by the production of destructive degrading corneal enzymes ('melting').

Clinical presentation

The cornea (especially superficially) is richly innervated, and therefore corneal ulceration is very painful. Deep corneal ulcers cause less pain, however, so the cat may appear to become more comfortable as the ulcer progresses. The affected cat typically has blepharospasm, ocular discharge (serous, mucoid or purulent), conjunctival hyperaemia, a protruding nictitating membrane, and a cloudy cornea due to oedema of the ulcerated area. Depending on how long the corneal ulcer has been there, a neovascularization response usually occurs.

Aetiology

The underlying cause should be identified to allow appropriate treatment. Causes include:

- Trauma
- Infectious disease, e.g. FHV, bacterial infection such as *Pseudomonas* keratitis, or opportunists such as *Staphylococcus* and *Streptococcus*
- Adnexal disease, e.g. entropion
- Lagophthalmos (inability to blink properly)
- Tear film abnormalities
- Miscellaneous, e.g. foreign bodies, chemical burns.

Investigation

The integrity of the epithelium is easily tested by the application of fluorescein dye. Any breach in the epithelium allows the hydrophilic corneal stroma to take up the dye; this is readily visible with the naked eye and can be enhanced with blue light. The depth of the ulcer is assessed using magnification, and the slit beam of an ophthalmoscope if available. Fluorescein staining may delineate dendritic corneal ulcers, which are pathognomonic for FHV infection (see Figure 8.2). A Schirmer tear test (see QRG 1.3) is indicated to check the volume of tears. The presence of a foreign body should be ruled out, by examining the dorsal and ventral conjunctival fornix, and protruding the third eyelid with a cotton-tipped swab or non-toothed forceps after application of topical anaesthesia.

A swab may be carefully taken from the corneal ulcer, to submit for bacterial culture and sensitivity testing. This is very useful if initial treatment is not successful but it does take time to receive the laboratory result. Cytology of a corneal scraping provides a much quicker result. The sample is stained with Diff-Quik or Gram stain; microscopic examination may reveal bacterial or fungal organisms and thereby help direct appropriate antibiotic therapy. Depending on the presentation of the ulcer, additional tests such as PCR for specific infectious agents (e.g. FHV), may be indicated (see Chapter 19).

Corneal scraping

1. A drop of topical anaesthetic (proxymetacaine or tetracaine) is applied to the cornea.
2. The blunt (handle) end of a scalpel blade is used to scrape the edge of the lesion.

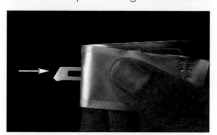

3. The fluid obtained is spread on to a microscope slide and stained with Diff-Quik or Gram stain as required.

Treatment

Treatment depends on the extent and depth of the ulcer and on the presence or absence of complicating factors such as infection or melting. If there is self-trauma, an Elizabethan collar should be fitted. If the underlying cause is identified and corrected, superficial corneal ulcers will heal rapidly. Frequent re-examinations are indicated for deep or complicated corneal ulcers, to check that healing is progressing rather than serious complications occurring, such as ulcer progression, globe rupture, endophthalmitis and glaucoma.

WARNING

Topical (and systemic) corticosteroids are contraindicated, as they may potentiate collagenolysis ('melting') by destructive corneal, bacterial and inflammatory cell enzymes.

Treatment may include the following:

- Simple ulcers are treated with a topical antibiotic such as fusidic acid q12h to prevent secondary infection
- If infection is present (suspected due to purulent discharge or confirmed by cytology or culture) an appropriate topical antibiotic is chosen, e.g. chloramphenicol for Gram-positive infections and gentamicin or ofloxacin for Gram-negative infections
- If secondary uveitis is present, topical treatment with tropicamide 0.5% q8h is indicated
- Antiviral treatment is indicated in the case of FHV infection. When ocular disease is the only sign, topical trifluorothymidine five times daily is indicated (see notes above re availability). However, this may be poorly tolerated as it may sting on application. If there are systemic signs of FHV infection, oral famciclovir may be more useful; a dose of 30–40 mg/kg q12h is the current recommendation
- Topical application of autologous serum is useful for melting corneal ulcers, as it has anticollagenolytic activity (Figure 8.5). It is

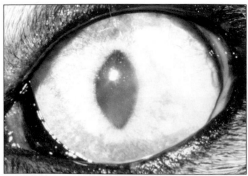

8.5 Appearance of the eye in Figure 8.4a six weeks later. The eye was treated with topical autologous serum and ofloxacin for 1 week, then topical fusidic acid for 2 weeks. This photograph is slightly over-exposed but it is possible to see that the cornea has regained much of its clarity, apart from some faint grey fibrosis visible throughout, and there is no visible neovascularization.

prepared by taking 10 ml of blood from the affected cat into a plain tube and allowing it to clot for at least 15 minutes (if this is not possible, blood from *another* animal can be used; dog serum is preferable to avoid transmission of infectious agents). The blood is then spun for 5 minutes at 5000 rpm. The resulting serum is decanted into an eye dropper bottle and stored in the fridge; it can be used for up to 7 days. The frequency of application depends on the extent of corneal melting: one drop per hour is usual initially until the melting is under control; thereafter the frequency can be reduced
- Surgery such as conjunctival pedicle graft placement (Figure 8.6) or corneo-conjunctival transposition is indicated for deep stromal ulcers or descemetoceles, but is usually carried out by specialists.

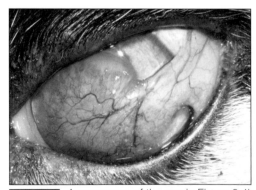

8.6 Appearance of the eye in Figure 8.4b six weeks after corneal pedicle graft placement from the lateral aspect. The conjunctival graft is well vascularized and incorporated nicely into the cornea; the epithelium of the cornea and conjunctiva are smooth and continuous.

Chronic indolent ulcers
Superficial chronic indolent ulcers are treated differently. If they do not resolve after 2 weeks of topical antibiotic ointment (e.g. fusidic acid), the loose epithelium at the edges of the ulcer should be debrided after application of topical anaesthetic. A dry sterile cotton-tipped swab is applied to the centre of the ulcer and firmly pushed radially to remove any epithelium which is not adherent to the underlying

stroma (several swabs may be required as it easier to do if the swab is dry; autoclaved cotton ear buds can work well). If the superficial ulcer does not heal with debridement, the cat should be referred for a superficial keratectomy.

> **WARNING**
>
> It is important *never* to perform a grid keratotomy in a cat because this may lead to corneal sequestrum formation (see below).

Corneal sequestrum

This condition is almost unique to cats. Cats of any breed may be affected, although there is a predisposition in Persians, Himalayans, Siamese, Burmese and Exotic Shorthairs. The sequestrum represents an area of stromal collagen degeneration, with accumulation of pigment.

Aetiology
A variety of factors contribute to the initiation of sequestrum formation. These include brachycephalic conformation, lagophthalmos, mechanical irritation such as trichiasis from entropion or distichia (see Figure 8.7a), chronic corneal ulceration, FHV infection, tear film abnormalities, corneal trauma, topical corticosteroid administration and primary corneal dystrophy. A combination of these predisposing factors causes corneal damage. It has been shown that cats subjected to a grid keratotomy for a chronic indolent ulcer are more likely to develop a corneal sequestrum, and for this reason the procedure should be avoided. FHV is frequently incriminated as a principal cause of corneal sequestration, but a definitive relationship has not been proven.

Clinical signs
The condition is typified by oval to round, tan to black focal discoloration of the central or paracentral cornea (Figure 8.7). The corneal staining intensity varies from a light tea-stain to a dark or black opaque plaque, and there is a varying degree of surrounding inflammation and vascularization. The depth of the necrotic

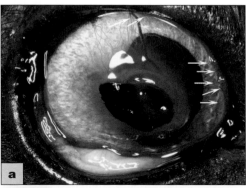

8.7 Corneal sequestrum. **(a)** A central black corneal sequestrum is surrounded by a rim of fibrovascular tissue (pink) and oedema (white) and has evoked a neovascularization reaction from the dorsal limbus. In this situation, the sequestrum appears to have been caused by multiple distichia from the upper eyelid (arrowed). (continues) ▶

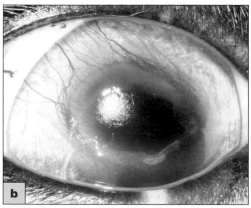

8.7 (continued) Corneal sequestrum. **(b)** A corneal sequestrum has developed in the stroma at the centre of a chronic corneal indolent ulcer that failed to heal despite topical antibiotic treatment. At the edge of the ulcer the epithelium is non-adherent, allowing fluorescein stain to under-run it. There is corneal neovascularization from the dorsolateral aspect and corneal oedema (white area) below the ulcer. The centre of the ulcer is black because it has become necrotic.

tissue within the stroma varies; it most commonly affects the anterior third of the stroma but may progress to extend to Descemet's membrane, where it can potentially lead to corneal perforation. Affected cats exhibit varying levels of discomfort, with blepharospasm and ocular discharge, which may be darkly staining. Some cases initially present with superficial corneal ulceration, within which an amber stain starts to become apparent. Once developed, uptake of fluorescein on top of the sequestrum cannot be appreciated, but uptake may be seen at the edges of the lesion and in adjacent cornea (Figure 8.7b).

Treatment

Sequestra may be treated medically or surgically. The decision as to whether to opt for medical or surgical treatment may be based on the present comfort of the patient, on the apparent risk of deepening disease with potential rupture and on finances available.

Medical treatment involves waiting for the sequestrum to loosen naturally and then slough off as it is extruded from the cornea, which can take weeks or months to occur. Topical antibiotics are indicated, e.g. fusidic acid q8–12h; the optical preparation Fucithalmic Vet also provides lubrication because of the carbomer component. Lubrication improves comfort, and the addition of topical artificial tears (e.g. carbomer gel or sodium hyaluronate drops) in between antibiotic applications is advisable if the cat is uncomfortable, and tolerates topical medications.

Surgery is often recommended, as it greatly reduces the duration of the condition. A keratectomy is carried out to excise the affected cornea. If the sequestrum is not superficial, a graft is required to fill the corneal deficit. This is normally carried out at a referral centre.

Prognosis

Recurrence is possible after both medical and surgical treatment; ongoing monitoring of the eye is therefore advised. This is initially carried out every 3 months after full healing, and then annually after the first year.

Eosinophilic (proliferative) keratoconjunctivitis

Clinical signs

Eosinophilic keratoconjunctivitis results in inflammation of the cornea and conjunctiva, but the cause is not known. Ultraviolet light is suspected to be a triggering factor. There may be an association with FHV infection, although the inflammation may also lead to recrudescence of pre-existing latent infection. Usually only one eye is affected initially, although it is not uncommon for the condition to progress to affect both eyes. Typically, there is conjunctival hyperaemia, corneal neovascularization and proliferative plaques with a white 'cottage-cheese' appearance, most often of the dorsolateral or the nasal quadrant (Figure 8.8).

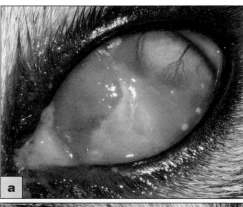
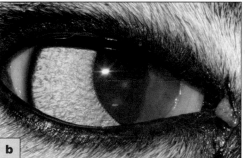

8.8 Eosinophilic keratoconjunctivitis. **(a)** There is white mucoid ocular discharge, a white corneal stromal infiltrate and corneal neovascularization; corneal cytology confirmed eosinophilic keratoconjunctivitis. **(b)** The other eye of the cat showed a whitish corneal infiltrate medially, which was probably an earlier stage of the disease process.

Diagnosis

The diagnosis may be confirmed using corneal and/or conjunctival cytology of a sample taken from the edge of the affected area using the blunt handle end of a scalpel blade or a cytobrush. This sample will contain eosinophils along with mast cells, neutrophils, lymphocytes and/or plasma cells. A cytologist will usually diagnose the condition, but the presence of any eosinophils at all is diagnostic if the clinician is confident with cytology.

Treatment

Topical corticosteroids (e.g. dexamethasone 0.1% or prednisolone 1% (Figure 8.9)) are typically used initially, although the condition may be chronic and recurrence is not uncommon when steroid treatment

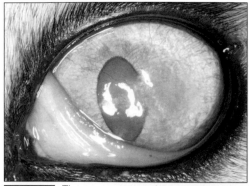

8.9 The appearance of the eye featured in Figure 8.8a six weeks after treatment with topical prednisolone three times daily. The cornea has markedly improved, but faint neovascularization and white stromal infiltrate remains, so treatment needs to continue though it can be reduced to once daily.

is stopped. Chronic cases may be best treated with topical ciclosporin q12h until the cornea appears clear and then q24h to prevent recurrence.

> **WARNING**
>
> Both topical steroids and ciclosporin are immunosuppressants, and therefore some caution is advised. Concurrent treatment with a topical antiviral medication (if available, see previously) may be wise. Careful monitoring during treatment is recommended.

Treatment may be stopped 3 months after the cornea is clear to assess whether ongoing medication is necessary. The eyes should be re-examined 2–4 weeks later and treatment restarted if there is any sign of recurrence. Some cases require lifelong treatment, in which case they should be monitored initially every 3 months and then every 6 months after a year. Refractory cases may be treated with oral megestrol acetate, although this drug has considerable systemic side effects and so should be used only as a last resort.

Anterior uveitis

Anterior uveitis is inflammation of the iris, ciliary body or both. The posterior uvea, the choroid, may also be involved. The condition is not uncommon and may affect one or both eyes, and cats of any age or breed. Undesirable consequences of uncontrolled uveitis include glaucoma, cataracts, lens luxation, posterior synechiae and retinal detachment. Long-term treatment and monitoring is required in some cases.

Aetiology

The most common causes are: idiopathic disease (lymphocytic–plasmacytic uveitis); immune-mediated disease such as lens-induced uveitis; neoplasia (primary uveal tumours such as melanoma and sarcoma, or secondary tumours such as lymphoma); trauma; and infectious conditions such as FIP, toxoplasmosis, FIV or FeLV infection. Other infectious agents that may be associated with uveitis include mycotic organisms (e.g. *Cryptococcus neoformans*), *Bartonella henselae* and FHV. Geographical location influences the diagnostic tests that will be undertaken, as certain infectious agents are more common in some locations.

Clinical signs

Uveitis results in disruption of the blood–aqueous barrier by chemical mediators of inflammation such as prostaglandins, leucotrienes and histamine. The immunological reaction causes increased permeability, which allows entry of plasma proteins and blood cellular components into the aqueous humour. Clinically, increased protein in the anterior chamber is visible as a diffuse haziness throughout the aqueous humour, termed 'aqueous flare'.

Possible clinical signs are:

- Red eye: due to conjunctival hyperaemia, peripheral corneal vascularization, episcleral congestion and occasionally hyphaema
- Cloudy eye: due to aqueous flare (turbid aqueous due to increased protein content), keratic precipitates (inflammatory cells on the corneal endothelium; Figure 8.10), hypopyon (inflammatory cells in the ventral aspect of the anterior chamber), fibrin in the anterior chamber or corneal oedema
- Moderate discomfort: there may be blepharospasm, ocular discharge and photophobia
- Changes to the iris:
  - Miosis
  - Altered contour due to swelling and nodules

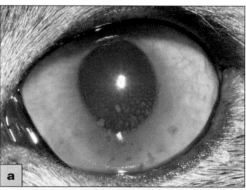

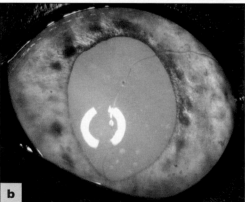

8.10 Anterior uveitis. **(a)** Multiple cream to brown opacities on the corneal endothelium (keratic precipitates) and loss of iris detail are visible in this kitten with FIP. **(b)** There are multiple keratic precipitates on the ventral aspect of the corneal endothelium, which appear white when silhouetted against the pupil and dark when silhouetted against the iris. A hair is present on the cornea. New blood vessel formation can be seen on the surface of the iris (rubeosis iridis). There are multifocal areas of increased pigmentation on the iris.

- Colour change from normal light colour to muddy brown colour
- Rubreosis iridis from neovascularization of the iris surface (Figure 8.10b)
- Posterior synechia to the anterior lens capsule
- Occasionally, other ocular changes are present such as cataract, lens luxation, glaucoma or retinal detachment.

Treatment

Treatment involves treating the underlying cause if that can be identified, along with symptomatic treatment. Topical corticosteroids are used unless there is concurrent corneal ulceration. Prednisolone acetate (Pred forte) is an appropriate choice as it has good intraocular penetration, and may be used initially 4–6 times daily, depending on the severity of the disease. Systemic steroids or NSAID drugs are indicated, and will have good intraocular penetration due to the breakdown of the blood–ocular barrier. A topical mydriatic/cycloplegic agent will improve comfort and reduce the likelihood of synechiae; usually tropicamide is given q8h or atropine q24h.

Glaucoma

Glaucoma is the damage that occurs to the retina and optic nerve as a result of sustained elevation of intraocular pressure (IOP). It is not as common in cats as it is in dogs, but is a very significant ocular disease as it results in discomfort and blindness.

The normal IOP in a cat is 15–25 mmHg. Low pressures indicate uveitis, and high pressures lead to glaucoma. Primary glaucoma in cats occurs uncommonly, and it is much more likely for secondary glaucoma to occur. This is most often in association with chronic uveitis (Figure 8.11), and may also occur with ocular neoplasia (such as uveal melanoma, lymphoma and intraocular sarcoma), blunt trauma, lens capsule laceration or lens luxation.

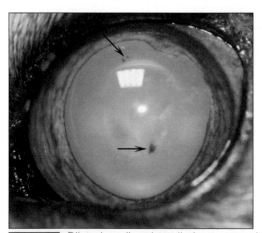

8.11 Dilated pupil and small pigment opacities (arrowed) on the anterior lens capsule due to glaucoma secondary to uveitis. There is a posterior synechia at the 1 o'clock position, making the pupil margin irregular.

Feline glaucoma normally has an insidious onset and there may be moderate blepharospasm, globe enlargement, conjunctival and episcleral congestion, corneal oedema and peripheral corneal vascularization. The pupil may be dilated, misshapen (dyscoria), or constricted (in the case of uveitis). Some vision may be retained despite chronically moderately raised IOP. The IOP should be measured by tonometry for diagnosis and to monitor response to treatment (see QRG 1.3).

Treatment

Treatment of the underlying cause may lower the IOP. Medications can be used to lower IOP but are not always effective in cats. Topical anhydrase inhibitors are most commonly used, e.g. dorzolamide q8–12h. Some surgical procedures to attempt to save the eye and also vision are available at referral clinics. Chronically blind and painful eyes are best enucleated (see QRG 8.1).

Lens luxation

Lens luxation or subluxation is the displacement of the lens from its normal location, either anteriorly or posteriorly. The abnormal position of the lens allows the edge of the lens to be seen (Figure 8.12), and an aphakic crescent can be seen on distant direct ophthalmoscopy (see QRG 1.3). Luxation occurs most often secondary to chronic uveitis, blunt trauma or globe enlargement associated with raised IOP (glaucoma). The IOP should be measured by tonometry (see QRG 1.3). If uveitis is the cause, this needs to be investigated and managed. Surgery to remove the displaced lens carries a good prognosis, although management of the predisposing factor will need to continue.

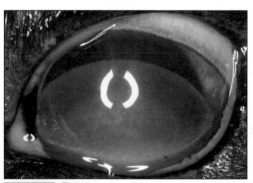

8.12 This lens has increased opacity and is sitting in the ventral aspect of the anterior chamber due to anterior lens luxation secondary to uveitis. Note the smooth round edge of the lens – never visible in a normal eye.

References and further reading

Barnett KC and Crispin SM (2002) *Feline Ophthalmology: An Atlas and Text*. Saunders Elsevier, Philadelphia
Gould D and McLellan G (in preparation) *BSAVA Manual of Canine and Feline Ophthalmology, 3rd edn*. BSAVA Publications, Gloucester
Maggs DJ, Miller PE and Ofri R (2008) *Slatter's Fundamentals of Veterinary Ophthalmology, 4th edn*. Saunders Elsevier, Philadelphia

QRG 8.1 Enucleation
by Natasha Mitchell

Approach

The subconjunctival approach is recommended, and outlined below. However, if there is orbital neoplasia or infection, the transpalpebral technique or orbital exenteration techniques are required; a surgery textbook should be consulted in these situations.

WARNING

Much care must be taken when performing enucleation, as the feline optic nerve is short and any traction exerted will be transmitted to the optic chiasma. The contralateral optic nerve could thus be damaged, which could result in blindness in the remaining eye.

Equipment

- Needle-holders
- Rat-toothed forceps (straight (shown) or curved)
- Stevens tenotomy scissors for conjunctiva
- Curved Metzenbaum scissors for tissue dissection
- Artery clamps (optional for haemostasis if required)
- Suture material, e.g. 0.7 metric (6/0 USP) lactomer (e.g. Polysorb)
- Swabs

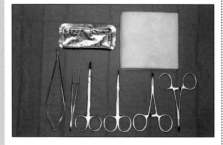

Patient preparation and positioning

The endotracheal (ET) tube is secured around the lower jaw so that the tie does not get in the way, and the head is positioned laterally, with the lateral and medial canthus level and parallel to the operating table. A vacuum cushion or a towel and sandbags may be used.

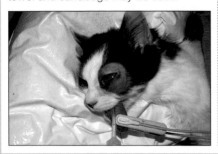

The periocular area is shaved, taking care not to traumatize the thin eyelid skin, and the area is surgically prepared with 1:10 concentration iodine solution.

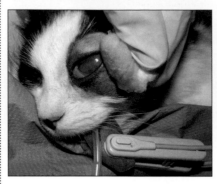

The surgical area is draped. The eyelids remain open for the procedure.

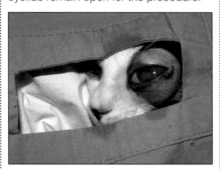

Procedure

1 A lateral canthotomy is performed using Stevens tenotomy scissors to increase exposure to the globe.

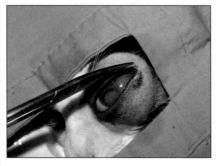

2 The third eyelid (nictitating membrane) is grasped and removed by cutting with the Stevens tenotomy scissors.

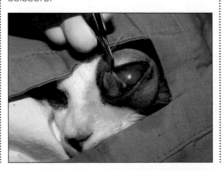

3 An incision is made in the conjunctiva 2–5 mm posterior to the limbus using Stevens tenotomy scissors.

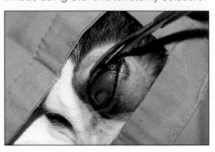

4 Keeping close to the globe, the conjunctiva is dissected from the globe for 360 degrees, along with the extraocular muscles. Traction on the extraocular muscles may result in bradycardia due to the *oculocardiac reflex*.

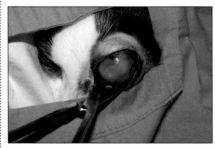

5 When the globe is almost free, the optic nerve is sharply cut approximately 2–5 mm from the globe. It is unnecessary (and ill advised) to clamp the optic nerve prior to resection.

6 The orbit is packed with a sterile swab, and pressure is applied for 5 minutes. Usually haemorrhage will have subsided at this point but, if not, pressure is applied for longer.

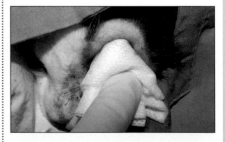

7 Visible remaining conjunctiva is removed.

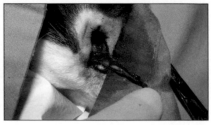

▶

QRG 8.1 *continued*

8 The edges of the upper and lower eyelids are removed, taking care to excise the eyelid completely at the medial canthus where it is more closely adhered to the bone.

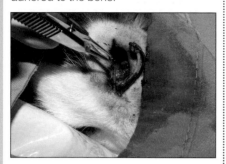

9 The orbit is closed, ideally in three layers using absorbable suture material such as 1 or 0.7 metric (5/0 or 6/0 USP) polyglactin 910 (e.g. Vicryl) or polyglycolic acid (e.g. Polysorb). First the tissue closest to the orbital rim is closed (it is normal for there to be a gap as there is not enough tissue to cover the orbit), then the adventitia under the conjunctiva (the pink tissue close to the cut eyelid edges), and the third layer may be either a subcuticular layer to appose the skin or external simple interrupted sutures.

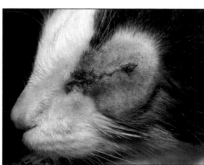

10 The removed globe and attached tissue (which will be minimal with this enucleation technique) should be fixed in 10% formalin and sent for histopathology, ideally to an experienced ocular pathologist.

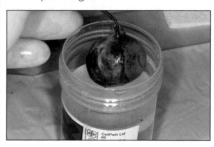

Postoperative care

Postoperatively, 5 days of antibiotics and anti-inflammatories are indicated, and an Elizabethan collar is recommended for 1 week.

Management of cardiovascular disorders

Luca Ferasin

This chapter will focus on the management of the most important cardiovascular disorders encountered in feline practice, notably primary cardiomyopathies, both asymptomatic and those presenting as congestive heart failure, and arterial thromboembolism. Management of respiratory disorders is discussed in Chapter 10.

Other information pertinent to cardiovascular disorders is included in relevant chapters throughout the Manual, including: collapse (Chapter 4.1), dyspnoea (Chapter 4.2), heart murmurs (Chapter 5.17) and hypertension (Chapter 5.18). Practical QRGs are provided for thoracic examination and auscultation (QRG 1.5), ECG (QRG 4.1.4), blood pressure measurement (QRG 5.18.1), thoracocentesis (QRG 4.2.4), oxygen supplementation (QRG 4.2.2) and emergency thoracic radiography (QRG 4.2.3).

There is a lack of evidence regarding many treatments used for heart disease in cats, and hence there may often be differences in specific treatment recommendations amongst cardiologists. Every individual cat is also different, and it is important that treatments are carefully tailored to the individual. Furthermore, this is a very dynamic field with precise treatment recommendations frequently changing as more evidence becomes available, or newer drugs enter the market. This chapter therefore provides generic advice but does not give prescriptive guidelines on when to use particular drugs and doses. The reader is encouraged to seek the latest information and advice from a cardiologist when managing these cases.

Cardiomyopathy and congestive heart failure

Classification and aetiology

Cardiomyopathy (CM) is a disease of the myocardium commonly observed in cats. It also represents the primary cause of congestive heart failure (CHF) in these patients. Several attempts have been made to classify feline cardiomyopathies over the years; however, the wide spectrum of structural and functional abnormalities observed in feline CM does not allow easy differentiation. Additional confusion may arise from overlapping structural changes, such as hypertrophy and dilation,

with functional abnormalities such as arrhythmia or a restrictive pattern of ventricular filling. Furthermore, some lesions may appear almost identical on echocardiographic examination even though they may have different aetiologies, such as valvular, ischaemic, inflammatory or arrhythmogenic disorders. This is due to the fact that structural remodelling may appear similar, even when it originates from different pathologies.

Traditionally, the classification of myocardial disorders is based on echocardiographic examination and clinicians should be aware of the substantial phenotypic variability within the same form of CM, as well as the inevitable subjective interpretations of images, especially by less experienced ultrasonographers. Sometimes, diagnosis is obtained after necropsy but this is obviously less relevant to practical clinical considerations.

The most commonly diagnosed form of feline myocardial disease is hypertrophic cardiomyopathy (HCM), which represents approximately two thirds of the CM cases seen in cats. The aetiology of feline HCM is not fully understood, although familial HCM has been described in different breeds. A causative mutation for HCM has been identified in the sarcomeric gene for the cardiac myosin binding protein C (MYBPC3) in the Maine Coon and Ragdoll. Genetic DNA tests for HCM exist for these two breeds; positive results identify cats with one copy of the defective gene (heterozygous) or two copies (homozygous). Interestingly, however, not all cats with this mutation will develop HCM, and HCM can still be diagnosed in cats that appeared negative on genetic testing, suggesting that other mutations or genetic influences can play a role. Therefore, results of genetic tests need to be interpreted with care.

Approximately 50% of feline HCM cases are accompanied by a dynamic obstruction of the left ventricular outflow tract, caused by an abrupt movement of the elongated anterior (septal) leaflet of the mitral valve towards the interventricular septum (systolic anterior motion, SAM). The degree of dynamic obstruction is usually related to the severity of hypertrophy and it could be speculated that such hypertrophy may not be solely a phenotypical manifestation of HCM but also a consequence of increased left ventricular pressure caused by the outflow obstruction itself. Indeed, several cases of SAM are observed in the absence of hypertrophy, indicating either an early stage of the disease not yet accompanied by hypertrophy, or a degree of ventricular pressure overload not sufficient to stimulate hypertrophy.

Clinical signs and diagnosis

Many cats diagnosed with feline CM are presented with clinical signs of CHF (e.g. lethargy, inappetence, dyspnoea, ascites (Figure 9.1a)) or limb paresis/paralysis secondary to an episode of arterial thromboembolism (ATE). Diagnosis of CHF is often supported by radiographic evidence of pulmonary oedema (Figure 9.1b) and/or pleural effusion (Figure 9.1c).

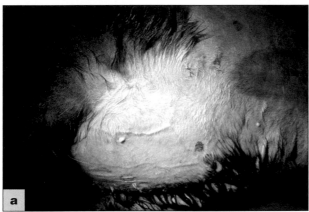

a

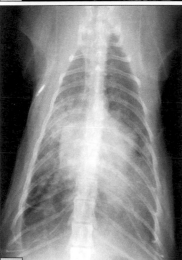

b

9.1

Three different presentations of CHF. **(a)** Ascites. **(b)** Pulmonary oedema. **(c)** Pleural effusion. Cytology and biochemistry of fluid obtained from the abdominal or pleural effusion in CHF is often compatible with a 'modified transudate' (see Chapter 5.1).

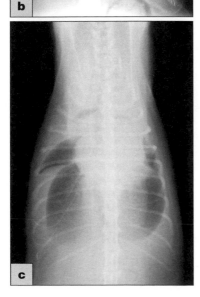

c

A diagnosis of CM may also be reached in asymptomatic patients that undergo echocardiographic examination for pedigree heart-screening programmes or following the discovery of an audible heart murmur (see Chapter 5.17) or a gallop sound on routine physical examination.

Clinical management

Unfortunately, with the exception of dietary taurine supplementation for cats with dilated CM secondary to taurine deficiency, there are no available treatments that have, to date, convincingly demonstrated increased survival and/or quality of life in feline CM.

The asymptomatic cardiac patient

Improvement of physical activity and general demeanour has been reported in asymptomatic cats with HCM after administration of heart-rate slowing agents, such as calcium-channel blockers (i.e. diltiazem) or beta-blockers (i.e. atenolol). The rationale of heart rate control lies behind the potential amelioration of coronary perfusion, reduction of perivascular collagen and decrease in renin–angiotensin–aldosterone system (RAAS) activation. Randomized placebo-controlled studies are lacking, however, and the clinical utility of heart-rate slowing agents in asymptomatic cats needs to be proven, especially in those cases accompanied by dynamic left ventricular outflow obstruction. Furthermore, the presence of CHF or systolic myocardial dysfunction should always be ruled out prior to initiation of beta-blocker therapy. ACE inhibitors and spironolactone, despite their widespread use in asymptomatic patients, have failed to demonstrate significant improvements in cats with subclinical forms of HCM.

Another common intervention observed in veterinary practice is the use of antithrombotic prophylaxis to reduce the risk of ATE, using aspirin (75 mg/cat orally q72h), clopidogrel (18.75 mg/cat orally q24h) or a combination of the two. This intervention has not been assessed by controlled clinical trials, and antithrombotic prophylaxis should probably be reserved for cases complicated by the presence of intracavitary thrombi, spontaneous echo-contrast ('smoke') or severe left atrial dilatation.

> **WARNING**
>
> Chronic diuresis (e.g. with furosemide) should always be avoided in the absence of CHF. Indeed, overzealous diuresis can potentially cause hypotension, dehydration and electrolyte depletion (especially hypokalaemia), as well as earlier RAAS activation.

Given the lack of clinical evidence to support pharmacological intervention in asymptomatic patients, the author would advise owner education and patient monitoring rather than early treatment in these patients. Sleeping respiratory rate (SRR) monitoring is becoming an increasingly accepted tool with which to detect early changes associated with the onset of CHF. Owners can easily count the respiratory rate of their cats while asleep and keep a diary of daily measurements. SRR in stable cats is believed to be <30–35/min. However, a progressive and consistent increase in SRR over sequential measurements may indicate an incipient pulmonary oedema or pleural effusion and may warrant thoracic radiography, ultrasonography or a response trial with furosemide.

The symptomatic cardiac patient

Many cases of CM are diagnosed after a sudden, and often unexpected, onset of CHF. Dyspnoea, lethargy and inappetence are the most common clinical signs, although ascites can be frequently observed in cases of right-sided or biventricular failure. The inception of clinical signs is often triggered by a stressful event, such as a long car journey, a noisy waiting room, or physical restraint to perform a diagnostic procedure or obtain a blood sample. Therefore stress should always be minimized (see Chapter 1) in cats with a suspected or previously recognized heart condition.

Immediate management: Cats presented with signs of CHF are extremely vulnerable and every attempt should be made to reduce their anxiety before any diagnostic test or therapeutic procedure. Effective sedation can be achieved with intramuscular acepromazine in combination with butorphanol or buprenorphine (see Chapter 3). Cage rest (in a quiet room away from dogs) and oxygen supplementation (see QRG 4.2.2) should follow until the patient appears less distressed. The patient should be maintained in a comfortable sternal recumbency, which facilitates respiratory movements, and chest percussion (see QRG 1.5) should be performed to identify the typical horizontal line of dullness of pleural effusion. The presence of fluid in the pleural space can also be easily confirmed by trans-thoracic ultrasonography, performed with the patient in a comfortable sternal position. Thoracocentesis (see QRG 4.2.4) can provide rapid removal of large volumes of pleural fluid and offer a rapid improvement of the respiratory function; bilateral drainage is often advocated by many clinicians, but the large fenestration in the feline mediastinum allows sufficient pleural drainage with a single unilateral access. In cases with ascites, abdominocentesis (see QRG 5.1.1) should be considered when the presence of ascitic fluid interferes with respiration or causes discomfort.

Pulmonary oedema is generally controlled by intravenous furosemide (1–2 mg/kg i.v. q3–6h) until a normal respiratory rate is achieved. Stabilization and control of acute CHF to the point of patient discharge would be expected to be achieved in 24–36 hours in the majority of patients. Systemic blood pressure should be monitored to avoid the risk of profound hypotension secondary to excessive dehydration, and renal parameters, as well as electrolytes (especially potassium, sodium and chloride) monitored, due to the disturbances that furosemide can induce (e.g. prerenal azotaemia, hypokalaemia).

Ongoing management: Once pulmonary oedema is clinically controlled, the patient can be discharged on oral furosemide (0.5–2 mg/kg q12h), gradually reduced to the lowest effective dose in order to reduce the risk of hypotension, prerenal azotaemia and hypokalaemia. Oral furosemide is usually given in tablet form, although human paediatric liquid formulations can be useful in some cats and allow more accurate dosing for those requiring low doses. If

hypokalaemia occurs, it can be treated effectively by concomitant administration of potassium supplementation and/or potassium-sparing agents such as spironolactone (2 mg/kg orally q24h; this takes a few days to have maximal effect), although sufficient data of clinical efficacy of spironolactone in symptomatic cats is currently unavailable. Furthermore, it should be noted that severe facial ulcerative dermatitis has been reported as an adverse effect in some Maine Coon cats treated with spironolactone.

Diltiazem (0.5–2.0 mg/kg orally q8h) is authorized in the UK for the management of HCM, due to its bradycardic, lusitropic (improving cardiac relaxation, so may be helpful if diastolic dysfunction is present) and coronary vasodilating properties. However, the clinical efficacy of diltiazem in feline CM has not been convincingly demonstrated with controlled randomized clinical studies. Furthermore, many cat owners struggle to comply with the three times daily administration scheduled for the authorized formulation.

Beta-blockers have been considered for the treatment of CHF secondary to feline CM but many clinicians have lost confidence in beta blockade following the results of a controlled study (Fox, 2003) that reported a shorter survival in cats receiving atenolol and furosemide when compared to cats receiving furosemide alone. The disappointing outcome of this study might have been because atenolol was given at full dose without titration, while guidelines from human cardiology indicate that patients should be haemodynamically stable when beta-blocker therapy is initiated and treatment should be started at a very low dose (e.g. 1–2 mg/cat q24h) and titrated to the full dose (6.25–12.5 mg/cat q12 or 24h) over a period of several weeks (e.g. 6–8 weeks). Furthermore, the presence of systolic myocardial dysfunction should be excluded prior to initiation of beta-blocker therapy, due to their negative inotropic properties.

Atenolol is usually preferred over propranolol because it does not pass through the blood–brain barrier and is less prone to inducing depression and lethargy. Furthermore, atenolol is a selective beta-1 receptor antagonist and the risk of bronchospastic reactions with atenolol is reduced compared to non-selective beta-blockers such as propranolol. Atenolol is also available as a liquid preparation that is easier to give to cats.

ACE inhibitors are not currently authorized for the treatment of CHF in cats and there are no clinical trials available to demonstrate their efficacy in these patients. However, ACE inhibitors are commonly used in veterinary practice to counteract the RAAS activation induced by furosemide. Side effects, such as hypotension, anorexia and vomiting, are rarely observed following administration of ACE inhibitors in cats with CHF; however, their administration can be prudently delayed in cases of inappetence or severe hypotension.

Similarly, pimobendan (a positive inotrope and vasodilator) is not authorized for use in cats, although small retrospective studies seem to demonstrate some improvement in appetite and demeanour in cats with CM accompanied by systolic dysfunction detected on echocardiography after administration of pimobendan at 1.25 mg/cat orally q12h. It has been recently demonstrated that absorption of pimobendan is more rapid in cats than in dogs, while plasma half-life is longer, suggesting that further studies are needed to identify the correct dosage and frequency of administration of pimobendan in cats.

Following these considerations, a prudent approach should be taken when recommending any of these drugs in addition to furosemide for the treatment of feline CM accompanied by clinical or radiographic signs of CHF, and specialist advice is always recommended.

Prognosis

Life expectancy depends mainly on the severity of the myocardial lesions, with a shorter survival in patients with severe cardiac remodelling and clinical signs of CHF.

Median survival time (MST) in symptomatic cats with HCM is 194 days, while life expectancy is significantly longer (>3000 days) in asymptomatic individuals. Other negative prognostic variables that should be taken into consideration include left atrial enlargement, presence of arrhythmias, gallop sounds, spontaneous echo-contrast observed in the left atrium ('smoke'), and reduced systolic function. Paradoxically, the presence of dynamic outflow obstruction seems to be associated with longer survival and this is likely attributable to the fact that such an obstruction produces an audible heart murmur and allows earlier identification of the disease. Prospective longitudinal studies are currently in progress and will soon provide additional prognostic information for HCM in cats.

Other non-hypertrophic forms of CM carry a less favourable prognosis, with an MST that varies from approximately 11 to 130 days, depending on the severity of cardiac dilatation and systolic dysfunction. It is believed that many of these severe CM forms may simply represent the end stage of any cardiac disease, including HCM.

Arterial thromboembolism

ATE is characterized by the embolization of a clot in an artery in the systemic circulation. The artery in which the clot will eventually lodge depends on the origin of the clot, its size, and the diameter of the artery. In most cases, the initial blood clot forms inside the cavities of the left heart, particularly in the left atrium. The clot, or a fragment of it, can subsequently flow to an anatomical location in the systemic arterial circulation, normally represented by a 'saddle' location at the aortic trifurcation, and subsequently compromising the blood flow in both external iliac arteries. Occasionally, emboli may travel into more distal arteries, compromising the blood flow to a single limb, including forelimbs. The compromise in blood flow results in ischaemic neuromyopathy (see Chapter 17). More rarely, ATE affects cerebral, renal and mesenteric arteries. The majority of cats presenting with ATE have underlying heart disease, although neoplasia and thyroid disease are also highly associated with ATE.

Clinical presentation

The classic clinical presentation is characterized by acute pain and paresis/paralysis of the affected limbs. The paws of the affected limb may appear pale

(Figure 9.2) or cyanotic, depending on the severity of the local ischaemia, and the limb extremity is generally colder than non-affected limbs. In most cases the 'saddle' thrombus obstructs the external iliac arteries and, consequently, femoral pulses are weak or absent. However, if the thrombus lodges across the internal iliac arteries (rather than external iliac arteries) femoral pulses may still be palpable despite the presence of pain and hindlimb paralysis/paresis (Figure 9.3). Conversely, the femoral pulse may be difficult to detect in cats with shock; therefore, the use of a Doppler transducer may assist the clinician in the identification of the arterial pulse in the affected limb.

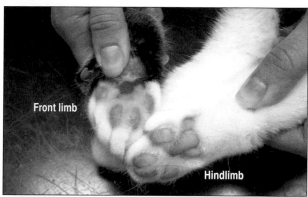

9.2 A 10-year-old male DSH cat presented with ATE and bilateral hindlimb paralysis. The metatarsal and digital pads of the hind foot are dramatically pale and were cold to the touch.

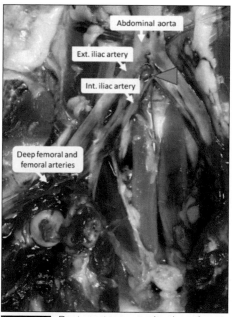

9.3 Post-mortem examination of an 8-year-old female DSH cat that had been euthanased following diagnosis of severe ATE. The cat presented with bilateral hindlimb paresis and echocardiographic evidence of myocardial disease. Both femoral pulses were palpable at presentation. A large thrombus (green arrowhead) was lodged at the trifurcation of the internal iliac and sacral arteries.

Diagnosis

Diagnosis of ATE can be challenging and it is usually based on history and clinical signs. In cats spending most of their time outdoors, the patient may be found recumbent on the ground, and the owner's initial thought is often towards a road traffic accident. Neurological disorders and musculoskeletal injuries are important differential diagnoses.

Marked elevations in AST and CK are highly suggestive of ischaemic damage to the limb skeletal muscles. In cats, both AST and CK have short half-lives, and their values peak at 6–12 hours, returning to normal within 24–48 hours after the acute ischaemic event.

Thoracic radiographs may reveal cardiomegaly and signs of CHF (pulmonary oedema and/or pleural effusion). Echocardiography allows identification of concomitant heart disease and sometimes confirms the presence of a thrombus or spontaneous echo-contrast (smoke) within the heart chambers. The localization of the thrombus can be deduced from the affected limb and, in many cases with hindlimb paralysis/paresis, where available (or via referral), colour-flow Doppler ultrasound examination of the descending aorta can be used to visualize the point of obstruction.

Clinical management

There is little scientific evidence and no consensus among clinicians regarding the ideal treatment of cats affected by ATE.

Surgical embolectomy would appear the most logical approach but is difficult due to the size of the affected vessels and the anaesthetic risks encountered in cardiac patients. It is also an extremely unrewarding technique due to the high mortality associated with rapid reperfusion (reperfusion injury). This complex phenomenon occurs when a large ischaemic area is acutely reperfused, accompanied by a violent inflammatory response within damaged tissues and leakage of cellular metabolic waste products into the circulation. Physical thrombolytic therapy may be performed by some referral centres, with pressurized saline jets that physically dissolve the thrombus, and has a clinical outcome comparable with that of conventional therapies. Medical thrombolytic therapy (urokinase, streptokinase and tissue plasma activator) has shown mixed results, especially because of complications due to rapid reperfusion. As with myocardial infarction in human patients, these expensive drugs are only effective if administered within hours of the occurrence of ischaemia, which is rarely possible in veterinary patients.

Conservative treatment is commonly recognized as acceptable management for cats with ATE, as long as pain is optimally controlled and the patients undergoing treatment are properly selected. The rationale of conservative treatment is to support the patient until collateral circulation develops to provide sufficient blood supply to the ischaemic areas. The time necessary for a satisfactory clinical improvement depends on the severity of the insult and the underlying cause, and may range from days to months.

Euthanasia should be considered in cases of non-responsive patients (lack of clinical improvement after 2–3 days or unsatisfactory pain control) or for those exhibiting signs highly associated with a negative prognosis (severe hypothermia, multiple limbs affected with complete loss of motor function, CHF).

The fact that feline ATE is a devastating clinical manifestation is undisputable. However, if euthanasia with no attempt to treat is excluded from survival analyses, the number of cats that may survive to discharge can increase up to 40–70%. Parameters that may indicate a more favourable prognosis are:

- Rectal temperature >37.2°C
- Presence of limb motor function (as evidenced by voluntary movement of limbs or positive withdrawal reflex)
- Absence of radiographic signs of CHF (e.g. pulmonary oedema, pleural effusion)
- Single limb affected (rather than two or more)
- Absence of tachycardia (i.e. heart rate <180 beats/min)
- Absence of hyperkalaemia (i.e. potassium <5 mmol/l).

Of all the above parameters, rectal temperature is the strongest survival predictor, indicating that hypothermia is most likely a reflection of compromised systemic haemodynamic status rather than just local hypoperfusion.

Short-term in-hospital conservative management

The goal of conservative treatment of ATE is to:

- Guarantee adequate rest and pain relief
- Reduce the risk of further thrombus formation
- Improve systemic perfusion and preserve the function of the affected limbs
- Control effusions in cases complicated by CHF
- Provide additional support where needed.

The ideal analgesic for cats affected by ATE probably depends on different patient responses, the individual clinician's experience, and drug availability. A variety of successful analgesics have been reported, including butorphanol, buprenorphine, morphine and fentanyl (see Chapter 3). A common protocol adopted in veterinary practice is intravenous or sublingual buprenorphine administration followed by application of a fentanyl patch to allow consistent and prolonged analgesia.

Intravenous or subcutaneous unfractionated heparin (UFH) treatment can be considered during the acute phase (hospitalization period) due to the rapid onset of its anticoagulation properties. Conversely, intramuscular UFH should be avoided due to the risk of injection-site haematomas. Low-molecular-weight heparin (LMWH) does not offer any practical advantage over UFH for short-term treatment. Cats absorb and eliminate LMWH very rapidly and therefore require higher doses and more frequent injections of the LMWH to achieve the therapeutic effects observed in human patients. It is also considerably more expensive than UFH.

Correcting systemic perfusion is a challenging task, especially in cats with signs of CHF who should never receive aggressive fluid therapy (see above). However, if patients are not in CHF and appear dehydrated, cautious fluid therapy would certainly be indicated. Acepromazine has been advocated for many years as a suitable drug to improve systemic perfusion in cats with ATE. However, its hypotensive effect can also exacerbate the signs of shock and many clinicians consider the use of acepromazine inappropriate for cats with ATE. Similarly, external physical warming should only be performed very cautiously to avoid the risk of peripheral vasodilatation and reduction of core perfusion. Little is known about the benefits of physiotherapy. Deep tissue massage of the affected areas and gentle forced movements of the affected limbs may be beneficial as long as the manoeuvre does not evoke pain or discomfort. Soft beds and gentle turning of the patient may also reduce pain and discomfort.

Cats affected by ATE are usually inappetent; nutritional support can easily be achieved via naso-oesophageal tubing (see QRG 5.5.2) in cats without respiratory distress.

Long-term at-home conservative management
When the patient appears sufficiently comfortable and is regaining its appetite, discharge can be discussed. The owner should be prepared to support the cat at home, including hand-feeding, grooming and toileting assistance.

Cats with an underlying cardiac disease and CHF should receive appropriate chronic treatment (see above). Similarly, appropriate treatment should be considered in cats affected by hyperthyroidism (see Chapter 14) or neoplasia (see Chapter 21).

Prophylactic anticoagulation therapy has been debated for several years. However, at present, there is not sufficient scientific evidence to support a specific medication or protocol. UFH treatment requires frequent parenteral administrations to achieve consistent anticoagulation and is not generally suitable for home treatment. Oral aspirin is frequently prescribed at 75 mg/cat ('baby aspirin') q72h. However, a lower dose (5 mg/cat q72h) seems associated with fewer side effects and similar recurrence rate of ATE when compared to the traditional dose, although a compounding pharmacy or dissolving soluble aspirin in water is necessary to obtain accurate low dosing. Nevertheless, very little is known about the pharmacokinetics and clinical efficacy of aspirin in preventing ATE. Clopidogrel (18.75 mg/cat orally q24h) is another inhibitor of platelet aggregation that seems to have few adverse effects in cats. It is commonly used in veterinary practice as a daily medication to prevent recurrence of ATE, often in association with aspirin. However, at present, the clinical efficacy of clopidogrel for ATE prevention has not been reported.

Prognosis
Long-term survival is negatively affected by the concomitant presence of CHF or neoplasia. Many survivors can experience a full recovery. However, a degree of neurological or muscular dysfunction of affected limbs may persist in some patients. Recurrence of ATE is relatively low (approximately 30%), although these episodes are often fatal or require prompt euthanasia. CHF represents the most common cause of death (or reason for euthanasia) in cats surviving acute episodes of thromboembolism (MST of 77 days in cats with concurrent CHF, compared to 223 days in cats with ATE without concurrent CHF).

References and further reading

Ferasin L (2009) Feline myocardial disease. 1: Classification, pathophysiology and clinical presentation. *Journal of Feline Medicine and Surgery* **11**, 3–13

Ferasin L (2009) Feline myocardial disease. 2: Diagnosis, prognosis and clinical management. *Journal of Feline Medicine and Surgery* **11**, 183–194

Fox PR (2003) Prospective, double-blinded, multicenter evaluation of chronic therapies for feline diastolic heart failure: interim analysis. *Journal of Veterinary Internal Medicine* **17,** 398 [abstract]

Luis Fuentes V, Johnson LR and Dennis S (2010) *BSAVA Manual of Canine and Feline Cardiorespiratory Medicine, 2nd edn.* BSAVA Publications, Gloucester

Pariaut R (2011) Heart. In: *BSAVA Manual of Canine and Feline Ultrasonography,* ed. F Barr and L Gasschen, pp. 37–71. BSAVA Publications, Gloucester

Payne J, Luis Fuentes V, Boswood A *et al.* (2010) Population characteristics and survival in 127 referred cats with hypertrophic cardiomyopathy (1997 to 2005). *Journal of Small Animal Practice* **51**, 540–547

Smith SA and Tobias AH (2004) Feline arterial thromboembolism: an update. *Veterinary Clinics of North America: Small Animal Practice* **34**, 1245–1271

Smith SA, Tobias AH, Jacob KA *et al.* (2003) Arterial thromboembolism in cats: acute crisis in 127 cases (1992–2001) and long-term management with low-dose aspirin in 24 cases. *Journal of Veterinary Internal Medicine* **17**, 73–83

Wess G, Schinner C, Weber K *et al.* (2010) Association of A31P and A74T polymorphisms in the myosin binding protein C3 gene and hypertrophic cardiomyopathy in Maine Coon and other breed cats. *Journal of Veterinary Internal Medicine* **24**, 527–532

Willis R (2010) Patients with cardiac disease. In: *BSAVA Manual of Canine and Feline Rehabilitation, Supportive and Palliative Care: Case Studies in Patient Management,* ed. S Lindley and P Watson, pp.268—288. BSAVA Publications, Gloucester

Management of respiratory disorders

10

Angie Hibbert

This chapter will focus on the management of the most important respiratory disorders encountered in feline practice, considered in order of anatomical regions of the respiratory tract: upper respiratory tract disorders (nasal neoplasia, nasopharyngeal stenosis, foreign bodies, stenotic nares, laryngeal paralysis, laryngeal neoplasia); lower respiratory tract disorders (bronchial disease, pneumonia); and pleural space disorders (pyothorax, chylothorax). The chapter also contains a practical QRG on administering inhalational treatments. A formulary at the end of the chapter (Figure 10.10) gives further details of drug use, including doses and side effects.

Other practical QRGs relevant to respiratory disorders that are included in other chapters include: thoracic auscultation (QRG 1.5); immediate management of severe dyspnoea (QRG 4.2.1); administration of oxygen (QRG 4.2.2); emergency thoracic radiography (QRG 4.2.3); thoracocentesis (QRG 4.2.4); inserting a chest drain (QRGs 4.2.5 and 4.2.6); bronchoalveolar lavage (QRG 5.10.1); assessing the nasopharynx (QRG 5.34.1); and nasal flush and biopsy (QRG 5.34.2).

Other chapters contain more information on the approach to specific presentations such as dyspnoea (Chapter 4.2), coughing (Chapter 5.10), and sneezing and nasal discharge (Chapter 5.34). Aspects of respiratory tract trauma, such as pulmonary contusions and diaphragmatic rupture, are included in the chapter on trauma and wound management (Chapter 4.10). Management of cardiovascular disorders is covered in Chapter 9. Respiratory endoscopy is not covered in this manual.

Upper respiratory tract (URT) disease

Management of chronic rhinosinusitis is discussed with management of infectious disorders (see Chapter 19).

Nasal neoplasia

The most commonly diagnosed nasal tumour is lymphoma; other types include adenocarcinoma, squamous cell carcinoma (SCC), undifferentiated carcinoma or sarcoma, osteosarcoma, fibrosarcoma and chondrosarcoma. The most common tumour of the nasal planum is SCC (see Chapter 21).

Clinical features

Nasal tumours are most often seen in mature to senior cats; however, young adults can also be affected. Nasal discharge is the most common clinical sign. The discharge may be unilateral or bilateral and can be variable in nature (serous, mucoid, mucopurulent or haemorrhagic). URT noise, sneezing, ocular discharge and dyspnoea with open-mouth breathing may also be seen. Additionally there may be facial deformity or exophthalmos (due to local extension of the tumour), weight loss and submandibular lymphadenomegaly. CNS signs, including seizures or depression, suggest extension of the tumour into the calvarium via the cribriform plate. A partial response to antibiotic treatment may feature in the case history, as superficial inflammation and secondary bacterial infection may be associated with a nasal tumour.

Diagnosis

Confirmation of neoplasia requires identification of malignant cells or tissue using cytology or histopathology.

- Fine-needle aspiration (see QRG 5.33.1) of enlarged draining submandibular lymph nodes may enable a rapid diagnosis without additional invasive diagnostic tests.
- Radiographs of the nasal chambers typically reveal increased soft tissue opacity and loss of the normal turbinate/vomer structure.
- Radiographs of the thorax should be obtained to look for evidence of distant metastasis (more common in epithelial or mesenchymal neoplasia).
- Cytology of a deep nasal flush (see QRG 5.34.2) sample may reveal neoplastic cells if the tumour is exfoliative, although the absence of neoplastic cells does not allow neoplasia to be excluded.
- Nasal biopsy (see QRG 5.34.2) should be performed, remembering that there may be superficial inflammation associated with a tumour on histopathology.
- Referral may be considered if a definitive diagnosis cannot be reached and the owners would consider pursuing treatment such as chemotherapy or radiotherapy:
  - CT and MRI (Figure 10.1) scans provide superior detail of the nasal chambers and sinuses

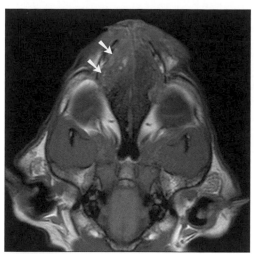

10.1 MRI (T1 scan dorsal plane) of a cat's skull, showing a nasal mass in the right nasal chamber (arrowed). The mass appears predominately hyperintense compared to the remainder of the tissue within the nasal chambers.

- Rhinoscopy enables detailed examination of the nasal chambers and directed biopsy of any masses or mucosal lesions.

Management

Nasal lymphoma can be treated successfully with multi-agent chemotherapy, radiotherapy or a combination of the two. Treatment with multi-agent chemotherapy may result in extended survival times (median survival time (MST) of 140 days for all cats, MST of 749 days for those achieving complete remission using various protocols (Taylor *et al.*, 2009)). A COP-based protocol (see Chapter 21 and *BSAVA Manual of Canine and Feline Oncology*) can be administered in practice; it is currently unknown whether addition of doxorubicin to a treatment protocol confers any advantage. A transient short response may be seen with prednisolone treatment alone.

Chemotherapy is currently not considered useful in other forms of nasal tumour, and radiotherapy appears to be the best option if owners wish to pursue treatment. If financial constraints prevent this, palliative treatment includes NSAIDs (for COX-2 inhibition), antibiotics (for any secondary bacterial infection) and nebulization (to encourage movement of nasal secretions).

Nasopharyngeal polyps

Polyps are inflammatory pedunculated masses arising from the mucosa of the tympanic bulla or eustachian tube, extending into the middle ear cavity, aural canal or nasopharynx and nose. There is currently no known cause or trigger for the development of polyps.

Clinical features

Nasopharyngeal polyps most commonly develop in young adult cats. Presenting signs depend upon the location of the polyp:

- An otic location is typically associated with aural discharge and head-shaking
- Involvement of the middle or inner ear cavity may cause vestibular signs (ataxia, head tilt, nystagmus), facial nerve paralysis and Horner's syndrome

- Growth of a polyp into the nasopharynx or nose may cause stertor, sneezing, dyspnoea, coughing and dysphagia.

Diagnosis

Some polyps may be identified by visual inspection of the auditory canal/tympanic membrane or nasopharynx, with or without palpation through the soft palate (see QRG 5.34.1). Lateral and ventrodorsal open-mouth skull radiographs allow examination of the entire nasopharynx and tympanic bulla, which can aid localization of a polyp (Figure 10.2) if not easily visualized or palpable through the soft palate. Endoscopic visualization of the nasopharynx and nose may be required; referral for this can be considered. A definitive diagnosis is reached with histopathological examination of any tissue removed; bacterial culture of resected tissue is also recommended.

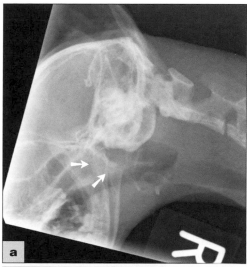

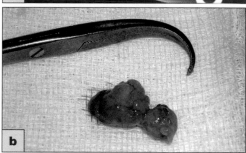

10.2 **(a)** A lateral skull radiograph showing a soft tissue opacity within the nasopharynx of a young DSH cat. The mass (arrowed) is seen dorsal to the soft palate. The mass was removed via traction and sectioning through the 'stalk'-like attachment and histopathology confirmed it to be a nasopharyngeal polyp. **(b)** Gross appearance of a nasopharyngeal polyp removed via traction from a young cat presented with stertor and sneezing.

Management

Traction and avulsion of nasopharyngeal or aural polyps can be performed as a first-line treatment, if the polyp is accessible. The polyp is grasped across the widest part of the mass and gently avulsed from the stalk using grasping forceps. Avulsion, followed by a 2–4-week course of anti-inflammatory prednisolone (e.g. 0.5 mg/kg orally q12h for 14 days, then 0.5 mg/kg orally q24h for 7 days, then 0.5 mg/kg orally on alternate days for five doses) was successful in resolving the condition in 59% of cases in one case series (Anderson *et al.*, 2000). A course of antibiotics (e.g. 14 days of amoxicillin/clavulanate) is also recommended following removal of aural polyps. Aural polyps removed by traction are more likely to recur compared to nasopharyngeal polyps. Transient Horner's syndrome is the most common complication following traction and avulsion.

Surgical treatment is indicated if there is regrowth of a polyp, or in aural cases where the tympanic bulla appears markedly abnormal radiographically (or with enhanced imaging such as CT or MRI) and there are associated signs of otitis media. Ventral bulla osteotomy is most commonly performed; referral should be considered for this. Possible postoperative complications include Horner's syndrome, facial nerve paralysis and vestibular signs, but these are usually transient. Return of hearing is unlikely if lost preoperatively.

Nasopharyngeal stenosis

Nasopharyngeal stenosis is a narrowing of the nasopharynx, which may be congenital (due to atresia of the choanae – the orifices between the caudal nasal chamber and nasopharynx) or acquired secondary to neoplasia or inflammation (e.g. URT infection or due to reflux of gastric material).

Clinical features

Typical presenting signs include stertor, gagging, coughing, nasal discharge and dyspnoea. The cat may have an obstructive respiratory pattern (increased phase of inspiration) and reduced nasal airflow. The principal differential diagnoses to exclude are foreign bodies, neoplasia, rhinitis and polyps (see Chapter 5.34).

Diagnosis

Diagnosis is made by visual inspection of the caudal nasopharynx (see QRG 5.34.1); one or both choanae will appear narrowed, with a sheet of mucosa-like tissue extending across the area where the normal orifices would be expected. More complete examination is achieved endoscopically using a flexible endoscope; referral for this can be considered.

Management

Mechanical dilation of the orifice can be achieved by opening curved artery forceps within the narrowed choanae. Alternatively, expandable balloons or mechanical stents can be used under endoscopic or fluoroscopic guidance; this is a referral procedure. Dilation is usually followed by a short course of anti-inflammatory steroids (e.g. prednisolone 0.5 mg/kg orally q12h for 14 days, then 0.5 mg/kg orally q24h for 7 days, then 0.5 mg/kg orally on alternate days for five doses) and broad-spectrum antibiotics (e.g. amoxicillin/clavulanate for 14 days) to try to prevent recurrence.

Nasal or nasopharyngeal foreign body

Foreign material may become lodged within the nasal chambers or nasopharynx following inhalation or reflux from the upper gastrointestinal tract. Grass blades are common nasopharyngeal foreign bodies.

Clinical features

Typically the cat has an acute onset of sneezing, facial irritation, gagging and coughing, with or without epistaxis. With chronicity there may be nasal discharge and halitosis.

Diagnosis

This is made by visual inspection of the nasal chambers and nasopharynx under anaesthesia (see QRG 5.34.1). With chronicity, nasal discharges may make visualization more difficult, and flushing with warmed saline (see QRG 5.34.2) will be required for visualization. The presence of a foreign body within the nasal cavity may induce local inflammation and secondary infection; radiographic changes may include a focal area of soft tissue opacity (due to the foreign material or associated exudate) with or without loss of local turbinates. Referral for a CT scan or specialist endoscopy should be considered if a foreign body is suspected but cannot be located.

Management

Nasopharyngeal foreign bodies can usually be retrieved using long curved artery forceps and retracting the soft palate (see QRG 5.34.1). Flushing the nose with sterile saline (see QRG 5.34.2) to dislodge secretions may actually remove foreign bodies; endoscopic removal is otherwise required. Following removal, a short course of broad-spectrum antibiotics is recommended (e.g. 5–7 days of amoxicillin/clavulanate).

Stenotic nares

This is a congenital breed-related anomaly most often seen in Persian and Himalayan cats. It forms part of the spectrum of anomalies associated with the brachycephalic conformation, which may also include an elongated soft palate, everted laryngeal saccules and nasopharyngeal turbinates.

Clinical features

Affected cats often have an extreme brachycephalic confirmation with marked narrowing of the nares. This may be associated with stertor, sneezing and dyspnoea, due to URT obstruction.

Diagnosis

Diagnosis is based upon visual inspection of the nares. Examination for other abnormalities of the brachycephalic conformation that may contribute to airway obstruction should be performed under anaesthesia. For example: the length of the soft palate relative to the larynx should be examined (it should terminate at the rostral aspect of the epiglottis); the nasopharynx can be examined for protruding turbinates extending beyond the choanae; and the laryngeal folds assessed for eversion.

Management

Surgical correction to widen the nares may be performed by wedge or punch alarplasty. If more extensive upper airway obstruction than that caused by the stenotic nares alone appears to be present, referral to a specialist soft tissue surgeon is recommended for evaluation of the soft palate and laryngeal saccules; surgical correction of an elongated soft palate or everted laryngeal saccules is, however, uncommonly required in cats. Prevention of obesity is important, as well as regular vaccination against URT infections (e.g. FHV, FCV). Severely affected cats should not be used for breeding.

Laryngeal disease

Laryngeal disease is relatively unusual in cats. The most common conditions include laryngitis or laryngeal oedema (e.g. acute due to URT infection or traumatic intubation; chronic associated with granulomatous inflammation), laryngeal neoplasia and laryngeal paralysis (idiopathic or acquired, e.g. secondary to surgery, neoplasia or trauma).

Clinical features

Laryngeal disease is usually associated with stridor, dysphonia, coughing and dyspnoea. Gagging and retching may also occur. Careful handling is required if laryngeal disease is suspected, to minimize stress and precipitation of a dyspnoeic crisis. Pre-oxygenation should be performed prior to any handling or an intervention such as venepuncture or induction of anaesthesia.

Diagnosis

Palpation of the larynx externally may identify local lesions, e.g. tumours infiltrating the recurrent laryngeal nerve. Radiography of the lateral cervical region may reveal soft tissue opacities over the larynx in cases of neoplasia.

Visual examination of the larynx under anaesthesia is required (endotracheal intubation may be difficult in cats with laryngeal abnormalities; see Chapter 3 for advice):

- Assess for paresis/paralysis: check that the movement of the larynx is coordinated with thoracic wall movement, i.e. abduction of the vocal folds should coincide with inspiration and outward excursion of the thoracic wall. Movement should be assessed under a light plane of anaesthesia; doxapram (0.5–1 mg/kg i.v.) can be used to stimulate movement
- Assess for inflammation, thickening or mass lesions.

Fine-needle aspirates or small pinch biopsy specimens (using small cup-tipped forceps such as endoscopic forceps) should be obtained if a thickening or mass is seen. The cat should not be recovered from anaesthesia until all haemorrhage has ceased; an anti-inflammatory dose of a short-acting steroid can be given to help reduce post-manipulation inflammation and swelling (e.g. dexamethasone sodium phosphate 0.1 mg/kg i.v.).

Management

In severe cases of laryngeal disease an emergency tracheostomy may, rarely, be required to alleviate dyspnoea (see *BSAVA Guide to Procedures in Small Animal Practice*).

Laryngeal paralysis: Depending on the underlying cause, bilateral laryngeal paralysis is managed surgically with arytenoid lateralization if there is associated dyspnoea; referral is recommended. The exception to this is in reversible neuropathies, such as tick paralysis, where laryngeal paralysis is a common presentation in cats.

Conservative management is appropriate for unilateral paralysis and cats that are only mildly affected by bilateral paralysis (e.g. stridor or respiratory compromise that is only evident upon marked exertion). Conservative management involves weight loss (if the cat is overweight), minimizing events that will increase respiratory effort (such as stress associated with travelling or handling) and treating any associated laryngitis (see below) or aspiration pneumonia.

Laryngeal neoplasia: Treatment is dependent upon tumour type. Extended survivals can be achieved using chemotherapy for lymphoma, which is the most common laryngeal neoplasm (see QRG 21.2).

Laryngitis: Management of laryngitis typically involves antibiotics (for any possible associated bacterial infection) and anti-inflammatory therapy (e.g. NSAID if known infectious cause, prednisolone in chronic sterile cases).

Lower airway disease

Bronchial disease: asthma and chronic bronchitis

Asthma and chronic bronchitis are both forms of inflammatory bronchial disease.

- **Asthma** is thought to be due to a type 1 hypersensitivity response to inhaled allergens, resulting in spontaneous and reversible bronchoconstriction, eosinophilic airway inflammation and remodelling.
- **Chronic bronchitis** is characterized by neutrophilic airway inflammation and remodelling; it is not typically associated with spontaneous bronchoconstriction and does not have an allergic basis. Chronic bronchitis is a diagnosis of exclusion; infectious disease and neoplasia have to be ruled out.

Distinguishing asthma from chronic bronchitis without examination of airway cytology is challenging; of clinical relevance is the reversible bronchoconstriction seen in asthma, meaning that asthmatic cats may benefit more from bronchodilator therapy than cats with chronic bronchitis. In the future, distinguishing asthma from chronic bronchitis may be more important if treatment can be directed towards the underlying allergy.

Clinical features

Asthma is more commonly diagnosed in young adult cats, with Siamese and Oriental breeds predisposed. Chronic bronchitis may develop at any age, and there are no breed predispositions.

Chronic bronchitis is associated with a frequent harsh cough. Often coughing is misinterpreted as vomiting, since many cats will terminate a paroxysm of coughing with a retch.

Asthma may also cause coughing, which may be paroxysmal, daily or intermittent, as the disease can wax and wane. There may also be associated lethargy, exercise intolerance and episodes of dyspnoea due to acute bronchoconstriction, with open-mouth breathing, hyperpnoea, tachypnoea, wheezing, pallor, cyanosis and collapse. Physical examination may reveal harsh respiratory sounds, wheezes/crackles and increased expiratory effort with an abdominal 'push'. The thorax may be hyper-resonant in asthmatic cats, due to chronic pulmonary over-inflation. Auscultation of the asthmatic cat between episodes of bronchoconstriction may be completely normal.

Diagnosis

Diagnosis is established through **cytology of BAL (bronchoalveolar lavage) samples** (see QRG 5.10.1) once the cat is stable enough to undergo general anaesthesia. Chronic bronchitis is characterized by neutrophilic inflammation, and asthma by eosinophilic inflammation (>25% of the total cell count) (Figure 10.3).

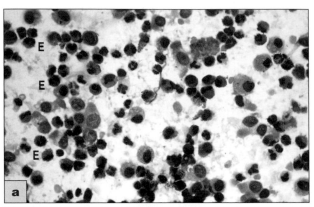

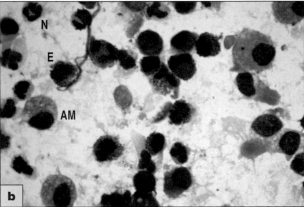

10.3 Cytology of a BAL sample demonstrating eosinophilic inflammation in a cat diagnosed with feline asthma. Eosinophils (E) are characterized by their red cytoplasmic granules; alveolar macrophages (AM) and neutrophils (N) are also present. Feline asthma is characterized by an increased percentage of eosinophils within the airways (>25% of the total cell count), as seen here. Modified Wright's stain; original magnifications: **(a)** X500, **(b)** X1000. (Courtesy of Kathleen Tennant)

WARNING

In acutely dyspnoeic cats, treatment for asthma should not be withheld. A positive response to a bronchodilator with or without short-acting steroids is supportive of the diagnosis.

Other investigations may include:

- **Radiography** (see QRG 4.2.3):
  - Asthmatic cats may have variable pulmonary patterns or even normal thoracic radiographs
  - The most common feature is a bronchial pattern, with bronchial wall thickening and mineralization ('tramlines and doughnuts')
  - Interstitial and focal alveolar patterns may also be seen, due to airway obstruction by mucus plugs, causing local atelectasis; the right middle lung lobe is most often affected
  - Asthmatic cats may have hyperinflation of the lungs, causing flattening of the diaphragm; there may be evidence of previously healed proximal rib fractures in the caudal thorax (Figure 10.4). Rarely, spontaneous pneumothorax may occur as a result of small airway obstruction causing increased alveolar pressure and emphysema
  - Airway inflammation cannot be excluded if the pulmonary fields appear radiographically normal
- **Haematology:** An inflammatory leucogram may be identified; peripheral eosinophilia is an inconsistent finding in asthmatic cats
- **Serum biochemistry:** Rarely helpful; hyperglobulinaemia may be identified
- **Faecal parasitology:** Faecal flotation and Baermann technique recommended on faeces submitted to an external laboratory, to search for *Aelurostrongylus abstrusus* and *Eucoleus aerophilus* (formerly *Capillaria aerophila*)
- **Serology:** For FeLV and FIV
- **Bacteriology:** Microbial culture of BAL samples should be performed (for aerobic, anaerobic and *Mycoplasma* spp.) ± PCR for *Mycoplasma felis* and *Bordetella bronchiseptica* to identify concurrent airway infection.

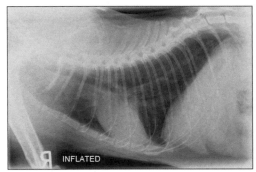

10.4 Lateral thoracic radiograph of a cat diagnosed with feline asthma. In this case there is a diffuse bronchial pulmonary pattern, which appears as bronchointerstitial in the cranial lobes. Note the proximal rib fracture lesions (T10–12) and barrel shape of the thorax, which are consistent with pulmonary hyperinflation. Other signs of hyperinflation to look for but not shown here include flattening of the diaphragm and extension of the tips of the caudodorsal lung fields to the 12–13th thoracic vertebrae during expiration (i.e. assessed on a non-inflated view).

Management

Emergency treatment of the dyspnoeic asthmatic cat

1. Provide supplemental oxygen (see QRG 4.2.2).
2. Administer a bronchodilator (terbutaline 0.015 mg/kg i.m.; can repeat dose after 30–60 minutes if partial response only, then q4–6h as required) and establish intravenous access.
3. Start a short-acting corticosteroid (e.g. dexamethasone sodium phosphate 0.1–0.2 mg/kg i.v. or s.c. once, or hydrocortisone 2 mg/kg i.v. q6h).

Once the cat has stabilized, diagnostic procedures can be pursued; a single dose of a short-acting corticosteroid will reduce airway inflammation but is unlikely to prevent a diagnosis being reached.

Longer-term management: Chronic bronchitis and asthma are both treated with anti-inflammatory steroids, ideally delivered by inhalation to reduce systemic absorption (see QRG 10.1). Fluticasone propionate is started at 125 µg/cat, one dose q12h, with gradual introduction of the spacer device, to help compliance. Fluticasone typically reaches therapeutic levels after 2 weeks, therefore oral prednisolone is started simultaneously and tapered off once therapeutic levels of fluticasone are achieved: e.g. 0.5 mg/kg orally q12h for 2 weeks, then 0.5 mg/kg orally q24h for 1 week then 0.5 mg/kg orally on alternate days for seven doses and then stop. The dose of inhaled steroid is gradually tapered after a period of stability (minimum 2–4 weeks); it is important to remember, however, that inadequate treatment of airway inflammation can be detrimental, due to ongoing airway remodelling.

All efforts should be made to exclude airway infection – on the basis of either airway culture or therapeutic trials (e.g. doxycycline at 10 mg/kg orally q24h for 3–6 weeks to exclude *Mycoplasma* spp. infection; topical imidacloprid/moxidectin or oral fenbendazole at 50 mg/kg q24h for 10 days to exclude airway parasites).

Asthmatic cats may benefit from continued use of a bronchodilator until the disease stabilizes; terbutaline and theophylline are both available in an oral form and suitable once a dyspnoeic crisis has resolved. Advice to improve airway hygiene is essential; this includes avoidance of exposure to smoke, aerosols, air fresheners and dust from litter trays, and restricting the cat from the bedroom. Steam nebulization may help to improve airway moisture levels and mucociliary clearance. Some cats may benefit from mucolytic treatment (e.g. bromhexine or acetylcysteine).

Pulmonary disease

Pneumonia

Pneumonia refers to inflammation of the pulmonary parenchyma. This may be due to infectious or non-infectious causes. Infectious causes include bacterial, viral, parasitic, protozoal and fungal disease. Bacterial infections may be primary (e.g. due to *Bordetella bronchiseptica* or *Mycoplasma* spp.) or secondary to aspiration of gastric contents, foreign material, viral infection, neoplasia, haematogenous spread or local extension of a pyothorax. Non-infectious conditions include lipid pneumonia and aspiration pneumonitis. Primary bacterial or viral pneumonia is more common in kittens than in adult cats.

Clinical features

In advanced stages there may be tachypnoea, dyspnoea and a soft cough. Lethargy, inappetence, weight loss, pyrexia and nasal discharge may also feature. Overt respiratory signs typically occur late in the course of pneumonia; hence, a lack of cough or tachypnoea does not exclude the possibility of pneumonia. Signs of systemic disease may be present depending upon the underlying cause, for example where aspiration pneumonia occurs secondary to vomiting, or in cats with FIP. Physical examination

may reveal increased adventitious respiratory noise (crackles and/or wheezes) or a loss of respiratory sounds if there is consolidation of pulmonary tissue. Pneumonia may be focal or generalized through the pulmonary fields.

Diagnosis

Diagnosis is based on consistent clinical signs, radiographic changes and, ideally, cytology of BAL samples with evaluation for infectious agents. In acute cases (e.g. acute cat 'flu with suspected secondary bacterial pneumonia), patients require stabilization first and are treated presumptively based on clinical signs with or without radiography. In stable patients, sampling of the airways enables a diagnosis to be confirmed and directs antimicrobial therapy based on culture and sensitivity testing.

Radiography: Thoracic radiography may reveal an interstitial ± alveolar pulmonary pattern. Radiographs may occasionally be normal, as the development of radiographic changes may lag behind the clinical course in acute disease. A nodular pattern may be seen with fungal, *Toxoplasma* and mycobacterial infections or FIP. A cranioventral distribution is often associated with aspiration pneumonia, but this may not always be seen and the diagnosis is then made based on a history of known vomiting, regurgitation or reflux in combination with an interstitial/alveolar pulmonary pattern (Figure 10.5).

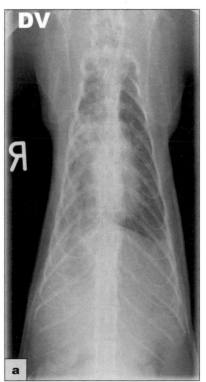

10.5 **(a)** Dorsoventral thoracic radiograph of a cat diagnosed with aspiration pneumonia secondary to vomiting and inhalation of gastric material. There is a marked alveolar pulmonary pattern in the right middle and caudal lung lobes; the other lobes appear to have a bronchointerstitial pattern on this view. The classic pulmonary change following aspiration is a cranioventral interstitial/alveolar pattern, with the right middle lung lobe frequently involved; however, radiographic changes may lag behind aspiration and development of clinical signs. (continues) ▶

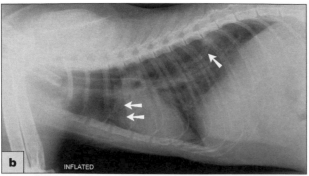

10.5 (continued) **(b)** In this left lateral thoracic radiograph of the same cat air bronchograms are now evident in the right cranial and caudal lung lobes (highlighted by the arrows), showing an area of lung with a focal alveolar pattern.

Infectious disease testing: This may include:

- Viral: Oropharyngeal swabs for FCV PCR or virus isolation and FHV PCR; cutaneous samples for cowpox PCR if crusting ulcerative skin lesions and a history of hunting; FeLV and FIV serology; feline coronavirus serology
- Bacterial: BAL samples for aerobic, anaerobic and *Mycoplasma* spp. cultures and for *Bordetella bronchiseptica* and *Mycoplasma felis* PCR; samples also examined for intracellular bacteria, including Gram staining (and Ziehl–Nielson stains if mycobacterial infection is suspected)
- *Toxoplasma gondii* serology (IgG and IgM)
- Fungal culture: Fungal infections are rare in the UK but more common in other parts of the world
- Faecal parasitology: For *Aelurostrongylus abstrusus* and *Eucoleus aerophilus;* faecal flotation and Baermann technique at an external laboratory is recommended.

Other tests:

- Airway cytology (BAL samples) typically demonstrates neutrophilic inflammation. A careful search for infectious organisms is made. Occasionally ultrasound-guided fine-needle aspiration of consolidated lung is performed, but this is generally a referral procedure.
- Haematology may reveal an inflammatory picture (neutrophilia ± left shift); in severe cases neutropenia with a degenerative left shift may occur. A mild non-regenerative anaemia of inflammatory disease may be found.
- Serum biochemistry is indicated to look for signs of systemic disease or complications of pneumonia, e.g. prerenal azotaemia or hypokalaemia secondary to inappetence and dehydration. Hyperglobulinaemia may feature.
- Consider whether an underlying cause for pneumonia requires specific investigation, e.g. where vomiting or regurgitation has led to aspiration pneumonia.

Management

Empirical antibiotic therapy is started pending culture results or in unstable patients where bacterial pneumonia is suspected. The most common bacteria cultured from the lower airways of cats are *Bordetella bronchiseptica, Pasteurella* spp., *Mycoplasma* spp., *Escherichia coli* and *Streptococcus* spp. For sick patients with dyspnoea or tachypnoea, parenteral treatment with amoxicillin/clavulanate or cefalexin is a reasonable first-line choice, with the addition of a fluoroquinolone if an inadequate response is seen. For stable outpatient treatment doxycycline can be used pending culture results.

Supportive treatment for sick cats includes intravenous fluid therapy, steam nebulization and coupage (see below) and nutritional support. Supplemental oxygen (see QRG 4.2.2) may be required. Bronchodilators such as terbutaline should be considered in severely compromised cats. Specific antimicrobial treatment is required if viral, fungal, *Toxoplasma* or mycobacterial infections are identified (see Chapter 19).

Nebulization and coupage

Steam nebulization and coupage can help to move airway secretions, increase mucociliary clearance and improve ventilation in the acute stages of pneumonia.

- Administer steam therapy for 10–15 minutes every 4 hours initially:
  - Deliver steam either via a paediatric nebulizer (using 0.9% sterile saline) or place the cat in a steamy environment under supervision (e.g. secure cat within a carrier, place a bowl of steaming water outside the cage door then cover the bowl and carrier with a towel).
- Following steam administration, perform coupage of the thorax for 5 minutes: using cupped hands tap the thoracic wall repeatedly and rapidly, moving in a caudal to cranial direction. This often causes coughing, which indicates a good response. Coupage is generally tolerated well by cats.
- Encouraging the cat to move around after nebulization and coupage has been performed is also helpful to move airway secretions, e.g. allow 5 minutes' free access to walk in a room, taking into consideration restrictions required to prevent infectious disease transmission.

Pleural space disease

Pleural effusions are a common cause of dyspnoea. The presence of a pleural effusion typically causes tachypnoea or hyperpnoea, and progresses to dyspnoea with an associated restrictive breathing pattern and abdominal effort or paradoxical respiration (Chapter 4.2). The first step in reaching a diagnosis is to obtain a sample of pleural fluid for analysis; thoracocentesis (see QRG 4.2.4) is usually both diagnostic and therapeutic. Fluid should be collected into EDTA tubes for cytology and into plain tubes for protein analysis and microbial culture (aerobic/anaerobic bacteria ± fungal). Characteristics of different pleural effusions are detailed in Figure 10.6.

Fluid	Gross appearance	Protein levels	Total nucleated cell count	Cell types	Differential diagnoses	Additional diagnostic tests to consider
Transudate	Translucent	<25 g/l	<1 cell $\times 10^9$/l	Macrophages, lymphocytes, mesothelial cells	Hypoalbuminaemia (e.g. in protein-losing nephropathy, protein-losing enteropathy, hepatic failure)	Serum biochemistry. Urinalysis (including UPC). Dynamic bile acids
Modified transudate	Slightly turbid; may be slightly sanguineous	25–35 g/l	0.5–10 $\times 10^9$/l	Macrophages, lymphocytes, mesothelial cells, neutrophils ± neoplastic cells	Congestive heart failure Neoplasia Diaphragmatic rupture Pericardial disease Lung lobe torsion	Thoracic radiography ± abdominal imaging after drainage. Echocardiography
Exudate: sterile	Turbid; cream or yellow; or pink if sanguineous	>30 g/l	>5 $\times 10^9$/l	Neutrophils, macrophages, lymphocytes, eosinophils ± neoplastic cells	FIP Neoplasia Pyothorax pretreated with antibiotics	Serum biochemistry, haematology, feline coronavirus antibody assays, alpha-glycoprotein levels. Immunocytochemistry of fluid
Exudate: septic	Turbid; cream or yellow; or pink if sanguineous	>30 g/l	5–50 $\times 10^9$/l	Degenerate neutrophils, macrophages, lymphocytes	Pyothorax	Gram staining of fluid; fluid culture. Thoracic imaging after drainage (radiography ± ultrasonography). Compare effusion and blood glucose (effusion glucose level usually lower than blood glucose)
Chyle	Milky white; pink if sanguineous	>25 g/l	>0.5 $\times 10^9$/l	Small lymphocytes predominate, neutrophils, macrophages	Idiopathic Congestive heart failure Neoplasia Trauma Lung lobe torsion Pericardial disease Heartworm infection	Compare triglyceride and cholesterol levels in fluid and fasted blood.[a] Thoracic radiography after drainage. Echocardiography. If history of travel, *Dirofilaria immitis* antibody and antigen testing and blood smear
Haemorrhagic [b]	Sanguineous	>30 g/l	>1 $\times 10^9$/l	Red blood cells predominate. Erythrophagocytes and lack of platelets if chronic haemorrhage	Trauma Coagulopathy Neoplasia Lung lobe torsion	Compare PCV of fluid and blood. Coagulation assessment – PT and APTT. Thoracic radiography ± ultrasonography after drainage

10.6 Characteristics of pleural effusions. APTT = activated partial thromboplastin time; PT = prothrombin time; UPC = urine protein: creatinine ratio. [a] In cases where the effusion fluid is chyle, effusion triglycerides are higher than serum triglycerides, and effusion cholesterol is lower than serum cholesterol; the ratio of effusion cholesterol to triglycerides is <1. [b] If grossly haemorrhagic fluid is aspirated, rapid distinction of haemothorax from a haemorrhagic effusion and iatrogenic contamination is required, since thoracocentesis is contraindicated if the patient has a coagulopathy and/or active cavitatory haemorrhage causing a haemothorax. A manual PCV assessment should be performed on the pleural fluid and compared to the PCV of the patient's blood. Recent haemorrhage due to a coagulopathy or trauma causing a haemothorax will result in the effusion having features similar to blood (e.g. high PCV ± platelets present) but the *fluid does not clot*. In contrast, if there is blood in the sample due to inadvertent puncture/sampling of an intercostal or pleural blood vessel, the sample will have a similar PCV to the patient but the *fluid will clot*. Haemorrhagic effusions have a PCV lower than that of the patient (often much lower despite their bloody appearance).

Pyothorax

Pyothorax is the accumulation of a purulent exudate within the pleural space. The most common cause of infection is aspiration of oropharyngeal bacteria leading to development of pneumonia, with extension into the pleural space (Barrs and Beatty, 2009). Other causes include bite wounds, haematogenous spread, a migrating foreign body, iatrogenic (e.g. following thoracocentesis), perforation of the oesophagus or airways and parasitic migration.

Clinical features

Pyothorax is most commonly diagnosed in young adult cats (mean 4–6 years), and cats from multi-cat households are at an increased risk. The clinical signs typically include tachypnoea progressing to dyspnoea (restrictive breathing pattern with or without abdominal effort or paradoxical pattern; see Chapter 4.2). Affected cats are usually lethargic, have lost weight, and may be inappetent and dehydrated. Coughing, pyrexia and hypersalivation may also occur. Some cats present with bradycardia and hypothermia, due to sepsis and advanced disease. Physical examination usually reveals muffled heart sounds and loss of pulmonary sounds in the ventral thorax due to the presence of a pleural effusion.

Diagnosis

Diagnosis is based upon analysis of pleural fluid and microbial culture (aerobic and anaerobic):

- Gross features – malodorous, turbid cream, pink or sanguineous fluid, sometimes with flocculent material
- Laboratory features – septic exudate with predominantly degenerate neutrophils and high protein levels
- The most common bacteria isolated are species of

Pasteurella, Clostridium, Fusobacterium, Bacteroides and *Actinomyces* (mixed species infections are common).

Following thoracocentesis, imaging of the thorax with radiography (or CT if available) with or without ultrasonography should be performed to search for an underlying cause of the pyothorax. Serum biochemistry, haematology and retrovirus testing are advocated. The most common biochemical abnormalities occur due to the exudative process and systemic effects of sepsis and include hypoalbuminaemia with hyperglobulinaemia, hypo- or hyperglycaemia, hyponatraemia, hypocalcaemia, hyperbilirubinaemia and increased AST. Haematology typically reveals a neutrophilia ± left shift, toxic changes, lymphopenia and mild nonregenerative anaemia (due to inflammatory disease).

Management

Immediate stabilization may require oxygen therapy (see QRG 4.2.2) and thoracocentesis (see Figure 10.9 and QRG 4.2.4). The principles of treatment thereafter are pleural space drainage using thoracostomy tubes, antibiosis and supportive care. Drainage via thoracostomy tubes is more effective than performing intermittent thoracocentesis and also permits lavage to be performed. Occasionally intermittent thoracocentesis is adequate, although the viscosity of the effusion often prevents complete drainage of the thorax.

- Initially intravenous broad-spectrum antibiotics are started pending culture and sensitivity testing; parenteral amoxicillin/clavulanate is suitable.
- Once stabilized (following thoracocentesis and fluid therapy) thoracostomy tubes are placed under anaesthesia (see QRG 4.2.5). A unilateral drain may be adequate if the mediastinum is no longer intact, indicated by complete evacuation of the pleural effusion by drainage from one hemithorax; bilateral drains are required if it is not possible to clear the entire pleural space from one side. Small-bore indwelling drains are well tolerated (e.g. Mila 14 G) and can be placed using a Seldinger technique (see QRG 4.2.6); however, if the pleural fluid is particularly flocculent, larger-bore drains may be required. Drain placement should be checked radiographically (Figure 10.7).
- Intermittent drainage via thoracostomy tube is performed (initially every 4 hours; Figure 10.8). Lavage using warmed saline or lactated Ringer's solution (10–20 ml/kg instilled aseptically over 5–10 minutes) once to twice daily can help debride the pleura and maintain drain patency. At least 75% of the instilled fluid should be recovered; altering the cat's position (e.g. lifting forelimbs up, changing from sternal to lateral recumbency for a few seconds) and then re-aspirating after 5 minutes may help fluid retrieval. Residual fluid that is not aspirated will be reabsorbed gradually across the pleural surface and for this reason large volumes of saline should not be instilled, due to the risk of inducing dyspnoea.
- Intravenous fluid therapy and nutritional requirements should be addressed.
- Opioid analgesia is recommended whilst thoracic drains are *in situ* (0.01–0.02 mg/kg buprenorphine q6–8h).

- Thoracic drainage and lavage is continued until the volume of accumulated fluid reduces to <2 ml/kg/day and there is cytological evidence of resolution of infection (absence of bacteria and reduction in the number of neutrophils and degenerate appearance). Often this may take 5–7 days.

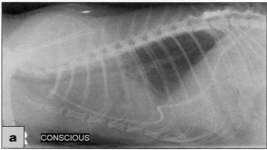

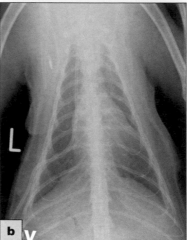

10.7 **(a)** Right lateral thoracic radiograph of a cat diagnosed with pyothorax, following a bite injury across the thoracic wall. A soft tissue opacity is present in the cranioventral thorax due to the presence of fluid and inspissated exudate. An indwelling small-bore thoracostomy tube is in place; a single drain was adequate to evacuate pleural fluid from both sides of the thorax in this case, indicating that the mediastinum was no longer intact.
(b) Dorsoventral thoracic radiograph following five days of antibiosis, thoracic lavage and drainage. There is significantly increased inflation of the cranial lung lobes, with residual opacity in the region of the right middle lung lobe. The thoracostomy drain was removed 7 days later, when the effusion volume had reduced to <2 ml/kg/day and there were reduced numbers of degenerate neutrophils and no intracellular bacteria present.

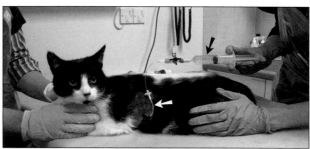

10.8 A cat with pyothorax undergoing thoracic lavage via a unilateral thoracostomy tube. Drainage was performed every 4 hours for 5 days, until the volume of effusion reduced, and lavage was performed twice daily. Further details on performing lavage are given in the text. Black arrow: Lavage solution – 10–20% ml/kg of warmed 0.9% sterile saline instilled over 5–10 minutes. White arrow: Indwelling drain – Mila 14 G.

Antibiotics should be continued for 4–6 weeks in total. Thoracic radiography is recommended at the 3-week point; if there are residual pulmonary abnormalities (e.g. evidence of pneumonia) or signs of persistent abnormal tissue or effusion within the pleural space, consideration should be given to repeating radiographs at the end of the antibiotic course to check for resolution of infection. A final physical examination is performed 1 week after completion of the antibiotic course.

Aggressive medical management, as above, is usually successful in resolving pyothorax and the prognosis is considered to be good. Rarely, exploratory thoracotomy is needed; indications include pulmonary or mediastinal abscessation, failure of the pleural effusion volume to reduce or the cytological appearance to improve with medical treatment, or repeated drain obstruction. Consideration of referral may be necessary for very sick septic cats, and where intensive care and close monitoring cannot be provided overnight or for exploratory thoracotomy.

Chylothorax

Chylothorax is the accumulation of chyle within the pleural space. Chyle normally drains via the thoracic duct into the left brachiocephalic vein. Any process that interferes with this drainage pathway can cause chylothorax. The most common aetiologies are: idiopathic; congestive heart failure (especially associated with thyrotoxicosis); and mediastinal neoplasia. Other less common causes include pericardial disease, heartworm infection, lung lobe torsion, fungal granulomas, cranial vena cava thrombosis and thoracic duct trauma.

Clinical features

Oriental breeds appear to have an increased incidence of chylothorax. The disease can be diagnosed in all ages of cats. Presenting signs typically include tachypnoea, dyspnoea (restrictive breathing pattern ± abdominal effort or paradoxical pattern), coughing (≤30% of cases, possibly due to the underlying aetiology or irritation of airways due to the effusion), lethargy, weight loss and inappetence. Physical examination may reveal signs typical of a pleural effusion, with muffled heart sounds and loss of ventral pulmonary sounds. Careful examination is required for signs of underlying causes, e.g. cranial rib spring to assess for mediastinal masses, and consideration of arrhythmia, heart murmur or gallop sounds indicating cardiac disease.

Diagnosis

Diagnosis is reached through confirming the presence of a pleural effusion (ultrasonographically, radiographically or by 'blind' thoracocentesis) and analysing the effusion (see Figure 10.6). Chyle is diagnosed by comparing lipid concentrations in the effusion and serum (fasted sample): triglyceride levels in the effusion are higher, and cholesterol levels lower than in the blood. Evaluation for possible underlying causes should be performed, including obtaining thoracic radiographs after thoracocentesis (to look for signs of mediastinal masses, cardiomegaly or lung lobe torsion) and echocardiography (assessing for cardiomyopathy and pericardial disease), when available (or consider referral). When

chylothorax is a chronic disease, fibrosing pleuritis may develop, which prevents full re-expansion of lung lobes; radiographically this may be recognized by rounded pulmonary lobar margins and lack of lung re-expansion following thoracocentesis.

Management

Immediate stabilization requires oxygen therapy (see QRG 4.2.2) and thoracocentesis (Figure 10.9 and see QRG 4.2.4). If an underlying cause has been diagnosed, treatment can be specifically prescribed (e.g. for congestive heart failure (see Chapter 9) or mediastinal lymphoma (see Chapter 21)) and the effusion managed in the interim with intermittent thoracocentesis.

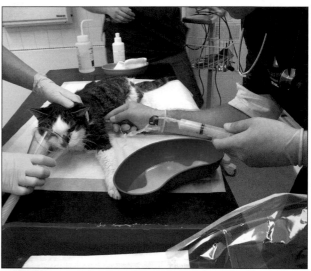

10.9 A cat with a chylothorax undergoing thoracocentesis. The aspirated fluid has a typical opalescent appearance. The chylothorax had developed secondary to congestive heart failure associated with severe thyrotoxicosis. Note the facemask providing supplemental oxygen and also the minimal restraint.

Idiopathic chylothorax is a challenging condition. Initially medical management is advised, using a combination of intermittent thoracocentesis, a reduced-fat diet (e.g. Hill's r/d) and rutin, a benzopyrone believed to increase macrophage uptake of lipids and increase proteolysis (50–100 mg/kg orally q8h); there is little evidence to know how effective this approach is, particularly as some cases resolve spontaneously.

Monitoring of electrolytes is required if repeat thoracocentesis is performed (hyponatraemia and hyperkalaemia may develop). If the effusion fails to resolve and thoracocentesis is required more than weekly, referral for surgery is recommended; typically thoracic duct ligation and pericardectomy with or without omentalization are performed. Variable success rates are described, with one group reporting that 80% of cats had complete resolution postoperatively following thoracic duct ligation and pericardectomy (Fossum *et al.,* 2004). The prognosis may be more guarded if the cat has developed severe fibrosing pleuritis.

Drug formulary

Drugs used in respiratory medicine are shown in Figure 10.10.

Drug	Type	Indications	Dose	Potential side effects	Notes
Antibacterials					
Amoxicillin/ clavulanate	Beta-lactam antibiotic	Bacterial URT infection; empirical treatment of pneumonia or pyothorax	20 mg/kg i.v. q8h, 12.5 mg/kg orally q12h or 8.75 mg/kg s.c. q24h	Nausea, vomiting, inappetence	Administer intravenous preparation slowly over 15 minutes
Doxycycline	Tetracycline	*Mycoplasma* spp. or *Bordetella bronchiseptica* infection	5–10 mg/kg orally q24h	Nausea, vomiting, hepatopathy	Must be followed with water or food to prevent oesophagitis and stricture development
Metronidazole	Nitroimidazole	Anaerobic infection (e.g. in pyothorax)	10 mg/kg i.v. or orally q12h	Neurological signs if excessive doses	Oral form has a bitter taste – disguise tablets in gelatine capsules (see QRG 3.1)
Cefalexin	Cephalosporin	Empirical treatment of pneumonia; effective against several Gram-+ve and –ve organisms	10–25 mg/kg s.c. q24h or orally q12h	Vomiting, diarrhoea	Increased risk of nephrotoxicity if given with furosemide
Clindamycin	Lincosamide	Chronic rhinosinusitis; toxoplasmosis	5.5 mg/kg orally q12h for routine use; 12.5 mg/kg orally q12h for toxoplasmosis	Vomiting, diarrhoea	Must be followed with water or food to prevent oesophagitis and stricture development
Marbofloxacin	Fluoroquinolone	Bacterial infection of respiratory tract; effective against Gram-+ve and –ve bacteria and *Mycoplasma* spp.	2 mg/kg orally, s.c. or i.v.	Nausea, vomiting	**Do not use higher doses**; unknown if higher doses could be associated with retinal toxicity. Second-line antibiotic. **Avoid in skeletally immature cats**
Pradofloxacin	Fluoroquinolone	Acute URT infection; authorized in UK for treatment of *Pasteurella multocida, Escherichia coli* and *Staphylococcus intermedius;* effective against Gram-+ve and –ve and anaerobic bacteria	5 mg/kg s.c. or orally q24h for 5 days	Vomiting	**Do not administer concurrently with antacids, sucralfate or multivitamins.** Use should be reserved as a second-line antibiotic due to extended spectrum of activity
Antiviral					
Famciclovir		FHV infection of URT	30–40 mg/kg orally q12h for 21 days	Little available information	Taper in response to clinical improvement
Bronchodilators					
Terbutaline	Beta-2 agonist	Bronchospasm	0.015 mg/kg i.v., i.m. or s.c. q4h or 0.3–1.25 mg/cat orally q8–12h	Tremors, tachycardia, hypokalaemia	Use with care if cat has cardiac disease, diabetes mellitus, hypertension, epilepsy or hyperthyroidism
Theophylline	Phosphodiesterase inhibitor	Bronchospasm (non-emergency)	10 mg/kg orally q24h using sustained release formula	Vomiting, diarrhoea, polyuria, polydipsia, agitation, hyperaesthesia, arrhythmias and tachycardia	Avoid concurrent use of terbutaline. Possible drug interactions with phenobarbital, cimetidine, diltiazem and fluoroquinolones
Salbutamol	Inhalational beta-2 agonist	Bronchospasm	100 µg (micrograms)/cat q6–12h or as required in acute crisis	Continued daily use may exacerbate airway inflammation	Reserve for emergency administration
Adrenaline		Use for refractory cases of status asthmaticus only	0.01–0.02 mg/kg i.v. or i.m. (1:10,000 dilution = 0.1 mg/ml)	Tachycardia, vasoconstriction and hypertension	Rescue therapy – rarely required
Atropine	Anticholinergic action	Use for refractory cases of status asthmaticus only	20–40 µg/kg i.v., i.m.or s.c.	Tachycardia	Rescue therapy – rarely required
Glucocorticoids					
Dexamethasone sodium phosphate	Short-acting	Emergency stabilization of bronchitis or asthma or URT inflammation	0.1–0.2 mg/kg i.v. or s.c. once		Avoid longer-acting preparations if further diagnostics are planned
Hydrocortisone	Short-acting	Emergency stabilization of bronchitis, asthma or URT inflammation	2 mg/kg i.v. or i.m. q6–8h		1–2 doses are unlikely to interfere significantly with interpretation of cytology of BAL samples
Prednisolone		Asthma or chronic bronchitis	Starting dose 0.5 mg/kg orally q12h; dose tapering required	Polyuria, polydipsia, polyphagia	
Fluticasone	Inhalational	Asthma or chronic bronchitis	50–125 µg/cat q12–24h. Starting dose of 125 µg/cat q12h, tapered to lowest dose required	Suppression hypothalamic–pituitary axis	

10.10 Drugs used in respiratory medicine, arranged by commonness of use within therapeutic class. (continues) ▶

Drug	Type	Indications	Dose	Potential side effects	Notes
Mucolytics					
Bromhexine		Chronic rhinosinusitis; chronic bronchitis	1 mg/kg orally q24h		
Acetylcysteine		Chronic rhinosinusitis; chronic bronchitis	30–60 mg/kg orally q8–12h		
Sedative					
Butorphanol	Opioid analgesic	Mild sedation for dyspnoeic cats	0.1–0.3 mg/kg i.v. or i.m. q4–6h		Can be combined with low-dose acepromazine (0.005–0.01 mg/kg) or midazolam (0.2–0.3 mg/kg) for short procedures (e.g. thoracocentesis)

10.10 (continued) Drugs used in respiratory medicine, arranged by commonness of use within therapeutic class.

References and further reading

Anderson DM, Robinson RK and White RAS (2000) Management of inflammatory polyps in 37 cats. *The Veterinary Record* **147**, 684–687

Barrs VR and Beatty JA (2009) Feline pyothorax – new insights into an old problem: Part 1. Aetiopathogenesis and diagnostic investigation. *Veterinary Journal* **179**, 163–170

Barrs VR and Beatty JA (2009) Feline pyothorax – new insights into an old problem: Part 2. Treatment recommendations and prophylaxis. *Veterinary Journal* **179**, 171–178

Beatty J and Barrs VR (2010) Pleural effusion in the cat: a practical approach to determining aetiology. *Journal of Feline Medicine and Surgery* **12**, 693–707

Fossum TW, Forrester SD, Swenson CL *et al.* (1991) Chylothorax in cats: 34 cases (1969–1989). *Journal of the American Veterinary Medical Association* **198**, 672–678

Fossum TW, Mertens MM, Miller MW *et al.* (2004) Thoracic duct ligation and pericardectomy for treatment of idiopathic chylothorax. *Journal of Veterinary Internal Medicine* **18**, 307–310

Taylor SS, Goodfellow MR, Browne WJ *et al.* (2009) Feline extranodal lymphoma: response to chemotherapy and survival in 110 cats. *Journal of Small Animal Practice* **50**(11), 584–592

Trostel TC and Frankel DJ (2010) Punch resection alaplasty technique in dogs and cats with stenotic nares: 14 cases. *Journal of the American Animal Hospital* **46**, 5–11

QRG 10.1 Inhalant asthma treatment
by Angie Hibbert

Inhalant treatment offers advantages for steroid administration, by reducing systemic absorption and the need to administer daily tablets. Inhalant treatment is best administered using a spacer specifically designed for cats (e.g. Aerokat).

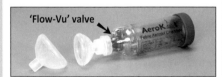

'Flow-Vu' valve

The Aerokat spacer (www.breatheazy.co.uk) comes with two different sizes of facemask to accommodate various sizes of patient.

Acclimatizing the cat prior to treatment

Training a cat to accept inhalant treatment requires patience and time on behalf of the owner, to ensure that the device is well tolerated and can be used in the longer term. Useful video resources are available online (e.g. www.fabcats.org/owners/asthma/inhalers.html, www.trudellmed.com/animal-health/aerokat).

1 The owner should first acclimatize the cat to the free facemask disconnected from the spacer unit. A few treats or catnip can be placed in the mask to encourage the cat to examine and investigate it.

2 A few days should be spent acclimatizing the cat to placement of the facemask over its nose and mouth. This should be done without rushing, in a quiet environment, and rewarding the cat with a treat (e.g. food treat, grooming, play). The mask is first held gently over the face for 2–5 seconds. The time can then be gradually increased over a few days to 30 seconds. Placing the cat on your lap facing away from you is often the easiest position; some owners may find this easier with the cat gently wrapped in a towel. Wiping the inside of the facemask with something that will leave a favourable smell may increase acceptance, e.g. catnip. The mask does not need to be held firmly against the face; a gentle seal is all that's required.

3 The cat is then acclimatized to the sound of actuation (pressing) of the metered dose inhaler (MDI) of fluticasone. The inhaler can make a hissing sound, which some cats object to. The MDI should be shaken before any actuation. The MDI can be actuated in the vicinity of the cat for a few days, to allow the cat to adjust to this sound, again rewarding the cat following this, to encourage a positive association to develop. The Aerokat spacer has a valve, and therefore actuation can be done just before placing the mask gently over the cat's face if it objects to the sound.

Administering treatment

1 The spacer with the MDI attached is placed over the cat's face and the device actuated.

2 Count 10–15 breaths to ensure inhalation of the drug.

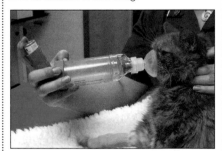

A veterinary nurse administering inhalant treatment via an Aerokat spacer. The 'Flow-Vu' valve allows the cat's breaths to be counted whilst the spacer is applied to the face.

PRACTICAL TIP

The facemask should be regularly washed in warm soapy water; disinfectant is not recommended as this may damage the plastic of the facemask.

Dietary modification and supplements

Cats should be fed an intact protein or hydrolysate elimination diet exclusively. This diet should be easily digestible, nutritionally balanced and palatable. If unsure whether an adequate dietary trial has yet been performed in the cat, feeding an elimination diet for at least 14 days should first be considered, with drug therapy introduced in addition if the cat fails to respond to dietary management alone. Some cats may respond differently to different hypoallergenic diets (for unknown reasons); it is therefore worth trying more than one type of diet, for at least 14 days per diet. Importantly, the superiority of either intact protein diets *versus* hydrolysate diets has not been demonstrated in clinical trials. In general, cats that fail to respond to two different elimination diets, where each has been fed exclusively for 14 days, may require drug therapy to induce clinical remission.

The diet should be supplemented with oral folate or vitamin B12 if serum concentrations are subnormal. Folate (0.004 mg/kg orally daily) or cyanocobalamin (250 mg/cat s.c. per week for 4 weeks) are given, as required, until serum concentrations normalize (retest one month after starting vitamin therapy) and clinical remission occurs. Cats with normal cobalamin concentrations but who continue to show gastrointestinal signs should receive drug therapy as described below.

Modulation of the enteric microbiota using prebiotics (e.g. psyllium, beet pulp, fructo-oligosaccharide (FOS)) and probiotics (e.g. Purina Fortiflora, Iams–Eukanuba Prostora Max, Nutramax Proviable-DC (proprietary synbiotic)) may be beneficial, but these agents have not been evaluated in feline IBD clinical trials. Additionally, supplementation with omega-3 fatty acids may also reduce the inflammatory products that drive chronic intestinal inflammation.

Drug therapy

Drug therapy can be combined with the dietary therapy described above.

- Metronidazole (20 mg/kg orally q12h) may reduce inflammation through antibacterial action or immunomodulation of cellular immunity. It can be used as single-drug therapy for mild IBD but it may be necessary to combine metronidazole with prednisolone for cats with moderate to severe clinical disease. The long-term strategy is to reduce administration of metronidazole gradually after 4–6 weeks of continuous therapy and to maintain the cat by diet alone.
- Suppurative (neutrophilic) colitis is an uncommon feline IBD variant that is most responsive to amoxicillin/clavulanate (62.5 mg/cat orally q12h for 14 days).
- Prednisolone (1–2 mg/kg orally q12h) can be used initially for 2–4 weeks and then be tapered as needed. This medication is useful as a single agent in cats with IBD of varying clinical severity.
- Chlorambucil may be used in cases refractory to steroids or when gastrointestinal lymphoma cannot be ruled out conclusively. Chlorambucil is administered at a dose of 2 mg/cat orally for four consecutive days every 3 weeks indefinitely (along with prednisolone) when treating for well differentiated lymphoma (see Gastrointestinal lymphoma, later).

Drug treatment for feline IBD is empirically based on disease severity at diagnosis and response to induction therapy. Clinical trials to date have not assessed the efficacy of single-drug therapy (prednisolone or metronidazole) *versus* combination drug therapy (metronidazole + prednisolone) for IBD in cats. Clinicians should strive to taper drug therapy as needed in an attempt to maintain clinical remission with diet alone.

The response to treatment in most cats with IBD is good with prolonged remission. However, owners should be informed that relapses may occur and are unpredictable in their occurrence.

Dietary/food hypersensitivity

Aetiology

Food allergy and food intolerance are recurring adverse reactions to dietary components that respond clinically to dietary exclusion trials. Food allergies represent an immune-mediated response to dietary constituents, while food intolerance is non-immunologically mediated. The pathophysiology for these disorders involves abnormal immune (e.g. IgE-mediated) responses, food allergens and an inadequate gut mucosal barrier, which leads to a breakdown of oral tolerance.

Clinical features

Most cats are middle-aged, since allergens must have been ingested for months or years for signs to develop. Both the skin and gastrointestinal tract may be affected in cats. Cutaneous signs predominate (see Chapter 6), with pruritus involving the feet and face along with otitis externa being observed. Symmetrical alopecia, miliary dermatitis and excoriation through self-trauma may predispose cats to secondary pyoderma and *Malassezia* spp. infections. Gastrointestinal signs are less commonly seen but may include vomiting, weight loss, and mild large-bowel diarrhoea.

Diagnosis

Dietary hypersensitivity is associated with negative results on routine diagnostic testing for gastrointestinal and dermatological conditions; accurate diagnosis is based on a positive response to an elimination dietary trial (e.g. attenuation or resolution of clinical signs). Feeding the elimination diet exclusively eliminates the provocative dietary ingredients found in the previous diet. Cats that fail an appropriately performed dietary trial should undergo additional diagnostic evaluation, including dermatology work-up, laboratory testing, diagnostic imaging and endoscopic biopsy, to determine the underlying gastrointestinal and/or dermatological disease process present.

Management

An intact protein or hydrolysate elimination diet should be fed exclusively for at least 2 weeks in cats with gastrointestinal signs. All commercial feline petfood manufacturers produce a number of excellent quality rations, and there is no reported superiority of one diet over another, regardless of the manufacturer. Resolution of clinical signs supports a working diagnosis of dietary hypersensitivity. (See QRG 6.1 for details of dietary trials for cats with cutaneous signs.)

A challenge with the original offending diet to confirm a diagnosis of dietary hypersensitivity (with recurrence of clinical signs) is necessary to confirm a definitive diagnosis. However, this is often impractical and many owners will be reluctant; it may therefore be unnecessary to do this if the cat is eating the new diet and the owner is willing to feed this diet long term.

Cats with dietary hypersensitivity may require lifelong treatment with the elimination diet. If this is not possible, then the gradual introduction of a controlled diet that does not contain a novel protein source may be attempted in an effort to reduce gastrointestinal signs. If gastrointestinal signs recur with use of a non-hypoallergenic diet, switching back to the elimination diet is recommended.

Gastrointestinal lymphoma

Aetiology

Gastrointestinal lymphoma (lymphosarcoma, LSA) is a malignant tumour of lymphoid cell origin. Lesions may occur within any portion of the gastrointestinal tract and may be composed of B, T or large granular lymphocytes (LGLs). Chronic IBD may be a risk factor for alimentary LSA, although the exact aetiology of these tumours is presently unknown.

Clinical features

Cats with gastrointestinal LSA are typically middle-aged (7–10 years) and present with chronic signs including vomiting, diarrhoea, anorexia and weight loss. Mucous membrane pallor is suggestive of blood loss (e.g. haematamesis, melaena) from the alimentary tract. Other abnormalities observed on physical examination may include loss of body condition, emaciation, hepatosplenomegaly, mesenteric lymphadenopathy and palpably thickened intestines. Clinical findings are influenced by the form (focal *versus* diffuse disease) and location of the lesions, as well as the duration of neoplastic disease. Intercurrent problems such as enteric blood loss and hypocobalaminaemia may contribute to disease morbidity.

Diagnosis

The diagnosis of gastrointestinal LSA requires histological confirmation of neoplastic cells from biopsy specimens collected either endoscopically, at laparoscopy or at laparotomy (see QRG 11.1). Referral to a specialist may be required for obtaining endoscopic/laparoscopic samples.

A minimum database consisting of a complete blood count, biochemical panel, urinalysis, faecal examination and FeLV/FIV testing is initially performed to exclude other causes for gastrointestinal signs. Evaluation of fTLI and fPLI will effectively screen for exocrine pancreatic insufficiency and chronic pancreatitis, respectively. Analysis of serum folate and cobalamin concentrations may indicate the presence of focal *versus* diffuse small-intestine disease, and determine whether supplementation is necessary.

Diagnostic imaging of the abdominal/thoracic cavities should be performed to identify organomegaly and potential thoracic metastasis. Abdominal ultrasound examination will detect mass lesions, intestinal wall thickening and/or mesenteric lymphadenopathy, and allow fine-needle aspiration of the gastrointestinal tract or mesenteric lymph nodes for cytological analysis. Immunohistochemical staining can confirm phenotypic characterization of B-cell, T-cell or LGL tumour subtypes; this phenotypic characterization may provide some prognostic information (e.g. T-cell phenotype may be less responsive to chemotherapy), although published evidence is currently lacking for feline cases. However, immunophenotyping of intestinal biopsy samples is of great value in differentiating alimentary LSA from severe IBD when this distinction cannot be made from H&E-stained tissues alone. Immunophenotyping using an anti-T cell or anti-B cell antibody serves to differentiate the homogenous (single clone) lymphoid population of alimentary LSA from the mostly heterogenous (multiple clones) lymphoid population characteristic of IBD.

Management

Treatment of all forms of gastrointestinal LSA is palliative, as no cure is possible; however, cats with low-grade gastrointestinal LSA may survive for years.

Focal neoplastic lesions may be surgically excised. Focal lesions with complete surgical excision need not undergo chemotherapy; in such cases thorough evaluation, including haematology and imaging, should have been performed to confirm that the tumour is indeed focal.

Most cats with diffuse mucosal disease can undergo multi-drug chemotherapy using either the Madison–Wisconsin or a COP-type protocol for high-grade disease, or prednisolone–chlorambucil protocol for low-grade disease. It is recommended that a specialist is consulted about the most appropriate protocol.

- The Madison–Wisconsin protocol (outlined in Vail *et al.*, 1998) uses five different drugs (cyclophosphamide, vincristine and prednisolone ± doxorubicin ± idarubicin) administered over 25 weeks. It is the treatment of choice for high-grade disease. In some instances, chemotherapy might result in perforation of transmural lesions (although this is believed to be uncommon) necessitating a staged and less aggressive multi-drug chemotherapy regimen; in such cases lower doses of the chemotherapeutic agents should be used at spaced intervals, and response to treatment assessed to determine continued chemotherapy. The advice of a specialist can be sought for discussion of the management of such cases if the reader is unfamiliar with this chemotherapy protocol.
- Prednisolone–chlorambucil protocols exist that are often effective in cats with low-grade (e.g. small mature lymphocytes) gastrointestinal lymphoma. One dose regime comprises prednisolone at 2 mg/kg orally q24h until clinical remission (then 1 mg/kg orally q48h as needed) plus chlorambucil at 2 mg orally q24h for 4 days every 3 weeks. Alternative dosing protocols for the prednisolone and chlorambucil combination exist (Barrs and Beaty, 2012).

More details on chemotherapy protocols can be found in Chapter 21 and in the *BSAVA Manual of Canine and Feline Oncology.*

Gastrointestinal infections

Protozoa

Giardiasis

Pathophysiology: *Giardia* is a flagellate protozoan parasite found in the gastrointestinal tract of humans and companion animals. Infection occurs through ingestion of faecal oocysts adherent to the haircoat or consumption of contaminated drinking water. Following faecal–oral transmission, the ingested oocyst localizes to the duodenum and subsequently trophozoites attach to the intestinal mucosa down to the level of the ileum. Trophozoites cause damage to the intestinal epithelia, resulting in villous atrophy which causes malabsorption. Following multiplication of trophozoites, infective oocysts are passed in the faeces and persist in the environment. Re-infection occurs commonly with overcrowding (e.g. catteries) and results in environmental contamination and a recurring cycle of infection. Abnormalities in immune competence may predispose individual cats to infection.

Clinical features: Most infections are asymptomatic, although some cats develop a spectrum of gastrointestinal signs ranging from mild, self-limiting acute diarrhoea to severe or chronic small intestinal diarrhoea with weight loss.

Diagnosis: *Giardia* infection is diagnosed by observing motile trophozoites on fresh faecal smears or oocysts by faecal zinc sulphate flotation. (Educational videos describing sample collection and the appearance of *Giardia* trophozoite movement are available at www.cvm.ncsu.edu/docs/personnel/gookin_jody.html.) Since infected animals shed oocysts intermittently, the sensitivity of detection is enhanced by examining multiple (2–3) faecal samples obtained serially. Immunoassays (e.g. ELISA and IFAT) that detect *Giardia* antigen are the most sensitive means of confirming the diagnosis.

Management: Management is directed at eliminating clinical signs, eradicating faecal shedding of infective oocysts and decontamination of the environment. It is important to note that drug resistance in *Giardia* can develop with any of the reported treatments, and appropriate control measures should be implemented (e.g. prevent overcrowding, minimize environmental contamination with infective faeces).

- Metronidazole (5–30 mg/kg orally q12h for 5 days) may be used to eliminate infection. The reported efficacy is only 70% and clinicians should be vigilant for potential adverse signs, including anorexia, vomiting and acute neuropathy characterized by generalized ataxia and positional nystagmus, especially at high dose rates.
- Fenbendazole (50 mg/kg orally q24h for 5 days) may also be effective and can be given as an alternative to metronidazole or if failure occurs with metronidazole treatment.
- A combination product of febantel + praziquantel + pyrantel offers the greatest efficacy for eradication of infection. For example, Drontal plus (Bayer) (15 mg/kg febantel + 1.5 mg/kg praziquantel) is administered orally q24h for 5 days.

- Decontamination is achieved by bathing and adequately disinfecting the environment using quaternary ammonium compounds.

> **WARNING**
>
> It should be borne in mind that *Giardia* is potentially zoonotic, although infection from cats to humans is extremely rare.

Tritrichomonas foetus

Pathophysiology: Infection of the ileocolic and colonic mucosa with this protozoan parasite may cause chronic large-bowel diarrhoea in susceptible cats. Young cats housed in shelters and catteries are at increased risk for *T. foetus* infection due to their age and the population density in these facilities. Infective trophozoites are passed in the faeces and are transmitted through the faecal–oral route. The protozoan parasite causes lymphocytic–plasmacytic and suppurative ileitis and colitis.

Clinical findings: Infected cats manifest chronic large-bowel diarrhoea that does not resolve with standard antibiotic or antidiarrhoeal therapy. Progression to watery and foetid small-intestine diarrhoea has been reported in some cats. Infected cats show no apparent systemic effects and thrive in spite of colonic colonization and mucosal inflammation. Physical examination often reveals no abnormalities.

Diagnosis: A diagnosis of *T. foetus* infection is based on positive identification of trophozoites in fresh faecal smears obtained from a cat with suggestive clinical signs (educational videos describing sample collection and the appearance of *T. foetus* trophozoite movement are available at www.cvm.ncsu.edu/docs/personnel/gookin_jody.html). However, episodic excretion of trophozoites in diarrhoeic faeces may make confirmation of infection difficult. Faecal culture using the *T. foetus* pouch (InPouch TF-Feline, Biomed Diagnostics Inc.) will improve the likelihood of trophozoite detection. PCR to amplify and detect *T. foetus* DNA in faeces is the most sensitive diagnostic tool and is increasingly available.

Management: There is no effective therapy for *T. foetus* infection. Ronidazole (related to metronidazole) has been used to treat *T. foetus* infection but it may be that the risks associated with treatment outweigh the inconvenience associated with the cat's diarrhoea, and careful consideration as well as consultation with a feline specialist is advised before embarking on treatment. See www.fabcats.org/breeders/infosheets/tritrichomonas.html for further details on treatment.

The clinical course in most cats that are untreated is prolonged (~2 years' duration), and chronic infection may persist despite resolution of gastrointestinal signs.

Other protozoal infections

Cystoisospora (formerly *Isospora*) spp. do not usually cause diarrhoea in adult cats but if they are identified on faecal examination in a younger cat with diarrhoea, treatment is warranted with sulfadimethoxine (50 mg/kg orally once, then 27.5 mg/kg orally q24h for 2–3 weeks).

Cryptosporidium parvum commonly infects cats but does not usually cause diarrhoea. If it is found in association with diarrhoea, treatment with tylosin (10–15 mg/kg orally q12h) or azithromycin (7.5–10 mg/kg orally q12–72h) can lessen oocyst shedding but it is unknown whether cats are cured.

> **WARNING**
>
> *Cryptosporidium* is potentially zoonotic, although transmission from cats to humans is extremely rare.

Enteropathogenic bacteria

Pathophysiology

Enteropathogenic bacteria including *Campylobacter jejuni*, *Salmonella* spp., *Escherichia coli* and *Clostridium* spp. may cause acute or chronic diarrhoea in cats. Disease incidence appears to be greatest in young, kennelled and/or immunocompromised animals. Other risk factors for infection include hospitalization in intensive care facilities (for *Clostridium perfringens*) and antibiotic administration (for *C. difficile*). Importantly, these bacteria may also be isolated from healthy animals; thus, some confusion exists about their significance when isolated from diarrhoeic cats. Only animals with suggestive gastrointestinal signs (diarrhoea) and laboratory evidence (e. g. positive faecal or blood cultures, suppurative inflammation on rectal cytology) of bacterial infection should be treated. Empirical therapy with antibiotics in asymptomatic cats is discouraged, may be harmful and may induce a carrier state.

Enteropathogenic bacteria may cause clinically significant intestinal disease via enterotoxin production or mucosal invasion. Enterotoxins may promote fluid and electrolyte secretion through interaction with mucosal receptors or can be directly injurious to intestinal epithelia. Other bacterial strains, including *Campylobacter jejuni* and *Salmonella* spp., invade the intestinal mucosa and cause bloody diarrhoea through disruption of the mucosal barrier.

Clinical features

Acute colitis or enterocolitis is most commonly observed. Affected cats with colitis present with classic large-bowel signs of tenesmus, haematochezia and/or mucoid faeces. Cats with enterocolitis may have watery diarrhoea (± blood) accompanied by vomiting, pyrexia and anorexia. Concurrent infection with nematodes, protozoan parasites (*Giardia* spp.,

see above), parvovirus or coronavirus leads to more severe disease.

Diagnosis

Diagnosis of bacterial enteritis is made in symptomatic cats following culture of fresh faeces. Faecal cytology is a useful, minimally invasive means of identifying bacterial organisms (e.g. slender seagull-shaped *C. jejuni*, 'safety-pin'-shaped *Clostridium* spores), or cellular evidence (neutrophils) of acute mucosal inflammation. More elaborate laboratory testing for bacterial antigens (via PCR) or bioassays for enterotoxin production are unnecessary.

Management

Bacterial pathogens are specifically treated based on the results of culture/susceptibility testing. *Campylobacter jejuni* infection is generally treated with erythromycin (15 mg/kg orally q12h for 10 days) while *Clostridium perfringens* infection is treated with metronidazole (10–15 mg/kg orally q12h) or amoxicillin (22 mg/kg orally q12h) and dietary fibre (psyllium at ½ tsp orally q24h for 7 days). Therapy for *Salmonella* spp. infection is only indicated in animals with fever, sepsis and bloody diarrhoea. Resistance to antibiotics may occur with some infections, making eradication of some species of enteropathogenic bacteria impossible.

> **WARNING**
>
> *Campylobacter jejuni*, *Salmonella* spp. and *Escherichia coli* are all potentially zoonotic, although transmission from cats to humans is rare.

References and further reading

Barrs V and Beatty J (2012) Feline alimentary lymphoma. 2. Further diagnostics, therapy and prognosis. *Journal of Feline Medicine and Surgery* **14**, 191–201

Ettinger SJ and Feldman EC (2010) *Textbook of Veterinary Internal Medicine, 7th edn.* Saunders Elsevier, St. Louis

Gaschen FP (2011) Chronic intestinal diseases of dogs and cats. *Veterinary Clinics of North America: Small Animal Practice* **41**, xi–xii. WB Saunders, Philadelphia

Greene CE (2006) *Infectious Diseases in the Dog and Cat.* Saunders Elsevier, St. Louis

Hall E, Simpson J and Williams D (2005) *BSAVA Manual of Canine and Feline Gastroenterology, 2nd edn.* BSAVA Publications, Gloucester

Jergens AE (2012) Feline idiopathic inflammatory bowel disease: what we know and what remains to be unraveled. *Journal of Feline Medicine and Surgery* **14**, 445–458

Vail DM, Moore AS, Ogilvie GK and Volk LM (1998) Feline lymphoma (145 cases): proliferation indices, cluster of differentiation 3 immunoreactivity, and their association with prognosis in 90 cats. *Journal of Veterinary Internal Medicine* **12**, 349–354

QRG 11.1 Gut biopsy
by Geraldine Hunt

Indications

Indications are intestinal disease causing chronic vomiting and/or small-bowel diarrhoea, most commonly inflammatory bowel disease and lymphoma. Since low-grade intestinal lymphoma can be difficult to distinguish from lymphocytic–plasmacytic enteritis, and because histological abnormalities can be patchy, collection of adequate samples from appropriate sites is very important. Infiltrative and inflammatory intestinal diseases may not affect all portions of the intestinal tract equally, and clinical signs may not provide enough information to guide decision-making as to the biopsy site. It is therefore usual to take biopsies from multiple sites, from the stomach to the ileum.

The colon is rarely sampled at exploratory laparotomy, due to the slower healing time of the colon and greater bacterial load (especially anaerobes); samples are usually obtained endoscopically. Full-thickness colon biopsy samples are occasionally required if colonoscopy is not available or has not been diagnostic, or if (focal) submucosal lesions are suspected (e.g. based on ultrasonography) that are very likely to be missed on colonoscopic biopsy. Consultation with a specialist is then advised.

- Gut biopsy samples are rarely taken from a healthy patient and most cats undergoing gut biopsy are thus likely to have some underlying local or systemic factor that may interfere with wound healing. The steps taken to reduce or avoid contamination and to secure closure of the biopsy site(s) are thus extremely important.
- The patient is unlikely to wake up after surgery with its primary problem resolved, and peri- and postoperative management are therefore critical to success.
- Surgery may be performed with the intention of collecting diagnostic samples from a known lesion, or an exploratory laparotomy might be visually negative and multiple biopsy samples are then taken as a 'scouting' exercise.

Patient evaluation prior to exploratory laparotomy

Haematology and biochemistry help rule out extra-intestinal causes of vomiting and diarrhoea and guide supportive therapy if a condition such as hypoproteinaemia or anaemia is discovered. Other diagnostic tests, such as faecal parasitology, abdominal palpation and imaging (radiography and ultrasonography if available) should be performed. Imaging in particular may be useful to identify a linear foreign body, intussusception or chronic partial obstruction due to intestinal adenocarcinoma or trichobezoars (see Chapter 5.14).

Type and number of samples

Gut biopsy samples taken at surgery are full-thickness, i.e. they should contain sufficient tissue for the pathologist to see tissue architecture from the inner mucosa to the outer serosa. The number of samples needed from each site is contentious but at least one sample should be taken from the gastric fundus, gastric pylorus, duodenum, jejunum and ileum. Some people take up to three biopsy samples from each site, but this prolongs surgical time significantly and may increase the risk of dehiscence. The location and number of any colonic samples will be dictated by the results of preoperative diagnostic tests such as ultrasound examination, but one is usually sufficient for a focal lesion.

Equipment

- 1.5 metric (4/0 USP) monofilament suture (polydioxanone (PDS) or poliglecaprone (e.g. Monocryl)) with a swaged-on taper needle
- Brown–Adson forceps
- Surgical suction with a Poole suction tip (B)

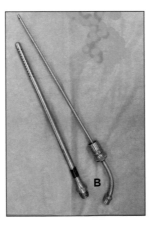

- Doyen bowel forceps if required
- No.11 or No.15 scalpel blades
- Metzenbaum scissors
- 4 mm skin biopsy punch

Patient preparation

The patient should be anaesthetized, and positioned and surgically prepared for laparotomy.

Procedure

1 Perform a laparotomy (coeliotomy) incision from the xiphoid to a point midway between the umbilicus and the pubis, to permit full exploration of the abdomen.

2 Conduct a full abdominal exploration prior to taking any samples, including palpation of the gastrointestinal tract from the oesophageal hiatus all the way down to the colon in the pelvic cavity.

3 Surgical suction should be available for both liquid ingesta and lavage fluid from the abdomen.

Gastric biopsy

1 Prepare the stomach for biopsy of the gastric fundus by exteriorizing a portion of the fundus of the stomach with minimal vascularity and stabilizing it with stay sutures (two shown). Pack the surrounding abdomen with moistened laparotomy sponges or swabs; these should always be counted as used, and attention paid to ensure all (counting again) are removed at end of surgery. Make a full-thickness stab incision into the stomach using a No.11 or No.15 scalpel blade.

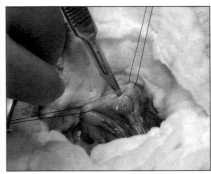

2 Grasp the stomach wall with Brown–Adson forceps and sharply excise a full-thickness wedge from the stomach wall, using Metzenbaum scissors.

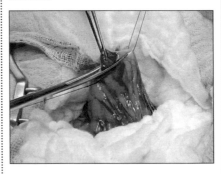

3 Place the biopsy specimen immediately into a labelled jar with formalin to submit for histopathology. ▶

QRG 11.1 *continued*

4 The stomach wall is closed in two layers:

a. A continuous pattern of 2 or 1.5 metric (3/0 or 4/0 USP) monofilament absorbable suture material is placed in the mucosa and submucosa of the stomach.

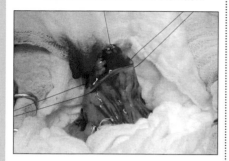

b. A Cushing suture (see Appendix) is placed incorporating the serosa and muscularis layers; note how the suture 'bites' are made parallel to the incision.

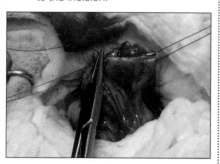

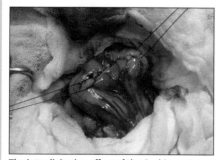

The interdigitating effect of the Cushing suture is shown. Taking bites parallel to the length of the incision, alternating from one side to the other, and overlapping by about 25% achieves this interdigitating effect.

Repeat steps 1 to 4 for collecting biopsy samples from the pyloric region of the stomach.

Intestinal biopsy

1 Prepare the duodenum for biopsy by exteriorizing the portion of intestine to be sampled and packing the surrounding area with surgical sponges moistened with saline (these should be counted in and out of the abdomen). An assistant should occlude the intestine between their fingers, or a pair of atraumatic forceps such as Doyen bowel forceps can be used.

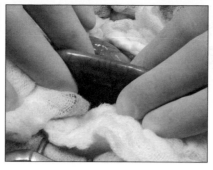

2 Harvest the duodenal biopsy from the antimesenteric (non-vascular) side of the intestine, using a 4 mm skin biopsy punch. Take care not to cut through the mesenteric side of the intestine deep to the biopsy site.

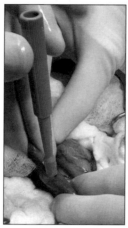

3 Place the biopsy specimen immediately into a labelled formalin jar to submit for histopathology.

4 Repair the duodenum with full-thickness single interrupted appositional sutures of 2 or 1.5 metric (3/0 or 4/0 USP) monofilament absorbable suture material. The suture should incorporate a generous amount of submucosa, as this layer is collagen-rich and has the best holding power. Avoid grasping too much mucosa, as this causes the mucosa to evert when the suture is tightened. Sutures are designed to be appositional, rather than inverting or everting, and can be full-thickness, as they will become embedded in the mucosa when tightened. Place sutures at 2–3 mm intervals.

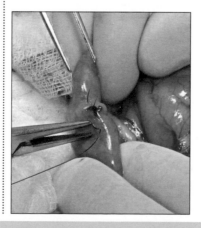

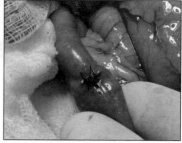

The duodenal biopsy site is closed perpendicular to the long axis of the intestine to avoid narrowing of the lumen.

5 Leak-test the duodenal biopsy repair site using a 20 ml syringe filled with saline, attached to a 25 G needle. Insert the needle into the duodenal lumen and inject the saline, looking for any leakage of saline from the biopsy site. If leakage occurs, additional full-thickness sutures must be placed at the location of leakage.

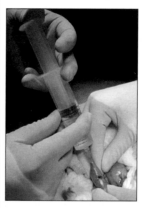

Repeat steps 1 to 5 for collecting biopsy samples from the jejunum and ileum. The duodenum is distinguished by its attachment to the pylorus cranially, the right limb of the pancreas (descending duodenum), and its attachment to the colon (duodenocolic ligament; caudal duodenal flexure). The jejunum is identified by its vasculature, which describes a number of arcades, sweeping from the root of the mesentery to the intestine and then back again. The ileum is distinguished by a straight antimesenteric vessel, rather than the arcade.

Colonic biopsy

The colonic biopsy technique is similar to that for the other intestinal segments. The location is dictated by whether lesions appear to be focal or diffuse. Be aware that the seromuscular layer and mucosal–submucosal layers separate easily from one another, with the seromuscular layer retracting away from the edge of the colotomy incision. Care must be taken to identify the cut edge of the seromuscular layer and incorporate it into each bite of the colotomy closure. Advice may be sought from a specialist to discuss this procedure.

▶

QRG 11.1 *continued*

Biopsy of the mesenteric lymph nodes

Lymph node biopsy is often very important in patients undergoing gut biopsy, and should be performed even if the structures are visibly normal, as lymphoma is usually a major differential diagnosis.

1 Perform blunt dissection of the mesenteric lymph node by gently dissecting the peritoneum over the lymph node to identify a portion suitable for biopsy. Choose a site that is not adjacent to a major blood vessel. Gently dissect the capsule from the lymph node in an avascular region, using Brown–Adson forceps and Metzenbaum scissors.

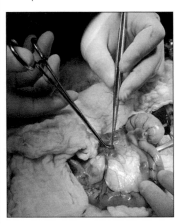

2 Pre-form a ligature of 1.5 metric (4/0 USP) polydioxanone or poliglecaprone (using a surgeon's knot) to slip over a portion of the lymph node to be sampled (usually around the base of the node).

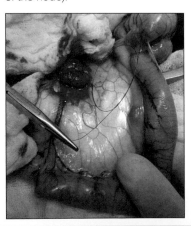

3 Tighten the ligature fully around the piece of lymph node to be removed and tie it using at least two square knots.

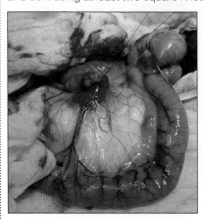

4 Remove the amputated portion of lymph node with fine Metzenbaum scissors, without damaging the pre-placed ligature. Ideally, 5 mm should remain between the ligature and the cut edge.

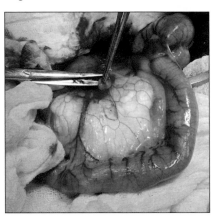

5 Place the biopsy specimen immediately into a labelled formalin jar to submit for histopathology. It may be wise to conserve a section of the specimen for potential future culture studies and/or PCR analysis (e.g. if tuberculosis or other infections are suspected); this can be done by taking an unfixed section of tissue and placing it on a sterile gauze swab moistened with sterile saline and into a plain pot before transferring the labelled pot into –20°C for conservation in the freezer.

6 Further haemorrhage is controlled using digital pressure on the cut edges of the lymph node; the peritoneum/lymph node capsule may be gently apposed using a cruciate or mattress suture (see Appendix) of 1.5 metric (4/0 USP) polydioxanone if additional haemostasis is required.

Laparoscopically assisted gut biopsy

Laparoscopically assisted gut biopsy is appropriate when the surgeon wishes to take samples from a defined portion of intestine, but it does not allow for as thorough an abdominal exploration as an open procedure. It should therefore only be used for cases in which biopsy is being performed simply to confirm a suspected diagnosis. Referral to a specialist practice is recommended.

Management of hepatic and pancreatic disorders

Andrea Harvey

This chapter will focus on the management of the most important hepatic and pancreatic disorders that are encountered in feline practice, notably inflammatory liver diseases, hepatic lipidosis and pancreatitis. This chapter also contains a practical QRG on liver biopsy at laparotomy. Other chapters contain more information on the approach to abnormalities such as jaundice (see Chapter 5.22) and elevated liver enzymes (see Chapter 5.31). Hepatic and pancreatic disorders are also commonly associated with gastrointestinal disease, which is covered separately in Chapter 11.

Neutrophilic cholangitis

Neutrophilic cholangitis was previously often known as suppurative cholangitis/cholangiohepatitis.

Aetiology

Neutrophilic cholangitis is caused by an ascending infection by bacteria from the gastrointestinal tract, such as *Escherichia coli*, streptococci and clostridia.

Clinical features

Neutrophilic cholangitis is more common in mature to senior cats, although it can occur at any age, particularly when there are other predisposing factors (e.g. biliary stasis, inflammatory bowel disease (IBD; see Chapter 11)). Most cases are presented with acute illness. The cats are usually jaundiced, pyrexic and anorexic, and may have abdominal pain. Neutrophilic cholangitis is often associated with pancreatitis and IBD ('triaditis'; see below). Cholelithiasis may occasionally occur concurrently, as a cause or consequence.

Diagnosis

History and clinical features may give important clues. ALT, ALP, GGT and bilirubin are elevated. There is a neutrophilia, often with a left shift with or without toxic neutrophils. Ultrasonography may reveal thickening of the gall bladder wall (>1 mm), distension of the bile duct (>5 mm) and the presence of sludge or inspissated bile within the gall bladder; there may also be a patchy echogenicity to the liver.

Histopathology is necessary for confirming the diagnosis but many cats are too ill for general anaesthesia at the time of presentation and therefore empirical treatment is often started based on other clinical findings. If complete recovery does not occur, liver biopsy should be performed once the cat is stable. Coagulation times should be assessed prior to biopsy; vitamin K should be administered if coagulation times are prolonged and can be given empirically if measurement is not possible (see Chapter 20). Samples of liver tissue should be submitted for bacterial culture and sensitivity testing, in addition to histopathology. If biopsy samples are obtained at laparotomy (see QRG 12.1), the patency of the bile ducts should also be evaluated, and bile aspirated for cytology and culture.

Management

Antibiotic therapy

Amoxicillin/clavulanate or cefalexin ± metronidazole should be given pending culture and sensitivity results, and treatment then adjusted as appropriate. Antibiotics should be administered parenterally until there is some improvement and the cat is eating. They can then be given orally and should be maintained for at least 4–6 weeks to reduce the risk of recurrence.

Supportive treatments

Intravenous fluid therapy: Saline (0.9%) should be administered, usually supplemented with potassium chloride depending on serum potassium concentration (see QRG 4.6.1). If potassium cannot be measured, fluid should be supplemented with 20 mmol/l KCl. A fluid rate of 2–4 ml/kg/h is usually appropriate, depending on the degree of dehydration (see also QRG 4.1.3).

Assisted feeding: If the cat is inappetent and vomiting is controlled, placement of a naso-oesophageal feeding tube for short-term assisted feeding should be considered (see QRG 5.5.2). If surgery for liver biopsy is being performed, placement of an oesophagostomy tube (see QRG 5.5.3) can be considered while the cat is under general anaesthesia.

Analgesia: Buprenorphine can be given at 0.01–0.2 mg/kg slowly i.v., i.m., s.c. or sublingually q8h.

Anti-emetics: If vomiting and/or nausea are present, maropitant (1 mg/kg s.c. or orally q24h for up to 5 consecutive days) and/or metoclopramide (CRI 1–2 mg/kg q24h) can be given (see also Chapter 5.35).

Additional treatments

Ursodeoxycholic acid (10–15 mg orally q24h) may be given, provided there is no evidence of extrahepatic biliary obstruction (markedly dilated biliary tree). *S*-Adenosylmethionine (SAMe) is available in various nutraceutical preparations and can be given as an adjunctive treatment (20 mg/kg orally q24h) to provide hepatic support during recovery.

Mixed inflammatory cholangitis

Occasionally, a mixed inflammatory infiltrate may be observed on histopathology of liver biopsy samples. This is usually considered to represent a chronic form of neutrophilic cholangitis. There may be a history of an initial acute illness, followed by a gradual loss of condition, inappetence and lethargy. In addition to histopathology, bacterial culture of liver biopsy samples and sensitivity testing are required.

Management

Broad-spectrum antibiotic treatment (as for neutrophilic cholangitis, see above) should be initiated while bacterial culture of liver tissue is pending. If bacterial cultures are positive, appropriate antibiotics should be continued for 4–6 weeks; if complete clinical improvement does not occur within 1–2 weeks, an anti-inflammatory dose of prednisolone (0.5 mg/kg orally q24h) should also be given. If bacterial cultures are negative, anti-inflammatory doses of prednisolone can be initiated earlier but antibiotics should be continued for 2–3 weeks (since negative cultures do not always exclude bacterial involvement).

Lymphocytic cholangitis

Aetiology

Lymphocytic cholangitis is believed to be an immune-mediated disease.

Clinical features

Lymphocytic cholangitis is seen most commonly in younger cats, 1–5 years old, and Persians may be over-represented. Animals are usually systemically well, with a normal to increased appetite, although significant weight loss may occur in some cases. Hepatomegaly can be marked, and mild generalized lymphadenopathy and ascites may be present.

Diagnosis

History and clinical features may give important clues. ALT, ALP, GGT and bilirubin are elevated. Neutrophilia is less common and does not feature a left shift or toxic neutrophils. There may be mild anaemia of inflammatory disease (see Chapter 5.4). Marked hyperglobulinaemia is often present. Diagnostic imaging confirms hepatomegaly, often with patchy echogenicity; mesenteric lymph nodes may be enlarged. If ascites is present, the fluid is usually highly proteinaceous, with a low mixed inflammatory cellularity (thus lymphocytic

cholangitis is a major differential for FIP). Histopathology is required for confirming the diagnosis.

Management

Prednisolone

Prednisolone should be given at immunosuppressive doses of 1 mg/kg q12h, gradually reducing the dose over 6–12 weeks if a good response is seen. If there is an inadequate response to treatment, alternative immunosuppressive drugs may need to be considered if the clinician is confident of the diagnosis. Specialist advice should be sought before instigating alternative treatments.

Additional treatments

The following may be considered:

- Ursodeoxycholic acid (10–15 mg orally q24h), provided there is no evidence of extrahepatic biliary obstruction (see above)
- SAMe is available in various nutraceutical hepatic support preparations (see earlier)
- Colchicine (0.03 mg/kg q24h) may be of benefit in an attempt to reduce fibrosis.

Hepatic lipidosis

Aetiology

The precise pathophysiology of hepatic lipidosis is unknown but proposed mechanisms include:

- Metabolic changes associated with anorexia and obesity
- Androgenic release during illness or stress
- Protein and nutrient (e.g. taurine) deficiency
- Relative carnitine deficiency
- Insulin resistance.

Hepatic lipidosis may be primary or (more commonly) secondary to another disease such as cholangitis, pancreatitis, neoplasia, gastrointestinal disease or endocrine disease.

Clinical features

There is often progressive lethargy and anorexia, sometimes accompanied by intermittent vomiting. As the disease progresses, jaundice develops and may be severe. Signs of encephalopathy such as depression and ptyalism can occur. In secondary hepatic lipidosis, there may be a history associated with the underlying disease. There may be a history of anorexia, and the cat may be overweight but show recent weight loss.

Diagnosis

History and clinical features may give important clues.

There are also characteristic biochemical and haematological changes:

- ALT and ALP are elevated; ALP is usually proportionately significantly more elevated than ALT (often increased more than five times as much)
- There is severe hyperbilirubinaemia (often >150–200 µmol/l bilirubin), although absence of jaundice does not exclude lipidosis
- GGT is often normal or only mildly elevated, unless there is underlying cholangitis
- There may be anaemia of inflammatory disease.

Ultrasonography often reveals hepatomegaly and diffuse marked hyperechogenicity of the liver.

Cytology of hepatic fine-needle aspirates demonstrates diffuse vacuolation of hepatocytes (Figure 12.1) and is usually diagnostic but does not distinguish between primary and secondary lipidosis (NB assessment of coagulation times is not essential prior to liver fine-needle aspiration but is essential prior to biopsy).

Once the patient is stabilized, further diagnostics may be required to look for an underlying disease.

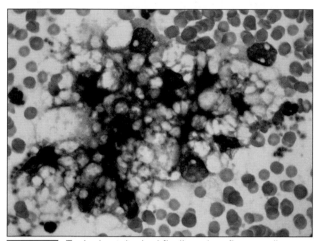

12.1 Typical cytological findings in a fine-needle aspirate from a cat with hepatic lipidosis. Red blood cells can be seen around the periphery of the image. In the centre are clumped hepatocytes with marked fatty vacuolation. (Wright's–Giemsa; original magnification X500.)

Management

Aggressive enteral assisted feeding

It is vital to initiate this immediately. Most cats will require enteral assisted feeding for at least a few weeks, often longer, and therefore oesophagostomy (see QRG 5.5.3) or gastrostomy tubes are the method of choice for the longer term. In the short term, until the cat is stable enough for general anaesthesia, naso-oesophageal tube feeding (see QRG 5.5.2) should be used.

A high-protein diet is required to treat hepatic lipidosis, unless the cat is initially showing signs of hepatic encephalopathy, in which case protein restriction may be indicated (but take care as there is a potential for developing hypoproteinaemia). Caloric intake should be approximately 60–80 kcal/kg/day (see QRG 1.1).

Nutritional supplements

These may include:

- L-Carnitine (250 mg/cat orally q24h) for potential effects in increasing mitochondrial fatty acid oxidation
- Taurine (250 mg/cat orally q24h) to prevent or treat taurine deficiency
- Vitamin E (50 mg/cat orally q24h) as an antioxidant
- Vitamin K1 (2 mg/cat orally q12h for 3 days, then 2 mg/cat weekly until recovered) to prevent (or treat) vitamin K deficiency-associated coagulopathies
- Vitamin B1 (100 mg/cat s.c. q24h)
- Vitamin B12 (250 µg/cat s.c. twice weekly until levels are normal)
- *S*-Adenosylmethionine (SAMe) (20 mg/kg orally q24h).

The importance of these in each case is difficult to ascertain and evidence is lacking; nutritional support is the most important aspect of treatment.

> **PRACTICAL TIP**
>
> Oral medications can be crushed and mixed with food/water to be given via the feeding tube (if oesophagostomy or gastrostomy tube) so are usually easy to administer.

Supportive treatments

Intravenous fluid therapy: Saline (0.9%) should be administered, usually supplemented with potassium chloride depending on serum potassium concentration (see QRG 4.6.1); if potassium cannot be measured, fluids should be supplemented with 20 mmol/l KCl. A fluid rate of 2–4 ml/kg/h is usually appropriate, depending on the degree of dehydration (see also QRG 4.1.3).

Patients with hepatic lipidosis are at particular risk of developing refeeding syndrome (see QRG 5.5.1), which may result in clinically significant hypophosphataemia (<0.3 mmol/l serum phosphate), so serum phosphate must be monitored closely (e.g. daily for the first few days of feeding), and supplementation with potassium phosphate initiated if required.

Anti-emetics/promotility drugs: If vomiting and/or nausea are present or there is evidence of gastric stasis (common), metoclopramide should be given at 1–2 mg/kg q24h as a CRI (see Chapter 5.35) as this acts as an anti-emetic and prokinetic agent. Maropitant (1 mg/kg s.c. or orally q24h for up to 5 consecutive days) is an alternative anti-emetic.

Pancreatitis

Aetiology

The cause of pancreatitis in cats is usually unknown. The role of diet is unclear: there is no evidence that feeding a high-fat diet precipitates pancreatitis, though it may still be important in some cats. Pancreatitis is often associated with neutrophilic cholangitis and/or IBD ('triaditis').

Clinical features

Clinical signs are often very vague and include lethargy/malaise and inappetence. Vomiting, nausea and abdominal pain may or may not be present. Diarrhoea may be a feature. Other disorders occurring secondary to pancreatitis are also common, e.g. hepatic lipidosis, diabetes mellitus and, occasionally with long-standing chronic pancreatitis, exocrine pancreatic insufficiency (EPI).

Diagnosis

Diagnosis of pancreatitis can be challenging, in view of the non-specific clinical signs, the frequent presence of concurrent disease and the limitations of diagnostic testing. Most laboratory findings are reflective of underlying disease. There is often mild hyperbilirubinaemia with normal liver enzyme levels (although liver enzymes may be increased if there is concurrent cholangitis). Hypocalcaemia may be present in severe cases.

Ultrasonography may show pancreatic enlargement with hypoechoic areas, and there may be hyperechoic fat surrounding the pancreas, but a lack of ultrasonographic abnormalities is common; abnormalities may be subtle and require expertise to identify.

Amylase and lipase assays are not useful in cats. Feline trypsin-like immunoreactivity (fTLI) may be elevated, but is often normal. Feline pancreatic lipase immunoreactivity (fPLI) is the most sensitive and specific test available for the diagnosis of feline pancreatitis, particularly in cats with moderate to severe disease. However a normal fPLI result does not completely exclude pancreatitis, particularly with chronic low-grade disease. An in-house fPLI test kit (SNAP fPL, Idexx) is available; this does not provide a quantitative result but registers as positive or negative. The test is sensitive but is less specific than the quantitative fPLI assay and therefore false positive results may be more frequently obtained. A positive test result should be followed up with a quantitative fPLI assay.

Cobalamin (vitamin B12) is often low in cases of pancreatitis and so should be measured and supplemented as necessary.

Management

Treatment priorities will vary, depending on the severity of clinical signs and whether pancreatitis is acute or chronic. However, treatment is largely supportive, consisting of:

- Intravenous fluid therapy and electrolyte (e.g. potassium, phosphate) supplementation (see QRGs 4.1.3 and 4.6.1)
- Anti-emetics, e.g. maropitant or metoclopramide (see Chapter 5.35 and above for doses). Maropitant can be especially useful as it also has visceral analgesic properties. Mirtazapine (see Chapter 5.5 for doses) can act against nausea as well as stimulating appetite, and so may be useful in some pancreatitis cases once analgesia has been adequately addressed.
- Analgesia, e.g. buprenorphine (see Chapter 3). Clinicians should be aware that abdominal pain is often hard to appreciate in these patients but is certainly likely to be present, and the response in demeanour and appetite to analgesia can often be dramatic
- Nutritional support (see Chapter 5.5). Generally, starving is not advised in cats. However, there are some cases that may benefit from a short period (e.g. 24 hours) of pancreatic rest. The ideal diet for cats with pancreatitis is not known but a low-fat highly digestible diet is advisable.

Pancreatic enzyme supplementation may be useful if there is evidence of malabsorption or demonstration of EPI. It is sometimes also advocated for reducing pain associated with eating, although there is no evidence for this. Supplementation of Vitamin B12 should be given if it is deficient.

There is some emerging evidence that Gram-negative intestinal bacteria may be involved in the aetiology in some cases and so there may be justification for antibiotic treatment, but currently this remains controversial. Use of corticosteroids is contraindicated in acute pancreatitis. They may have a role in the treatment of chronic pancreatitis, particularly if there is associated IBD.

Any concurrent disease such as IBD and/or cholangitis also needs to be managed accordingly. Concurrent diseases can commonly result in conflicting treatments (e.g. choice of diet, whether to use corticosteroids), and decision-making in choosing treatments is frequently not straightforward. Indeed, these cases in general can be very difficult to manage. Readers are encouraged to seek further specialist advice regarding optimal management in such cases.

References and further reading

Harvey AM (2009) Inflammatory liver disease. *In Practice* **31**, 414–422

Hitt ME (2010) Inflammatory liver diseases. In: *Consultations in Feline Medicine 6*, ed. JR August, pp. 213–223. Saunders Elsevier, St. Louis

Warman S and Harvey AM (2007) Feline pancreatitis: current concepts and treatment guidelines *In Practice* **29**, 470–477

Watson P (2005) Diseases of the liver. In: *BSAVA Manual of Canine and Feline Gastroenterology, 2nd edn*, ed. EJ Hall *et al.*, pp. 240–268. BSAVA Publications, Gloucester

Watson P (2010) Patients with gastrointestinal, liver or pancreatic disease. In: *BSAVA Manual of Canine and Feline Rehabilitation, Supportive and Palliative Care: Case Studies in Patient Management*, ed. S Lindley and P Watson, pp. 338–364. BSAVA Publications, Gloucester

Williams DA (2005) Diseases of the exocrine pancreas. In: *BSAVA Manual of Canine and Feline Gastroenterology, 2nd edn*, ed. EJ Hall *et al.*, pp. 222–239. BSAVA Publications, Gloucester

QRG 12.1 Liver biopsy
by Geraldine Hunt

Indications

Liver biopsy samples are obtained for the purposes of histopathology and microbiology.

Considerations prior to biopsy

- A decision must be made as to how much liver is required and how it should be stored after collection; usually a piece of liver is placed in formalin for histopathology and another piece is kept fresh (in a plain pot) for culture.
- The site of liver biopsy should also be considered:
  - If diffuse changes are present (e.g. hepatic lipidosis), a lobe that is large and mobile is usually chosen
  - If focal changes are present (e.g. metastatic liver disease), samples should be taken from both abnormal and more normal-appearing liver.
- Bile should also be collected for cytology if cholangitis is suspected (elevated ALP, GGT), and microbiology if a bacterial infection is suspected (based on previous cytology and/or the presence of a peripheral neutrophilia and/or pyrexia, etc.).
- A coagulation panel (prothrombin and activated partial thromboplastin times) should be performed before liver biopsy in cats with hepatopathies; vitamin K treatment (1.0 mg/kg s.c. q12h, 2–3 doses) should be given for 24–36 hours before surgery if any coagulation abnormalities are found (or pre-emptively pending results), and repeat coagulation time assays performed to confirm correction prior to surgery (see Chapter 20). If vitamin K treatment has no effect, a blood transfusion (or ideally a transfusion of fresh plasma) before surgery should be considered.

Biopsy techniques

Various techniques exist for liver biopsy; these should be considered on a case-by-case basis. Patients with a normal coagulation profile may be tolerant of a Tru-cut biopsy performed under ultrasound guidance, or a punch biopsy performed surgically; whereas for patients with proven or suspected coagulopathy a technique that provides suture haemostasis should be used, such as wedge biopsy. The suture amputation technique for liver biopsy is appropriate for diffuse lesions in a liver lobe that has a projecting part of its free edge, enabling a ligature to be placed across the base. This is the most common technique used for liver biopsy in the cat.

Suture amputation technique

Equipment

A basic surgical pack is required, containing:

- Towel clamps (A)
- Brown–Adson thumb forceps (B)
- Needle-holders (C)
- No.3 scalpel handle (D)
- No.15 scalpel blade (E)
- No.10 scalpel blade (F)
- Mosquito forceps (G)
- Metzenbaum scissors (H)
- Mayo scissors (I)
- Blunt–sharp suture scissors (J)
- Gauze surgical swabs (K).

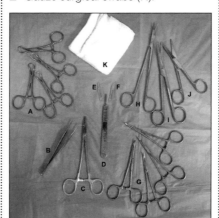

Procedure

The tip of the quadrate lobe is routinely removed in cats with normal-appearing livers or those with diffuse liver disease.

1 A length of monofilament absorbable suture material of 1.5 or 2 metric (4/0 or 3/0 USP) is preformed into a ligature, slipped over a protruding piece of liver and tightened.

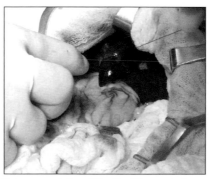

Suture amputation of the tip of the quadrate lobe (this lobe is identified by its close association with the gall bladder) in a cat undergoing multiple biopsy of abdominal organs due to suspected triaditis.

2 After the ligature is pulled tight, the protruding tip of the liver lobe is amputated using Metzenbaum or Mayo scissors, leaving at least 3 mm between

the cut edge and the suture, thus avoiding any risk of cutting the ligature at its base.

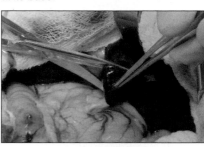

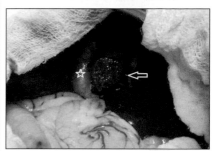

The cut surface of the liver can be seen. The stump of the ligature is just visible on the right-hand side (arrowed). The gall bladder (starred) is visible to the left of the liver biopsy site.

3 The biopsy site is checked for haemorrhage; if hepatic haemorrhage continues, steps should be taken to stop it using the techniques described below.

- The main surgical products available to assist with haemostasis after liver biopsy are cellulose gel foam, which can be packed into defects or laid on top of them, and cellulose fabric (e.g. Surgicell) that can be wrapped over a bleeding site. These are both designed to be implanted and break down gradually over time and therefore do not need to be removed.
- Small pieces of fat or muscle can also be cut from the body wall and used to similar effect.
- Surgical staples are also useful for haemostasis.

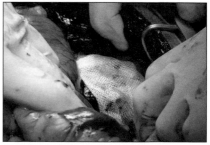

Surgicell used to assist haemostasis after surgical liver biopsy.

If there is no haemorrhage, the abdomen is closed routinely (as for caesarean section; see QRG 15.1).   ▶

QRG 12.1 *continued*

Punch biopsy

A 4 mm skin biopsy punch is used to obtain a core of liver tissue. The core may be separated from the base either by turning the biopsy punch on its side to cut across the tissue, or by carefully lifting the tissue core and cutting its base with fine scissors.

Haemostasis is achieved by applying digital pressure for at least 2 minutes. If bleeding continues, a plug of gel foam (see above), muscle or fat may be placed into the deficit. If this does not halt the haemorrhage, a single mattress or cruciate suture (1.5 metric (4/0 USP) monofilament absorbable) (see Appendix) is placed across the defect. Note that feline liver tissue is usually extremely friable, and the main aim of a suture is to exert gentle pressure from one side of a defect to the other, pressing the cut edges together and assisting haemostasis. Thicker sutures or ligatures are only effective when applied to the hilus of a liver lobe during lobectomy, or when amputating the tip of a liver lobe.

Wedge biopsy

The wedge biopsy technique for obtaining a liver biopsy is most useful for focal lesions deep within the liver lobes, or for patients requiring larger pieces of liver to be taken from the liver edge, or patients with a coagulopathy. The wedge sample is removed from the liver using sharp excision.

A continuous mattress suture (see Appendix) of 1.5 or 2 metric (4/0 or 3/0 USP) monofilament absorbable suture material is placed, in a through-and-through pattern if at the liver edge (i.e. entering the capsule of the liver on one side of the lobe and exiting through the capsule on the other side of the lobe), or taking large bites of tissue on either side of the defect if it is closer to the hilus. Once the suture has traversed the defect in one direction, it is reversed and continued back to its origin. The suture arms at the beginning and end (A and B in diagram below) may then be tied to one another in a square knot, and gently tightened until the edges are apposed and the haemorrhage is controlled. Take care not to pull this suture too tight as it will tear out of the liver parenchyma. Care must also be taken during suture placement and tying of the final knots not to pull the suture too much and risk pulling it out.

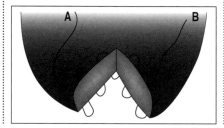

If a bile sample is required, it is collected using a fine needle (no larger than 22 G) inserted through liver parenchyma and into the gall bladder. Insertion through the liver parenchyma reduces the risk of leakage from the gall bladder following aspiration. First ask your pathologist how much bile they will require for cytology (likely needed in an EDTA tube) and microbiology (plain tube).

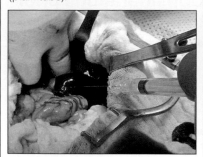

Management of urinary tract disorders

13

Samantha Taylor

This chapter will focus on the management of the most important urinary tract disorders that are encountered in feline practice; notably chronic kidney disease, acute kidney injury, urinary tract infections, feline idiopathic cystitis and urolithiasis. The chapter also contains practical QRGs on subcutaneous fluid therapy and strategies for increasing water intake by cats. *Other relevant practical QRGs are included in other areas of the book*, including cystocentesis (QRG 4.11.4), urinalysis (QRG 4.11.3), radiographic contrast studies (QRG 5.21.1), treatment of hyperkalaemia (QRG 4.11.1), unblocking urethral obstruction (QRG 4.11.2) and bladder rupture repair (QRG 4.10.2). Other Chapters contain more information on the approach to specific urinary tract problems such as inappropriate urination, dysuria and pollakiuria (Chapter 5.21), urethral obstruction (Chapter 4.11) and azotaemia (Chapter 5.7). Additional information relevant to urinary tract disorders is also contained in Chapters 4.9, 5.11 and 18.

Chronic kidney disease

Chronic kidney disease (CKD) was previously termed chronic renal failure/insufficiency. The condition was renamed by the International Renal Interest Society (IRIS) to improve communication with owners and facilitate the creation of standardized treatment guidelines and scientific study.

Aetiology
The majority of cases of CKD are caused by chronic, progressive tubulointerstitial disease, where the inciting cause is unidentified. However, other causes of renal damage that may result in CKD, and influence management, include:

- Pyelonephritis (see Urinary tract infection (UTI), later)
- Neoplasia (commonly lymphoma)
- Hypercalcaemia and nephrocalcinosis
- Sequelae to hydronephrosis due to ureteral obstruction
- Primary glomerulonephropathies (often resulting in protein-losing nephropathy)
- Sequelae to acute kidney injury (AKI)
- Renal ischaemia (due to hypotension, thrombosis)

- FIV-related nephropathy
- Feline infectious peritonitis (FIP) with renal involvement
- Polycystic kidney disease (PKD) (seen in Persian cats and related breeds).

CKD is a progressive condition with irreversible loss of function, since nephron regeneration cannot occur. However, treatment aimed at slowing progression of disease and management of the consequences of CKD are recommended, and can result in very long periods of good quality of life.

Clinical features and examination
CKD is most commonly diagnosed in older (especially senior and geriatric) cats but may be seen in younger cats as a result of the conditions listed above. Patients are usually presented with a history that includes a combination of: polyuria and polydipsia (PU/PD) (note that PD can be difficult to appreciate in cats and PU may be unobserved if, for example, the cat urinates outside); weight loss; inappetence; and vomiting. Affected cats often have a poor hair coat and may have concurrent geriatric diseases (e.g. osteoarthritis, dental disease or hyperthyroidism). An ammonia-like smell to the breath may have been noted by owners of cats with severe uraemia.

Patients may have clinical signs specific to the primary disease. For example: a Persian cat with PKD or a cat with renal lymphoma may present with bilateral renomegaly, whereas a cat with AKI may be oliguric/anuric.

Cases can present acutely with sudden-onset deterioration and collapse, during a uraemic crisis that can occur pre-diagnosis or during treatment (often termed 'acute on chronic' kidney disease).

Small, firm kidneys can be noted on physical examination along with loss of body condition and dehydration. Complications due to CKD may include acute vision loss and hyphaema with hypertension; and dysuria/pollakiuria with urinary tract infection. Blood pressure should be measured (see QRG 5.18.1) in all cases of CKD, as approximately 20% of affected cats are hypertensive. Treatment of the hypertension may slow the progression of CKD as well as preventing hypertensive complications.

Diagnosis

Signalment (older cats), history and physical examination may suggest CKD.

Clinical pathology

Biochemical results may reveal azotaemia; they must be combined with measurement of urine specific gravity (USG; see QRG 4.11.3) demonstrating loss of urine-concentrating ability (i.e. USG <1.035) to exclude pre-renal azotaemia (see Chapter 5.7). Patients with early renal disease may have reduced urine-concentrating ability without azotaemia (IRIS stage I CKD, see later). Ideally urine samples are obtained by cystocentesis (see QRG 4.11.4).

Other clinical pathology abnormalities that may be noted in cats with CKD include:

- Hyperphosphataemia
- Hypercalcaemia (usually elevated total calcium but normal/low ionized calcium)
- Hypokalaemia
- Non-regenerative anaemia
- Proteinuria may be present in some cases. Urine dipsticks can identify the presence of protein but an additional quantitative test should also be performed, as the USG will affect the amount of protein detected. Determination of the urine protein:creatinine ratio (UPC) is recommended.

Proteinuria can be categorized as follows:

- **Pre-renal:** Excessive plasma proteins (e.g. haemoglobin, myoglobin or Bence–Jones proteins (found in multiple myeloma)) leak into the urine and overwhelm tubular reabsorptive mechanisms
- **Renal:** Physiological proteinuria (e.g. as a result of seizures or fever and usually mild and transient) or pathological (glomerular, tubular or interstitial abnormalities). Note that CKD in cats is predominantly a tubulointerstitial disease and therefore proteinuria (UPC >0.4) is uncommon. Glomerular disease often results in marked proteinuria (e.g. UPC >3.0)
- **Post-renal:** Entry of protein into the urine after glomerular filtration and tubular reabsorption (e.g. urogenital tract disease, UTI, urolithiasis). Note that these causes of proteinuria are often accompanied by haematuria and/or an active sediment (see QRG 4.11.3).

Imaging

Normal kidney size ranges on imaging are as follows:

- Radiography: Normal kidney is 2.4–3 times the length of the second lumbar (L2) vertebra on a VD abdominal radiograph
- Ultrasonography: Normal kidney length is 3.0–4.3 cm.

Radiography and ultrasonography may demonstrate small kidneys (with a hyperechoic ultrasound appearance). If CKD is the result of another cause of renal injury (see above) then the renal appearance will vary (e.g. PKD, hydronephrosis, nephrocalcinosis (Figure 13.1)).

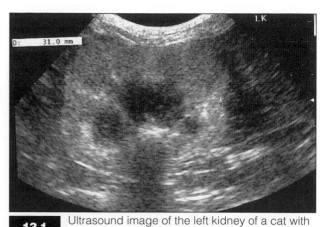

13.1 Ultrasound image of the left kidney of a cat with CKD as a result of idiopathic hypercalcaemia. Shadowing from the renal pelvis can be seen due to a calcium oxalate nephrolith. This cat presented for investigation of polydipsia and weight loss. Hypercalcaemia and IRIS stage II CKD were identified. Medical management of both the hypercalcaemia and renal disease resulted in a clinical improvement. The nephroliths were monitored and remained a similar size until the cat's death one year later due to recurrence of hypercalcaemia and progression of CKD. Removal of the nephroliths was not indicated in this case, as monitoring showed they were not causing an obstruction and management of the underlying cause (hypercalcaemia) was initially successful. Note that feline upper urinary tract (renal, ureteral) uroliths are more likely to be calcium oxalate than any other type.

Renal biopsy

Renal biopsy is not usually required for diagnosis of CKD. There are significant risks of haemorrhage and further decline in renal function, and results will rarely alter management. Biopsy is therefore only recommended in cases where an underlying alternative pathology is suspected that would change treatment, e.g. lymphoma (most cases of lymphoma will, however, be diagnosed on cytology of a renal fine-needle aspirate rather than by tissue biopsy).

Differentiating AKI from CKD

Differentiation of AKI from CKD (Figure 13.2) is important for treatment and prognosis. Cats with AKI are usually very unwell for their level of azotaemia, whereas cats with CKD compensate well with severe azotaemia.

Acute kidney injury	Chronic kidney disease
History	
No history of clinical signs consistent with renal disease	History consistent with CKD (e.g. PU/PD, weight loss, inappetence)
History of toxin/drug exposure	Usually polyuric
May be oliguric or anuric	
Physical examination	
Good body condition	Reduced body condition
Kidneys may be painful	Kidneys firm and small and not usually painful
Possible renomegaly	Urine usually present in bladder
May have very small bladder	
Biochemistry and haematology	
Hyperkalaemia	Hypo- or normokalaemia
Metabolic acidosis (marked, particularly in ethylene glycol toxicity)	Non-regenerative anaemia
Haematology usually normal	

13.2 Comparative diagnostic features of AKI and CKD. (continues) ▶

Acute kidney injury	Chronic kidney disease
Urinalysis	
Isosthenuria (USG 1.008–1.015) Cylinduria (casts in the urine); calcium oxalate monohydrate crystals in ethylene glycol toxicity; cell debris May be proteinuric Occasionally glycosuric	Isosthenuria or loss of urine-concentrating ability (USG <1.035) Sediment usually benign but can have active sediment if UTI present Not usually proteinuric (but may be at higher IRIS stages or if glomerular disease present)

13.2 (continued) Comparative diagnostic features of AKI and CKD.

Cats with CKD may present acutely with 'acute on chronic' kidney disease (also termed decompensated chronic kidney disease) if a uraemic crisis occurs in a cat with previously stable CKD. Common causes of acute on chronic kidney disease include:

- Conditions resulting in fluid volume loss (e.g. vomiting, diarrhoea) or reduced fluid intake (e.g. pain causing decreased eating/drinking, lack of water through accidental confinement)
- UTI or pyelonephritis
- Hypertension
- Other concurrent diseases resulting in clinical deterioration (e.g. diabetes mellitus, neoplasia, dental disease).

IRIS staging of CKD

Staging of renal disease is important, as it allows monitoring of disease progression and formation of treatment protocols according to stage; it also provides prognostic information. The IRIS staging and substaging of CKD is described below (more details can also be found at www.iris-kidney.com).

Initial evaluation – serum or plasma creatinine

The initial stage is determined by serum creatinine levels (Figure 13.3). Creatinine should be measured once the patient has been rehydrated (where

IRIS stage	Creatinine concentration (µmol/l)	Comments
I (non-azotaemic CKD)	<140 (within reference range)	Another abnormality present indicating renal disease (e.g. renomegaly; renal proteinuria (UPC >0.4); poor urine-concentrating ability (USG <1.035)). Note that loss of urine-concentrating ability in non-azotaemic patients was commonly previously termed 'renal insufficiency'
II (mild CKD)	140–250	The lower end of this range may be within some laboratory's reference ranges
III (moderate CKD)	251–439	
IV (severe CKD)	≥440	

13.3 IRIS stages of CKD.

necessary), to reduce any pre-renal component that could influence the allocated stage. Ideally, serial creatinine measurements are taken, as staging should be performed on patients with *stable* CKD (ideally indicated by obtaining two similar readings).

Substage

Once a stage has been allocated based on serum creatinine, measurement of urine protein and systolic blood pressure allows allocation of substages. Substaging of CKD is important for monitoring of disease and identification of treatment targets. Proteinuria has also been shown to influence prognosis for survival in CKD.

Urine protein: Proteinuria is a negative prognostic indicator in CKD, and should be targeted during treatment. Measurement of urine protein and determination of the urine protein:creatinine ratio (UPC; Figure 13.4) is therefore recommended. Pre-renal proteinuria and post-renal proteinuria (see earlier) should be excluded. Initially a dipstick examination can be performed and a UPC requested if protein is evident. A negative dipstick result allows classification as non-proteinuric (NP).

Substage	UPC
Non-proteinuric (NP)	<0.2
Borderline proteinuric (BP)	0.2–0.4
Proteinuric (P)	>0.4

13.4 IRIS substages of CKD based on UPC.

Blood pressure: Cats with CKD may be hypertensive, resulting in progression of CKD and other clinical signs associated with the hypertension (see Chapter 5.18). Blood pressure should therefore be measured in all cats with CKD and a blood pressure substage allocated (Figure 13.5). Assessment for end-organ damage (also called target-organ damage) should be performed.

Substage	Systolic blood pressure (mmHg)
Minimal or no risk of end-organ damage (N)	<150
Low risk of end-organ damage (L)	150–159
Moderate risk of end-organ damage (M)	160–179
Severe risk of end-organ damage (H)	≥180

13.5 IRIS substages of CKD based on blood pressure.

Management

Specific treatment of the underlying cause of the CKD is rarely achievable, as the inciting cause is usually unknown. Therefore, management of CKD most often centres around slowing progression and managing the consequences of CKD. Once a stage and substage have been allocated to each cat, this should be recorded in the patient records and stage-appropriate treatment given (Figure 13.6).

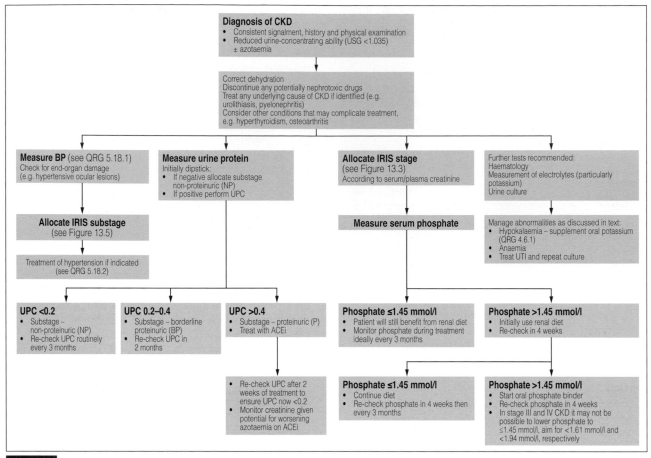

13.6 Approach to staging and management of chronic kidney disease. ACEi = ACE inhibitors.

Initial steps
Initial management steps include:

- Discontinuation of any potentially nephrotoxic drugs (for cats that require analgesia for a concurrent disease such as osteoarthritis, see Chapter 3).
- Correction of dehydration and/or electrolyte imbalances (see QRGs 4.1.3 and 13.2)
- Exclusion of treatable conditions that may result in or perpetuate CKD, e.g. urolithiasis (ultrasonography), pyelonephritis (urine culture)
- Management of complicating concurrent conditions (Figure 13.7); most cases of CKD occur in older cats and therefore comorbid disease is common. Failure to manage these conditions can reduce the effectiveness of strategies to manage CKD; for example, dental disease may reduce intake of food, including renal prescription diets.

- Cardiac disease
- Osteoarthritis/degenerative joint disease
- Hyperthyroidism
- Diabetes mellitus
- Dental disease
- Neoplasia

13.7 Examples of concurrent diseases that may influence treatment of CKD.

Specific management
Specific management of CKD uses a multimodal treatment approach:

1. Dietary management.
2. Management of the complications of CKD.
3. Management of factors that may cause progression of CKD (e.g. proteinuria, hypertension, renal secondary hyperparathyroidism).

Additionally, preventing dehydration is an important aspect of long-term management and involves increasing oral water intake (see QRG 13.1) ± subcutaneous fluid therapy (see QRG 13.2).

Dietary management: Several features of renal prescription diets make them desirable for use in managing CKD, including:

- Reduced protein (but of high digestible quality)
- Reduced phosphate
- Reduced sodium
- Increased B vitamins
- Increased calorific density, i.e. usually increased fat
- Increased potassium
- Non-acidifying
- Antioxidants
- Polyunsaturated fatty acids (PUFAs).

Dietary intervention is appropriate for IRIS stage II and upwards. It is best introduced when the cat has a reasonable appetite rather than during a period of nausea/anorexia, so consideration should be given to including this as part of the diet for cats in IRIS stage I. A renal prescription diet is beneficial, but reduced calorie intake or starvation (if the prescription diet is refused) is more detrimental than eating the old familiar diet. A cat with CKD will benefit even if the renal diet only makes up a proportion of the diet as a whole.

Tips to improve the acceptance of a renal (or other prescription) diet are given in Figure 13.8.

- Do not offer the new diet during hospitalization or the initial stabilization period, as the presence of nausea or pain could result in food aversion and a negative association with the new diet.
- Manage nausea or pain as appropriate.
- Try more than one brand if initial brand is refused; and try wet and dry formulations, as tastes and textures vary.
- Some older cats will change their food preference every few days or weeks, so owners can stock a variety of flavours/brands of renal diet and rotate them.
- Although a slow transition via mixing a component of the old diet with the new diet is often recommended, some cats dislike a mixture of flavours. It is often better to offer the new diet and the old diet separately at the same time, slowly reducing the volume of the old diet and increasing that of the new diet as it becomes accepted.
- Warm the new diet to increase odour.
- Ensure that older cats in particular have an accessible, quiet area in which they can eat.
- Appetite stimulants may be used when initially changing diet.

13.8 Tips to improve the acceptance of a renal (or other prescription) diet. (See also Chapter 5.5.)

Management of complications of CKD: As CKD cannot itself be reversed, the consequences of CKD need to be monitored for, and managed as they arise (Figure 13.9). Some complications also result in progression of CKD (see later).

Management of factors causing progression of CKD: Factors that cause progression of CKD have been identified as hyperphosphataemia, proteinuria and hypertension (possibly via an increase in urine protein loss). These complications should be a priority to identify and treat, as described below. Undiagnosed urinary tract infections may also result in further renal damage and certainly reduce quality of life; regular urinalysis and culture for cats with CKD is therefore recommended.

Hyperphosphataemia: Hyperphosphataemia will result in hyperparathyroidism, which has a detrimental effect on the cat's quality of life and may contribute to progression of renal disease. Early effective management of hyperphosphataemia is important. A renal prescription diet is the first step but if this is refused, or the cat remains hyperphosphataemic despite the diet, then a phosphate binder should be added into treatment.

Complication	Management	Ongoing monitoring
Dehydration	Initial intravenous fluid therapy. Home management includes increasing oral fluid intake (see QRG 13.1). Subcutaneous fluid administration at home may be performed by owners in some cases (particularly for higher IRIS stages) (see QRG 13.2)	Monitor hydration status on clinical examination at each re-check. Monitor azotaemia during initial treatment. NB Do not perform IRIS staging until dehydration is corrected
Hyperphosphataemia (phosphate >1.45 mmol/l) *Note that hyperparathyroidism may contribute to progression of CKD and clinical signs, so management is a priority*	Initially give renal diet, with reassessment of serum phosphate after 4 weeks. If phosphate remains >1.45 mmol/l, add a phosphate binder (see text for options)	All phosphate binders should be titrated to effect and their dose adjusted according to serum phosphate level (see text)
Hypertension	Anti-hypertensive agents include calcium channel blockers (e.g. amlodipine) and ACE inhibitors (see text and Chapter 5.18.2)	All patients with CKD should have systolic blood pressure (SBP) assessed at each check-up. Hypertensive cats should have SBP rechecked 1 week after starting amlodipine and after a dose change
Proteinuria *Note that proteinuria at higher levels is a negative prognostic factor so detection and treatment are desirable*	Proteinuric cats (UPC >0.4) should be treated with ACE inhibitors (e.g. benazepril 0.5–1 mg/kg orally q24h) (see text for further discussion)	Monitor for hypotension and worsening azotaemia. Borderline proteinuric cats should have UPC reassessed after 2 weeks
Inappetence, nausea or vomiting	The appetite stimulant mirtazapine (3.75 mg/cat q72h; reduce to 1.875 mg/cat for IRIS stage II or above) also has an anti-emetic effect. Other anti-emetics include maropitant (1 mg/kg orally q24h for up to 5 days) and metoclopramide (1–2 mg/kg i.v. as an infusion over 24 h; or 0.25–0.5mg/kg i.m., i.v. or orally q12h). H2 blockers (e.g. ranitidine: 2.5 mg/kg slow i.v. q12h or 3.5 mg/kg orally q12h) or proton pump inhibitors (e.g. omeprazole: 0.75–1 mg/kg orally q24h) may help with uraemic gastritis. Some anorexic cats may be best managed with feeding tubes	Monitor appetite and frequency of vomiting, as well as bodyweight and condition
Anaemia	If non-regenerative, normocytic, normochromic and if PCV <20% and cat exhibits clinical signs relating to anaemia (e.g. lethargy), treatment with erythropoietin (EPO) or darbepoietin can be considered after excluding/treating other causes of anaemia (see text for further discussion)	Iron supplementation required when EPO or darbepoetin given. Monitor PCV and stop treatment with EPO or darbepoietin if PCV falls. Also discontinue if erythrocytosis occurs. Monitor blood pressure and adjust dose or stop treatment if hypertension results. Adjust dose according to effect, with target PCV at lower end of reference range
Hypokalaemia	During hospitalization i.v. supplementation may be indicated, particularly in dehydrated patients on fluids. Oral potassium supplementation (potassium gluconate 2–6 mEq (mmol)/cat/day in divided doses) indicated if cat is eating (see also QRG 4.6.1)	Monitor serum potassium concentration

13.9 Management and monitoring of complications of CKD. (continues) ▶

Complication	Management	Ongoing monitoring
Urinary tract infection	Treatment is ideally based on bacterial culture results. In their absence, or if financial limitations, it should be noted that most isolates are *Escherichia coli* sensitive to amoxicillin/clavulanate. As UTIs in cats with CKD are considered 'complicated urinary tract infections', a 4-week course of antibiotics is recommended. Fluoroquinolones should be reserved for resistant cases (see Chapter 3)	Ideally, repeat culture during therapy with antibiotics and 2 weeks after completion of course. If financial limitations, examination of sediment in house may suggest resolution, as most (though not all) cases have an active sediment. Note that some UTIs are clinically silent: cats with CKD should ideally have a sediment examination ± culture every 3–6 months

13.9 (continued) Management and monitoring of complications of CKD.

Several phosphate binder products are available, including:

- Chitosan with calcium carbonate (a powder preparation): 0.5 g/kg on food, twice daily (serum calcium levels should be monitored due to the potential for development of hypercalcaemia)
- Lanthanum carbonate octahydrate (a liquid preparation): 400–800 mg orally per day, divided and given at each meal
- Aluminium antacids (contain aluminium hydroxide in tablet or gel preparation): 10–30 mg/kg orally with food.

Note that efficacy of sucralfate as a phosphate binder is uncertain and palatability may be an issue in cats.

All phosphate binders should be titrated to effect and their dose adjusted according to serum phosphate level. Once a phosphate binder is introduced, serum phosphate should be measured at least 4 weeks after introduction or dosage change.

Targets for phosphate in cats with CKD are as follows:

- IRIS stage II: ≤1.45 mmol/l
- IRIS stage III: <1.61 mmol/l
- IRIS stage IV: <1.94 mmol/l

Hypertension: Amlodipine, a calcium channel blocker, is most often used for the treatment of hypertension in cats with CKD (see QRG 5.18.2).

ACE inhibitors in CKD

Angiotensin-converting enzyme (ACE) inhibitors are often prescribed for cats with CKD. They have been shown to vasodilate the efferent arteriole preferentially, so reducing intraglomerular pressure, and also reduce proteinuria. However, studies in cats have not shown a definitive clinical and/or survival benefit in non-proteinuric CKD (IRIS substage NP), which includes the majority of cats seen in practice with naturally occurring CKD. Therefore, the use of ACE inhibitors should be carefully considered and in the majority of cases of CKD other treatments (e.g. diet, phosphate binders) are usually prioritized.

Indications for the use of ACE inhibitors in CKD are as follows:

- Persistent proteinuria (cats with a persistent UPC of >0.4 following exclusion of pre- and post-renal proteinuria) ▶

- As an adjunctive treatment for hypertension if amlodipine alone is not fully effective (note that ACE inhibitors will only lower blood pressure by approximately 10 mmHg and are therefore usually ineffective as a sole treatment for hypertension).

Contraindications to the use of ACE inhibitors in CKD include:

- Any cat with fluid deficits (e.g. dehydration)
- Unstable azotaemia
- Hypotension
- Hyperkalaemia
- Cats receiving NSAIDs.

If ACE inhibitors are prescribed, serum urea and creatinine plus blood pressure should be checked after 1 week for evidence of deterioration.

Anaemia: Anaemia in CKD is likely to be multifactorial. Causes include:

- Erythropoietin (EPO) deficiency
- Gastrointestinal blood loss
- Reduced red blood cell survival time
- Iron deficiency due to chronic inappetence
- Anaemia of inflammatory (chronic) disease.

Treatment with exogenous EPO is only indicated if other causes of anaemia are excluded and the anaemia is severe (PCV <20%). Treatment with human recombinant EPO can result in worsening anaemia (due to the production of antibodies that interact with the cat's own EPO), and complications such as hypertension and erythrocytosis can occur. A new EPO analogue called darbepoetin shows promise as an effective treatment with reduced side effects (see Figure 13.9). Consultation with a specialist prior to treatment is recommended.

Monitoring

Due to the tendency for cats to conceal illness, regular reassessment of cats with CKD is desirable (Figure 13.10). How often cases are examined should

Check approximately every 3 months

- Bodyweight and body condition score (see Chapter 1)
- Systolic blood pressure
- Free-catch urine sample for in-house USG, dipstick and sediment examination

Check approximately every 6 months

- Biochemistry and haematology (minimum: urea, creatinine, phosphate, calcium, potassium, PCV)
- Urinalysis and culture (minimum: dipstick and in-house sediment examination) from cystocentesis sample

13.10 Suggested minimum monitoring for cats with CKD.

be based on IRIS stage, clinical stability and owner wishes/finances.

Prognosis

Factors affecting prognosis include IRIS stage, proteinuria (UPC) and serum phosphate level. Weight loss may also be an indication of deteriorating renal function.

Median survival times with appropriate management and treatment are estimated as follows:

- IRIS stage II: 1151 days
- IRIS stage III: 679 days
- IRIS stage IV: 35 days.

Acute kidney injury

To align veterinary medicine with human medicine, 'acute renal failure' is now correctly termed 'acute kidney injury (AKI)' to cover the whole spectrum of this condition (i.e. reversible and irreversible renal damage). AKI is uncommon in cats but often fatal when it does occur. However, with prompt and aggressive treatment, irreversible renal damage is sometimes avoidable.

Aetiology

The most common causes are nephrotoxins (particularly lilies, see Chapter 4.9) and pyelonephritis. A list of causes of AKI can be found in Chapter 5.7.

Clinical signs and diagnosis

Prompt recognition and treatment of AKI is vital; however, ingestion of toxins is rarely witnessed and clinical signs are often non-specific (lethargy, collapse, vomiting). Enlarged, painful kidneys may be noted on physical examination. Severe uraemia and ethylene glycol intoxication (see Chapter 4.9) can result in neurological signs. Hyperkalaemia (see QRG 4.11.1) may result in bradycardia and ECG abnormalities. Many cats with AKI are anuric or oliguric (urine production <0.5 ml/kg/h). Cats presenting with AKI may be in good body condition, previously healthy and now severely unwell, often with only moderate levels of azotaemia (with the exception of cats with CKD undergoing an acute decompensation, which are usually severely azotaemic; see Chronic kidney disease, above).

Management

> Consultation with a specialist is strongly recommended early in the management of AKI. Referral should be considered, as close monitoring and intensive care will be required.

Treatment priorities when managing AKI are as follows:

- **Specific therapy to eliminate the cause of AKI:**
  - Specific treatment should be instituted if the causative agent is known (e.g. ethylene glycol toxicity)
  - Appropriate antibiotic therapy should be started if pyelonephritis is suspected
  - Ureteral obstruction may require surgical treatment or urinary diversion procedures. Consultation with a specialist is recommended

- **Correction of fluid volume deficits and restoration of renal perfusion:**
  - Fluid therapy is the mainstay of AKI management. Most cats with AKI are hypovolaemic and dehydrated on presentation. Intravenous boluses of 0.9% NaCl (10–20 ml/kg over 20 minutes) should be given, followed by reassessment of vital parameters and repeat boluses as required (see QRG 4.1.3)
  - Monitor urine production and avoid volume overload (see below)

- **Restoration of urine output:**
  - Ideally, an indwelling urinary catheter with a closed urine collection system (Figure 13.11) is placed to monitor urine output every 30–60 minutes and maintain output at >0.5 ml/kg/h
  - If a catheter cannot be placed, the bladder should be regularly palpated or measured using ultrasonography to estimate urine production
  - Correction of volume deficits may be adequate to restore urine output. If not, a fluid challenge can be administered (10 ml/kg crystalloid fluid over 20 minutes). Monitor for hypervolaemia via respiratory rate and chest auscultation, as well as monitoring systolic blood pressure
  - If the cat remains oliguric/anuric after correction of volume deficits and a fluid challenge, or develops volume overload, administer furosemide (2 mg/kg i.v.) and repeat after 30–60 minutes if no effect

- **Correction of acid–base and electrolyte abnormalities:**
  - Hyperkalaemia may resolve with restoration of urine output; see QRG 4.11.1 for specific treatment of hyperkalaemia
  - Acidosis is common in AKI (particularly in ethylene glycol toxicity) but specific treatment with sodium bicarbonate is rarely needed and requires close monitoring of blood pH
  - Hypokalaemia often occurs after initial treatment of AKI (during so-called post-obstructive diuresis) and may require potassium supplementation

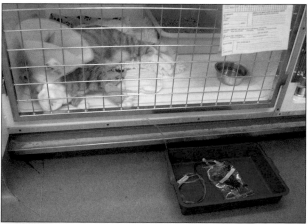

13.11 A cat with AKI with a 'homemade' closed urine collection system. This system includes a giving set and clean, empty intravenous fluid bag. Removal of the giving set's 'chamber' section (as shown here) can reduce resistance to urine flow. It is preferable, however, to use a commercially available small animal closed collection system. All components of the system should be handled in a sterile fashion.

■ *Additional treatments:*
  • Anti-emetics and gastroprotectants may be needed, along with attention to nutrition
  • In cases of pyelonephritis, appropriate antibiotics (ideally based on bacterial culture and sensitivity results) should be administered
  • Peritoneal dialysis may be indicated for severely affected patients (particularly toxicity cases) and may be available at referral centres; but rarely is there a good outcome when the AKI is so severe as to require this
  • Haemodialysis may be effective in the treatment of AKI but availability is extremely limited.

Prognosis

The prognosis for cats with AKI depends on the cause, time period to presentation and response to treatment. Cats with ethylene glycol toxicity have a poor prognosis. It is important to note that the level of azotaemia is not prognostic for reversibility of AKI and that complete recovery is possible with early and aggressive treatment. Recent research suggests that a failure to improve azotaemia with 3 days of treatment is a negative prognostic indicator. Sequelae may include development of CKD.

Urinary tract infections

Urinary tract infections (UTIs) are uncommon in otherwise healthy cats and occur in <2–3% of cats with feline lower urinary tract disease. Cats with adequate urine-concentrating ability and in good physical health are protected from UTIs by multiple defence mechanisms (e.g. length of urethra, supersaturated very hypersthenuric urine). Risk factors for UTIs are listed in Figure 13.12. Cats in 'at risk' groups should be regularly monitored for UTIs as these can be clinically silent; routine sediment examination and bacterial culture should be considered.

■ Older cats. This patient group is more likely to have conditions resulting in polyuria (e.g. CKD) and pain/reluctance to move/void regularly (e.g. osteoarthritis)
■ Any cat with a disease reducing urine-concentrating ability (e.g. CKD, hyperthyroidism)
■ Cats with diabetes mellitus
■ Any cat that has, or has had, urethral catheterization
■ Cats that have had perineal (or other types of) urethrostomy
■ Immunosuppressed cats (e.g. receiving corticosteroids or chemotherapeutics)
■ Female cats in all above categories are at greater risk than males

13.12 Cats at risk of urinary tract infections.

Clinical signs and diagnosis

A UTI is usually associated with clinical signs of dysuria, haematuria, stranguria and pollakiuria. However, inappropriate urination may be the only indication and it is important to note that some UTIs are clinically silent. Pyelonephritis may be associated with AKI and CKD, and affected cats may show signs of renal pain, pyrexia, lethargy, vomiting and inappetence. Low-grade pyelonephritis may be asymptomatic.

Cystocentesis (see QRG 4.11.4) and bacterial culture should be performed. Urine sediment examination will usually demonstrate pyuria, haematuria and bacteriuria (see QRG 4.11.3). The majority of UTIs are caused by *Escherichia coli,* with *Staphylococcus*, *Streptococcus* and *Proteus* spp. making up the majority of remaining isolates.

Treatment
Antibiotic selection should be based on bacterial culture and sensitivity if possible (see Chapter 3).

■ Simple acute bacterial cystitis is rare in cats. If no underlying cause is found then treatment for 7–14 days is indicated.
■ Complicated UTIs (pyelonephritis, urolithiasis, immunosuppression) are more common and require 4–6 weeks of therapy.
■ Ideally, urine bacterial culture is repeated a week after completion of the antibiotic course to confirm resolution. If financial limitations are present, in-house sediment examination is useful to demonstrate an inactive sediment indicating effective treatment.

FLUTD

FLUTD (feline lower urinary tract disease) is a spectrum of diseases with common clinical signs (e.g. dysuria, pollakiuria, haematuria, stranguria and periuria). The multiple potential underlying causes require consideration and investigation. The most common cause is feline idiopathic cystitis (FIC, below), followed by urolithiasis (see later), urethral obstruction (e.g. mucous plug, spasm) (see Chapter 4.11), bacterial cystitis, anatomical defects, neoplasia and behavioural problems (see Chapter 18).

Feline idiopathic cystitis

FIC is the most common cause of FLUTD and is commonly seen in young to middle-aged cats. FIC may be obstructive or non-obstructive. Obstructed cats require emergency treatment (see Chapter 4.11); management strategies to prevent recurrence should follow. FIC is a diagnosis of exclusion made following a logical investigation excluding other causes of FLUTD.

Aetiology
FIC by definition is a disease of unknown aetiology. However, evidence from a number of studies demonstrates various physiological abnormalities in cats with FIC. These include: an inappropriate hormonal and sympathetic nervous system response to stress; alterations in bladder neurons ('neurogenic inflammation'); depletion of the protective glycosaminoglycan (GAG) layer lining the bladder; and compounds within (often highly concentrated) urine exacerbating bladder wall inflammation. This evidence suggests that FIC is the result of complex interactions between the urinary and nervous systems, and certain cats will be predisposed when in a provocative environment (e.g. exposed to acute or chronic stress).

Risk factors for the development of FIC are listed in Figure 13.13.

- Inactivity
- Indoor housing
- Low water intake and concentrated urine
- Higher bodyweight and body condition score
- Use of an indoor litter tray
- Chronic stress (e.g. multi-cat household with conflict between cats; inappropriate litter tray environment – location, hygiene, media, number; conflict outside the home with neighbouring cats)
- Acute stress (e.g. house move, new baby, new pet, building work)

13.13 Risk factors for the development of FIC.

Management

Successful management of FIC is complex. As mentioned above, FIC cases that present with urethral obstruction require emergency treatment of the obstruction and possibly anti-spasmodic treatments (see Chapter 4.11), but management strategies to prevent recurrence, as for non-obstructed cases, should follow. Given the known risk factors and current evidence on the aetiology of FIC, the lifestyle of the cat must be considered for treatment to be successful. A full history should be taken and will in most cases necessitate a longer than routine consultation.

A 'multimodal' approach to management is most effective, encompassing behavioural therapy, medication and dietary manipulation to increase water intake. Client education is vital to educate owners and emphasize the potential recurrent nature of the condition without appropriate management. Use of printed material can help motivated clients to educate themselves about the condition (e.g. Caney and Gunn-Moore, 2009).

Decrease stress

Through taking a full history and looking at the affected cat's lifestyle, points of stress can be identified. A questionnaire may be useful (see the *BSAVA Manual of Canine and Feline Behavioural Medicine*). Attention should be paid to: relationships between cats inside and outside the house, availability or access to resources, litter tray factors, and sources of acute stress (see Chapter 18).

Based on the history, a plan to decrease stress can be formulated, to include:

- Appropriate litter tray facilities
- Measures to reduce cat-to-cat conflict inside and outside the home
- Use of a pheromone diffuser at appropriate locations in the home
- Prediction of stressful events (e.g. house moves) and efforts to reduce their impact. Remember that visits to the veterinary practice are stressful and can result in acute exacerbation of FIC, so the practice should be 'cat-friendly' (see Chapter 1).

Referral to, or consultation with, a veterinary behaviourist is recommended for complex cases.

Increase water intake

Together with stress reduction, this is the most important factor for preventing recurrence of FIC. Increasing water intake will result in more dilute urine and may reduce neurogenic bladder inflammation. The easiest way to do this is with a wet diet; for further methods see QRG 13.1. A gradual diet change is indicated, as diet change itself may result in stress in susceptible cats. Creation of an information sheet for clients on methods to increase water intake can be useful. The goal is to produce urine with a specific gravity of <1.035.

Dietary management of FIC – misconceptions
Historically, cats with FIC have been treated with acidifying diets, particularly if struvite crystals have been identified in the urine. However, crystalluria is no more common in cats with FIC than in normal cats, and there is no evidence that crystalluria contributes to the development of FIC. It is also important to note that crystals form in urine shortly after collection and sediment should be examined within 1–2 hours of urine collection and stored at room temperature (i.e. not in the fridge). The most important factor in dietary management of FIC is increasing water intake and NOT reducing/eradicating crystalluria, which is considered a normal finding in some cats.

Encourage weight loss and increase activity

Decreased activity is a risk factor for FIC, and contributes to the development of obesity (again client education literature can be helpful, e.g. Harvey and Taylor, 2012). Techniques to increase activity should be discussed with owners and this is particularly important for indoor cats where environmental enrichment will also improve quality of life (see Chapter 2). A weight loss diet may be required but should only be introduced once an episode of FIC has resolved. As mentioned, a wet diet may be more suitable than a dry diet.

Drug therapy

Multiple medications have been assessed in attempts to manage FIC. Controlled studies are lacking and response to treatment is difficult to assess, as the condition resolves spontaneously in 3–7 days in most cases. Currently no interventional medical therapy has been shown to be of significant benefit. Short-term use of drugs should be considered in severe cases and long-term medication reserved for recurrent forms of FIC when environmental and dietary therapy have failed. The following medications may be considered.

Analgesia and anti-inflammatory drugs: FIC is a painful condition and treatment of pain may reduce the severity and duration of episodes of FIC. Analgesia is therefore a very important component of therapy. Control of bladder pain may also reduce urethral spasm and therefore functional urethral obstruction. Analgesia is also essential for all hospitalized cats with urethral obstruction. NSAIDs may be useful in cats with normal renal function. Buprenorphine can be administered via the buccal mucous membranes by owners, if indicated or if NSAIDs are contraindicated.

Glycosaminoglycan (GAG) replacers: GAG replacers (e.g. glucosamine, pentosan polysulphate) may benefit some individuals with FIC, although no significant reduction in recurrence of episodes has been reported in published studies. Trial therapy is warranted in recurrent or refractory cases. Consider method of supplementation, as administration of large tablets may result in stress (for both cat and owner).

Amitriptyline: The tricyclic antidepressant amitriptyline has effects on the central nervous system and also potentially reduces neurogenic bladder inflammation. Given current lack of evidence of benefit, despite several studies, and the potential side effects (e.g. sedation, reduced grooming, constipation) amitriptyline is generally not advised for FIC.

Others: Many other drugs have been used to manage FIC but currently studies on efficacy are lacking. Note that short-term prednisolone has been shown NOT to be of benefit, and acid solutions for use intravesicularly are contraindicated. Nutraceuticals such as alpha-casozepine, and some diets, are used with the aim of having anxiolytic effects (see Chapter 18) and may be a useful adjunctive treatment for some cats. It should be emphasized, however, that in the management of FIC the **priority** is increasing water intake and the management of the underlying cause of stress.

Prognosis

Most cases of FIC resolve spontaneously within 3–7 days. With adequate attention to environmental manipulation and increasing water intake, recurrence can be avoided in most cases.

A small percentage of cats suffer chronic or recurrent FIC. Such cats may benefit from drug treatment (e.g. GAG replacers) and referral to a behaviourist. In a few cases, where sources of stress cannot be avoided, rehoming may be the only way to avoid recurrence. Owner prediction of stressful events should be encouraged and, in cases of recurrent obstructive FIC, early use of analgesia and anti-spasmodics (see Chapter 4.11) may prevent a severe episode.

Prognosis is in some cases dependent on owner motivation to comply with recommendations.

Urolithiasis

Urolithiasis is the second most common cause of FLUTD but it can also affect the upper urinary tract.

- Struvite and calcium oxalate uroliths are those most commonly seen in cats.
- Other uroliths consist of:
  - Ammonium biurate – in cats with portal vascular anomalies and other hepatopathies
  - Calcium phosphate – in hypercalcaemic cats
  - Cystine – associated with congenital renal tubular abnormalities
  - Dried solidified blood calculi – presumed the result of urinary tract inflammation/haemorrhage.

Risk factors for the development of urolithiasis include increasing age, obesity, inactivity and certain breed predispositions (Figure 13.14). Clinical signs will depend on location of the urolith and include haematuria, dysuria, periuria and stranguria/urethral obstruction (bladder or urethral stones). Nephroliths may be clinically silent or result in AKI or haematuria. Ureteroliths can cause hydronephrosis and AKI. Diagnosis is based on clinical signs, imaging (radiography and

Struvite urolithiasis	Calcium oxalate urolithiasis
Risk factors	
Oriental and foreign shorthairs Female>male Prime to mature cats Concentrated urine	Burmese, Persian, Himalayan, Ragdoll Male>female Prime to mature cats Concentrated urine Hypercalcaemia
Diagnostic features	
Urinalysis: alkaline pH Radiopaque	Urinalysis: acidic pH Radiopaque
Management	
May dissolve with diet producing undersaturated urine. Monitoring with repeat imaging to confirm dissolution is recommended; diet should be continued for a month beyond apparent dissolution of uroliths *Prevention of recurrence*: increase water intake (see QRG 13.1) to achieve USG <1.035; increase activity; manage any obesity; dietary management should produce urine with pH 6.2–6.4 and reduced magnesium and phosphate	Cannot be dissolved; surgical resection indicated. Management of hypercalcaemia (see Chapter 4.3) if present *Prevention of recurrence*: increase water intake (see QRG 13.1) to achieve USG <1.035; increase activity; manage any obesity; dietary management should produce urine with pH 6.6–6.8

13.14 Struvite and calcium oxalate urolithiasis: risk factors, diagnosis and management.

ultrasonography) and urinalysis. Crystalluria may be present and reflect urolith type but some cases will have no crystalluria or have crystals of a different mineral composition to the urolith; therefore, all removed uroliths should be submitted for analysis.

Management of struvite and calcium oxalate urolithiasis is described in Figure 13.14. Ureteroliths or nephroliths causing AKI require surgical management. Advice from a specialist on specific management of nephrolithiasis and ureterolithiasis is recommended.

References and further reading

Barrett E (2011) Bladder and urethra. In: *BSAVA Manual of Canine and Feline Ultrasonography*, ed. F Barr and L Gaschen, pp. 155–164. BSAVA Publications, Gloucester

Buffington CAT (2011) Idiopathic cystitis in domestic cats – beyond the lower urinary tract. *Journal of Veterinary Internal Medicine* **25**, 784–796

Buffington CAT, Westropp JL, Chew DJ and Bolus RR (2006) Clinical evaluation of multimodal environmental modification (MEMO) in the management of cats with idiopathic cystitis. *Journal of Feline Medicine and Surgery* **8**, 261–268

Caney S and Gunn-Moore D (2009) Caring for a cat with lower urinary tract disease. Available at: www.catprofessional.com

Elliott J and Grauer G (2007) *BSAVA Manual of Canine and Feline Nephrology and Urology, 2nd edn.* BSAVA Publications, Gloucester

Elwood C (2010) Patients with urogenital disease. In: *BSAVA Manual of Canine and Feline Rehabilitation, Supportive and Palliative Care: Case Studies in Patient Management,* ed. S Lindley and P Watson, pp. 289–308. BSAVA Publications, Gloucester

Graham JP (2011) Kidneys and proximal ureters. In: *BSAVA Manual of Canine and Feline Ultrasonography*, ed. F Barr and L Gaschen, pp. 110–123. BSAVA Publications, Gloucester

Harvey A and Taylor S (2012) Caring for an overweight cat. Available at: www.catprofessional.com

Hotston Moore A (2009) The bladder and urethra. In: *BSAVA Manual of Canine and Feline Abdominal Imaging*, ed. R O'Brien and F Barr, pp. 205–221. BSAVA Publications, Gloucester

Larson MM (2009) The kidneys and ureters. In: *BSAVA Manual of Canine and Feline Abdominal Imaging*, ed. R O'Brien and F Barr, pp. 185–204. BSAVA Publications, Gloucester

QRG 13.1 Increasing water intake
by Samantha Taylor

Indications

- Any cat with an underlying disease resulting in reduced urine-concentrating ability (USG <1.035), as they will be more prone to dehydration. Examples are chronic kidney disease (CKD), diabetes mellitus and hyperthyroidism.
- Cats with lower urinary tract disease (see Chapter 13), particularly feline idiopathic cystitis (FIC), as diluting the urine has been shown to prevent recurrence.
- Cats with urolithiasis, as increasing water intake will reduce urine saturation and decrease the risk of stone formation in some cases.
- Cats receiving NSAIDs. Cats with osteoarthritis that are being treated with NSAIDs are often older cats prone to dehydration for various reasons (e.g. undiagnosed CKD, reluctance to move and therefore visit the water bowl).

Considerations to increase water intake

- **Type of food:**
  - Feeding a wet diet is the most effective way of increasing water intake and diluting urine
  - Adding water to food (although this can reduce palatability for some cats)
  - Some diets contain higher levels of sodium chloride, which has been shown to result in increased water intake and reduced USG
  - Making a 'soup' of favourite food (i.e. mashing with water) can encourage drinking
  - The water from a tin of tuna in spring water can be offered
  - Using the broth or cooking water from cooking fish or chicken
  - Small amounts of preferred flavouring (e.g. tuna water, chicken broth) can be frozen in ice cube or baby weaning food trays, easily allowing a cube to be added to a bowl of water each day.
- **Type of bowl:**
  - Many cats prefer ceramic or glass bowls over plastic, which can taint the taste of the water
  - Some cats do not like to see their reflection in metallic bowls
  - Some cats like drinking from a full water glass
  - Wide brimmed bowls are preferred over tall, narrow receptacles, as cats do not like the sensation of their whiskers touching the sides of the bowl
  - Bowls should be filled right to the brim and topped up regularly, as cats prefer to drink from the surface to avoid putting their head into the bowl.
- **Location:**
  - Water bowls should be positioned away from food bowls and litter trays (avoid 'double' bowls with food adjacent to water)
  - Water should be provided in more than one location (e.g. on each floor of the house) and preferably also outdoors for indoor/outdoor cats (and allowed to fill with rainwater if preferred by the cat)
  - In a multi-cat household, resources (including water) should be in more than one accessible location to avoid conflict and guarding by other cats.
- **Other water sources:**
  - Water fountains are popular with some cats, and many types are commercially available
  - A tap can be left dripping into a bath, shower or sink
- **Alternative strategies:**
  - Diluted 'cat milk' is popular with some cats (but the added calories should be included in any weight management plans; note that cow's milk should be avoided)
  - Some cats do prefer bottled or filtered water to tap water, whilst others prefer rain water. Rain water can be collected and then used indoors.

PRACTICAL TIP

- Make changes to food gradually.
- Do not move an existing water source until the cat is observed using the new sources.

QRG 13.2 Subcutaneous fluid therapy
by Samantha Taylor

Indications

- Mild dehydration (≤8%; see Chapter 5.11) such as in chronic kidney disease (CKD) or from mild fluid losses due to vomiting/diarrhoea.
- Fluid therapy at home in cases of chronic low-grade dehydration (CKD is the most common cause).
- Prevention of dehydration in inappetent patients (NB management of inappetence should be prioritized; see Chapter 5.5).

Contraindications

- Subcutaneous fluid therapy is not suitable for cats with moderate or severe (>8%) dehydration, ongoing significant fluid losses, hypovolaemia or hypothermia.
- Hypertonic solutions (e.g. glucose solutions >5% or hypertonic saline) should not be given subcutaneously.

Equipment

- Appropriate fluid (crystalloids: 0.9% saline, Hartmann's solution) which should be warmed to body temperature by placing in a warm water bath.
- Needles: maximum 18 G (18 G and 21 G shown).
- Giving set.
- Potassium can be added to the fluid if indicated but only to a maximum concentration of 30 mEq/l to avoid irritation.
- The amount of fluid required can be removed from the fluid bag into a large syringe but it is simpler (and more appropriate for owners at home) to weigh the fluid bag plus giving set at the start and reweigh them during administration to see how much fluid has been administered.

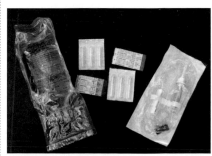

(Courtesy of the Feline Advisory Bureau)

QRG 13.2 continued

The following technique uses a giving set and needle but subcutaneous catheters are available to facilitate frequent subcutaneous fluid administration. There is limited experience of such catheters in cats and, anecdotally, problems can be encountered such as frequent blockage, infection and local discomfort. However, for some patients the catheters have been successful and well tolerated. For suitable cases contact a specialist for further advice.

Patient restraint

Only gentle restraint by an assistant is needed in most cases. For more fractious cats the fluids can be given with the cat in a cat basket.

Procedure

1 The skin between the shoulder blades is tented and the needle inserted.

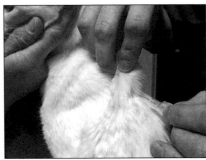

(Courtesy of the Feline Centre, Langford Veterinary Services, University of Bristol)

2 The giving set is raised to allow fluid to flow into the subcutaneous space and form a large pocket.

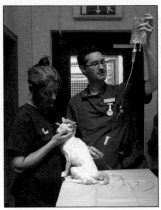

(Courtesy of the Feline Centre, Langford Veterinary Services, University of Bristol)

3 The cat can be allowed to relax/rest during the administration, with minimal restraint.

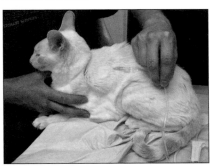

(Courtesy of the Feline Centre, Langford Veterinary Services, University of Bristol)

The fluid can be given into just one site, but if the skin over the fluid pocket is becoming tense, or the patient is uncomfortable, then the needle can be repositioned in a different location and administration continued. Regular palpation of the fluid pocket for distension and discomfort is recommended, as different cats will tolerate different volumes of fluid. The pocket of fluid will naturally disperse quite quickly (within an hour) after administration.

Approximately 10 ml/kg (usually around 50 ml in total) should be given into one site (although tolerance levels vary from cat to cat) and the procedure may be repeated at different sites as required to provide an adequate volume of fluid. The total amount given will be dependent on the degree of dehydration (see Chapter 5.11) and frequency of administration. For home management of CKD this is usually twice weekly, although more frequent administration may be required in some cases.

Motivated owners can be taught the procedure at home and many cats are tolerant of the procedure, sitting on the owner's lap or on a bed/sofa with a little training and provision of rewards (e.g. food treats). A detailed step-by-step guide for owners is available at www.fabcats.org/owners/kidney/subcutaneous/info.html.

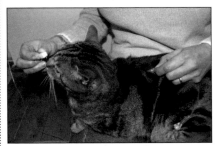

(Courtesy of the Feline Advisory Bureau)

Management of endocrine disorders

Nicki Reed

This chapter will focus on the management of the most important endocrine disorders encountered in feline practice: hyperthyroidism and diabetes mellitus (including diabetic ketoacidosis). It also contains practical QRGs on ear vein blood sampling for blood glucose measurement, and performing thyroidectomy. Other sections of the book contain more information on the approach to specific presenting problems that can be associated with endocrine disorders, such as hypercalcaemia (Chapter 4.3), hypocalcaemia (Chapter 4.4), hypoglycaemia (Chapter 4.5), hypokalaemia (Chapter 4.6), dehydration (Chapter 5.11), hypertension (Chapter 5.18), hyphaema (Chapter 5.19), polyphagia (Chapter 5.28), polyuria and polydipsia (Chapter 5.29) and weight loss (Chapter 5.36). Emerging endocrine disorders (e.g. primary hyperaldosteronism and acromegaly) and more unusual endocrine disorders (e.g. hyperadrenocorticism, diabetes insipidus, hyper- and hypoparathyroidism, hypothyroidism) are not covered in this book; the reader is referred to the *BSAVA Manual of Canine and Feline Endocrinology* for information about these disorders.

Hyperthyroidism

Aetiology
Hyperthyroidism is caused, in the majority of cases (98%), by a functional adenoma, which may be unilateral (~30%) or bilateral (~70%). The remaining 2% of cases are due to thyroid carcinoma.

Clinical features

- **Signalment:** Occurs in older cats (95% >10 years old). No sex or breed predilection, although Siamese and Himalayan cats appear under-represented.
- **History:** Weight loss, polyphagia, polyuria, polydipsia, intermittent vomiting and/or diarrhoea, altered behaviour including increased irritability/aggression, decreased or excessive grooming. Apathetic hyperthyroid cats may be lethargic with a decreased appetite, but this presentation is less common.
- **Physical examination:** Poor body condition and muscle condition score, palpable goitre (Figure 14.1), tachycardia, gallop sounds, cardiac murmur,

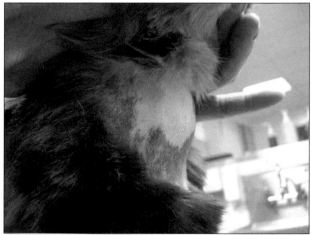

14.1 Goitre: there is an obvious cervical swelling due to an enlarged, cystic thyroid gland. Not all goitres will be as obvious as this one. Palpation of an enlarged thyroid is most readily performed with the cat sitting in front of you and facing away. The cat's head is elevated slightly and the cervical groove palpated with the thumb and first two fingers, from the larynx ventrally to the thoracic inlet. In most cases, the thyroid gland is felt as a small round or oval structure slipping below the fingers. Some people find it easier to palpate alternate sides with different hands.

tachypnoea, plantigrade stance or cervical ventroflexion from muscle weakness, and matted, unkempt coat or alopecia.
- **Systolic blood pressure:** May be elevated due to the increased sympathetic output associated with hyperthyroidism
- **Routine clinicopathological findings:**
  - Routine haematology: Non-specific but mild erythrocytosis and/or lymphopenia may be seen
  - Routine biochemistry: Elevated liver enzymes (ALT, ALP) and elevated inorganic phosphate can arise directly due to the hyperthyroid state; azotaemia and hypokalaemia may be variably seen in association with concurrent chronic kidney disease (CKD), but elevated urea may also be seen as a result of polyphagia and increased protein catabolism
  - Urinalysis: This is not specific for the diagnosis of hyperthyroidism, but may help identify

concurrent disease (e.g. CKD, diabetes mellitus). Urinary tract infections may also occur in hyperthyroid cats
- Main use for routine haematology/biochemistry/urinalysis is for identifying concurrent diseases that could influence treatment choice, and to provide baseline parameters for monitoring during treatment, e.g. evaluating any development or worsening of CKD or development of side effects of medical therapy.
■ Differential diagnoses are given in Figure 14.2.

Clinical signs	Primary differential diagnoses
Weight loss (with good appetite) (see Chapter 5.36)	Diabetes mellitus, inflammatory bowel disease, exocrine pancreatic insufficiency, intestinal neoplasia, inappropriate diet, endoparasitism
Polyuria/polydipsia (see Chapter 5.29)	Chronic kidney disease, diabetes mellitus, acromegaly, hypercalcaemia, pyelonephritis
Altered behaviour (see Chapter 5.24)	Hypertension, cognitive dysfunction, intracranial disease (e.g. meningioma, toxoplasmosis, FIP), pain
Cervical mass	Lymphadenopathy, enlarged parathyroid gland, thyroid cyst
Tachycardia and heart murmur (see Chapter 5.17)	Hypertrophic cardiomyopathy, secondary cardiac hypertrophy, restrictive cardiomyopathy, unclassified cardiomyopathy, dilated cardiomyopathy, physiological (increased sympathetic tone), anaemia (compensatory tachycardia and decreased blood viscosity)
Unkempt coat	Ectoparasitic disease, arthritis, malabsorption, vitamin B12 deficiency
Muscle weakness	Diabetes mellitus, hypokalaemia (chronic kidney disease, anorexia, hyperaldosteronism), hypercalcaemia, polymyopathy
Elevated liver enzymes (see Chapter 5.31)	Lymphocytic cholangitis, neutrophilic cholangitis, hepatic lipidosis, FIP, toxoplasmosis, sepsis

14.2 Primary differential diagnoses for clinical findings associated with hyperthyroidism.

Diagnosis

Elevated total T4 (thyroxine) is the most useful definitively diagnostic finding, being highly specific for the diagnosis of hyperthyroidism, and is adequate as a sole diagnostic test in the majority of cases. Measurement of total T4 by radioimmunometric assay is considered the gold standard.

In some hyperthyroid cats with concurrent illness, total T4 can be lowered into the (upper half of the) normal range. Free T4 should then be measured by equilibrium dialysis. This should not be used as an initial diagnostic test as it is not as specific as the total T4 assay (i.e. it may give a false positive diagnosis of hyperthyroidism) but it is less susceptible to influence by concurrent illness and so may be used in combination with total T4 assay where there is a high index of suspicion for hyperthyroidism but total T4 is within the upper half of the reference range.

Although other diagnostic tests such as thyroid-stimulating hormone (TSH) suppression and scintigraphy are available, these are rarely required in routine practice, and further information or specialist advice should be sought before use. See the *BSAVA Manual of Canine and Feline Endocrinology* for details of these diagnostic tests.

Management

Options for management include medical (drug) management, dietary management, surgery and radioactive iodine treatment. The decision as to which of these options to pursue may be based on a number of considerations (Figure 14.3).

Patient considerations
- Concurrent medical problems
- Compliance with regard to medication
- Age
- Adverse reactions to drugs

Owner considerations
- Finances
- Commitment to lifelong medication
- Willingness to have cat hospitalized or referred

Other considerations
- Availability of I[131] (see Figure 14.5)
- Dietary management: a restricted-iodine diet for control of hyperthyroidism has recently been launched. This needs to be fed exclusively and the iodine content of water provided for the cat needs to be considered to ensure the effect of iodine restriction in the diet is not compromised. Further work is required to investigate the long-term suitability of this for sole management of hyperthyroidism

14.3 Considerations that must be taken into account before deciding upon a management option for hyperthyroidism.

Medical management

Medical therapies act by inhibiting the enzyme thyroid peroxidase, which is involved in a number of steps in the formation of T4 and T3. Medical management may be used before other forms of therapy as it can stabilize the patient prior to surgery (tachycardia, hypertension), and may also enable identification of underlying renal disease previously masked by hyperthyroidism. It is often perceived to be the cheapest option for management; however, drug and monitoring costs over several years may be cumulatively more expensive than surgery or radioactive iodine therapy. It should be borne in mind that medical management will not treat the adenoma (the goitre remains). Over time the adenoma and associated thyroxine production may increase, leading to an increased drug requirement.

Methimazole: A veterinary product (Felimazole) is authorized in the UK for twice-daily dosing, initially at a rate of 2.5 mg orally q12h. Side effects associated with its use occur in up to 18% of cats and include gastrointestinal signs (vomiting and diarrhoea), haematological abnormalities (thrombocytopenia, neutropenia, aplastic anaemia), hepatopathy, facial pruritus (Figure 14.4) and, rarely, myasthenia gravis. *Side effects with methimazole are the same as for carbimazole (see below); therefore, cats that have exhibited side effects with carbimazole (especially serious ones) should generally not be changed to methimazole.* In some countries transdermal formulations of methimazole are available; the carriers used for such formulations vary, as does absorption, so consultation with a local specialist is recommended before using them for the first time.

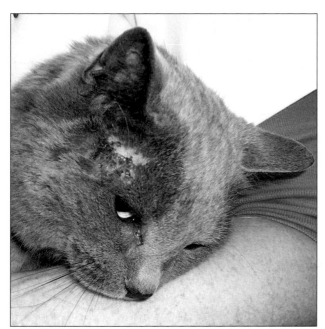

14.4 Facial erythema and pruritus following 4 weeks' medication with methimazole therapy. This side effect can be extremely severe, causing severe self-trauma and necessitating immediate cessation of treatment. These signs resolved within 3 weeks of ceasing therapy.

Carbimazole: Carbimazole is metabolized to methimazole. A sustained-release carbimazole formulation (Vidalta) is authorized for cats in the UK, facilitating owner compliance by allowing once-daily dosing. For mild cases (T4 50–100 nmol/l) a starting dose of 10 mg/day is recommended, but for cats with T4 >100 nmol/l, a dose of 15 mg/day (equivalent to 7.5 mg methimazole) is recommended. Lack of efficacy is anecdotally reported in some cats, possibly due to erratic absorption in the hyperthyroid state. Prior to veterinary authorized products being available, human carbimazole was used at a dose of 5 mg q8–12h. The author sometimes finds this successful (as an 'off-licence' treatment) in cases difficult to control with sustained-release carbimazole, or in cats that are difficult to medicate, as the pills are taken more readily in the food than are other formulations. *Side effects with carbimazole are the same as for methimazole; therefore, cats that have exhibited side effects with methimazole (especially serious ones) should not be changed to carbimazole.*

Monitoring: Routine haematology and biochemistry, along with urinalysis and measurement of total T4, should be repeated approximately 2 weeks after initiation of therapy. Specific attention should be paid to: platelet count (beware automated machines; see QRG 5.4.2); newly identified or increasing azotaemia; and increasing liver enzymes. The dose can be titrated upwards if the cat does not respond to the initial dose. Once euthyroidism is achieved, the dose of medical therapy should be adjusted to maintain this state, using the lowest dose possible.

If severe renal disease is present, maintaining these cats in a slightly hyperthyroid state to maintain glomerular filtration rate was previously thought to be beneficial. This approach is now questioned, as the hyperthyroid state may further exacerbate renal damage; so euthyroidism is usually recommended with concurrent management of any CKD (see Chapter 13). The hypothyroid state must, however, be avoided, as this is detrimental to any underlying CKD. Continued monitoring of blood pressure is recommended, as many hyperthyroid cats may be normotensive at the time of presentation but develop hypertension several months after successful management.

Dietary management

Very recently an iodine-restricted diet has become available for control of hyperthyroidism. The severely restricted iodine within the diet limits thyroxine production. If used, the diet must be fed exclusively and therefore cats must be kept indoors to prevent access to other iodine sources. In addition, deionized water may need to be provided, especially in areas with iodine-rich water. This option may not be suitable for multi-cat households, or where cats require a specific medical diet for another reason. Successful control can be obtained where the necessary criteria can be met and where palatability is not an issue, although long-term studies are limited.

Radioactive iodine

Radioactive iodine (I^{131}) is considered the best therapy for hyperthyroidism as:

- It is safe
- It is successful (>90% of cases only require one treatment)
- Recurrence is rare
- It does not require general anaesthesia
- It can address ectopic thyroid tissue
- It can address thyroid carcinoma more effectively than surgery or medical management.

The I^{131} is typically administered by subcutaneous injection and the patient is then held in isolation for a period of time specified by the local radiation protection authority. Previously, periods of isolation up to 4 weeks were required; much shorter times are now being allowed at certain sites.

I^{131} therapy is not always suitable for patients with concurrent medical problems that require either medication (e.g. diabetes mellitus) or close monitoring, due to the restricted handling allowed during the period of isolation. In addition, some owners do not like the thought of their cat not being able to interact with them for a period of time, or they are put off by the costs or lack of availability. Given the costs that may be involved in medicating and monitoring a hyperthyroid cat long term, I^{131} may well be cost-effective. Withdrawal of medical management is usually recommended shortly (4–9 days) before I^{131} therapy, as methimazole may reduce the organification of iodine within the thyroid gland, thereby reducing its efficacy, but advice should be sought from the centre offering this therapy, as individual guidelines vary. Contact details for current providers (at December 2012) within the UK are given in Figure 14.5; the service may be more widely available in other countries.

Surgical management

Ideally, patients should be stabilized medically prior to surgery, as the hyperthyroid cat is at higher anaesthetic risk due to the potential for cardiac arrhythmias.

Provider	Address	Telephone	Website	Email/enquiries
Barton Veterinary Hospital and Surgery	34 New Dover Road, Canterbury, CT1 3BH	01227 765522	www.barton-vets.co.uk	Online enquiry form on website
Bishopton Veterinary Group	The Surgery, Mill Farm, Studley Road, Ripon, HG4 2QR	01765 602396	www.bishoptonvets.co.uk	admin@bishoptonvets. co.uk
Rowe Veterinary Group	Bradley Green, Wotton under Edge, Gloucestershire, GL12 7PP	01453 843295	www.rowevetgroup.com	Online enquiry form on website
Royal Veterinary College	Hawkshead Lane, North Mymms, Hatfield, Hertfordshire, AL9 7TA	01707 666 333	www.rvc.ac.uk	qmhreception@rvc.ac.uk
University of Bristol	The Feline Centre, Langford Veterinary Services, University of Bristol, Langford House, Langford, BS40 5DU	0117 928 9447	www.felinecentre.co.uk	sah@langfordvets.co.uk
University of Edinburgh	Hospital for Small Animals, Easter Bush Veterinary Centre, Roslin, Midlothian, EH25 9RG	0131 650 7650	www.ed.ac.uk/schools-departments/vet/services/small-animals/vets/services/thefelineclinic/services/radioactiveiodinetherapy	Feline.Clinic@ed.ac.uk
University of Glasgow	Faculty of Veterinary Medicine, University of Glasgow, Bearsden Road, Glasgow G61 1QH	0141 330 5700	www.gla.ac.uk/schools/vet/smallanimal hospital	webmaster@vet.gla.ac.uk

14.5 Contact details for current providers known to author of radioactive iodine treatment within the UK. (Data current as of February 2013.)

Surgical options comprise:

- Unilateral thyroidectomy – increased risk of recurrence
- Bilateral thyroidectomy – increased risk of postoperative hypocalcaemia
- Staged bilateral thyroidectomy – may be recommended if calcium cannot be closely monitored
- Intracapsular technique (see QRG 14.1) – decreases the risk of damage or removal of the associated parathyroid gland; increases the risk of recurrence of clinical signs from residual thyroid tissue
- Extracapsular technique – more likely to remove the thyroid gland completely, but increases the risk of damage to the parathyroid gland or its blood supply.

Owners should be advised of the potential for recurrence of clinical signs at a later period, due to either remnant thyroid tissue or ectopic thyroid tissue (often within the thorax). For management of postoperative hypocalcaemia see Chapter 4.4.1.

Diabetes mellitus

Aetiology

Diabetes mellitus (DM) results when there is inadequate insulin to maintain blood glucose within the normal range. In cats, this is primarily due to peripheral insulin resistance rather than inadequate insulin production by the beta cells of the islets of Langerhans in the pancreas. Peripheral insulin resistance is most commonly the result of obesity, particularly in association with feeding of high-carbohydrate diets. It can also be due to elevated levels of growth hormone, cortisol or progesterone (endogenous or exogenous), which prevent the intracellular uptake of glucose. The hyperglycaemia from insulin resistance stimulates production of more insulin from the beta cells, until eventually insufficient insulin is produced to meet the increased demand. The resulting hyperglycaemia itself can contribute to reduced insulin responses due to the negative effect of glucose toxicity on the beta cells. Pancreatitis is commonly identified in association with DM, and may contribute to the development of the disease due to loss of pancreatic islet cells.

Clinical features

- **Signalment:** Middle-aged to older cats are typically affected. Males are more commonly affected than females. The Burmese breed is predisposed.
- **History:** Polyuria and polydipsia are consistent findings, although they may not be noticed by owners, particularly in cats that drink outside. Polyphagia and weight gain may be reported. Hindleg weakness and plantigrade stance (diabetic neuropathy) may be noted by some owners. A history of recurrent infections is occasionally reported. Other signs (e.g. anorexia, vomiting, diarrhoea) may relate to concurrent illnesses such as pancreatitis.
- **Physical examination:** Often unremarkable in the uncomplicated diabetic cat.
- **Routine clinicopathological findings:**
  - Routine haematology: May be unremarkable, although dehydrated patients may show haemoconcentration
  - Routine biochemistry: Hyperglycaemia is a consistent finding, with glucose usually >20 mmol/l. Increases in ALT and ALP (1.5–2 times the upper limit of the reference range) may be present
  - Urinalysis: Glycosuria indicates that the degree of hyperglycaemia is above the renal threshold (i.e. blood glucose >12–15 mmol/l). Ketonuria may also be detected, particularly in sick patients. The presence of glycosuria will

increase urine specific gravity (by approximately 0.004 for each + on the dipstick). Culture should be performed, even in the presence of inactive sediment, as cats with DM may have impaired neutrophil function and are predisposed to urinary tract infections.

- **Differential diagnoses:** Primarily relate to polyuria/polydipsia (see Chapter 5.29). The main differential diagnosis to consider is stress hyperglycaemia; care should therefore be taken to minimize stress when blood sampling (see QRG 1.7).

Diagnosis

The diagnosis of DM requires documentation of sustained hyperglycaemia and glycosuria. While the degree of hyperglycaemia may give some indication of whether DM or stress hyperglycaemia is present, blood glucose values up to 20 mmol/l may be found in stressed patients. Finding hyperglycaemia without concurrent glycosuria suggests stress hyperglycaemia. Fructosamine (glucose bound to a plasma protein) assay indicates the average glucose values over approximately 2 weeks prior to sampling. Elevated fructosamine therefore indicates sustained hyperglycaemia consistent with DM compared to stress hyperglycaemia.

Management

Newly diagnosed diabetic cats

Insulin: Insulin should be administered to decrease the demand on the pancreas and to reverse the glucose-intolerant state. Insulin options for the management of feline DM are given in Figure 14.6. In the UK the only authorized veterinary product is porcine lente suspension and therefore this has to be the first treatment of choice. This requirement will be variable in other countries. Lente insulins should be administered twice daily, usually at a starting dose of 0.25 IU/kg; in practical terms this usually means 1 IU/cat, although insulin pens can facilitate administration of smaller doses. Obtaining a blood glucose value 6–8 hours after administration of the initial insulin dose can help assess whether there is a response to the insulin, and whether the patient is at risk of hypoglycaemia. Incremental increases of 0.5 IU per dose every 7–10 days are reasonable until clinical signs are controlled. Insulin doses should not be adjusted too rapidly (i.e. leave at least 5 days between dose alterations), as it can take a period of time before the full effect of a new dose is seen. In some cats the duration of action of lente insulin is inadequate; therefore changing to a longer-acting preparation such as protamine zinc insulin (PZI) or glargine may be required (Figure 14.7).

Trade name	Type of insulin	Onset of action	Peak action	Duration of action	Comments
Caninsulin	Porcine: 30% amorphous; 70% crystalline	30–60 minutes	2–8 hours	6–14 hours	This porcine lente formulation is the only authorized veterinary insulin product in the UK
Hypurin lente	Bovine	30–60 minutes	2–8 hours	6–14 hours	
Hypurin PZI	Bovine	1–4 hours	3–12 hours	6–24 hours	May be used twice daily where duration of action of Caninsulin is inadequate
Lantus	Glargine: synthetic insulin analogue	1–4 hours	3–14 hours	12–24 hours	Precipitates at site of injection and is released slowly. Generally considered to be a 'peakless' insulin. Used differently to other insulins (see Figure 14.7). May be used where duration of action of Caninsulin is inadequate

14.6 Insulin options for the management of feline diabetes mellitus.

Starting dose

- If blood glucose (BG) is >20 mmol/l start glargine at 0.5 IU/kg; if <20 mmol/l start at 0.25 IU/kg
- Use a 0.3 ml insulin syringe – DO NOT DILUTE the insulin
- Administer every 12 hours
- Do not increase the dose during the first week

Initial management

- Typically, there is no response for the first 10 days but then a response should be seen
- Perform a 12-hour BG curve at 10 days, 2 weeks and 4 weeks after starting the insulin; earlier urine glucose monitoring or BG curves can be performed if any concerns arise
- Sampling every 4 hours is adequate as glargine is very long-acting

Changing the dose

- If pre-insulin BG is >20 mmol/l and/or trough is >10 mmol/l, increase the dose by 0.5 IU
- If pre-insulin BG is 14–20 mmol/l and/or trough is 5–10 mmol/l, keep to the same dose
- If pre-insulin BG is <10 mmol/l and/or trough is <3 mmol/l, reduce the dose by 1 IU
- **If clinical signs of hypoglycaemia occur, reduce the dose by 50%**
- If pre-insulin BG is <10 mmol/l, continue reducing the dose until only giving 1 IU once daily
- If pre-insulin BG is still <10 mmol/l after 2 weeks, withhold insulin and continue monitoring
- If BG starts increasing again, restart insulin at 1 IU q12h
- Insulin should not be withdrawn within 2 weeks of starting glargine because the beta cells need time to recover

Monitoring urine glucose

Once the appropriate dose of glargine is being administered there should be minimal glycosuria, so longer-term control can be monitored using urine glucose assessments

14.7 Basic guidelines for insulin glargine use. (More detailed information can be found at http://www.uq.edu.au/ccah/docs/diabetesinfo/link4.pdf and www.thecatclinic.com.au/info-for-vets/using-glargine-in-diabetic-cats-2/)

Oral hypoglycaemic agents: The use of these drugs (e.g. glipizide) is generally no longer recommended. Resolution of diabetes is possible with insulin injections, as these reverse glucose toxicity; in contrast, oral hypoglycaemic drugs merely stimulate more insulin production from the pancreas, which is often associated with amylin deposition in the pancreas, leading to an irreversible state.

Diet: Cats have different nutritional requirements from dogs, and this also translates into different dietary management of the feline diabetic patient compared to the canine diabetic patient (Figure 14.8); wet prescription high-protein, low-carbohydrate diets are most appropriate for diabetic cats. Dry diets tend to be higher in carbohydrate than wet diets; therefore if the cat will not tolerate a high-protein, low-carbohydrate diet, changing from a proprietary dry diet to a wet food may be of some benefit.

Dietary management	Rationale
Dogs	
Feed two meals per day	Fed just before insulin therapy to enable maximal insulin effect at time of post-prandial peak in blood glucose
Feed a high-fibre diet	High-fibre diet slows intestinal transit time, thereby slowing glucose absorption from gut; fibre should be insoluble or mixed solubility
Cats	
'Graze' meals throughout day	More natural feeding behaviour for cats; several small meals maintains a more stable glucose throughout day. Disadvantage: cats may over-eat, contributing to obesity
Feed a high-protein, low-carbohydrate diet (wet preferable to dry)	Cats do not find high-fibre diets palatable. Cats are less likely to develop postprandial hyperglycaemia; cats have low levels of glucokinase enzymes involved in carbohydrate utilization. Cats have a higher requirement than dogs for dietary protein; arginine and other amino acids act as insulin secretagogues. Wet diets are lower in carbohydrate than the equivalent dry diets

14.8 Differences in the dietary management of diabetes in cats and dogs.

Concurrent disease management: Any concurrent diseases that have been identified should be treated. If patients are taking potentially diabetogenic drugs (e.g. glucocorticoids, progestogens) for concurrent illnesses, these should be withdrawn, or reduced to as low a dose as possible. Change of formulation, e.g. changing asthmatic cats on to inhaled steroids, may reduce systemic effects.

Monitoring: Decreasing thirst and urination, and normalization of appetite, may be monitored by the owner; indeed, improvement in clinical signs associated with DM is a good indicator of treatment efficacy. In addition, bodyweight should be optimized. Owners should be aware of the potential for resolution of DM in cats, which may manifest as episodes of weakness, ataxia, stupor or lethargy, associated with hypoglycaemia (see QRG 4.5.1 for treatment of hypoglycaemia).

Fructosamine can be assessed after 2–3 weeks on insulin. Ideally, fructosamine measurements should be within the reference range, but values slightly above the reference range usually indicate good diabetic control.

Blood glucose curves may be employed in management, but the reasons for obtaining them and the associated problems should be borne in mind (Figure 14.9). Teaching the owner to obtain a blood glucose curve at home may be more reliable in cats that become very stressed. Ear vein blood sampling can help with this, both in the hospitalized cat and for the owner at home (see QRG 14.2).

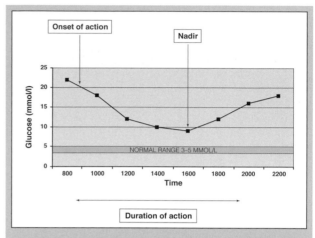

- Onset of action = The point at which blood glucose starts to fall in response to the effect of insulin (usually 30–120 minutes after insulin administration).
- Nadir = The lowest blood glucose value (equates to peak effect); should not be <5 mmol/l.
- Duration of action = Time from onset of effect of insulin to point at which blood glucose >15 mmol/l; should be 8–14 hours for insulin that is administered twice daily.

Limitations
- Sample points should not really be joined together as it is not known what is happening between these times.
- Day-to-day variation is a recognized problem.
- Continuously high values may represent:
  - Stress hyperglycaemia
  - Insulin resistance
  - Failure to administer insulin correctly
  - Somogyi overswing – this is a rebound hyperglycaemia following either a rapid fall in blood glucose levels or the development of hypoglycaemia. It is often sustained for more than 36 hours, and occasionally for up to 3 days. If suspected, insulin should be withdrawn and then reinstated at a lower dose, e.g. 50% of previous dose or 0.5 IU/kg.

Information that can be gained
- Is there a response to insulin?
- Is the nadir too low? Patient at risk of hypoglycaemia.
- Is the duration of action too short? Change to a longer-acting insulin.
- Is the duration of action too long? Risk of a Somogyi overswing with cumulative dose; change to a shorter-acting preparation or decrease frequency of administration.

14.9 Blood glucose curves.

Monitoring of urine may be helpful to identify the presence of ketones (e.g. unstable patients), or consistently low or negative glucose results that may indicate the onset of diabetic remission or too high an insulin dose. However, urine glucose levels should *not* be used to adjust the insulin dose.

Ketoacidotic diabetic cats

Diabetic ketoacidosis (DKA) is diagnosed by demonstrating the presence of hyperglycaemia and ketonuria/ketonaemia together with acidosis and the presence of accompanying clinical signs such as anorexia, vomiting, lethargy, dehydration and shock. DKA must be distinguished from ketosis (without acidosis), where the cat has ketonuria/ketonaemia but is clinically well. Such cats are treated as 'normal' unstable diabetics, whereas cats with DKA require aggressive treatment. A detailed discussion of the management of the ketoacidotic diabetic is beyond the scope of this book, but a basic summary of the management considerations is given in Figure 14.10.

Further information can be found in the *BSAVA Manual of Canine and Feline Endocrinology*.

Unstable diabetic cats

Management of the unstable diabetic cat, requiring >2 IU/kg insulin per dose, is beyond the scope of this book, but primarily centres around ensuring adequate insulin storage and administration and ruling out concurrent disease states (e.g. urinary tract infections, hyperadrenocorticism, acromegaly, hyperthyroidism,

---

Fluid therapy

Initially, 0.9% sodium chloride at 2–3 times maintenance rate, depending on hydration status. If severely dehydrated, replace 50% of the estimated deficit over 2–4 hours, then the remainder over the following 24 hours, in addition to meeting the ongoing requirements (with the inevitable increased requirements resulting from the obligatory polyuria).

Potassium

Despite cats often having normal serum potassium concentrations, whole-body potassium is usually depleted and, once therapy for DKA is started, there is usually a dramatic drop in blood potassium levels (as insulin pushes potassium into cells). If serum potassium concentration is <3.5 mmol/l, supplement intravenous fluids with potassium chloride. The amount of potassium supplementation required depends on serum potassium concentration, which should be monitored every 4 hours.

Serum K+	KCl required in 1 litre of 0.9% NaCl
<2.0 mmol/l	80 mmol
2.0–2.5 mmol/l	60 mmol
2.5–3.0 mmol/l	40 mmol
3.0–3.5 mmol/l	30 mmol

If serum potassium concentration is unable to be measured, 30 mmol/l potassium chloride can be added safely when starting DKA therapy, since a drop in serum potassium will be expected. Rate of potassium administration should not exceed 0.5 mmol/kg/h (see QRG 4.6.1).

Phosphate

Serum phosphate concentrations often dramatically reduce when DKA treatment is started (severe reduction may cause intravascular haemolysis). Serum phosphate concentration should be monitored carefully every 6 hours, and fluids supplemented if necessary. A dose of 0.01–0.03 mmol/kg/h potassium phosphate in 0.9% saline can be infused, but supplementation is most practically achieved by administering 50% of potassium requirements as potassium chloride and 50% as potassium phosphate (e.g. 15 mmol/l KCl and 15 mmol/l K_3PO_4).

Acid–base status

If facilities are available, acid–base status should be monitored every 4–6 hours. If pH is <7.1 following rehydration, sodium bicarbonate can be carefully administered to correct the acidosis but this is rarely required; further details on bicarbonate therapy can be found in the *BSAVA Manual of Canine and Feline Endocrinology*.

Insulin therapy

Regular/neutral/soluble insulin is usually only started after 2–4 hours of fluid therapy, as fluid therapy alone may reduce glucose concentrations and affect electrolyte concentrations. Insulin may be given as an intravenous CRI (prepared and administered in a different fluid bag and port to that providing fluid for rehydration/potassium/phosphate) or by intermittent intramuscular or intravenous injection.

Constant rate infusion	Intermittent injection
1.1 IU/kg in 250 ml 0.9% NaCl Flush 50 ml through drip line Rate dependent on blood glucose: 　>14 mmol/l = 10 ml/h 　11–14 mmol/l = 7 ml/h 　5.5–10.9 mmol/l = 5 ml/h 　<5.5 mmol/l = stop insulin Administer separately from fluid therapy Change insulin solution q6h	0.2 IU/kg i.m. or i.v. as an initial dose Then 0.1 IU/kg i.m. or i.v. every hour until blood glucose approaches 14 mmol/l Then change to 0.1–0.3 IU/kg i.m. or i.v. q4–6h

The aim of the insulin therapy is to cause a gradual decline in blood glucose concentration by about 3–4 mmol/l per hour until it is <14 mmol/l. When BG is <14 mmol/l, the intravenous fluids should be changed from saline to 5% dextrose saline, continuing to provide insulin as described above.
Once the patient is well hydrated, eating, and the acidosis has resolved, the insulin can be changed to a subcutaneous formulation with a longer duration of action (e.g. Caninsulin; see Figure 14.6). This will only need to be administered q8–12h.

Additional treatment

DKA may be precipitated by a concurrent disorder causing insulin resistance (e.g. pancreatitis, glucocorticoid administration, bacterial infections). Bacterial infections are common and it is therefore advisable, after collecting urine for culture, to initiate broad-spectrum antibiotics if no other precipitating cause is evident.

14.10 Management of diabetic ketoacidosis.

pancreatitis) causing insulin resistance. Further information can be found in the *BSAVA Manual of Canine and Feline Endocrinology*.

References and further reading

Fleeman L and Rand J (2006) Options for monitoring diabetic cats. In: *Consultations in Feline Internal Medicine, Volume 5*, ed. JR August, pp. 183–190. Elsevier Saunders, St. Louis

Graves T (2010) Hyperthyroidism and the kidneys. In: *Consultations in Feline Internal Medicine, Volume 6*, ed. JR August, pp. 268–273. Elsevier Saunders, St. Louis

Lurye J (2006) Update on treatment of hyperthyroidism. In: *Consultations in Feline Internal Medicine, Volume 5*, ed. JR August, pp. 199–205. Elsevier Saunders, St. Louis

Mooney C and Peterson M (2012) *BSAVA Manual of Canine and Feline Endocrinology, 4th edn*. BSAVA Publications, Gloucester

Peterson M (2006) Diagnostic methods for hyperthyroidism. In: *Consultations in Feline Internal Medicine, Volume 5*, ed. JR August, pp. 191–198. Elsevier Saunders, St. Louis

Peterson M (2009) Radioiodine for feline hyperthyroidism. In: *Kirk's Current Veterinary Therapy XIII*, ed. JD Bonagura and DC Twedt, pp. 180–184. Elsevier Saunders, St. Louis

Rand J (2009) Feline diabetes mellitus In: *Kirk's Current Veterinary Therapy XIII*, ed. JD Bonagura and DC Twedt, pp. 199–204. Elsevier Saunders, St. Louis

Reusch C and Sieber-Ruckstuhl N (2010) Home monitoring of blood glucose in cats with diabetes mellitus. In: *Consultations in Feline Internal Medicine, Volume 6*, ed. JR August, pp. 274–285. Elsevier Saunders, St. Louis

Rios L and Ward C (2008) Feline diabetes mellitus: diagnosis, treatment and monitoring *Compendium on Continuing Education for Veterinarians (Small Animal)* **30**, 626–640

Rios L and Ward C (2008) Feline diabetes mellitus: Pathophysiology and risk factors. *Compendium on Continuing Education for Veterinarians (Small Animal)* **30(12)**, E1–E7 [available at www.vetlearn.com/compendium]

Scott-Moncrieff JC (2010) Insulin resistance in cats. *Veterinary Clinics of North America: Small Animal Practice* **40(2)**, 241–257

Shiel R and Mooney C (2007) Testing for hyperthyroidism in cats. *Veterinary Clinics of North America: Small Animal Practice* **37(4)**, 671–692

Syme H (2007) Cardiovascular and renal manifestations of hyperthyroidism *Veterinary Clinics of North America: Small Animal Practice* **37(4)**, 723–744

Trepanier L (2007) Pharmacologic management of feline hyperthyroidism *Veterinary Clinics of North America: Small Animal Practice* **37(4)**, 775–789

QRG 14.1 Intracapsular thyroidectomy with preservation of the cranial parathyroid gland
by Geraldine Hunt

Surgical excision may be the best treatment option available to many hyperthyroid patients. The frequency with which it is performed varies substantially from one part of the world to another, being more frequently performed where availability of radioactive iodine is lower.

Advantages of surgery:
- Can be performed in general veterinary practice
- Provides a high chance of long-term cure.

Disadvantages:
- Requires general anaesthesia in patients that may have compromised cardiac and renal function. Patients requiring removal of both thyroid glands will experience hypoparathyroidism if at least one of the parathyroid glands is not preserved
- The thyroid glands are also situated close to the carotid artery, vagosympathetic trunk and recurrent laryngeal nerve; so care must be taken to avoid damaging these structures
- There is a risk that euthyroidism may not be achieved if ectopic hyperfunctional thyroid tissue is present, which may be the case in as many as 10–15% of hyperthyroid cats.

Preoperative evaluation

Patients undergoing surgical thyroidectomy should be carefully evaluated for cardiovascular and renal disease. Ideally, they should be placed on methimazole or carbimazole (see main chapter text) in order to stabilize their condition prior to the procedure, and attenuate the effects of hyperthyroidism that might increase anaesthetic risk.

Equipment

- A delicate instrument pack:
  - Babcock forceps (A)
  - Sterile Q-tips (B)
  - Small Metzenbaum scissors (C)
  - Small Debakey forceps (D)
  - Right-angled dissection forceps (E)
  - Gelpi retractors (F)

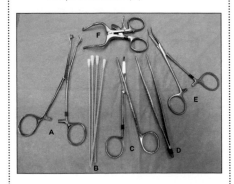

- Specialized instruments:
  - A flat spay hook
  - Small haemoclip applicator and cartridge (A)
  - Small Poole suction nozzle (B)

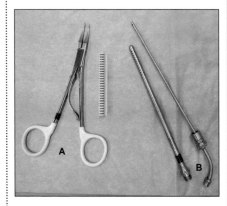

Patient preparation

Anaesthetize the cat and set up anaesthesia monitoring equipment (see Chapter 3). Clip and surgically prepare the ventral neck from the chin to the manubrium sternum.

▶

QRG 14.1 *continued*

Procedure

1 Position the patient in dorsal recumbency with the neck extended over a small sandbag. Start the surgery by making a ventral midline skin incision, starting 1 cm caudal to the hyoid bone and finishing 2 cm cranial to the manubrium sternum, and incise the platysma muscle (as shown) with fine scissors.

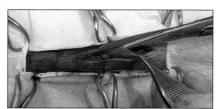

The cat's head is to the left.

2 Continue the dissection through the loose connective tissue between the paired bellies of the sternohyoideus muscles, using Metzenbaum scissors.

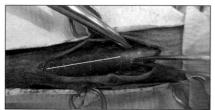

The white line demonstrates the position of the incision between the paired sternohyoideus muscles.

3 Continue the dissection through the loose peritracheal fascial connective tissue on either side of the trachea, using right-angled dissecting forceps. Dissection should be in a craniocaudal plane, rather than a transverse plane, to avoid damaging the delicate recurrent laryngeal nerve.

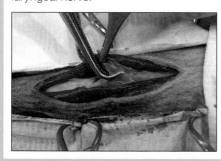

4 Retraction of the tissues is achieved with Gelpi forceps retractors (shown cranial and caudal to the site being dissected). The tissues should be moistened regularly with sterile saline. Retract the trachea using a flat spay hook. The loose connective tissue around the thyroid gland will then become apparent.

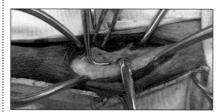

5 Careful dissection reveals the external (cranial) parathyroid gland as a pale, disk-like structure (arrowed) attached to the cranial capsule of the darker (red) thyroid gland. A small branch from the cranial thyroid artery penetrates the cranial parathyroid, and this must be identified and preserved.

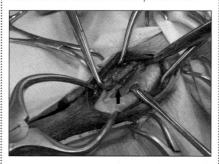

6 Dissect the cranial parathyroid gland from the thyroid capsule, while maintaining its vascular attachment (arrowed).

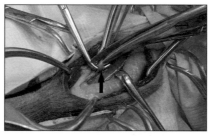

7 The blood supply to the thyroid gland is then ligated cranially and caudally with 1.5 metric (4/0 USP) monofilament absorbable suture material, or surgical haemoclips, and the thyroid is separated from the parathyroid gland and removed. The parathyroid gland is returned to its original position.

For thyroid carcinomas, where local invasion is accompanied by ingrowth of blood vessels, it may be necessary to use bipolar cautery or to ligate additional blood vessels, but for cats with thyroid adenomatous hyperplasia there should only be two vessels for which haemostasis is required.

8 The surgeon may choose either to remove both thyroids at once, or to perform this procedure in two stages. Results for a single-stage procedure are very good, as long as one of the cranial parathyroid glands can be preserved. The excised thyroid gland(s) should be submitted for histopathology. Calcium monitoring in the postoperative period is critical if bilateral thyroidectomy is undertaken.

9 Check the surgical site for haemorrhage; apply lavage and suction to the site and remove the retractors.

10 Re-appose the paired bellies of the sternohyoideus muscles using a continuous pattern and 1.5 metric (4/0 USP) polydioxanone, and suture the subcutis likewise. Subcuticular or skin sutures may be placed to complete the closure, according to the surgeon's preference.

Postoperative considerations

Postoperative analgesia should be provided; 24–48 hours of an opioid such as buprenorphine is usually adequate (see Chapter 3).

Cats should be monitored postoperatively for at least 3 days for hypocalcaemia if bilateral thyroidectomy has been performed, even in the absence of clinical signs of hypocalcaemia (e.g. muscle twitches/tremors, hypersensitivity to stimuli (sound/touch), ataxia, tetany, seizure, dullness/disorientation; see Chapter 4.4). Blood calcium concentrations should be measured once to twice daily.

Total T4 concentration, renal function (urea, creatinine, urine SG), blood pressure and cardiovascular status should be rechecked at 2 weeks and 6 months after surgery.

QRG 14.2 Ear vein sampling for blood glucose determination

by Nicki Reed

Indications

- Evaluation of blood glucose in the hospitalized patient.
- Evaluation of blood glucose at home by the owner.

Contraindications

Ear vein sampling is contraindicated in patients with very bruised ear veins.

Advantages over cephalic/jugular venepuncture

- A smaller volume of blood is obtained, which is beneficial in anaemic patients or where frequent sampling is required.
- Sampling can often be performed single-handed.
- Cephalic/jugular veins are preserved.

Equipment and preparation

Gather together the glucometer and test strips, petroleum jelly (e.g. Vaseline) and a needle or stylet for venepuncture. Although a 25 G hypodermic needle can be used, owners particularly may find a stylet (shown here) easier to use. Any glucometer can be used, but an example of a veterinary glucometer that has been calibrated for animal use is the Alphatrak glucometer. Abbot also supply boxes of stylets, for use with the Alphatrak glucometer, as shown.

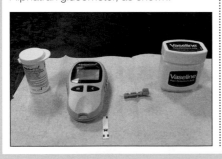

Position the cat so it is sitting on a towel or blanket, either on a table top or on the owner's lap.

Procedure

1 Identify the lateral ear vein. Clipping the fur from the lateral margin of the ear (using small, quiet clippers) may help with visualizing the vein (as shown) but is not usually necessary. Applying warm swabs to the ear may cause vasodilation, assisting with vein identification.

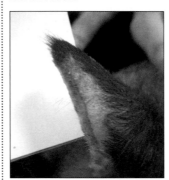

2 Apply a small amount of petroleum jelly; this will prevent the bleb of blood dissipating once obtained.

3 Prepare the glucometer: Insert a strip into the glucometer, ensuring codes are compatible if applicable.

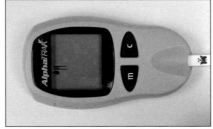

4 Immobilize the vein by applying pressure at the basal and proximal ends with your fingers; a swab may be wrapped around the fingers if there are concerns about piercing them with the

stylet. Pierce the vein with the stylet (as shown here) or small-gauge needle. A small bleb of blood should appear on the surface of the ear.

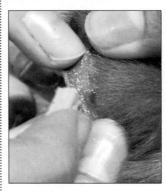

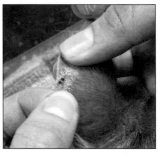

5 Touch the glucometer strip to the bleb of blood until the glucometer registers it has drawn up the blood sample. The glucometer and strip can then be moved away.

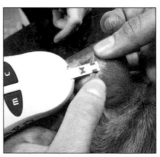

6 While waiting for the result, apply digital pressure to the lateral ear vein with a swab to stop the bleeding.

Management of reproduction and related disorders

Susan Little

This chapter will focus on the management of the most important issues related to reproduction in feline practice; notably, suppression of oestrus, and management of pregnancy, parturition and postpartum problems in the queen. Care of the neonate and management of common neonatal disorders are also discussed. The chapter finishes with a consideration of other disorders of the reproductive tract, such as ovarian remnant syndrome, mammary fibroadenomatous hyperplasia and pyometra. A practical QRG is provided on managing dystocia, and caesarean section is briefly described. Other sections of the book deal with aspects of preventive healthcare (see Chapter 2) including prepubertal neutering techniques. The reader is referred to the *BSAVA Manual of Canine and Feline Reproduction and Neonatology* for further detail.

Control of reproduction in the queen

Surgical neutering (ovariohysterectomy (OHE) and ovariectomy (OE)) is well described for the queen and is safely performed at or before the age of 16 weeks (see Chapter 2). In breeding animals, temporary control of reproduction may sometimes be desirable. Currently the safest and most effective method for non-surgical contraception in the queen is not known. The practitioner should select the method with the best safety profile from among the choices available.

Suppression of oestrus

Induction of ovulation

The simplest method of controlling oestrus is to induce ovulation; this delays return to oestrus by causing a pseudopregnancy that lasts on average 40–50 days.

- Mechanical stimulation of the vagina, using an instrument such as a glass rod or cotton-tipped swab, will induce ovulation in a queen in oestrus; this may need to be performed two or three times over an hour or two to be successful, and the operator should be aware that a post-coital response may be seen (vocalization, excessive and energetic grooming).
- A teaser tom (a vasectomized male or a castrated male with intact libido) can also be used to induce ovulation in queens in oestrus.
- Pharmacological treatment options for induction of ovulation (see Figure 15.1) include chorionic gonadotrophin (hCG) and gonadotrophin-releasing hormone (GnRH), which must be administered *during oestrus*.

> **WARNING**
>
> Repeated induction of pseudopregnancy by mechanical or pharmacological methods to induce oestrus may predispose queens to cystic endometrial hyperplasia (CEH)/pyometra.

Drugs suppressing oestrus

Drugs used for control of oestrus and reproduction in the queen, such as progestins, melatonin and deslorelin, are listed in Figure 15.1. Not all of these drugs are authorized for use in the cat and many either have undesirable side effects or have not been extensively evaluated in the cat so that their potential adverse effects are not well understood.

Drug	Dose	Comments
Chorionic gonadotrophin (hCG)	250–500 IU/cat i.m.	Administered in oestrus; effect lasts about 40–50 days
Gonadotrophin-releasing hormone (GnRH)	25 µg/cat i.m.	Administered in oestrus; effect lasts about 40–50 days
Megestrol	In pro-oestrus: 5 mg/cat orally q24h for 5 days, then q2wk In anoestrus: 2.5–5 mg/cat orally q1–2wk	Progestin; significant adverse effects (see text); best administered in anoestrus; oestrous suppression lasts for duration that treatment is given, but time to return to oestrus following cessation of treatment is very variable. If breeding is desired, wait for second oestrus following cessation of treatment

15.1 Drugs used for control of oestrus and reproduction in the queen. (continues) ▶

Drug	Dose	Comments
Medroxyprogesterone	25–100 mg/cat i.m., given no more frequently than every 3 months; alternatively, lower doses of 5 mg/cat can be given orally q7d	Progestin; significant adverse effects (see text); best administered in anoestrus; effect lasts 6–12 months for intramuscular injection, and for the duration of treatment with oral administration. Time to return to oestrus following cessation of treatment is very variable
Proligestone	100 mg/cat s.c., repeated after months 3 and 4, then every 5 months	Progestin; best administered in anoestrus; effect lasts about 6.5 months
Delmadinone	0.25–0.7 mg/kg orally q7d	Progestin; best administered in anoestrus; not widely used
Chlormadinone	2.5–5 mg/kg s.c. or i.m, every 6 months or 2 mg/cat orally q7d	Progestin; best administered in anoestrus; not widely used
Melatonin	18 mg subcutaneous implant beside umbilicus	Mimics decreasing photoperiod; effect lasts 2–4 months, longest when administered during interoestrus
Deslorelin	4.7 mg subcutaneous implant beside umbilicus	GnRH analogue; may be administered before puberty to delay onset; if administered during anoestrus, an initial stimulation of oestradiol release may occur; duration of effect variable

15.1 (continued) Drugs used for control of oestrus and reproduction in the queen.

Progestins:

- Megestrol is effective for suppressing oestrus in queens when started in *anoestrus*.
- Medroxyprogesterone is also most effective when started in *anoestrus*, and is a long-acting injectable progestin that is effective at suppressing oestrus when given every 6–12 months.
- Proligestone is another long-acting injectable progestin with weaker progestational activity than the other available drugs; at the authorized dose, oestrous suppression lasts about 6.5 months. While proligestone appears to be safer than other progestins, there are reports of adverse effects, such as hair loss and calcinosis circumscripta at the injection site.
- Chlormadinone and delmadinone have been reported as safe and effective for prevention of oestrus in queens when given by subcutaneous or intramuscular injection, or by mouth. These drugs are not widely available and information is scant.

Adverse effects of progestins are well known and include diabetes mellitus, uterine disease (CEH/pyometra) and infertility, adrenocortical suppression, polyuria, polydipsia, mammary hyperplasia and mammary neoplasia. In general, progestins are safest when started in anoestrus. Prolonged use should be avoided.

Drug implants: Melatonin implants, available in many countries in different strengths for treatment of adrenal disease in ferrets and for alopecia X in dogs, have been used for suppression of ovarian activity in cats. A single subcutaneous implant containing 18 mg melatonin has been shown to suppress oestrus effectively and reversibly for 2–4 months without adverse effects. The duration of effect is longer when treatment occurs during interoestrus than during oestrus.

Deslorelin is a GnRH agonist. Subcutaneous implants (4.7 mg/cat) are effective in inducing reversible suppression of oestrus, but the duration of suppression varies widely from cat to cat (ranging mostly from 5 to 14 months, but sometimes longer). If administered during anoestrus to a mature queen, an initial stimulation of secretion of luteinizing hormone (LH) and follicle-stimulating hormone (FSH) may induce oestrus before suppression. Deslorelin has also been shown to be effective in male cats. When male and

female kittens are implanted at 2–4 months of age, puberty may be delayed. No adverse effects have been noted.

While no guidelines have been developed to determine the best location for these implants, most commonly the implant is placed beside the umbilicus rather than between the scapulae in order to make removal easy should it be desired. Small animal formulations of melatonin and deslorelin implants may be placed without sedation in most patients.

Pregnancy

In cats, gestation normally lasts 65–67 days.

Diagnosis

Clinical signs

The failure of a queen to return to oestrus after breeding is one of the most obvious signs of pregnancy, but pseudopregnancy will produce the same effect. Pseudopregnancy may be caused by administration of progestins (see above) or by ovulation without conception, especially in queens >3 years. One of the first physical indications of pregnancy is 'pinking' of the nipples (Figure 15.2), which occurs around day 15–18 after mating. This change in the nipples, which become noticeably pinker and easier to see as the hair around them recedes somewhat and they increase in size, is most obvious in maiden queens.

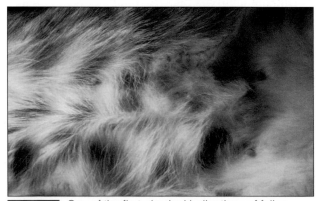

15.2 One of the first physical indications of feline pregnancy is 'pinking' of the nipples, which occurs approximately 15–18 days after ovulation.

Abdominal palpation

The developing fetuses can be palpated in the abdomen as early as 14–15 days after mating, but most easily at about 21–25 days. They remain distinctly palpable up to about 35 days, when the fetuses and placentas become large enough that they cannot easily be distinguished individually.

Hormonal assay

The hormone relaxin is produced primarily by the placenta and is therefore a useful marker for pregnancy. Relaxin levels increase in pregnancy but not in pseudopregnancy. An in-clinic test kit is available (Witness Relaxin, Synbiotics) that uses a small volume of plasma, and results are available in about 10 minutes. The kit is first able to detect pregnancy between days 20 and 25 of gestation. The test is estimated to have 100% sensitivity and 91% specificity after day 25 of gestation, with a positive predictive value of 93%. False positive results have been reported in queens with large ovarian cysts.

Radiography

Radiography may be used to detect pregnancy once fetal bones begin to mineralize, as early as 25–29 days before parturition. Until this time, only uterine enlargement (which may be due to other causes, such as pyometra) may be detected. There is a predictable sequence of radiographic fetal bone mineralization in cats, which is similar to that in dogs but begins about a week earlier in gestation. Prediction of the date of parturition to within 3 days is possible using references for bone mineralization. The most reliable indicators are mineralization of the femur (19–23 days before parturition) and the humerus (20–24 days). Radiography may also be used to determine the number of fetuses by counting the number of skulls present (Figure 15.3).

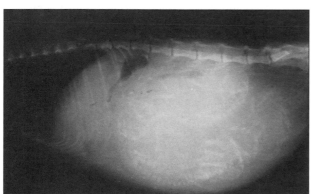

15.3 Radiography is useful for determining the number of fetuses present, by counting the number of skulls visible. This late-gestation queen is carrying five fetuses. (Reprinted from Little S (2012) *The Cat: Clinical Medicine and Management* with the permission of Elsevier.)

Ultrasonography

Ultrasonography is more sensitive than radiography in early pregnancy.

> ### PRACTICAL TIPS
> - The hair coat should be clipped prior to scanning. ▶

> ### PRACTICAL TIPS
> - Ideally, the queen should have a full bladder to move the bowel out of the way and also to move the uterine body out of the pelvic canal so that it is more readily imaged.
> - It also helps to fast the queen for 12 hours before the examination so that intestinal gas is less likely to obscure the views, especially in early pregnancy.

The gestational sac, a spherical anechoic structure slightly compressed at the pole, can be detected at 11–14 days post-mating, and the embryo at 15–17 days post-mating. Pregnancy diagnosis with ultrasonography is 99% accurate at 28 days post-mating. From day 30, it is possible to identify fetal organs. Details on the time of ultrasound appearance of various fetal and extrafetal structures in the cat have been published (Zambelli *et al.*, 2002).

A benefit of ultrasonography is the ability to determine fetal viability by detecting a beating heart (about 16 days post-mating) and fetal movement (about 32 days post-mating). Early fetal death is also identifiable, as scans performed on consecutive days will show that the gestational sacs decrease in size. However, ultrasonography may not be as good as radiography for determining the number of fetuses present. Prediction of gestational age and date of parturition are possible, to within 1–2 days, using ultrasonogram measurements (in centimetres) of fetal head diameter (HD) or body diameter (BD). This can be performed by practitioners with good ultrasonographic skills and equipment, or by a board-certified radiologist or theriogenologist.

> - Gestational age (GA) in days =
>   - $25 \times HD + 3$
>   - *or* $11 \times BD + 21$
> - Days before parturition = $61 - GA$

Care of the pregnant queen

> - The mean length of pregnancy in the queen is 65–67 days, but it is highly variable.
> - Length of pregnancy is influenced by:
>   - Breed (longest in Siamese and Oriental breeds)
>   - Litter size (larger litters are associated with shorter gestations).
> - Normal pregnancies lasting <54 days or >74 days are rare and are often associated with high neonatal mortality.

Unlike most other mammals, the queen gains weight linearly from conception to parturition; mean weight gain during pregnancy is approximately 40% of the cat's bodyweight pre-breeding. Energy intake also increases linearly. At parturition, only 40% of the total weight gained during pregnancy is lost; the remainder is used for milk production. High-quality diets designed for growth or reproduction and lactation are appropriate for the pregnant queen; excessive weight gain should be avoided both before and during pregnancy (see QRG 2.1).

During pregnancy the queen should not be exposed to new or sick cats, to prevent transmission of infectious diseases. There is no need to restrict activity, although most queens become less active and eat smaller meals more frequently during the last trimester, due to rapid uterine enlargement. During the last 2 weeks of gestation, the queen should be isolated from all other cats and provided with a safe, quiet maternity area for delivery. Stressors (e.g. small children, other pets) should be avoided due to detrimental effects on normal labour and delivery and on maternal behaviour. A nest box should be provided that is lined with absorbent material that can be laundered (e.g. towels or blankets) or that is disposable (e.g. disposable nappies or pads).

WARNING

The use of medications in a pregnant or lactating cat must be carefully considered in light of potential benefits *versus* potential risks. Most medications have not been specifically tested in pregnant or lactating queens, so information may be scant about the safety of a given drug.

Signs of impending parturition

Monitoring rectal temperature twice daily, starting at day 61, can be used to detect impending labour, although it may not be completely reliable. Labour typically begins within 12–24 hours of a temperature drop of one full degree Celsius (usually to about 37.5°C or less).

Another sign that active labour will begin within 24–48 hours is the presence of milk in the mammary glands, although in some queens milk comes in up to 8 days before delivery of the litter.

Some queens may not eat for up to 24 hours before active labour begins.

In contrast to puppies, the heart rate of fetal kittens is stable throughout pregnancy.

Parturition

Stages of normal labour

Stage 1: The cervix dilates and the uterus starts contracting. This stage may last for a few hours or for as long as 24 hours. Queens may be restless, exhibit overgrooming, pacing, panting, or even vomiting. No visible contractions are seen, although there may be a clear mucous discharge from the vagina. As the end of stage 1 approaches, most queens will settle in the nest box, purr loudly and scratch around to prepare the box. The location where the queen will give birth should be warm enough to prevent chilling of neonatal kittens (i.e. 27–32°C). ▶

Stage 2: The kitten is delivered. The time from the start of active stage 2 labour to the birth of the first kitten is usually <60 minutes. Strong, visible uterine contractions deliver each kitten from its uterine horn, into the uterine body and through the cervix and vagina. The queen can be seen bearing down, but crying out is uncommon. Both head-first (2/3 of births) and hindquarters-first (1/3 of births) presentations are normal. Presentation of the tail and rump before the hindlegs is a more difficult delivery but can still be accomplished without intervention. Kittens are typically born within the amniotic sac, and the queen will bite through the amniotic membrane and the umbilical cord and lick the kitten to stimulate breathing.

Stage 3: The placenta is delivered. The queen may or may not eat the placentas; there is no evidence that this is necessary.

The delivery of the litter is a series of stage 2 and stage 3 labours. Once delivery begins, kittens are generally born every 30–60 minutes. Average delivery time for an entire litter is highly variable (range 4–42 hours) although <2% of queens require >24 hours. In extended deliveries, the queen may rest and nurse the kittens already born for a period of time before delivery resumes. Since stage 2 and 3 labours happen concurrently in the queen, delivery of kittens is interspersed with delivery of placentas.

Problems during parturition

If kittens are born in rapid succession, the queen may not be able to clear membranes from each kitten or sever the umbilical cords promptly. This may also be a problem for inexperienced queens delivering their first litter. Occasionally, kittens may die while they are still inside the amniotic sac, or several kittens may become entwined via the umbilical cords as they crawl around the nest box. Entrapment of a distal limb by umbilical cord can result in significant injury.

Gentle, calm intervention is necessary to ensure survival and prevention of injury in these situations. The amniotic membranes should be removed by hand and each kitten should be carefully cleaned and dried using a clean towel. The umbilical cord may be clamped, ligated and transected about 2 inches from the kitten's body wall. Kittens should be kept warm and safe until the queen can attend to them.

Dystocia is defined as a painful, slow, or difficult delivery. It is not always easy to differentiate normal parturition from dystocia in the queen, as prolonged time between the births of kittens is normal in a small percentage of cases. Veterinary surgeons may intercede in some cases where queens would have delivered normally if left alone; thorough evaluation of the queen and fetuses can help avoid unnecessary intervention. Diagnosing and managing dystocia, including caesarean section, is discussed in QRG 15.1.

Postpartum care of the queen

Most queens begin eating within 24 hours of delivery and should be fed a diet intended for reproduction and lactation, or growth. Fresh water should be provided *ad libitum*. Many queens are reluctant to leave the nest box for more than a few minutes at a time during the first week. The owner should ensure that the queen has easy access to a litter box as well as to food and water, and the queen should be monitored for adequate nutritional intake.

Postpartum discharge (lochia) is typically scant in the queen. Since the queen cleans her vulva frequently, it may not even be noticed by the owner. Uterine involution is virtually complete by 28 days postpartum (earlier than in the bitch). The queen should be monitored for signs of abnormal vulvar discharge (which could indicate metritis) or mammary discharge (which could indicate mastitis), fever, anorexia or neglect of the kittens (all of which could be signs of any systemic illness).

Management of postpartum problems

Metritis

Metritis, a bacterial infection of the postpartum uterus, is caused by bacteria ascending from the vagina into a compromised uterus and is most likely to occur in the first week postpartum. Risk factors include dystocia, obstetric manipulation, dead fetuses and retained placentas. Clinical signs include fever, anorexia, lethargy, purulent or sanguineous vaginal discharge and neglect of kittens. Haematology typically shows leucocytosis with a left shift (although occasionally leucopenia is seen). The most common bacteria involved are *Escherichia coli*, staphylococci or streptococci. Cytology of the vaginal discharge shows degenerate neutrophils with intracellular bacteria. Abdominal radiographs or ultrasound images can detect dead fetuses, retained placentas or an enlarged uterus.

Prompt and aggressive treatment is indicated. Broad-spectrum antibiotic therapy should be initiated for all patients and can be adjusted based on the results of culture and sensitivity testing of vaginal discharge. Appropriate initial choices include a combination of amoxicillin/clavulanate and a fluoroquinolone. *If the queen is nursing kittens, it is safest to avoid fluoroquinolones and use only amoxicillin/clavulanate.* However, the queen may be too ill to nurse kittens and hand-rearing may be required. If the queen is not intended for breeding, OHE can be performed once she is stable or the kittens are weaned. Antibiotic therapy should be continued for up to 4 weeks, or for at least 10 days if OHE is performed as treatment.

For breeding queens, uterine evacuation is indicated if the uterus is not friable and thin-walled and no retained fetuses or fetal membranes are present on ultrasound examination. If there is doubt about the integrity of the uterine wall or if retained fetal tissues are present, OHE may be the best treatment option.

Oxytocin (0.5–1.0 IU/cat i.m. q30min for 1–2 doses) is only effective within 24 hours postpartum. After that time uterine oxytocin receptors are no longer present and other drug choices for uterine evacuation should be used; these include prostaglandin F2α (dinoprost tromethamine, 0.1–0.2 mg/kg s.c.) or cloprostenol (1–2 µg/kg s.c.) every 12–24 hours to effect (it can take several days to evacuate the uterus). *Uterine evacuation is not recommended in severely ill queens.*

The queen's condition should be stabilized with fluid therapy and broad-spectrum antibiotic therapy before either medical treatment or OHE.

Mastitis

Mastitis is inflammation and infection of lactating mammary glands and is typically caused by *E. coli*, staphylococci or streptococci. Bacteria most commonly ascend into the gland via the nipple due to poor hygiene or trauma, although haematogenous spread is possible. Clinical signs include swelling and pain in one or more glands, fever, anorexia, depression, and neglect of kittens. In severe cases, abscessation and necrosis of skin and tissue may occur. Cytology of milk from an affected gland will show degenerate neutrophils containing bacteria. Broad-spectrum antibiotic therapy for 2–4 weeks using drugs that are safe for neonates (e.g. amoxicillin/clavulanate or cefalexin) is recommended. Analgesia can be accomplished with an opioid such as buprenorphine. Warm compresses may also be helpful. If abscessation has occurred, surgical lancing and flushing with saline to establish drainage is required. Large ruptured abscesses are managed as open wounds. If the mastitis is diagnosed early, kittens may be allowed to continue nursing, as long as the queen is not too uncomfortable. In more severe cases the kittens must be removed from the queen and hand-raised.

Managing neonatal problems

The neonatal period is often defined as the first 4 weeks of life.

Normal neonates

- Normal body temperature for newborn kittens is 36–37°C; rectal temperature rises slowly thereafter, reaching 38°C by about 4 weeks of age. For the first 2 weeks of life kittens are essentially poikilothermic and lack a shiver reflex. They then become homeothermic but are still susceptible to environmental conditions and may become hypothermic easily.
- Neonates have a higher heart rate than adult cats; normal neonatal heart rate is >200 beats/min (range 220–260).
- Normal respiratory rate is 10–18 breaths/min in the first week of life and 15–35 breaths/min in kittens aged 1–4 weeks.
- The typical kitten birth weight is 90–110 g (range 80–140 g), although there is considerable variation between and within pedigree breeds. Healthy neonates have a strong suckle reflex, though less vigorous that that of a neonatal puppy. Normal kittens gain 50–100 g per week (10–15 g/day) and should double their birth weight before 2 weeks of age.
- The deciduous incisors (I) and canines (C) appear at 3–4 weeks of age, and the deciduous premolars (PM) erupt at about 5–6 weeks. The dental formula for deciduous teeth is 2 [I3(upper)/3(lower), C1/1, PM3/2]; there are no deciduous molars.

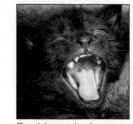

Deciduous incisors and canines appear at about 3–4 weeks of age. (Courtesy of Chantal Bourdon)

- Important developmental milestones include:
  - Umbilical cord remnant falls off at 3 days
  - Eyes open at an average of 7–10 days (range 2–16 days)
  - Crawling starts at 7–14 days
  - Voluntary elimination starts at 3 weeks
  - Uncoordinated walking by 21 days; coordinated walking by 28 days
  - Menace and pupillary light reflexes develop after 28 days
  - Adult eye colour appears at 4–6 weeks.

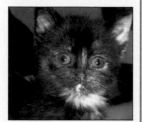

Kittens have blue irises until the adult eye colour appears at 4–6 weeks of age. (Courtesy of Chantal Bourdon)

Congenital defects

Congenital defects are abnormalities of structure, function or metabolism that are present at birth. Many congenital defects are cosmetic or minor, while others may cause serious impairment of health or death. Congenital defects may be of various types:

- Obvious at birth, e.g. cleft palate
- Found only with diagnostic testing or at necropsy, e.g. diaphragmatic hernia
- Subtle abnormalities found only with sophisticated testing, e.g. lysosomal storage diseases.

Common congenital defects in kittens that may be detected at birth include:

- Umbilical hernia
- Gastroschisis (abdominal hernia)
- Tarsal hyperextension
- Syndactyly
- Chest wall defects (e.g. flat chest, pectus excavatum)
- Cryptorchidism
- Cleft palate
- Atresia ani and anogenital fistula.

Congenital defects may be heritable, and the inheritance pattern or mutation(s) responsible may or may not be known. Non-heritable causes of congenital defects include:

- Infectious disease (e.g. feline panleucopenia virus infection as a cause of cerebellar hypoplasia)
- Drugs (e.g. griseofulvin as a cause of cleft palate)
- Inadequate intrauterine environment for the fetus, such as the presence of CEH/pyometra complex
- Nutritional factors (e.g. taurine deficiency as a cause of neurological abnormalities)
- Chromosomal abnormalities (e.g. pseudohermaphroditism)
- Chemicals, environmental toxins.

In some cases defects may be caused by interplay of both environmental and genetic factors. When pedigree breeders encounter a congenital defect where no information is available on heritability, several factors can be evaluated. A defect is more likely to be heritable if there is evidence of a breed or familial predisposition and the problem has a consistent age of onset and clinical course. A defect is less likely to be heritable if more than one abnormality occurs in a kitten or a litter or there is potential exposure to teratogens. A fact sheet ('What to do if your cat produces a deformed kitten') has been produced by the Feline Advisory Bureau to advise breeders on steps to take when a defect is observed (available at www.fabcats.org).

Common clinical problems of young kittens

Rapid identification of illness and prompt intervention are necessary for treating sick kittens. It is important to note that there is no 'fading kitten syndrome'. Rather, the specific cause of illness should be identified whenever possible to allow for more effective, targeted treatment.

Common causes of illness in young kittens include:

- Low birth weight
- Congenital defects
- Neonatal isoerythrolysis (see Chapter 5.4)
- Maternal neglect
- Environmental effects (e.g. inappropriate temperature and humidity, poor ventilation, overcrowding)
- Trauma
- Infectious diseases
- Inadequate nutrition.

Every sick kitten should be evaluated for three common clinical problems: hypothermia; hypoglycaemia; and dehydration.

Hypothermia

Severe hypothermia (rectal temperature <34.4°C) is associated with depressed respiration, impaired immune system function, bradycardia and ileus. Warming should occur slowly, over at least 3 hours, to a maximum rectal temperature that is age-appropriate (see box above). Rapid warming may cause increased metabolic demand and result in dehydration, hypoxia and loss of cardiovascular integrity. Various methods can be used for warming kittens, such as an incubator, oxygen cage, warm-air blower (e.g. Bair-Hugger), hot water bottle or heating lamp. Careful monitoring is always necessary. Severely hypothermic and dehydrated kittens can be treated with intravenous fluids warmed to 35–37°C.

> **WARNING**
>
> Feeding should be delayed until the kitten is warmed, as hypothermia causes gastrointestinal hypomotility that could result in regurgitation and aspiration pneumonia.

Hypoglycaemia

Hypoglycaemia (blood glucose <3 mmol/l) occurs easily in young kittens due to immature liver function and rapid depletion of glycogen stores. Causes of hypoglycaemia include vomiting, diarrhoea, sepsis, hypothermia, and inadequate nutritional intake (see Chapter 4.5). Clinical signs include weakness, lethargy, and anorexia.

Treatment: For kittens that are not dehydrated or hypothermic, 5–10% dextrose may be given by gastric tube (0.25–0.50 ml per 100 g bodyweight). When the kitten is stronger, it can be returned to the queen or fed with milk replacer. Critically ill kittens may be given an intravenous bolus of 10% dextrose (made by taking 0.2 ml of 50% dextrose and making it up to 1 ml with saline) slowly over 5–10 min (0.1–0.2 ml per 100 g bodyweight), followed by a constant rate infusion of 1.25–5% dextrose in a balanced electrolyte solution. Hypertonic dextrose solutions should not be administered subcutaneously as tissue sloughing may occur.

Dehydration

Dehydration may be caused by hypothermia, diarrhoea, vomiting, or inadequate nutritional intake. Young kittens have immature kidney function and poor compensatory mechanisms, coupled with higher fluid requirements than adults.

- Skin turgor is not always a reliable test of hydration in kittens <6 weeks of age, as their skin has decreased fat and increased water content compared with adult cats, so is less likely to tent.
- A well hydrated kitten has moist mucous membranes that are either slightly hyperaemic or pink. Pale mucous membranes and a slow capillary refill time (>3 seconds) indicate at least 10% dehydration.
- In dehydrated kittens, urine specific gravity will be >1.020; this is lower than that expected in a dehydrated adult cat (≥1.035), due to the kitten's immature renal function.

Fluid therapy:

> **Maintenance fluid rate for neonates =**
> 8–12 ml per 100 g bodyweight per day for oral, subcutaneous, intravenous and intraosseous routes.

Subcutaneous/oral: For kittens that are not hypothermic nor in shock or cardiovascular collapse, warmed subcutaneous fluids (e.g. lactated Ringer's solution) may be given, although absorption may be slow in young kittens. Warmed oral fluids may be given if there is no vomiting or diarrhoea. Amounts of fluids for subcutaneous or oral administration should be calculated on the basis of replacing losses plus ongoing maintenance needs.

Intravenous: Kittens that are moderately or severely dehydrated may be treated with warmed intravenous fluids. A slow (over 10–15 minutes) bolus of 1 ml per 30 g bodyweight is given, followed by maintenance plus replacement of ongoing losses. A balanced electrolyte solution should be used and 1.25–5% dextrose may be added if needed. A mini-set (60 drops/ml) is used with a fluid or syringe pump or a burette. The cephalic or jugular vein can be catheterized with a 24 G ¾-inch or 22 G 1-inch catheter.

Intraosseous: An alternative route for fluid administration in larger kittens (e.g. 4 weeks of age and older) if intravenous access is not possible is the intraosseous route, using the trochanteric fossa of the proximal femur. A 20–22 G 1-inch spinal needle or 18–25 G ⅝–1½-inch hypodermic needle can be used as an intraosseous catheter.

1. Clip and aseptically prepare the skin over the trochanteric fossa; local anaesthesia can be achieved with lidocaine or bupivacaine injected into the subcutaneous tissue and periosteum over the insertion site, medial to the trochanteric fossa.
2. Make a small skin incision using a No.11 scalpel blade and insert the intraosseous catheter. This is done with a to-and-fro rotary motion in line with the long axis of the femur and is usually relatively easy due to the soft nature of the bones. Resistance will lessen when the catheter is through the bone cortex and in the marrow cavity.
3. Advance the needle until the hub meets the skin. Verify correct positioning by moving the leg; the catheter will move with the femur.
4. Withdraw the stylet if using a spinal needle and attach an intravenous extension set.
5. Attempt to infuse 1 ml of heparinized saline to check patency. If infusion is not possible, try rotating the catheter 90 degrees as this will alleviate any blockage due to apposition of the catheter bevel to the inner bone cortex.
6. Apply antibiotic ointment and a light sterile dressing. Bandaging is typically not required.

Fluid administration in neonates and young kittens can be done using gravity flow or an infusion pump. Pain may be caused if cold fluids are administered, if a large volume is administered in a short time, or if alkaline or hypertonic solutions are administered (such as some drugs). Complications of intraosseous administration include infection, extravasation, and bone and soft tissue trauma.

Intraosseous catheters can be left in place for 72 hours (flush regularly q6h with heparinized saline to help avoid blockage) but they are rarely in place for long. Intravenous access should be established as soon as possible if ongoing fluid support will be required.

Monitoring: Fluid therapy should be monitored closely as it is easy to overhydrate young kittens due to immature renal tubular function. Monitoring methods include weighing the kitten three or four times per day and serial measurement of PCV and total protein. Electrolyte (e.g. sodium, chloride and potassium) and blood glucose status should also be monitored and deficits corrected. For venepuncture, position the kitten in dorsal recumbency with the forelegs drawn back toward the abdomen and the head and neck extended (see QRG 1.2). Blood can be drawn from the jugular vein using a 1 ml syringe with a 25 G or 26 G needle. Slow aspiration of blood is essential to avoid collapsing the vein. A small volume (0.5 ml) of blood in a microtainer tube can be used for the most critical tests.

Anaemia

Blood transfusions (see Chapter 20) may be required in kittens with anaemia due to fleas or intestinal parasites, or blood loss due to trauma. Indications for blood transfusion include weakness, tachycardia, pale mucous membranes, and PCV <15%. Blood from a compatible donor is diluted 9:1 with a citrate anticoagulant and given with a millipore filter. It may be administered either intravenously or intraosseously at a rate of 20 ml/kg over at least 2 hours.

Orphan kittens

Successful treatment of orphan kittens requires knowledge of the particular needs of these often fragile patients. If a foster queen is not available, the caregiver must replace the care normally provided by the queen, such as providing warmth and nutrition, facilitating elimination of urine and faeces, and ensuring cleanliness. Social stimulation should be provided by regular but brief periods of handling.

Accommodation

The ideal housing for orphan kittens is an incubator, but any warm and safe enclosure will suffice, such as a pet carrier or cardboard box. Bedding should be absorbent, soft, warm and either readily cleaned or disposable. The environmental temperature for kittens in the first week of life should be 30–32°C but this can be gradually lowered to 24°C over the next few weeks. If a heat source is used in a box or carrier, it should be placed so that a temperature gradient is created, allowing the kittens to move away from the warmest areas when needed. Humidity should be maintained at 55–60% to prevent dehydration and maintain the health of mucous membranes.

Protection against infectious diseases

This is important, especially if failure of passive transfer (FPT) of immunity is possible due to failure to ingest colostrum. Kittens with uncorrected FPT start to produce IgG at about 4 weeks of age; they are therefore most vulnerable to infection from birth to at least 6–8 weeks. Young orphans should not be exposed to older kittens or adults for social interaction until they are immunized. All bedding and equipment should be kept clean and caregivers should wash their hands before handling neonates. Vaccination of orphan kittens is often started between 6 and 8 weeks of age, with booster vaccinations every 3–4 weeks until 16 weeks of age. The earliest age for vaccination is generally recommended as 4 weeks. The choice of vaccine type (e.g. killed *versus* modified live) will be dependent on the environment, level of endemic disease, and risk of serious disease. In high-risk environments such as shelters, modified live vaccines are preferred.

Feeding

If a litter of kittens is orphaned, they will often try to nurse on each other; skin trauma or genital trauma, especially of the penis and prepuce, may occur if the kittens are not separated.

- The energy requirement for kittens in the first few weeks of life is approximately 20 kcal ME per 100 g bodyweight per day.
- The maintenance water requirement is about 180 ml/kg per day (range = 130–220 ml/kg/day).

Milk replacers: Orphan kittens should be fed a commercial milk replacer specifically designed for kittens to approximate the composition of the queen's milk. Homemade formulas are best reserved for short-term

or emergency use. The manufacturer's directions should be followed for mixing, storage and feeding quantities. Strict hygiene is necessary, and if milk replacer must be reconstituted, no more than a 48-hour supply should be prepared at a time. The reconstituted milk replacer can be divided into individual feedings and refrigerated until use. Reconstituted milk replacer should be warmed to 35–38°C before feeding by immersing the container in a warm water bath. Initially, only 50% of the recommended amount of milk replacer should be fed, to avoid inducing diarrhoea. Extra water or an oral electrolyte solution can be added to make up volume and provide fluid needs. Over several feedings, the concentration of the milk replacer can be increased to that recommended by the manufacturer.

> **WARNING**
>
> Never microwave milk replacer as overheating or uneven heating may result.

Bottle-feeding: Vigorous orphans with a good suck reflex may be bottle-fed or syringe-fed while in sternal recumbency with the head elevated, simulating a normal nursing position (Figure 15.4). The hole or slit in the nipple should be made large enough to allow a drop of milk to form when the bottle is held upside down. A drop of milk is expressed from the bottle on the kitten's tongue to help initiate feeding.

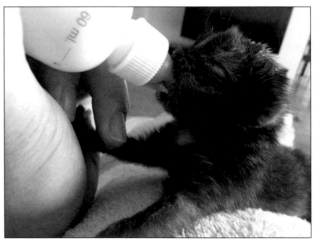

15.4 Kittens should be placed in sternal recumbency, with the head elevated to simulate a normal nursing position, when bottle-fed. (Courtesy of Chantal Bourdon)

> **WARNING**
>
> - Milk should never be forced out of the bottle while it is in the kitten's mouth, to avoid aspiration.
> - Care should be taken to ensure that no air is ingested while bottle-feeding, by keeping the bottle inverted.

Tube feeding: Weaker kittens are best fed using a gastric tube. Tube feeding is also more efficient if more than one kitten must be hand-raised. Feeding tubes should be selected according to the size of the kitten: 5 Fr for kittens <300 g; 8 Fr for kittens >300 g.

1. Measure from the tip of the kitten's nose to just before the last rib and mark this position on the feeding tube. The tube will have to be re-measured and marked weekly as the kitten grows.
2. With the kitten in a sternal position, the lubricated tube should pass easily down the left side of the mouth into the oesophagus, and is advanced to the mark. If resistance is felt or coughing occurs, the tube should be removed and repositioned. Kittens do not have a gag reflex until about 10 days of age.
3. Proper placement of the tube can be confirmed by instilling a small volume of saline first and assessing the response; if coughing occurs, remove the tube and start again.
4. The milk replacer is drawn up in a 3 or 10 ml syringe, which is then attached to the feeding tube. The tube is then filled with milk replacer warmed to about 38°C. The milk replacer is slowly infused over several minutes. Avoid overfeeding; the maximum stomach capacity for kittens is about 4–5 ml/100 g bodyweight.
5. Before withdrawing, the tube should be kinked to prevent aspiration of formula.
6. All tube feeding equipment should be cleaned thoroughly after use.

Feeding frequency, monitoring and other care: Kittens should be fed every 2–4 hours during the first week of life, and then every 4–6 hours until weaning. Diarrhoea is the most common problem seen in kittens fed milk replacer. It can be treated by temporarily reducing the amount fed and by diluting the formula by 50% with water or oral electrolyte solution for a few feedings. Orphan kittens should be weighed every 12 hours in the first 2 weeks of life, and at least daily thereafter to ensure that nutrition is adequate to support growth. Daily records should be kept of weight, feedings, elimination, and general behaviour.

Orphans <3 weeks of age must have the anogenital area stimulated after every feeding to induce defecation and urination. At least twice a week, orphan kittens should be cleaned gently with a soft moistened wash cloth.

Weaning: At 3–4 weeks of age, kittens can first be taught to drink milk replacer from a shallow saucer. Then solid food can be introduced by mixing a small amount of canned kitten food with milk replacer. Once the kitten has learned to eat from a saucer, the amount of formula fed can be slowly decreased until only solid food is being ingested. By 5–6 weeks of age, kittens are able to chew dry food. Weaning is usually completed by 6–8 weeks of age.

Disorders of the reproductive system

Ovarian remnant syndrome

Aetiology
Ovarian remnant syndrome (ORS) is the presence of functional ovarian tissue with signs of oestrus, caused by failure to remove all or part of an ovary at OHE or OE, or by revascularization of ovarian tissue inadvertently dropped into the abdomen during surgery.

Exposure of a pet to exogenous oestrogen via an owner's topically applied hormone product may produce similar clinical signs and should be ruled out.

Clinical features
Signs of oestrus may occur weeks to many years after surgery and include lordosis, vocalizing, rolling on the ground and receptivity to intact males.

Diagnosis
Diagnosis is most commonly made by observing signs of oestrus in a spayed cat, with vaginal cytology consistent with oestrus (Figure 15.5).

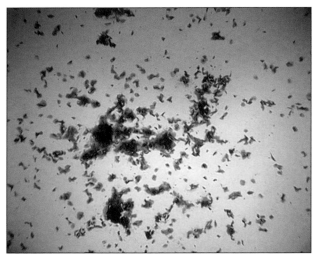

15.5 Cells for vaginal cytology are collected by gently rotating a saline-moistened cotton-tipped swab on the dorsal wall of the vagina about 1 cm from the vulvar entrance. A human urethral swab is smaller and often easier to use in the queen than a standard cotton-tipped swab. The procedure is brief and painless and does not require sedation. The swab is then rolled on a microscope slide to deposit the cells and the smear is air-dried. It can then be stained with any product used to stain blood films. Use of a trichrome stain will colour cells containing keratin red and cells without keratin will appear blue. Superficial cells predominate in this vaginal cytology smear, made during oestrus in the queen. These cells have been stained with Harris–Schorr stain, which colours keratin red. (Courtesy of Elise Malandain; reprinted from Little S (2012) *The Cat: Clinical Medicine and Management* with permission from Elsevier.)

Documentation of elevated serum oestradiol levels (>20 pg/ml; >73.4 pmol/l) while signs of oestrus are occurring is also consistent with ORS, although the diagnosis cannot be ruled out if oestradiol levels are not elevated. A better option is to induce ovulation of mature ovarian follicles during oestrus by injecting gonadotrophin-releasing hormone (GnRH) (25 µg/cat i.m.) with subsequent documentation of elevated serum progesterone (>2 ng/ml; >6.4 mmol/l), signifying the luteal phase, 2 weeks later.

Management
Once ORS is confirmed, the ovarian tissue should be surgically removed during an exploratory laparotomy. A thorough search of the peritoneal cavity is necessary, starting at the most common location for remnants, the ovarian pedicles. Other common sites for ovarian remnants are the omentum and the peritoneal walls. Remnants may be unilateral or bilateral. Surgery is most rewarding if performed when the cat is in the

luteal phase, which starts shortly after natural breeding or induction of ovulation, and lasts about 6 weeks, and is documented by an elevated serum progesterone level (see above). The corpora lutea are visible as yellow/orange structures against the red background of ovarian tissue. Excised tissue should be submitted for histopathology to confirm that ovarian tissue has been removed.

Mammary fibroadenomatous hyperplasia

Approximately 20% of feline mammary masses are benign and these are predominately mammary fibroadenomatous hyperplasia (MFH; also called fibroepithelial hyperplasia or mammary hyperplasia).

Aetiology

MFH is most commonly seen in young cycling queens, but may also be seen in pregnant queens, and in male or female cats treated with progestins (e.g. megestrol, medroxyprogesterone, proligestone, delmadinone). The cause is suspected to be an exaggerated response to natural progesterone or synthetic progestins, but the disease is also rarely reported in sterilized male or female cats with no history of progestin therapy. In spayed queens, ORS (see above) may be the initiating cause.

Clinical features

Typically most or all of the mammary glands are affected. The hyperplasia can be severe and may develop rapidly, leading to tissue necrosis, ulceration and infection (Figure 15.6). It is often mistaken for neoplasia on gross appearance. Histologically, MFH lesions show benign unencapsulated fibroglandular proliferation.

Diagnosis

The diagnosis is made on the basis of clinical signs, patient signalment and history. Biopsy of affected tissue and histopathology will confirm the diagnosis but surgical biopsy of markedly swollen mammary glands may create incisions that are difficult to heal due to wound tension, so surgery is best avoided if possible.

Management

Intact queens with MFH that are not intended for breeding should be spayed; a flank approach is most appropriate. Recovery usually takes 4–5 weeks following OHE/OE.

Treatment with progestins should be discontinued immediately. The drug of choice for treatment of MFH is aglepristone (10–15 mg/kg/day s.c. on days 1, 2 and 7). This may be used either as sole treatment in cats where OHE/OE is not desired, or to reduce the size of mammary tissue before surgery in cats that will be undergoing OHE/OE. Total remission of clinical signs with aglepristone treatment takes around 4 weeks in cats that have not had progestins and around 5 weeks in cats treated with long-acting medroxyprogesterone. Although aglepristone may cause abortion in pregnant queens, successful pregnancy has also been reported after aglepristone treatment. Another option when aglepristone is not available is the dopamine agonist cabergoline (5 µg/kg/day orally for 5–7 days), though this can also cause abortion.

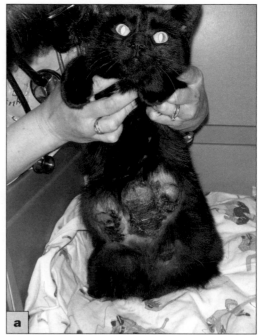

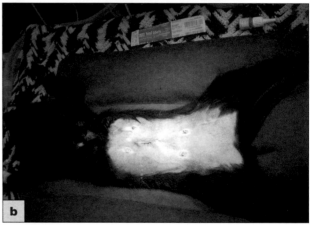

15.6 **(a)** Mammary hyperplasia in a young late-gestation pregnant queen. A litter of kittens was born 12 days later. The queen was initially treated with amoxicillin/clavulanate and a fluoroquinolone, as well as tramadol, until the kittens were born. Therapy with cabergoline was then initiated and the tramadol was replaced by a fentanyl patch. The kittens were hand-reared, both because the queen refused to allow nursing due to pain and because cabergoline caused the milk supply to dry up within a few days. **(b)** The same queen approximately 2 months later, after OHE, showing normal mammary tissue. (Courtesy of Dr Shelagh Morrison; reprinted from Little S (2012) *The Cat: Clinical Medicine and Management* with permission from Elsevier.)

Infections, as indicated by signs such as inflammation/heat, purulent discharge and/or pyrexia, should be treated for a minimum of 2 weeks with broad-spectrum antibiotics (e.g. amoxicillin/clavulanate) or as indicated by culture and sensitivity testing or a swab sample of affected tissue.

Pyometra

Pyometra is a form of CEH associated with inflammation and secondary bacterial infection and accumulation of purulent exudate in the uterine lumen.

Aetiology

CEH/pyometra is a luteal phase disease, where progesterone is the dominant hormone. Progesterone induces hyperplasia of the surface or glandular epithelium and cystic dilatation of the uterine glands. Fluid present in cystic structures and free in the uterine lumen readily supports bacterial growth. Progesterone also inhibits local leucocyte responses and decreases myometrial contractility, which increases the risk of ascending bacterial infection. The uterus may be chronically exposed to progesterone during pseudopregnancy or during treatment with progestins (e.g. megestrol) for control of oestrus, whereas pregnancy appears to protect the uterus against pathological changes.

Clinical features

Older queens (2.5–7.5 years) and maiden queens >3 years of age have the highest risk for CEH/pyometra. Clinical signs of pyometra include sanguineous to mucopurulent vulvar discharge, lethargy, anorexia, abdominal distension, dehydration, polyuria, polydipsia and pyrexia. Pyometra may produce either segmental or diffuse uterine enlargement (Figure 15.7), both of which may be mistaken for pregnancy on abdominal palpation. Queens with closed cervix pyometra have abdominal enlargement with no vulvar discharge and may be severely ill due to septicaemia.

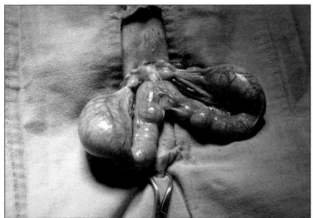

15.7 Pyometra may produce segmental uterine enlargement. In this case each uterine horn contains a large pocket of fluid. This could mimic a fetus on abdominal palpation but not on ultrasonography. (Reprinted from Little S (2012) *The Cat: Clinical Medicine and Management* with the permission of Elsevier.)

Diagnosis

Diagnosis of pyometra is based on history, signalment, clinical signs and physical examination findings. An intact queen with vulvar discharge should be assumed to have pyometra until proven otherwise. Laboratory abnormalities include mild anaemia of inflammatory disease (normocytic, normochromic, non-regenerative), thrombocytopenia, leucocytosis with neutrophilia, as well as hyperproteinaemia, hyperglobulinaemia, hypokalaemia, elevated ALT and ALP, and azotaemia. Many of the changes are related to endotoxaemia and dehydration. Radiography may demonstrate uterine enlargement (Figure 15.8). Typical ultrasonographic findings are an enlarged uterus with convoluted tubular horns filled with flocculent material of variable echogenicity (Figure 15.9). Ultrasonography is preferred over radiography for diagnosis and to rule out pregnancy. The most common bacterial species isolated on culture of vulvar discharge is *E. coli*.

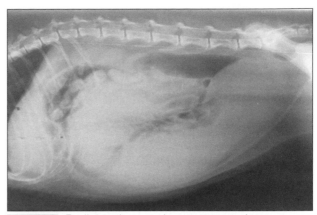

15.8 Radiography may demonstrate uterine enlargement in queens with pyometra, though it may not rule out pregnancy. In this case the uterus is severely enlarged and fills most of the abdomen but no fetal mineralization is seen as would be expected for the size of the uterus, suggesting that it is enlarged due to fluid accumulation and possible pyometra. (Reprinted from Little S (2012) *The Cat: Clinical Medicine and Management* with the permission of Elsevier.)

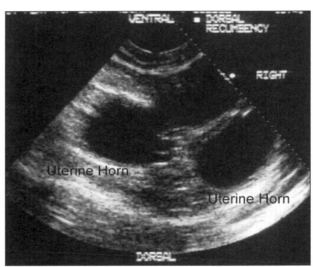

15.9 Typical ultrasonographic findings in queens with pyometra are an enlarged uterus with convoluted tubular horns, as in this case. The uterine horns may also be filled with flocculent material of variable echogenicity. (Reprinted from Little S (2012) *The Cat: Clinical Medicine and Management* with the permission of Elsevier.)

Management

Initial management depends on the status of the patient.

> **WARNING**
>
> Cats with closed cervix pyometra should be treated as emergency patients requiring urgent stabilization and surgical intervention.

Cats with open cervix pyometra (diagnosed by the presence of vulvar discharge) are typically more stable and not in need of urgent intervention. Intravenous fluid therapy with crystalloids and correction of hypokalaemia may be necessary for some patients. Broad-spectrum antibiotic therapy (e.g. a fluoroquinolone plus ampicillin) is initiated for all queens with pyometra and can be adjusted based on the results of culture and sensitivity testing of vulvar discharge. Antibiotic therapy should be continued for at least 3 weeks.

Antibiotic therapy alone will not resolve pyometra in the majority of queens. Therapeutic decisions should be based on the health status and age of the queen, as well as reproductive value. Queens that are not required for a breeding programme should undergo ovariohysterectomy. Young (<5 years), otherwise healthy queens with open cervix pyometra and reproductive value may be managed medically with treatments such as antiprogestins and/or prostaglandins in addition to broad-spectrum antibiotics, in an attempt to preserve fertility.

Antiprogestins such as aglepristone are synthetic steroids that bind to progesterone receptors but lack the effects of progesterone. Intrauterine progesterone concentrations are reduced, allowing for increased myometrial contractility and opening of the cervix. Aglepristone is administered at 10 mg/kg/day s.c. on days 1, 2, 7 and 14. Response to treatment is assessed by clinical signs, laboratory data and ultrasonographic findings 2 weeks after completion of treatment. Aglepristone can also be used in combination with prostaglandins, although no guidelines have been developed to determine which cases are best treated in this way. Therefore, clinical judgement based on the severity of disease is used to determine the best treatment approach.

Prostaglandin F2α (PGF2α) is a naturally occurring prostaglandin that, in the form of dinoprost tromethamine, can be administered to induce luteolysis and evacuation of uterine contents. The most commonly recommended dose is 0.1 mg/kg s.c. q12–24h for 3–5 days, although smaller doses given more frequently may reduce side effects and increase the frequency of uterine contractions (e.g. 0.02–0.05 mg/kg s.c. three to five times daily). The endpoint for treatment is reached when ultrasound examination shows a decrease in uterine size and no remaining fluid in the uterine lumen, and the serum progesterone concentration is <2 ng/ml (<6.4 mmol/l). Side effects (e.g. restlessness, panting, vomiting, defecation, tenesmus, salivation, vocalizing) are common but short lived. Risks associated with administration (e.g. uterine rupture) are few when appropriate patients are chosen for treatment. Queens should be re-evaluated 1–2 weeks after therapy by physical examination, uterine ultrasonography, haematology and serum biochemistry. A clear vulvar discharge may be present for several days after successful treatment.

Breeding queens that have recovered from pyometra should be bred at the next oestrus. Fertility rates after treatment with either aglepristone or dinoprost tromethamine are about 90%. Delaying breeding until after the next oestrus may result in a relapse of pyometra or in infertility.

References and further reading

England GCW and von Heimendahl A (2010) *BSAVA Manual of Canine and Feline Reproduction and Neonatology, 2nd edn*. BSAVA Publications, Gloucester

Haney DR, Levy JK, Newell SM, Graham JP and Gorman SP (2003) Use of fetal skeletal mineralization for prediction of parturition date in cats. *Journal of the American Veterinary Medical Association* **223**, 1614–1616

Little S (2011) Feline reproduction: problems and clinical challenges. *Journal of Feline Medicine and Surgery* **13**, 508–515

Zambelli D, Caneppele B, Bassi S and Paladini C (2002) Ultrasound aspects of fetal and extrafetal structures in pregnant cats. *Journal of Feline Medicine and Surgery* **4**, 95–106

Zambelli D and Prati F (2006) Ultrasonography for pregnancy diagnosis and evaluation in queens. *Theriogenology* **66**, 135–144

QRG 15.1 Diagnosing and managing dystocia
by Susan Little and Geraldine Hunt

Causes of dystocia

Maternal factors

- Primary or secondary uterine inertia:
  - Primary uterine inertia is complete failure of initiation of effective uterine contractions. Causes include obesity, inadequate uterine stimulation from small litters, overstretching of the myometrium from large litters, hypocalcaemia and uterine disease (e.g. infection, torsion, tear)
  - Secondary uterine inertia occurs due to uterine fatigue and is typically seen after part of a large litter has been delivered. It may also occur during dystocia from another cause, such as obstruction due to fetal malpresentation
  - Although not strictly a type of inertia, delivery may be interrupted if a queen is disturbed or stressed and will not resume until she feels calm and secure
- Familial predisposition
- Stressors
- Advanced age
- Obesity
- Systemic disease
- Uterine overdistension (e.g. large litter size, large fetuses)
- Uterine underdistension (e.g. small litter size, small fetuses)
- Narrow pelvic canal, typically due to previous trauma
- Uterine abnormalities (e.g. torsion, tear, rupture, prolapse)

Fetal factors

- Malpresentation
- Cephalopelvic disproportion occurs when the shape or size of the fetal head makes normal passage through the queen's pelvis difficult, such as in brachycephalic (e.g. Persian) and dolichocephalic breeds (e.g. Siamese)
- Death of one or more kittens
- Large fetuses
- Congenital defects

Diagnosis

Dystocia may be diagnosed when:

- Normal delivery is interrupted (obstruction or secondary uterine inertia):
  - A kitten and/or membranes are visible at the vulva for over 15 minutes with no progress
  - >3 hours have passed between delivery of individual kittens
  - No kittens have been produced after 3–4 hours of stage 2 labour
  - Strong contractions are present for >60 minutes with no kitten delivered ▶

QRG 15.1 *continued*

- Failure to deliver all kittens within 36 hours (the vast majority of normal parturitions are complete by 24 hours, although very rarely normal parturition can take up to 42 hours)
- Normal labour is not initiated at term (primary inertia) – queen is >1 week overdue
- Maternal health is compromised:
  - Queen is distressed and biting at the vulvar area
  - Serious systemic illness in the queen
  - Abnormal vulvar discharge (e.g. profuse haemorrhage, green discharge with foul odour)
- Fetal distress is diagnosed (heart rate <150–160 beats/min; normal fetal heart rate is 193–263 beats/min).

Accurate diagnosis of the cause of dystocia is necessary to determine whether medical or surgical intervention is most appropriate.

Diagnostic plan for dystocia

The diagnostic plan for dystocia should include:

- Collection of a reproductive and medical history (current health status, concurrent diseases, drugs or supplements being administered, details of previous pregnancies, etc.)
- Physical examination (including abdominal palpation for uterine size and position, palpation of the pelvis via the rectum to detect obstruction, vaginal examination for the presence of a kitten)
- Laboratory testing (minimum data required: haematology, serum calcium and glucose to determine if supplementation is necessary)
- Abdominal radiographs (evaluate fetal size, number and position)
- Evaluation of fetal condition with ultrasonography (fetal movement, fetal heart rates) or Doppler probe applied to the abdomen (heart rates only), when available.

Treatment

Manual assistance in the delivery of a kitten visible at the vulva

1 Apply copious amounts of sterile lubricant around the kitten using a syringe and soft catheter (e.g. feeding tube).

2 If the head is visible, clear the nose and mouth of membranes and fluid with a nasal bulb syringe or a catheter with a mucus trap designed for resuscitation of human neonates.

3 Grasp the kitten around the head and neck, or around the pelvis and hindlimbs if presented backwards, with a clean dry cloth. Never grasp an extremity as avulsion may occur.

4 Apply traction in a posterior–ventral direction, coordinated with the queen's contractions.

5 Gently twist or rock to help free the kitten, using a lubricated finger to free trapped extremities if necessary.

Pharmacological treatment

This is likely to be most effective in queens that have already delivered at least one kitten and where the litter size is not larger than average. It is indicated when:

- The queen is in good condition
- There is no obstruction to delivery (based on radiographs, rectal palpation and vaginal examination)
- The fetuses are not in distress
- Hypocalcaemia and hypoglycaemia, if present, have been corrected.

Oxytocin

Oxytocin promotes myometrial contractions, uterine involution and expulsion of retained placentas. Smaller, more frequent doses of oxytocin (0.5–2.0 IU/cat i.m. every 30 minutes, for a maximum of 2–3 doses) are recommended to avoid prolonged myometrial contractions, ineffective contractions, placental separation and disruption of blood flow to the fetus that can be associated with higher doses.

Calcium

Calcium therapy is used less commonly in the queen than the bitch as it may stimulate very strong uterine contractions. Calcium increases the strength of uterine contractions. Criteria for use include:

- Weak and ineffective contractions
- Poor response to oxytocin alone
- The presence of hypocalcaemia.

Calcium is given by diluting 10% calcium gluconate 1:1 with normal saline and giving 2–3 ml (of the diluted solution) by slow intravenous infusion (over 10–20 minutes), monitoring heart rate for bradycardia (by concurrent auscultation or electrocardiography); slow or stop if bradycardia occurs. Some queens may also benefit from administration of dextrose if hypoglycaemic (0.2 ml 50% dextrose diluted to 1 ml in sterile water or saline (thus 1:4 dilution) by slow intravenous infusion over 5–10 minutes).

Surgery

Indications for surgical intervention by caesarean section include:

- Failure of manual assistance or medical therapy (see above)
- Complete primary uterine inertia
- Secondary uterine inertia with a large litter
- Systemic illness in the queen (e.g. metritis, impending sepsis)
- Evidence of serious fetal distress (e.g. fetal heart rate <130 beats/min)
- Fetal death
- Obstructive dystocia (e.g. malpresentation, narrow pelvic canal, large fetuses) that cannot be corrected manually (see below)
- Uterine torsion, tear or rupture, or prolapsed uterus.

Dystocia requiring caesarean section is thankfully uncommon in the general cat population, but when it occurs it is an emergency. Veterinary surgeons should know the appropriate steps ahead of time, so as to best advise clients and institute treatment as quickly as possible. Occasionally a caesarean may be performed in the absence of dystocia but as a pre-planned (elective) procedure, e.g. when a queen has experienced dystocia in a previous pregnancy or in breeding cats with a known dystocia problem (e.g. brachycephalic breeds). In other cases, the breeding history of the queen and the expected date of parturition may be unknown, making it difficult to ascertain whether clinical signs are due to impending parturition or other causes.

Presurgical considerations

Prior to any surgical intervention, it is important to establish whether the cat is indeed pregnant and how many fetuses are present (see also main text).

- Abdominal radiography provides an opportunity to count skulls or vertebral columns, or confirm that the last fetus has been born.
- Ultrasonography also permits evaluation of the fetal heartbeat.
- Abdominal palpation can be misleading, especially when the uterus contains fragments of placenta or fluid, or is firmly contracted.
- Fetuses may be positioned within the pelvic canal, or very cranial in the abdomen. Vaginal examination should always be performed to establish whether a fetus is present in the pelvic canal, and this should be repeated following caesarean section to ensure that the fetus has been removed.

Preparation

The anaesthetic protocol should be chosen to allow rapid recovery of the queen and minimal impact on the fetuses (see Chapter 3).

If possible, the queen should be clipped and a basic surgical kit organized prior to induction of anaesthesia. The surgical kit should include:

- Towel clamps (A)
- Brown–Adson thumb forceps (B)
- Needle-holders (C)
- No. 3 scalpel handle (D) ▶

QRG 15.1 *continued*

- No. 15 scalpel blade (E)
- No. 10 scalpel blade (F)
- Mosquito forceps (G)
- Metzenbaum scissors (H)
- Mayo scissors (I)
- Blunt–sharp suture scissors (J)
- Gauze surgical swabs (K).

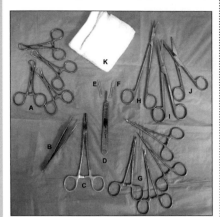

Procedure

1 A ventral midline skin incision is made swiftly but carefully, taking care not to penetrate the uterus and damage the kittens.

2 The uterus is exteriorized and packed off with moist laparotomy pads.

3 A longitudinal incision is made in the ventral surface of the uterine body or portion of the uterine horn close to the bifurcation.

4 The fetuses are milked out, inside their membranes if possible. Gentle traction can be applied to remove the placenta, which will come out easily if parturition has been underway for some time, but may be more difficult and result in more bleeding with an elective caesarean. The fetus and placenta are handed to a non-sterile assistant who breaks the membranes, clamps and cuts the umbilical cord, and commences stimulation/resuscitation of the kitten (see later). Care should be taken not to place undue traction on the umbilical cord,

and it should be ligated and the clamp removed as soon as possible.

If the placenta is more firmly adhered to the uterus: The surgeon breaks the fetal membranes and delivers the fetus separately, clamps and cuts the umbilical cord then hands the kitten to the non-sterile assistant before returning to the uterus to remove the fetal membranes and the placenta. The placenta is often still attached to the uterine wall and should be gently detached by traction.

5 The remaining kittens are milked down their respective uterine horns and delivered through the same incision.

6 The reproductive tract is palpated from each ovary to the cervix, and an assistant performs a vaginal examination to confirm that all fetuses have been removed.

7 Oxytocin (0.5–2.0 IU/cat i.m.) is then given to facilitate uterine contraction and haemostasis.

8 The uterus is then closed in two layers:

- Mucosa and submucosa – Continuous suture of 2 metric (3/0 USP) monofilament absorbable suture (e.g. polydioxanone, proligicaprone)
- Seromuscular layer – Continuous suture (simple continuous or Cushing (see Appendix)) using the same type of suture material.

9 The abdominal wall is then closed in three layers:

- Linea alba/external rectus sheath – Take full-thickness bites at least 5 mm from the incision and make sure you incorporate either the linea alba or the external rectus sheath. The rectus abdominus muscle on its own does not provide a strong enough closure. Use single interrupted sutures or continuous suture of a monofilament absorbable synthetic suture (e.g. 2 metric (3/0 USP) polydioxanone)
- Subcutaneous tissue – Continuous suture using 1 metric (4/0 USP) poliglecaprone 25

- Skin – subcuticular sutures (1 metric (4/0 USP) poliglecaprone 25) are preferable to skin sutures to reduce interference by the sucking kittens.

Postoperative management

Antibiotics are not routinely required for an uncomplicated caesarean. Analgesia should be provided as required to the queen; 24–48 hours of an opioid analgesic such as buprenorphine is usually adequate.

The kittens are returned to the queen as soon as possible and, assuming the queen does not experience any anaesthetic complications or undue amounts of postoperative bleeding, she and her litter can be sent home within a few hours, once her condition is stable.

Care of neonates

- As soon as each kitten is born, it should be rubbed with a towel to dry it and stimulate respiration.
- If necessary, the airways should be cleared with a nasal bulb syringe or a catheter with a mucus trap designed for resuscitation of human neonates.
- Weak kittens with poor body tone may benefit from a few drops of 50% dextrose solution under the tongue. 'Swinging' kittens and puppies to clear airways of fluids is no longer recommended due to the risk of potentially lethal cerebral trauma.
- Oxygen may be administered using the open end of a Bain circuit without an attached mask.

If initial attempts at resuscitation are not successful:

- Intubate for oxygen administration and ventilation with a large-bore catheter (12–16 G) or a size 1 uncuffed endotracheal tube. The normal respiratory rate for newborn kittens is 10–18 breaths/min.
- Resuscitation can be attempted using the Renzhong acupressure point (GV26). A 25 G hypodermic needle is inserted into the nasal philtrum at the base of the nose until bone is felt; the needle is gently rotated and then removed.

Management of fractures and orthopaedic disease

16

Sorrel J. Langley-Hobbs

This chapter will focus on brief discussion of the important fractures and orthopaedic diseases that are encountered in feline practice, notably: pelvic and sacroiliac fractures/luxation; skull fractures including mandibular symphyseal separation; hip luxation and dysplasia; femoral fractures; cruciate rupture; patellar luxation and fractures; stifle derangement; tibial, humeral and radial fractures; carpal and metacarpal injuries; and degenerative joint disease (DJD). The investigative approach to lameness is covered in Chapter 5.23. Information pertaining to the investigation and management of trauma cases presenting with fractures is given in Chapter 4.10. Further information on management of chronic pain in relation to DJD is given in Chapter 3.

This chapter is not intended to be exhaustive; rather, it gives a summary of conditions that the reader should consider, with brief options for management to provide enough information for a pertinent discussion with clients. In most cases, referral or extensive further reading will be required before definitive treatment can be given.

Axial fractures and luxations

Pelvic fracture and sacroiliac fracture/luxation

Pelvic fractures are common in cats. These fractures will heal without surgical intervention as they are well splinted and vascularized by surrounding musculature. The bone will heal as a malunion but this will usually be functional, with the exception of cases that heal with significant narrowing of the pelvic canal. This can result in problems for the cat, including constipation or obstipation (see Chapter 5.9), which may require surgical intervention such as pelvic osteotomy or colectomy. Constipation is likely if there is narrowing of the pelvic canal by 50% or more (Hamilton *et al.*, 2009). Comparison of the intersacral distance with the interacetabular distance is used to assess for narrowing (Figure 16.1). However, narrowing may progress and worsen during the healing period if it is not corrected, so this value can only be used to determine which cats definitely need surgery (if ≥50% narrowing); if there is <50% narrowing on initial

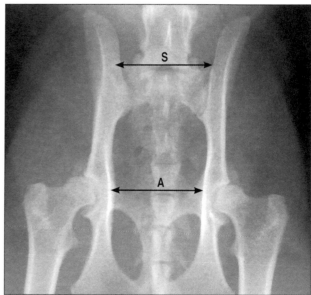

16.1 Using a ventrodorsal radiograph of the cat's pelvis, the intersacral distance (arrowed and labelled S) can be compared to the interacetabular distance (arrowed and labelled A). The S:A ratio in this radiograph of a normal cat is 1:0.97 (in practical terms this can be considered to be 1:1).

radiographs this does not mean that surgery is not necessary on this factor alone, however.

Conservative management

Cats can be managed conservatively if they are ambulatory and have minimal fragment displacement, and pain that is easily controlled. This entails cage rest until fracture healing is demonstrated radiographically or the cat has improved clinically. Analgesia should be given during the rehabilitation. Nursing is essential, ensuring the cat is eating, drinking, defecating and urinating. Physiotherapy can be beneficial if there are neurological injuries, to prevent tendon contracture (see *BSAVA Manual of Canine and Feline Rehabilitation, Supportive and Palliative Care*). Follow-up radiographs are usually taken after 4 weeks and at this stage, if it is progressing well, the cat can be allowed to exercise in the house (avoiding jumping and climbing) and can be eventually allowed access to the outside again after approximately 8 weeks (Figure 16.2).

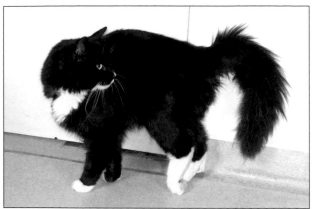

16.2 This cat sustained a pelvic fracture in an RTA and has mild proprioceptive deficits in the left pelvic limb. The fracture fragments were minimally displaced and the injury was treated conservatively: strict cage rest for 3 weeks followed by supervised limited exercise (no jumping) outside the cage for a further 3 weeks, before allowing unsupervised activity and a return to being allowed outside. There was a complete recovery from the neurological deficits within 2 weeks.

Surgery

Surgical intervention for pelvic fractures will generally give a quicker and less painful return to function and should be considered if the following are present:

- Loss of the weight-bearing axis on radiography due to sacroiliac fracture/luxations, iliac body fractures or acetabular fractures
- Narrowing of the pelvic canal diameter due to iliac body fractures or ischial fractures (remembering that narrowing can progress during healing). If narrowing is approaching 50% of the intersacral distance (see Figure 16.1) then surgery is recommended, to prevent constipation and obstipation. If narrowing is less severe initially, there is still the possibility that the degree of narrowing could worsen during healing
- Articular fractures such as acetabular fractures
- Nerve impingement – usually seen with iliac body fractures; cats can be hyperpathic (in more pain than expected and perhaps biting or looking at their back end) due to the impinged nerve.

Surgical options available include the following:

- Sacroiliac luxation can be treated with a variety of options, including a 2.0 or 2.7 mm lag screw, possibly combined with a transilial pin or bolt if bilateral or significant displacement of the hemipelvis medially
- Iliac body fractures can be treated with bone plate and screws (or occasionally lag screws or pins if fracture is long oblique)
- Acetabular fractures can be treated with a bone plate, or screws and tension band wire, or treated conservatively, performing a femoral neck and head excision if pain persists.

Areas of skin necrosis may occur after pelvic fracture, due to avulsion and damage to the dermal vascular plexus.

Pelvic fracture repair requires a reasonable level of orthopaedic surgical experience, and referral may therefore be considered.

Skull fractures

Cats are prone to injuries of the skull after falls or road traffic injuries. Concussion, brain trauma and concurrent cranial nerve injuries can occur (see Chapter 17); cats may present as dull or comatose, with an obviously asymmetrical jaw, bleeding from their nostrils and/or conjunctival contusions. Examination should include a neurological examination (see QRG 1.6) and an oral examination (see QRG 1.4), which should include a check that the hard palate is not split and that dental occlusion is correct.

Mandibular symphyseal separation

Mandibular symphyseal separations are common in cats and, when simple, are relatively easy to repair, even for those inexperienced with orthopaedic surgery. Repair is with a cerclage wire (Figure 16.3). It is important to use wire of a large enough gauge (22 G or 0.8 mm) to achieve good stability and allow healing, and to ensure that the wire is not overtightened as that could cause distortion of the canine teeth and result in malocclusion or inability to close the mouth.

1. A small skin incision is made in the midline on the ventral aspect of the jaw.
2. A 16 G hypodermic needle that has been bent into a curve is placed through the incision and along the lateral aspect of the bone to penetrate the oral mucosa just caudal to the canine tooth where the labial and buccal mucosa meet.
3. A 0.8 mm piece of orthopaedic wire is threaded into the tip of the needle.

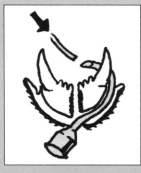

4. The needle is then withdrawn, pulling the wire with it.
5. The needle is inserted on the other side of the jaw, to exit just caudal to the other mandibular canine tooth.
6. The other end of the wire is directed through the tip of the needle, and the needle withdrawn back to the ventral chin skin incision, again pulling the wire with it.
7. The wire ends of the cerclage are twisted ventrally, while reduction is controlled manually. The wire must be tightened sufficiently, until no motion can be elicited between the two mandibles.

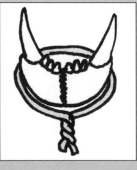

8. The wire twist is left protruding from the ventral aspect of the chin for ease of removal after healing.

16.3 Cerclage wiring of a mandibular symphyseal separation. (Adapted from Montavon *et al.* (2009), with permission.)

Mandibular fractures

Fractures of the mandibular body (Figure 16.4) can be more problematical, particularly if the fracture involves the caudal part of the body or the temporomandibular joint (TMJ), as there is minimal bone available for implant placement. There are a huge variety of techniques described for stabilization of mandibular fractures in cats. The priority is to restore dental alignment so the cat can open and close its mouth and prehend food. The surgical option chosen depends on a wide variety of factors, including location of fracture, availability of implants, experience of the surgeon and facilities for observation of the cat after surgery; the route for feeding, such as placement of a naso-oesophageal, oesophagostomy or gastrostomy feeding tube, should also be taken into consideration. Mandibular fracture repair can be challenging in the cat and requires some level of expertise with orthopaedic surgery.

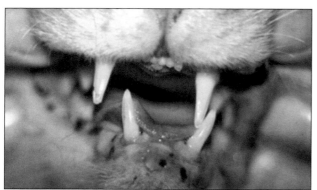

16.4 This cat sustained a fracture of the mandibular body following an RTA, which resulted in dental malocclusion. Surgical reduction and stabilization are required to restore good function. These fractures can be challenging to repair, and referral to a specialist should be considered.

Conditions of the appendicular skeleton

Pelvic limb

Hip luxation

Dislocation of the hip is the most common joint dislocation seen in the cat. It is caused by trauma, the type of which is often unknown.

The hip usually dislocates in a craniodorsal direction. Cats will have marked pelvic limb lameness and the affected limb will appear to be relatively shorter than the unaffected leg on orthopaedic examination. Concurrent injuries and fractures may be present. There is palpable asymmetry of the pelvis, with the greater trochanter displaced craniodorsally.

Radiographs should be taken to confirm the diagnosis, the direction of luxation and whether there are concurrent injuries such as hip dysplasia (shown on the radiograph by periarticular osteophytosis and subluxation of the contralateral hip) or an avulsion fracture of the femoral head, which would preclude closed reduction.

Treatment options include closed reduction (Figure 16.5), open reduction and surgical stabilization using techniques such as the iliofemoral suture or transarticular pin (Sissener *et al.*, 2009) or a salvage procedure such as femoral head and neck excision or total hip replacement (THR). The author's preference is for transarticular pinning (Figure 16.6), which has a good success rate, although it does have the disadvantage that the cat needs a second period of anaesthesia for pin removal. Femoral head and neck excision would be recommended for a chronic dislocation where there is damage to the articular surface of the femoral head, if there is hip dysplasia or if there is a fracture of the femoral head that involves more than about a quarter of the head.

Closed reduction of a luxated hip joint is performed under general anaesthesia. The aim of the manipulation is to bring the femoral head across the acetabular rim and back into the acetabular fossa, without causing additional iatrogenic damage.

1. The cat is placed in lateral recumbency, with the affected limb uppermost.
2. The femoral head is first externally rotated and pulled caudally and ventrally by exerting manual traction on the stifle.
3. Once the femoral head is assumed to be located at the level of the acetabulum, it is internally rotated. A satisfying clunk should occur if closed reduction is successful.
4. The femoral head is then pressed into the acetabular fossa with the thumb, and the hip joint is manipulated carefully, through a full range of motion, to aid removal of soft tissue out of the acetabular fossa. The leg is held in inward rotation during this manipulation.
5. Stability is tested by putting the hip joint through its range of motion. Excessive outward rotation of the hip and adduction of the leg are avoided, as they will cause reluxation in most cases.
6. Correct reduction is confirmed on a lateral radiograph.
7. Consideration can be given to placing an Ehmer sling following reduction but most cats will either not tolerate this bandage or it will slip off the leg.

16.5 Closed reduction of a craniodorsal coxofemoral luxation. (Adapted from Montavon *et al.* (2009) with permission.)

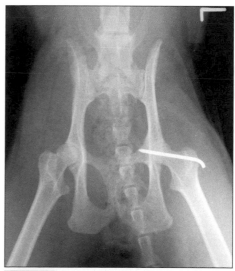

16.6 Ventrodorsal radiograph showing a temporary 1.6 mm transarticular pin, which was placed after a left hip dislocation. This technique can be used with good success for dislocated hips in cats and is the author's preferred method as it has a good success rate in maintaining reduction of the hip even if other techniques have failed. Pin placement must be central in the femoral head and the pin must be large enough to be stiff so that it will not break. The pin does need removal, necessitating a second period of anaesthesia, after 2–4 weeks. In simple cases, where the only injury is a hip luxation, the pin can usually be removed after 2 weeks; in more complicated cases, where there are additional injuries, other legs affected or neurological deficits, then it is recommended that the pin is left *in situ* for 4 weeks.

Hip dysplasia

Hip dysplasia causes stiffness and difficulty in jumping in affected young cats. Some publications intimate an increased predisposition in certain pedigree breeds such as the Maine Coon, Himalayan, Siamese, Abyssinian, Devon Rex and Persian.

Treatment should initially be conservative, with weight reduction, pain medication and nutraceuticals (appropriate for arthritis). Cats are difficult to rest without cage confinement, so this does not tend to be a good long-term option but it could be considered in the short term to alleviate an acute exacerbation. In severely affected animals or those that do not respond to conservative management, surgical options include femoral head and neck excision or THR. Osteoarthritis will also develop subsequent to hip dysplasia, and this can cause problems of lameness, stiffness, inactivity and difficulty in jumping, particularly in older cats (see later).

Capital femoral fractures

Two types of capital femoral fractures are seen in cats.

True traumatic capital femoral fracture: This condition is seen in young (<12 months) male or female cats that have suffered trauma; they may have sustained other fractures, and the onset of the lameness is usually acute. Radiographs show a separation of the capital epiphysis at the physis from the proximal femoral neck (Figure 16.7a). Treatment is usually by parallel pinning with very small implants (Figure 16.7b) or by femoral head and neck excision.

Slipped capital femoral epiphysis: This pathological/atraumatic fracture is usually seen in male cats aged 12–24 months, with one study suggesting that overweight Siamese cats are predisposed. The lameness usually has an insidious onset. Cats have unilateral pelvic limb lameness, with muscle atrophy and pain on hip extension. Radiographs show a capital femoral fracture (Figure 16.8); in early cases, the fracture line may be imperceptible and several views, including ventrodorsal extended and 'frog leg', may be required to confirm the diagnosis. In chronic cases there is remodelling and resorption of the femoral neck, giving it an 'apple core' appearance. The condition can be bilateral, although that is usually sequential rather than concurrent. Treatment is femoral head and neck excision or THR. There is no known prevention for the contralateral capital femoral epiphysis undergoing the same disease.

Femoral diaphyseal fractures

The femur is a commonly fractured bone in the cat; as for most long bone fractures in cats, the cause is usually trauma. Femoral diaphyseal fractures in cats are often comminuted and fissured, as the bones are quite brittle. There are many stabilization options available, depending on the level and bone affected. The bone is straight and this lends itself to stabilization by a variety of implants, including intramedullary pinning with cerclage wiring for simple long oblique fractures in young cats. Comminuted, short oblique or transverse fractures can be stabilized with an intramedullary pin combined with external skeletal fixation or with plate and screw fixation, alone or with pins. Interlocking nails are also ideal for diaphyseal fractures in medium to large cats (Figure 16.9).

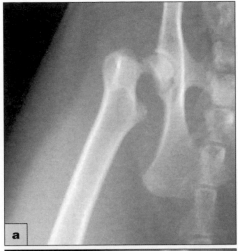
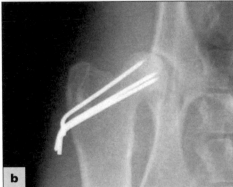

16.7 **(a)** A traumatic femoral capital physeal fracture is shown on this craniocaudal view of the femur; the fracture occurs through the capital physis. This occurred after an RTA in which the 8-month-old cat also sustained a distal femoral fracture and a comminuted tibial fracture on the same leg. **(b)** Craniocaudal radiograph of the femur showing stabilization of the femoral capital physeal fracture with three small stainless steel arthrodesis wires (0.9 mm diameter).

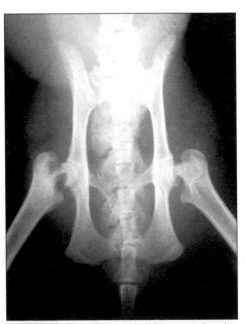

16.8 This 18-month-old neutered male cat presented with bilateral pelvic limb lameness and hip pain over a duration of 4 weeks. The ventrodorsal radiograph shows bilateral capital physeal fractures, with resorption (seen as lucency) and narrowing of the femoral necks. These changes are consistent with slipped capital femoral epiphyses (atraumatic fractures).

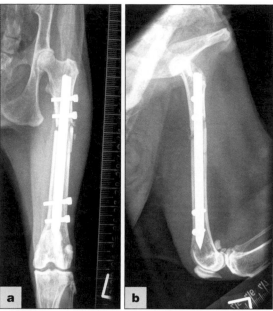

16.9 This 14-year-old hyperthyroid cat sustained a femoral diaphyseal fracture of unknown cause. **(a)** Craniocaudal and **(b)** mediolateral radiographs show the interlocking nail repair of the proximal third femoral fracture, using a 4.0 mm nail. This repair method was chosen as it was anticipated that the fracture would take a long time to heal in this elderly cat with osteopenia (seen as a double cortical line). The interlocking nail implant is placed inside the bone and is therefore very resistant to bending forces; and the interlocking nature of the bolts prevents rotation and shear of the fracture fragments. Plate and screw fixation could have been used but there was limited space in the proximal fragment for placement of many screws (ideally requires a minimum of three). External skeletal fixation was not considered optimal in this cat as it has osteopenia and it was therefore anticipated that pin-holding might be poor in the bone, which could result in premature pin loosening. This would not be good in a cat where fracture healing was anticipated to be slow.

Distal femoral condylar fractures

Condylar fractures of the distal femur are common in young cats, usually due to a fall or similar trauma. The distal femoral condyle displaces in a caudoproximal direction (Figure 16.10a). These fractures require surgical stabilization with dynamic intramedullary pins, a single intramedullary pin or cross pins (Figures 16.10b,c). The tendency at surgery is for the condyle

to remain displaced in a caudal direction, so every effort should be made to obtain and maintain correct reduction of the fracture.

Quadriceps contracture

Quadriceps contracture (see Figure 5.23.7) is a potential complication after any type of femoral fracture, particularly if fracture treatment is delayed more than a few days, if the leg is particularly swollen and/or if the fracture repair is unstable. To have any chance of successful treatment, the condition must be recognized and treated rapidly (i.e. preferably within days of its occurrence). A cat that is developing a quadriceps contracture has a tendency to walk with the stifle in extension and is initially reluctant to flex the stifle; this reluctance progresses to an inability to flex the stifle over days to weeks, as the muscle undergoes contracture. Treatment of quadriceps contracture once it has started to occur is very challenging and the prognosis for success is guarded. Multiple different treatment options have been tried in individual cases. The aim of treatment is to prevent the contracture worsening and to maintain stifle flexion, so treatment is aimed at keeping the stifle in a flexed position temporarily or intermittently, by bandaging, or external skeletal fixation or pins and elastic bands (Montavon et al., 2009).

Cruciate ligament rupture

Rupture of the cranial cruciate ligament (CCL) is seen most commonly in older overweight cats as a degenerative condition. Partial ruptures and meniscal tears are also seen but are not common. Radiographs may show intra-articular mineralization, which usually affects the fat pad and joint capsule (as well as the meniscus in some cases).

Conservative treatment can be tried (cage rest for 4–6 weeks) but surgical stabilization will give a quicker return to function and should be considered in all cases that do not improve with conservative treatment. Conservative treatment for the older cat with a suspected degenerative rupture can be tried as the first line of treatment, only resorting to surgery if the cat does not improve and remains lame.

Surgery should be considered, and recommended, as the initial treatment method in cats with a high degree of instability (marked positive cranial draw) as it will be likely to give a faster return to function and, by stabilizing the joint, there may be less severe development of DJD. If the rupture is suspected to

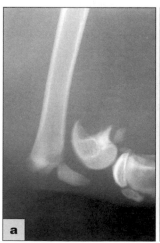

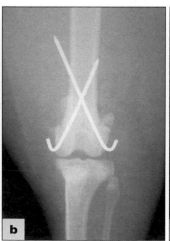

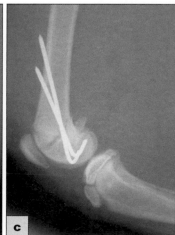

16.10

A 5-month-old male cat presented after unknown trauma with severe lameness of the right hindlimb. **(a)** Mediolateral radiograph showing a distal femoral condylar fracture with proximocaudal displacement of the femoral condyle. **(b)** Craniocaudal and **(c)** mediolateral radiographs after the fracture had been reduced and stabilized with two small arthrodesis wires placed as cross pins.

be traumatic rather than degenerative, then surgery would also be recommended. Mineralized tissue should be resected carefully so as not to damage the menisci and their ligaments. Stabilization is usually achieved by extra-articular stabilization with a suture. Sutures should be placed at the isometric points of the joint so there is minimal change in length when the joint is taken through its full range of movement and the suture will not break or become lax when moved through the normal range of motion (ROM). The most challenging parts of the surgery are correct placement of the suture behind the lateral fabella and positioning the hole in the tibial tuberosity in an appropriate place, to try and mimic the anatomy of the CCL.

Patellar luxation

Due to their active natures and ability to jump, cats have a high level of laxity in their joints as a normal finding, so it is important to compare the contralateral joint before diagnosing ligament laxity, although some conditions can be bilateral. Patellar luxation is a manifestation of a higher than normal level of joint laxity. Clinically normal cats can have incidental laxity that allows movement of the patella out of the groove (grade I luxation). Patellar luxation of a higher grade is one of the recognized causes of pelvic limb lameness in young cats and the patella usually displaces in a medial direction (Figure 16.11).

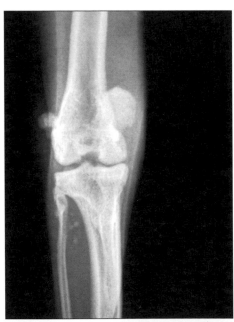

16.11 Craniocaudal radiograph showing a medial patellar luxation in a 9-year-old male cat. There is also synovial osteochondromatosis, with joint mice that have migrated into the extension of the joint capsule around the long digital extensor tendon; this condition can be seen in osteoarthritic joints. A wedge recession sulcoplasty had been performed for a previous luxation of the same patella when the cat was 1 year old. He had not then shown any lameness until there was an acute deterioration with marked lameness 2 days prior to referral. The patella was permanently luxated; although it was possible to reduce it into the groove, it reluxated almost immediately on release (grade III). Revision surgery was performed on the cat and the groove was found not to be wide enough for the patella to sit in, so it was deepened by performing a block recession sulcoplasty. The cat recovered well after surgery and it was walking well at a 4-week postoperative check.

Surgical stabilization, involving deepening of the groove by wedge or recession sulcoplasty (trochleoplasty), is usually beneficial. The patella is flat and wide in the cat and it is important that this is taken into consideration when considering the width of the trochlear groove to create. It is not always necessary to transpose the tibial tuberosity, as there is not usually much displacement or rotation of this bony prominence. If a tibial tuberosity transposition is performed, care must be taken as the bone is quite brittle and liable to fracture further if too small a piece of bone is cut when osteotomizing the tuberosity. If bony correction is performed then the success rate is usually good. If only soft tissue procedures such as imbricating (tightening and overlapping the joint capsule) are done then the chance of reluxation is very high.

Patellar fractures

The commonest patellar fractures in cats are transverse and affect the mid or proximal bone. They are usually seen in young cats (1–3 years of age) with no history of direct trauma. They are thought to be stress fractures (incomplete fractures, typically due to overuse) and the contralateral patella will often fracture subsequently after a median of 3 months (Langley-Hobbs, 2009). The patella is brittle, and repair using pins and tension band should not be attempted as failure is very likely, with further fracturing or breakdown of the repair. Conservative treatment, circumferential wiring or tension-band wiring of the patella (without pins) could be tried. The surgery is not especially difficult, although achieving reduction of the articular surface can be the most challenging aspect. Fractures rarely heal, however, and the bone usually forms a functional non-union, so conservative management may be preferable. Underlying pathology is suspected, the cause of which is undetermined but may be a type of osteogenesis imperfecta, which is an inherited brittle bone disease. A proportion of cats will also subsequently suffer from other stress fractures (Figure 16.12), including avulsion of the ischial tuberosity, proximal tibia or humeral condyle, and owners need to be warned of this possibility (Langley-Hobbs et al., 2009). Unfortunately there is no known preventive treatment.

Traumatic patellar fractures can also occur; injuries or other fractures of the femur and tibia occur concurrently in this situation.

Stifle derangement

Stifle derangement, disruption or luxation occurs when the cat ruptures several ligaments around the stifle joint. There is usually rupture of one of the collateral ligaments (most commonly the medial) and both cruciate ligaments. This serious injury is most usually seen in cats over 3 or 4 years of age (younger cats are more likely to sustain a fracture of the femoral condyle or proximal tibia). The tibia displaces cranially and there is significant instability of the stifle in either a lateral or medial direction, depending on which ligament is ruptured. These injuries need surgical stabilization through repair of the individual ligaments, and postoperative support with transarticular skeletal fixation or by use of a temporary transarticular pin; cases can be quite challenging.

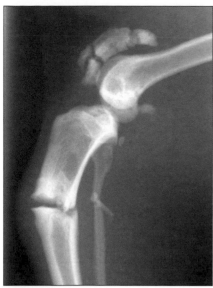

16.12 Mediolateral radiograph of a transverse tibial stress fracture and a proximal fibular fracture in a 10-year-old female cat with a chronic patellar non-union fracture. There is sclerosis of the tibia around the fracture and thickening of the cranial tibial cortex, which is characteristic of these fractures. The patella has enthesophytosis (bone or mineral deposition at the sites of soft tissue, such as ligaments, inserting on to bone) affecting the proximal and distal aspects, and there is pronounced metaplastic bone formation, which is a characteristic of some chronic patellar fractures in cats. This cat also had a history of atraumatic humeral condylar fractures and a contralateral tibial and patellar fracture, all at different times in the past.

Tibial diaphyseal fractures

Tibial fractures are common in cats. Options for stabilization include:

- External coaptation (see Figure 16.17), particularly for minimally displaced spiral tibial fractures when the fibula is intact in young cats
- Intramedullary pinning combined with cerclage wiring for long oblique fractures
- External skeletal fixation, alone or with a small intramedullary pin (linear and circular) and plate-and-screw fixation.

Distal tibial fractures in adult cats are prone to delayed union or non-union, taking as long as 6 months to heal. Bone grafting should be considered. Spiral fractures of the tibia with an intact fibula are relatively easy to repair using a simple unilateral external skeletal fixator (ESF), even if the surgeon is relatively inexperienced. Comminuted tibial fractures and particularly distal tibial fractures are challenging cases and would benefit from an experienced surgeon.

Distal tibial physeal fractures

The distal tibial epiphysis is a very thin piece of bone, so fractures can be challenging to stabilize. If the fracture is minimally displaced, external coaptation (see Figure 16.17) or cage rest may be sufficient to allow uncomplicated healing. If the fracture is displaced, after reduction the position is maintained by placement of two small Kirschner wires (Figure 16.13). Postoperatively, the repair needs support through external coaptation or a transarticular external skeletal fixator (TESF).

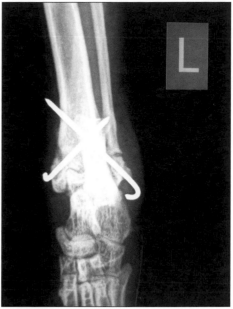

16.13 Craniocaudal tarsal radiograph showing a distal tibial epiphyseal fracture in an 8-month-old male cat, stabilized with two cross pins. The repair is usually protected by external coaptation or a TESF for 4 weeks postoperatively.

Malleolar fractures

The hock joint in the cat is supported by the distal fibula laterally (lateral malleolus) and the medial malleolus medially. Injury to these structures is common following trauma. Fracture of one or both malleoli will result in a very unstable joint, and tension-band repair of the fractures to restore stability to the joint is required. As the malleolar fracture fragments are small, surgery involves the use of very small implants and requires accurate positioning of the pins to avoid penetrating the joint. Open degloving injuries, where the malleolus is removed by friction with a road for example, are best stabilized with a TESF. The wounds can then be managed as open wounds and a free skin graft carried out once granulation has occurred. If damage is severe, with >30% of the articular surface of the talus or distal tibia destroyed, or if there are concurrent talar fractures, then a tarsal arthrodesis should be performed rather than trying to salvage the joint.

Thoracic limb

Humeral diaphyseal fractures

These fractures most commonly affect the distal to middle third of the bone; humeral condylar fractures are very uncommon in cats. The medullary canal of the humerus in the cat rarely extends beyond the distal quarter of the bone, which has implications for very distal humeral fractures; intramedullary pins cannot easily be placed into the distal bone without penetrating the elbow joint by exiting through the supratrochlear fossa, so intramedullary pinning cannot be relied upon to provide much stability for distal humeral fractures. Fractures can be stabilized with intramedullary pinning combined with external skeletal fixation for transverse, oblique or comminuted fractures. Plate-and-screw fixation can also be used for a variety of feline humeral fractures, and the plate can be applied to the lateral, medial or cranial surface of the bone. Humeral fractures can be challenging to repair, particularly if comminuted and distal; referral should be sought unless the surgeon is a competent experienced orthopaedic surgeon.

Olecranon fractures and Monteggia lesions

Fractures of the olecranon are avulsion fractures displaced by the pull of the triceps tendon. They are very disabling, as cats are unable to bear weight or extend their elbows. Surgical repair is required to restore weight bearing, using a tension-band repair (pins and figure-of-eight wire or a caudal or lateral plate).

Olecranon or proximal ulnar fractures that occur in association with dislocation of the radial head are known as Monteggia lesions; they often occur after a fall or if cats sustain a caudal blow to the proximal antebrachium when the elbow is extended. There are two main types (Schwarx and Schrader, 1984):

- Proximal to the annular ligament, so that the relationship between the radial head and ulna is maintained. Ulnar repair alone is sufficient
- Distal to the annular ligament (more common) (Figure 16.14): the annular ligament is ruptured and the radial head and ulna separate. The ulna should be repaired and then the contact between the two bones restored, using a screw or wire, to mimic or replace the function of the annular ligament and prevent reluxation of the radial head.

Simple fractures can be relatively easy to repair if the basic principles of orthopaedic surgery (and particularly tension band application) are applied. Comminuted fractures are more challenging and experience is required before undertaking such repairs.

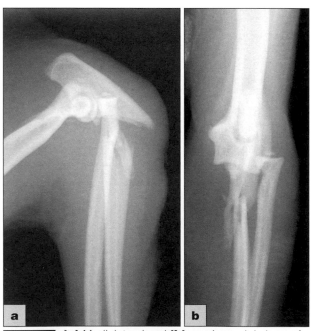

16.14 (a) Mediolateral and (b) craniocaudal views of the elbow and proximal antebrachium of a 5-year-old cat that had suffered a fall. There is a mildly comminuted fracture of the proximal ulna and cranial luxation of the radial head, with significant soft tissue swelling. This injury is known as a Monteggia lesion. It is important that both the ulnar fracture and the radial head luxation are repaired, and that the annular ligament that holds the radius and ulna in close contact is replaced with a prosthetic ligament or suitable alternative such as a screw placed between the radius and ulna.

Antebrachial fractures

Radial fractures in cats commonly affect the mid to proximal aspect of the bone. Surgery should be considered for the majority, although stable minimally displaced fractures in young cats may be successfully treated with external coaptation. Complications after surgery occur, particularly with the more proximal fractures. If both the radius and ulna are fractured, repair of both tends to result in better outcomes and fewer complications (Wallace *et al.*, 2009). The ulna in the cat can be pinned in a retrograde fashion, in combination with stabilizing the radius by either plate or free-form external skeletal fixation (Figure 16.15). Stabilizing both bones helps maintain the supination and pronation movement of the antebrachium that is important to the cat.

A simple fracture of the radius and ulna could be stabilized by a surgeon with some orthopaedic experience of bone plating and pinning. It is essential that small screws and pins are used; 2.0 mm or smaller screws would be used in most average-sized cats.

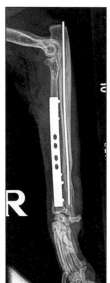

16.15 Mediolateral radiograph of an 8-year-old cat presented with a simple distal ulnar fracture and a comminuted radial fracture; the type of trauma that caused the injury was unknown. The fracture healed after reduction and stabilization (intramedullary pin in the ulna, placed in a retrograde fashion from the ulnar fracture site; a 2.0 mm dynamic compression plate applied craniomedially to the radius) and a cancellous bone graft.

Carpal injuries

Traumatic hyperextension injuries are very rare in the cat; when they do occur carpal arthrodesis is usually indicated. Carpal luxations usually occur after falls, and reduction and ligament repair may be sufficient to restore function without always needing arthrodesis. These injuries are challenging to repair, however.

Metacarpal (and metatarsal) fractures

If there is fracture of two or more of the metacarpal or metatarsal bones (meta-bones), surgical stabilization may be required. If only one or two bones are fractured, the adjacent intact bones may act as splints and external coaptation alone may be all that is needed. The decision depends on the degree of displacement, the level of fracture and the age of the cat:

- In a young cat with minimally displaced fractures, external coaptation (see Figure 16.17) for two fractures may be a very successful option
- In an older cat with displaced fracture fragments, even if only two bones are affected, surgery will restore alignment, give some additional pain relief and result in faster healing

- If the fractures are very proximal, and particularly if there is involvement of the lateral aspect of the 5th metatarsal or metacarpal, there is likely to be instability of the carpometacarpal or tarsometacarpal joint, and surgery would be indicated (either to repair the avulsed fragment with a pin and tension-band wire or to arthrodese the joint).

In cats, the easiest method of stabilization is by fracture reduction with toggle or dowel pinning, followed by external coaptation to support the repair (Degasperi *et al.*, 2007; Zahn *et al.*, 2007). This is a relatively easy procedure that can be performed by someone with minimal orthopaedic surgery experience.

External coaptation: bandages, splints and casts

Some injuries, including certain fractures and luxations, will benefit from external coaptation. Bandages can be used for protection of clean wounds and for treatment of contaminated wounds with dressings, for temporary stabilization before surgery, and for additional support or protection of the repair after surgery. A splinted bandage is generally preferable to a pressure bandage such as a Robert Jones for stabilization of a distal limb fracture prior to surgery, as it will provide better stabilization of the broken bone. Other indications for splinted bandages and cylinder casts are given in Figure 16.16.

Splinted bandage
- Immobilization of joints (especially carpus, tarsus, toes; elbow with spica splint)
- Metacarpal, metatarsal, and phalangeal fractures
- Protection of tendon sutures (e.g. digital tendon or Achilles tendon)
- Neurological deficits (e.g. peroneal nerve deficit)
- Protection of suboptimal surgical fracture repair (radius/ulna, tibia/fibula)
- Greenstick fracture in very young cats

Cylinder cast

- Fractures of the lower limb – radius/ulna and tibia in immature cats
  - Closed
  - Simple
  - Reducible
  - Transverse/interdigitating

- On orthogonal radiographs there should be at least 50% of the fracture ends in contact
- Fractures of the radius when the ulna is intact
- Fracture of the tibia when the fibula is intact

16.16 Indications for splints and casts. (Adapted from Montavon *et al.* (2009), with permission.)

Cats do not always tolerate bandages, slings, splints and casts, and they can be adept at removing them. The use of stirrups – adhesive tape placed on the fur and then incorporated into the bandage – can help prevent slippage and premature removal. Slings in particular are not easy to keep in place in cats, but in some cases they can be useful (Figure 16.17).

When using any type of external coaptation, it is essential that it is not placed too tightly as this could cause pressure sores or even necrosis, and in the most severe cases this can result in loss of a limb.

Function	Indications	Duration
Tape muzzle		
Interarcuate stabilization of mandibular fracture	After closed reduction of temporomandibular luxation; for conservative treatment of selected mandibular fractures	1–2 weeks
Velpeau sling		
Flexion of shoulder, elbow and carpus; prevents weight bearing	For conservative treatment of selected scapular fracture/dislocation; after open or closed reduction of medial shoulder luxation	7–10 days
Carpal sling		
Prevents weight bearing	To prevent weight bearing while maintaining elbow and shoulder mobility, after closed reduction or surgical repair of elbow and shoulder fractures or luxations	7–10 days
Ehmer sling or Robinson sling		
Internal rotation and slight abduction of femur (Ehmer); prevent weight bearing	After closed reduction of craniodorsal/caudodorsal hip luxations (although not usually well tolerated or slips off the leg)	7–10 days
Hobble		
Prevents abduction of hindlimbs	For conservative treatment of pelvic floor fractures; after closed reduction of a ventral hip joint luxation	1–3 weeks

16.17 Function, indication, and suggested duration of application for selected orthopaedic slings and miscellaneous bandages. (Adapted from Montavon *et al.* (2009), with permission.)

Degenerative joint disease

Degenerative joint disease (DJD) or osteoarthritis is being increasingly recognized in cats; the elbows, hocks, hips and stifles of older cats are most commonly affected.

Clinical features

On clinical examination, if the cat is cooperative, stiffness, lameness or a reluctance to jump may be seen in the consulting room. Affected joints will have a decreased ROM, and pain at extremes of ROM; in chronic cases there may be joint enlargement due to fibrosis and/or effusion and crepitus. Certain behavioural changes are commonly reported by owners of cats with DJD (Figure 16.18); these vary depending on which joints are affected.

- Reluctance to jump up on to objects (e.g. on to a bed) or to jump down
- Unwillingness to play
- Reduced activity
- Reduced grooming
- Aggression
- Altered toileting habits, e.g. if a litter tray has high sides which make it difficult to access, cats may stop using the litter tray altogether or may 'miss' the litter tray
- Reduction in hunting behaviour
- Increased sleeping

16.18 Behavioural changes associated with DJD in cats.

Investigation

As affected cats are often elderly, a full general examination with haematology, serum biochemistry and urinalysis should be performed on initial presentation, to assess for concurrent disease. Radiographs of affected joints should be taken if there is any doubt about the diagnosis, mainly to rule out other conditions that might require different management. In some circumstances, surgery may be appropriate for joints affected with DJD, such as femoral head and neck excision for hip osteoarthritis or elbow arthroscopy for debridement and lavage.

Management

If investigations do not reveal any contraindications, the cat can be started on a short course (e.g. 7 days) of NSAIDs. It would be advisable to re-examine the cat regularly to see if there has been an improvement; if there has, NSAIDs can be continued for another 2–3 weeks before another reassessment. If the cat does not show an improvement, or NSAID administration is contraindicated, then alternative drugs that could be considered include gabapentin, tramadol, amitriptyline and buprenorphine (see Chapter 3). Another pain management option to consider would be acupuncture. Polysulphated glycosaminoglycans are not authorized for use in cats but they may be an option for a cat that is not amenable to being given oral medication. Nutritional supplements are available for cats and include substances such as glycosaminoglycans, chondroitin sulphate, manganese, evening primrose oil, omega-3 fatty acids and green-lipped mussel; these may have some analgesic and anti-inflammatory effects in addition to purported chondroprotection and repair.

Environmental modifications that can be beneficial for cats with DJD

- Low-sided litter tray or ramp up to litter tray
- Warm comfortable bed that is easily accessible
- Low position to cat flap or provision of a litter tray if the cat is unwilling to go outside
- Pheromone diffusers may help decrease anxiety
- Introduce play sessions of gradually increasing duration, with toys that encourage movement

---

Long-term management of cats with chronic degenerative orthopaedic disorders also includes prevention of obesity (see also Chapter 2). The aim of the weight loss plan in overweight cats should be to enable modest reductions in bodyweight. Even subtle reductions in bodyweight may improve mobility, decrease pain and improve quality of life. Weight control will require calorie restriction and frequent monitoring of body condition to guide further alterations to the feeding regimen; weighing the daily intake of food is the most accurate tool rather than using a scoop. Implementation of meal-feeding strategies, use of an automatic feeder in a cat that is used to *ad libitum* feeding can help to spread the availability of food out evenly over 24 hours. *Ad libitum* feeding should be discouraged; this type of feeding contributes to obesity. A purpose-formulated diet, designed for feeding during weight management, is ideal. Activity can also be increased in other ways; for example, if the cat has a dry-food diet, a feeding toy can be used to increase activity at meal times (see Figure 1.4). Some dry food (part of the ration) can be fed in different places to encourage the cat to move around. Finally, outdoor cats may spontaneously increase activity, and should be encouraged to do so. The cat should be weighed regularly on the same set of scales to monitor weight loss. It is vital that weight loss is gradual in cats to avoid hepatic lipidosis; they should not lose more than approximately 1% of bodyweight per week (see QRG 2.1).

Owners are best placed to monitor changes in pain severity when the cat is in the home environment. The use of client-specific outcome measures (CSOM) has been recommended for monitoring changes in the severity of pain following initiation of analgesic therapy in cats with DJD (Lascelles and Robertson, 2010). DJD management is a life-long commitment. This must be explained to the owner.

References and further reading

Coughlan A and Miller A (2006) *BSAVA Manual of Small Animal Fracture Repair and Management [revised reprint]*. BSAVA Publications, Gloucester

Degasperi B, Gradner G and Dupré G (2007) Intramedullary pinning of metacarpal and metatarsal fractures in cats using a simple distraction technique. *Veterinary Surgery* **36**, 382–388

Hamilton MH, Evans DA and Langley-Hobbs SJ (2009) Feline ilial fractures: assessment of screw loosening and pelvic canal narrowing after lateral plating. *Veterinary Surgery* **38**, 326–333

Houlton JEF, Cook JL, Innes JF and Langley-Hobbs SJ (2006) *BSAVA Manual of Canine and Feline Musculoskeletal Disorders*. BSAVA Publications, Gloucester

Langley-Hobbs SJ (2009) Survey of 52 fractures of the patella in 34 cats. *Veterinary Record* **164**, 80–86

Langley-Hobbs SJ (2010) Patients with orthopaedic disease. In: *BSAVA Manual of Canine and Feline Rehabilitation, Supportive and Palliative Care: Case Studies in Patient Management*, ed. S Lindley and P Watson, pp. 194–231. BSAVA Publications, Gloucester

Langley-Hobbs SJ, Ball S and McKee WM (2009) Transverse stress fractures of the proximal tibia in 10 cats with non-union patellar fractures. *Veterinary Record* **164**, 425–430

Lascelles BDX and Robertson S (2010) DJD-associated pain in cats: what can we do to promote patient comfort? *Journal of Feline Medicine and Surgery* **12**, 200–212

Montavon PM, Voss K and Langley-Hobbs SJ (2009) *Feline Orthopaedic Surgery and Musculoskeletal disease*. Elsevier Saunders, Edinburgh

Roch SP, Stork CK, Gemmill TJ *et al.* (2009) Treatment of fractures of the tibial and/or fibular malleoli in 30 cats. *Veterinary Record* **165**,165–170

Schwarz PD and Schrader SC (1984) Ulnar fracture and dislocation of the proximal radial epiphysis (Monteggia lesion) in the dog and cat: a review of 28 cases. *Journal of the American Veterinary Medical Association* **185**, 190–194

Sissener TR, Whitelock R and Langley-Hobbs SJ (2009) Long term results of transarticular pinning for surgical stabilisation of coxofemoral luxation in 20 cats. *Journal of Small Animal Practice* **50**, 112–127

Wallace A, De La Puerta B, Trayhorn D *et al.* (2009) Feline combined diaphyseal radial and ulnar fractures: a retrospective study of 28 cases. *Veterinary Comparative Orthopaedics and Traumatology* **22**, 38–46

Zahn K, Kornmeyer M and Matis U (2007) Dowel pinning for feline metacarpal and metatarsal fractures. *Veterinary Comparative Orthopaedics and Traumatology* **20**, 256–263

Management of neurological and neuromuscular disorders

Laurent Garosi

This chapter will focus on the management of the most important neurological/neuromuscular disorders that are encountered in feline practice, notably head and spinal trauma, brachial plexus avulsion, ischaemic neuromyopathy, hypokalaemic polymyopathy, myasthenia gravis, vestibular disease and cognitive dysfunction syndrome. Other sections of the book contain more information on the approach to specific problems such as seizures (Chapter 4.7), sudden-onset blindness (Chapter 4.8), toxicities (Chapter 4.9), trauma and wound management (Chapter 4.10), ataxia (Chapter 5.6), head tilt (Chapter 5.16), mentation and behavioural changes (Chapter 5.24), lameness (Chapter 5.23). Ophthalmic and neurological examinations are described in QRGs 1.3 and 1.6. Orthopaedic conditions are described in Chapter 16. A practical guide to tail amputation following tail-pull injury is provided in QRG 17.1. The reader is referred to the *BSAVA Manual of Canine and Feline Neurology* for more in-depth information on all conditions.

should be evaluated to determine whether it is stable, requires treatment of immediate life-threatening conditions (e.g. shock, haemorrhage) and/or requires appropriate monitoring, so that potential problems can be anticipated and prevented. The four major organ systems (respiratory, cardiovascular, urinary and neurological) should be evaluated as part of the primary survey. The 'ABC' (airway, breathing and circulation) rule of triage should be observed (see Chapter 3).

The aims of the neurological examination are to:

- Determine whether the nervous system is affected
- Obtain an anatomical diagnosis (forebrain, brainstem, cerebellar, with/without spinal cord involvement, multifocal)
- Gain information about the prognosis using the modified Glasgow coma scale (modified GCS).

Head trauma

(See also Chapter 4.10 for a general approach to trauma cases.)

Pathophysiology

Head injuries can produce primary and secondary brain injury. Primary injuries, which are not treatable or reversible, describe the direct tissue damage that occurs at the time of initial impact. Secondary injury is the additional insult imposed on the neural tissue following the primary impact, resulting in ischaemia, infarction, brain oedema and subsequent elevations in intracranial pressure (ICP).

Clinical features

Initial physical assessment should focus on any imminently life-threatening abnormalities and evaluation of vital functions, all of which can influence not only interpretation of the neurological examination but also the prognosis for the patient. Primary survey assures identification and immediate treatment of conditions that are life-threatening. Upon arrival, every animal

> **Modified Glasgow coma scale**
> The modified GCS is a quantitative measure that has been shown to be associated with survival to 48 hours in dogs with traumatic brain injury. It provides a score that can be used to assess both initial neurological status and progression of signs. Although no study has evaluated this modified scale system in cats, the modified GCS provides an objective way for the clinician to grade the patient on admission and follow any response to treatment. The scale incorporates three domains:
>
> - Posture and limb motor function
> - Pupillary size/response to light and oculocephalic reflexes
> - Level of consciousness.
>
> A score of 1 to 6 is assigned to each domain. The final score ranges from 3 to 18, with lower scores indicating more severe neurological deficits. ▶

Parameter	Score
Motor activity	
Normal gait, normal spinal reflexes	6
Hemiparesis, tetraparesis or decerebrate activity	5
Recumbent, intermittent extensor rigidity	4
Recumbent, constant extensor rigidity	3
Recumbent, constant extensor rigidity with opisthotonus	2
Recumbent, hypotonia of muscles, depressed or absent spinal reflexes	1
Brainstem reflexes	
Normal pupillary light reflexes and oculocephalic reflexes	6
Slow pupillary light reflexes and normal to reduced oculocephalic reflexes	5
Bilateral unresponsive miosis with normal to reduced oculocephalic reflexes	4
Pinpoint pupils with reduced to absent oculocephalic reflexes	3
Unilateral, unresponsive mydriasis with reduced to absent oculocephalic reflexes	2
Bilateral, unresponsive mydriasis with reduced to absent oculocephalic reflexes	1
Level of consciousness	
Occasional periods of alertness and responsive to environment	6
Depression or delirium, capable of responding but response may be inappropriate	5
Semicomatose, responsive to visual stimuli	4
Semicomatose, responsive to auditory stimuli	3
Semicomatose, responsive only to repeated noxious stimuli	2
Comatose, unresponsive to repeated noxious stimuli	1

The initial neurological examination should be interpreted in light of the cardiovascular and respiratory systems, since shock can have a significant effect on neurological status.

Neurological assessment should be repeated every 30–60 minutes in patients with severe head injury, to assess for deterioration and to monitor the efficacy of any therapies administered. Advice from a specialist and/or referral should be considered early on in cases with neurological signs, since intensive management and monitoring can be required.

Diagnosis

Initial database
Because of the likelihood of multisystemic injury associated with head trauma, an initial emergency database should focus on:

- Packed cell volume (PCV) and total solids to assess for haemorrhage
- Blood glucose
- Blood pressure
- Ventilation
- Oxygenation
- Acid–base status and arterial blood gas, where available, to assess perfusion (arterial samples are usually only performed at specialist centres).

Imaging
Brain imaging is recommended for patients with moderate-to-severe neurological deficits that do not respond to aggressive extracranial and intracranial stabilization (see below), and those with progressive neurological signs. When this situation arises, if/when the cat is stable enough to travel and finances allow, referral to a specialist should be considered at the earliest opportunity. Skull radiographs are usually of limited value, but can sometimes identify fractures of the calvarium.

The two other imaging modalities of choice are magnetic resonance imaging (MRI; Figure 17.1) and computed tomography (CT) of the brain. Both have their advantages but CT seems to be the most suitable modality for cats with head trauma; it is faster, less expensive, produces better resolution of bone details and acute haemorrhage, and does not require general anaesthesia as it can often be performed under sedation.

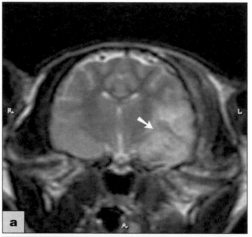

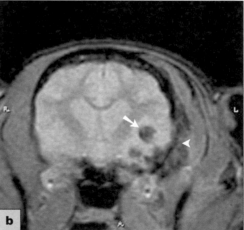

17.1 MR images of a cat with head trauma caused by a road traffic accident. **(a)** Transverse T2-weighted image showing marked oedema (arrow) within the left piriform lobe. **(b)** T2-gradient echo with areas of hypointensity in the left piriform lobe (arrow), suggestive of haemorrhage and comminuted calvarial fracture (arrowhead).

Brain imaging is an important step in the decision-making process when dealing with a head trauma patient, as it will help to decide on either medical or possible surgical treatment (required for depressed skull fractures, intra- or extra-axial haemorrhage, leaks of cerebrospinal fluid (CSF), etc.).

Management

The most important considerations in the treatment of head injuries are the maintenance of cerebral perfusion and oxygenation, together with the management of ventilation. Cerebral blood flow (CBF) is tightly controlled by alterations in vasomotor tone, regulated according to changes in partial pressures of arterial oxygen (P_aO_2) and carbon dioxide (P_aCO_2) and in systemic blood pressure. P_aCO_2 is one of the most potent regulators of CBF, with elevated P_aCO_2 levels causing vasodilation of cerebral vasculature and a subsequent increase in cerebral blood volume and ICP. Hypovolaemia and hypoxaemia must be recognized and treated immediately. Circulatory shock as a result of hypovolaemia causes a significant reduction in organ perfusion. During the compensatory phase of the shock syndrome, blood pressure is maintained by the body's responses to reduced tissue perfusion (e.g. increased heart rate, peripheral vasoconstriction, shifts in fluid from the interstitial space to the intravascular space and reduced urine production). Once the fluid deficit exceeds the ability of the body to compensate (decompensatory shock), decreases in blood pressure occur. Monitoring of blood pressure (see QRG 5.18.1) is therefore essential to ensure adequate arterial and cerebral perfusion pressures are maintained. The initial approach should therefore focus on extracranial stabilization (oxygen therapy, management of ventilation, fluid resuscitation and support of mean arterial blood pressure), closely followed by therapies directed toward intracranial stabilization (e.g. hyperosmolar therapy, hyperventilation) and, where indicated, surgical decompression.

Extracranial stabilization

This includes:

- Primarily, oxygen therapy (see QRG 4.2.2), aiming to have $S_pO_2 \geq 95\%$ or $P_aO_2 \geq 80$ mmHg
- Management of ventilation, aiming to have $P_{ET}CO_2$ = 30–35 mmHg (if measurements of end-tidal carbon dioxide are possible; see Chapter 3) or P_aCO_2 = 35–40 mmHg
- Fluid resuscitation
- Support of mean arterial blood pressure, aiming to have MABP = 80–100 mmHg.

In the recumbent cat, the head should be kept slightly elevated above the horizontal to assist in lowering ICP by increasing venous return from the brain.

Intracranial stabilization

Intracranial stabilization is indicated in: cats with moderate to severe head injury that are refractory to aggressive extracranial stabilization; and cats with progressive neurological signs.

- Following adequate volume resuscitation, the use of mannitol (0.25–1.0 g/kg i.v. over 10–20 minutes up to q8h) is the next most useful therapeutic modality to reduce ICP in severe brain injury. Mannitol should be avoided in hypovolaemic patients, however, in which intravenous hypertonic saline (7%) 3–5 ml/kg over 15 minutes may be used as an alternative.

- Corticosteroids should not be administered to cats with traumatic brain injury.
- The use of furosemide has been called into question because of the potential for intravascular volume depletion and systemic hypotension, ultimately leading to decreased cerebral perfusion pressure. It should be reserved for cats with pulmonary oedema or oligoanuric renal failure.

Exogenous spinal trauma

(See also Chapter 4.10 for a general approach to trauma patients.)

Aetiology

Exogenous spinal trauma is an important cause of spinal cord dysfunction in cats. In general, spinal trauma can be due to an event directly injuring the spinal cord (contusion, concussion, laceration) or to a condition affecting the surrounding structures (meninges, vertebrae, intervertebral disc) with secondary compression of the spinal cord. Approximately 20% of cats with traumatic spinal injuries also have acute intervertebral disc extrusion secondary to the trauma. Although all segments of the spine are susceptible to trauma, the cervicothoracic, thoracolumbar, lumbosacral and sacrococcygeal junctions are the most common sites of avulsion, fractures and luxation.

Clinical features

Nociception (perception of a noxious stimulus, tested by compression of the skin at the base of a digit or compression of a fold of skin on the body surface using forceps) in affected limbs is the most important prognostic indicator following spinal trauma. Lack of nociception associated with luxated or fractured vertebrae implies a complete absence of sensory perception, suggesting a poor prognosis due to the likely functional transection of the spinal cord.

In sacrococcygeal subluxation/luxation, transection of the nerves forming the caudal part of the cauda equina (pudendal and sciatic nerve roots) is frequently reported. In these patients, particular attention should be paid to the perineal reflex (stimulation of the perineal region with a cotton bud or haemostat should result in anal contraction and flexion of the tail) and nociception in genital, anal and tail structures, together with the presence of potential urinary and faecal incontinence.

Diagnosis

Survey spinal radiography will assist with initial evaluation of the patient (Figure 17.2). Approximately 20% of patients with thoracolumbar fractures have a second spinal column fracture/luxation; radiographs of the whole spine should therefore be performed in any cat with spinal trauma, together with survey chest radiographs and abdominal ultrasonography to look for concurrent injuries such as diaphragmatic and bladder rupture (see Chapter 4.10). Sedation may be required to obtain well positioned radiographs, and caution should be used during manipulation of the patient if this is the case (a board can be used), due to the ensuing relaxation of the epaxial musculature and the potential for further destabilization of the spine.

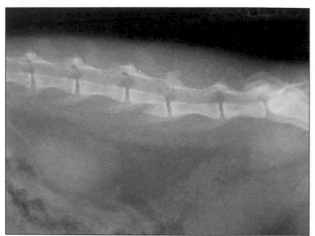

17.2 Lateral radiograph of a lumbar spine in a cat with fracture of the caudal part of the body of L5. (Courtesy of Cristian Falzone)

While there are different methods of predicting instability, the most commonly used method divides the spine into three compartments:

- The first compartment contains the ventral three-quarters of the vertebral body and disc, and the ventral longitudinal ligaments
- The second compartment consists of the dorsal quarter of the vertebral body and disc, and the dorsal longitudinal ligaments
- The third compartment includes the articular facets, lateral pedicles, dorsal laminae, interarcuate ligaments and dorsal spinous processes.

Disruption of any two of the three compartments is suggestive of instability. Advanced imaging, including myelography, CT–myelography and MRI, is needed to evaluate spinal cord compression and to search for other lesions not visible on radiographs (Figure 17.3); referral can be considered for these procedures.

Management

Management of a cat with spinal trauma should focus first on systemic stabilization. In a case of external trauma, such as car-associated injury, evaluation of the 'ABC' of trauma management is mandatory before performing a neurological examination. It is important to keep the cat immobilized, which can be achieved by securing it to a flat board.

Blood testing (a minimum of PCV, total protein, urea, creatinine and electrolyte assays), should be performed as soon as possible. Fluid therapy is important to maintain spinal cord perfusion; depending on the severity of hypotension, isotonic crystalloids, hypertonic saline, colloids or blood products can be used (see QRG 4.1.3).

Use of corticosteroids in acute spinal trauma is controversial. Although still routinely used in human medicine to reduce the secondary effects of ischaemic and reperfusion injury lesions, in veterinary medicine the use of corticosteroids in spinal trauma may lead to secondary side effects such as infections and gastrointestinal signs.

When spinal instability is detected, surgical stabilization of the spine is required. When neurological deficits are present in any trauma case, once the cat has

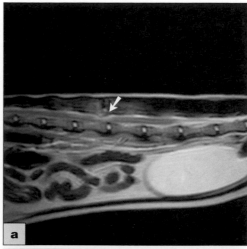

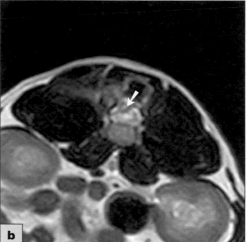

17.3 Sagittal **(a)** and transverse **(b)** T2-weighted MR images of the caudal lumbar spine of a cat shot by an air gun pellet. Note the fracture of the caudal part of the dorsal lamina (arrow) of L3, causing compression of the spinal cord.

been systemically stabilized and concurrent injuries addressed, referral to a specialist for further assessment of the spinal trauma should be considered at the earliest opportunity.

Nerve injury and brachial plexus avulsion

Aetiology

Common causes of nerve injury in cats include road traffic accidents (RTAs), gunshot wounds, bites, lacerations, stretching (Figure 17.4), fractures, and iatrogenic damage from surgical procedures or injection injuries. Three types of nerve damage are distinguished, depending on the degree of structural damage:

- Neurapraxia – transient physiological conduction block of nerve transmission in the absence of structural damage
- Axonotmesis – disruption of the axons, with the endoneurial and Schwann cell sheaths remaining intact
- Neurotmesis – complete severance of all structures of the nerve.

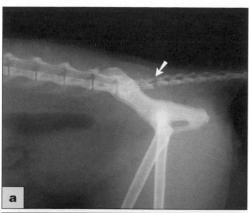

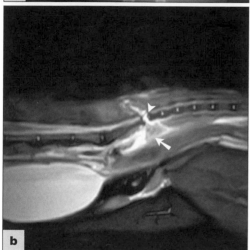

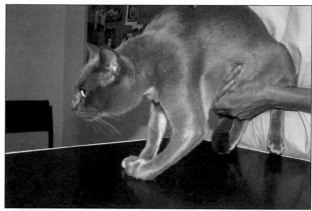

17.5 Brachial plexus paralysis in a cat secondary to trauma. There is marked neurogenic muscle atrophy in addition to the obvious lack of strength and extensor tone.

17.4 Images of a cat with tail-pull injury. **(a)** Lateral radiograph, showing the sacrocaudal dislocation (arrow). **(b)** Short tau inversion recovery (STIR) MR image, showing transection at the level of the origin of the pelvic and pudendal nerves (arrowhead) and soft tissue damage (arrow) ventral to the tail. (See QRG 17.1 for a guide to tail amputation.)

Both axonotmesis and neurotmesis are followed by Wallerian degeneration (degeneration of a nerve distal to the site of injury and away from the cell body) and carry a guarded to poor prognosis. Avulsion of the nerve roots forming the brachial plexus, as a result of an RTA or a fall from height, is the most common traumatic neuropathy in the cat. The damage occurs at the level of the spinal roots, where resistance to stretch is less than that of peripheral nerves due to the lack of perineurium.

Clinical features
Neurological signs associated with brachial plexus avulsion depend on which nerve roots are affected:

- Avulsion of the cranial plexus roots (C6–C7 nerve roots) causes loss of shoulder movement and elbow flexion, although the animal can still bear weight on that limb as the extension of the elbow is spared. Cutaneous sensation may be lost in the dorsum of the paw and in the cranial and lateral antebrachium
- Avulsion of the caudal plexus roots (C8–T2 nerve roots) results in carriage of the limb with the elbow and shoulder flexed and an inability to bear weight due to paralysis of the triceps brachii muscle (elbow extension) (Figure 17.5). The elbow is dropped and knuckling of the carpus is marked on

evaluation of the gait. Cutaneous sensation may be lost distal to the elbow
- Complete avulsion of all plexus roots (C6–T2 nerve roots) causes a flaccid limb with inability to bear weight and loss of the cutaneous sensation in the entire limb.

Many cats with brachial plexus avulsion will also present with:

- Ipsilateral Horner's syndrome – involvement of the preganglionic neuron of the sympathetic supply to the eye, which originates in thoracic spinal cord segments T1–T3
- Loss of cutaneous trunci reflex – stimulation of the skin along the thoracolumbar area (one side at a time) with haemostats should elicit contraction of the cutaneous trunci muscle, seen as a skin twitch. If absent, either the sensory supply from spinal nerves is affected or the motor supply to the cutaneous trunci muscle, which originates from C8–T1 spinal cord segment and hence is affected by brachial plexus avulsion.

Diagnosis
Diagnosis is mostly based on a history of trauma and neurological evaluation of limb function. If referral to a specialist is an option, electromyography can help to document the extent of muscle denervation and confirm the distribution of nerve injury, although electromyographic changes may not be seen for 7–10 days after the injury. Serial evaluation of radial nerve motor conduction velocity has been suggested as a useful prognostic indicator, with early decreased conduction velocity indicating a poor prognosis.

Management
Treatment of brachial plexus injury is conservative and mainly revolves around aggressive physiotherapy. Advice should be sought regarding appropriate physiotherapy techniques. Pancarpal arthrodesis, to prevent carpal collapse secondary to loss of radial nerve function, is rarely appropriate since, in most cases, elbow function is also absent.

Prognosis is good for cats with cranial brachial plexus avulsion that retain the ability to bear weight and have intact cutaneous sensation. Cats with complete or caudal brachial plexus avulsion have a guarded to poor prognosis, especially if cutaneous sensation has been lost. If no improvement is seen during the first 2 months, recovery is considered to be unlikely to occur. Gabapentin (10–20 mg/kg orally q8–12h) or pregabalin (5–10 mg/kg orally q12h) can be considered for control of neuropathic pain if self-mutilation from paraesthesia is seen. Amputation is recommended in these cases, especially if complications develop, such as self-mutilation refractory to medical management, joint contractures or trophic ulcers.

Ischaemic neuromyopathy

Ischaemic neuromyopathy occurs particularly in cats with cardiomyopathy (especially cardiomyopathies associated with left atrial enlargement), when thrombosis of the caudal aorta or of its main branches typically occurs. Arterial thromboembolism (ATE) also occurs as a complication of hyperthyroidism and neoplasia. Clinical signs are typically acute and include:

- Paresis/paraplegia with cold extremities
- Weak or absent femoral pulses
- Firm painful muscles
- Loss of nociception.

In most cats, ATE will affect both pelvic limbs, although a single limb (thoracic or pelvic) can be embolized. The diagnosis, management and prognosis of ATE are discussed in Chapter 9.

Hypokalaemic myopathy

Aetiology
Hypokalaemic myopathy is a metabolic disorder of older cats that has been linked most commonly with chronic kidney disease (CKD) and excessive urinary potassium loss, and less commonly with primary hyperaldosteronism. Cats on potassium-deficient diets were also shown to have cyclical disease, with episodes of polymyopathy recurring after periods of spontaneous clinical recovery. A similar syndrome with a hereditary basis has been reported in Burmese cats (genetic test available). Hypokalaemia causes an increase in resting membrane potential and hyperpolarization of muscle membrane.

Clinical features
Hypokalaemia (see Chapter 4.6) can manifest as generalized weakness of acute-onset apparent muscular pain and persistent ventroflexion of the neck.

Ventroflexion of the neck
This can be associated with:

- Hypokalaemia (e.g. CKD, primary hyperaldosteronism, Burmese cats)
- Myasthenia gravis
- Polymyopathy (including idiopathic and toxoplasmosis-associated myositis)
- Severe cervical spinal cord disease affecting grey matter
- Thiamine deficiency
- Polyneuropathy.

Diagnosis
Serum potassium concentrations are low (usually 1.5–3 mmol/l) and creatine kinase activity is often markedly increased (500–10,000 IU/l).

Management
Myopathic signs resolve after parenteral and oral administration of potassium (see QRG 4.6.1).

Myasthenia gravis

Aetiology
Myasthenia gravis (MG) results from either a congenital deficiency of nicotinic acetylcholine receptors on the postsynaptic membrane of the neuromuscular junction or an acquired immune-mediated destruction of these receptors, mediated by specific autoantibodies (anti-acetylcholine receptor antibodies). The mechanism that triggers such antibody production is usually unknown but it can occur in association with methimazole therapy and thymoma or cystic thymus. Breed predisposition for the acquired form is recognized in Abyssinians and Somalis. Acquired MG in cats is often associated with other neuromuscular diseases such as polymyositis or polyneuritis.

Clinical features
Affected cats tire easily and are reluctant to exercise. Collapse may occur after a few steps. Dyspnoea and an altered 'miaow' have been described, and some cats show dysphagia and regurgitation (see Chapter 5.32).

Diagnosis
A presumptive diagnosis of MG can be achieved by a positive response to edrophonium chloride (a short-acting cholinesterase inhibitor) at 0.22 mg/kg i.v. once. A positive response is an immediate and dramatic increase in muscle strength for a short period of time (2–10 minutes), although some cats with non-MG-associated myopathy may show a partial response and some cats with MG may show no response at all. Edrophonium chloride can cause cholinergic side effects (urination, lacrimation, vomiting, defecation, salivation, bradycardia, bronchospasm); if severe, atropine should be administered (0.04 mg/kg i.v. once).

Definitive diagnosis of acquired MG is achieved by measuring antibodies to the acetylcholine receptor. This test is negative in cases of congenital MG.

Management
Treatment is with long-acting anticholinesterase therapy (oral pyridostigmine 0.5–3.0 mg/kg q8–12h). If oral therapy is not possible initially, intramuscular neostigmine can be given at 0.04 mg/kg q8h, starting at the low end to avoid cholinergic crisis (bradycardia, salivation, diarrhoea, dyspnoea, miosis, limb tremor). If limb muscle strength has not returned to normal following anticholinesterase treatment and if there is no evidence of aspiration pneumonia, alternate-day low-dose corticosteroid therapy should be initiated (0.5 mg/kg orally q48h) and slowly increased over 5–7 days to an immunosuppressive dose (2 mg/kg q24h)

if necessary. It is advisable to seek advice before initiating corticosteroids, as treatment is not always straightforward; alternative immunosuppressive treatments may sometimes be advised.

Vestibular disease

Aetiology

Clinical signs of vestibular disease (VD) may be a result of: lesions involving the receptor organs in the inner ear or the vestibular portion of cranial nerve VIII (i.e. peripheral VD); or lesions involving the brainstem, vestibular nuclei or vestibular centres in the cerebellum (i.e. central VD). Idiopathic vestibular syndrome and middle ear disease (otitis and/or nasopharyngeal polyps) are the most common causes of peripheral VD. Caudal fossa tumours and inflammatory/infectious CNS diseases are the most frequently encountered conditions in cats presented with central VD.

Clinical features

VD may result in any or all of the following clinical signs:

- Head tilt (see Chapter 5.16)
- Falling
- Rolling
- Leaning
- Circling
- Abnormal nystagmus (Figure 17.6)
- Positional strabismus
- Ataxia (see Chapter 5.6).

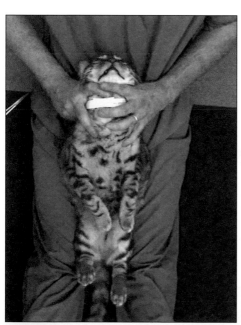

17.6 Testing for positional nystagmus should be considered as part of the neurological evaluation of any cat with ataxia. Extending the head and neck while the cat is in dorsal recumbency – here lying along the legs of the vet seated on the floor – can help in detecting a positional nystagmus by challenging the vestibular system.

Cats with acute VD may additionally display vomiting associated with disequilibrium. Facial paralysis and Horner's syndrome can be seen with peripheral VD due to the proximity of cranial nerve VII (facial nerve) and the sympathetic nerve supply to the eye to the vestibular nerve in the region of the petrous temporal bone.

Bilateral VD is characterized by a head sway from side to side, loss of balance on one side and symmetrical ataxia, with a crouched posture closer to the ground surface. A physiological nystagmus usually cannot be elicited.

Diagnosis

The first step is to determine whether the patient has evidence of peripheral or central VD, as the differential diagnoses, diagnostic and treatment considerations, and prognoses differ.

Correctly identifying central VD requires identification of clinical signs that cannot be attributed to diseases of the peripheral vestibular system. However, even if such signs are not present, a central lesion cannot be excluded. Lesions that affect the central vestibular system typically have additional clinical signs suggestive of brainstem involvement. Therefore, abnormal mental status (depression, stupor, coma), ipsilateral upper motor neuron (UMN) hemiparesis and general proprioceptive (GP) ataxia, and conscious proprioceptive deficits are commonly associated with central VD. Deficits of cranial nerves V through XII (other than VII and VIII) can also be associated with central VD. Vertical nystagmus and nystagmus that changes in direction on changing position of the head (i.e. variable nystagmus) are features of central VD.

Diagnostic tests for evaluation of peripheral VD should include:

- Otoscopic and pharyngeal examination under general anaesthetic
- Swabs for cytology and culture (aerobic, fungal and yeast) from the middle ear if the tympanic membrane is ruptured (see QRG 5.15.1)
- Myringotomy with a 20 G spinal needle to obtain samples for cytology and culture if the tympanic membrane is intact but bulging or of an abnormal colour (advice should be sought before doing this if the clinician does not have experience with this technique)
- Imaging of the tympanic bullae with radiographs, CT or MRI to assess for otitis media/interna and polyps.

If central VD is suspected, some basic evaluations can be performed in practice to evaluate for causes of potential cerebrovascular accident, but for most cases of central VD, advice or referral should be sought. Advanced imaging of the brain (CT or MRI), CSF analysis, and serum and CSF serology and PCR for various infectious agents (e.g. feline coronavirus, *Toxoplasma, Cryptococcus*) are indicated to evaluate central VD.

Further investigations may be required in cases of suspected:

- Brain tumour – tissue biopsy by surgical or stereotactic biopsy, thoracic and abdominal imaging to investigate metastatic disease
- Thiamine deficiency – urinary organic acids excretion screening or transketolase activity in fresh erythrocytes
- Cerebrovascular accident – routine hematology

and serum biochemistry, clotting profile, evaluation of arterial blood pressure, thyroid, kidney, adrenal and heart function.

Management

Treatment is determined by the underlying cause. No treatment has been proven to be beneficial for idiopathic vestibular syndrome, but this usually resolves without treatment in 1–3 weeks from onset, although some cats may be left with episodic ataxia or a persistent head tilt. Recurrence occasionally happens after a variable period of weeks to months. Meclizine (6.25 mg orally q12h) or diazepam (1–2 mg orally q12h; though rarely associated with idiosyncratic hepatotoxicity which can be fatal) are sometimes helpful in decreasing signs associated with acute vestibular disorder (nausea, anorexia, anxiety and, in some instances, the severity of the head tilt and ataxia).

Cognitive dysfunction syndrome

Cognitive dysfunction syndrome (CDS) describes an age-related decline of cognitive abilities, which is characterized by behavioural changes unattributable to other medical conditions plus increasing brain pathology.

Aetiology

The pathophysiology of feline brain ageing still requires considerable study. Age-related brain pathology in cats includes cerebral atrophy, beta-amyloid accumulation within the cerebral blood vessels, atrophy of the cholinergic system in the locus coeruleus, and abnormal tau protein accumulation within individual neurons. Functional changes include a depletion of catecholamine neurotransmitters, a decline in the cholinergic system, an increase in monoamine oxidase B (MAOB) activity and a reduction of endogenous antioxidants. While the brains of older cats show many of these changes, it is not yet clear which of them may be directly associated with cognitive dysfunction.

Clinical features

While the exact age of onset is not established, studies suggest that age-related behavioural changes consistent with CDS may be found in cats from as early as 10 years of age but that prevalence increases significantly in older cats. The most commonly seen behavioural changes in CDS in cats include:

- Spatial or temporal disorientation
- Altered interaction with owners
- Changes in sleep–wake cycles
- Inappropriate urination (see Chapter 5.21)
- Inappropriate defecation (see Chapter 5.20)
- Inappropriate vocalization.

Diagnosis

The diagnosis of CDS requires the identification of geriatric behavioural changes that are not caused by other medical problems, although the two may not be mutually exclusive. A thorough medical and behavioural history must be obtained from the owner. Diagnostic investigations should begin with evaluation for metabolic disease (haematology, serum biochemistry, thyroxine levels, urinalysis and assessment of systemic blood pressure) and, depending on findings, may go on to include evaluation for structural brain disease (head MRI, CSF analysis, serological testing for FeLV, FIV, *Toxoplasma* and feline coronavirus). Where appropriate and indicated from initial findings, further investigations may also include thoracic, abdominal or skeletal radiography, abdominal ultrasonography, echocardiography, electrocardiography, intestinal endoscopy and biopsy.

Management

Treatment currently centres around diets enriched with antioxidants (e.g. those designed for joint disease in cats) and other supportive compounds (e.g. vitamin E, L-carnitine, beta-carotene and omega-3 fatty acids), combined with environmental stimulation (e.g. toys, company, food-hunting games; see Chapter 2) and drugs such as selegiline (0.25–1 mg/kg orally q24h), propentofylline (one-quarter of a 50 mg tablet q24h) and anti-inflammatory medications (oral prednisolone at 0.5 mg/kg/day).

References and further reading

Platt SR and Olby N (2013) *BSAVA Manual of Canine and Feline Neurology, 4th edn.* BSAVA Publications, Gloucester
Platt SR, Radaelli ST and McDonnell JJ (2001) The prognostic value of the modified Glasgow Coma Scale in head trauma in dogs. *Journal of Veterinary Internal Medicine* **15**, 581–584

QRG 17.1 Tail-pull injuries and tail amputation
by Geraldine Hunt

Tail-pull injuries

Tail-pull (traction) injuries causing fracture/luxation at the sacrocaudal (sacrococcygeal) junction result in neurological signs associated with injury to the sensory and motor nerves of the lumbar plexus (sciatic, pelvic and pudendal nerves). While the cat may often walk well, the tail is flaccid with poor or no pain perception, and the cat has faecal and urinary incontinence. Faecal retention can also occur as a result of pain, poor perineal muscle tone and absence of reflexes stimulating defecation.

The fracture/luxation usually occurs between the sacral and caudal vertebrae, leaving the tail dangling and producing more traction on the already damaged nerve roots. Diagnosis is made on the basis of clinical signs and radiographs. Some improvement may occur in the days to weeks following injury, but in most instances the nerves are too badly damaged to permit re-innervation and the author usually recommends surgery to amputate the tail within 4 weeks of injury.

Damage to the surrounding soft tissues is variable, depending on the severity of the initial injury. In most cases, the soft tissue injuries heal ▶

QRG 17.1 continued

with conservative management, but in some cases avulsion of the perineal musculature from the sacrotuberous ligament and sacrum occurs, tearing the perineal diaphragm and leading to problems with defecation (similar to a perineal rupture). This should be suspected if a faecal ball forms in an area of rectal sacculation just cranial to the anus; the diagnosis is confirmed by rectal examination. If perineal rupture is suspected, cases should be referred for a specialist opinion as such soft tissue injuries should be explored and repaired.

Tail amputation

Although repair of the vertebral fracture/luxation may be considered in tail-pull injuries, the tail may never regain function and exerts a strong lever-arm effect on the fracture site, increasing the risk of repair failure. Hence direct repair is not often undertaken and tail amputation is usually performed.

The main purposes of tail amputation in this clinical setting are to:

- Avoid injury to the insensitive tail
- Reduce traction on the nerve roots
- Reduce pain associated with the fracture/luxation and nerve root traction.

The tail amputation is usually performed between the 2nd and 3rd, or 3rd and 4th, caudal vertebrae. This leaves a short tail stub to protect the anus. It is easier to perform than a high amputation at the level of the sacral or caudal fracture/luxation, and reduces most of the traction effect, even though two or three caudal vertebrae remain. It also requires less soft tissue dissection, which is beneficial in reducing further trauma to the area.

Equipment

A basic surgical kit is required, containing:

- Towel clamps (A)
- Brown–Adson thumb forceps (B)
- Needle-holders (C)
- No.3 scalpel handle (D)
- No.15 scalpel blade (E)

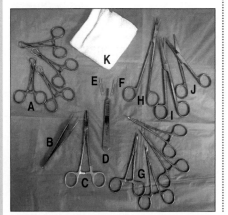

- No.10 scalpel blade (F)
- Mosquito forceps (G)
- Metzenbaum scissors (H)
- Mayo scissors (I)
- Blunt–sharp suture scissors (J)
- Gauze surgical swabs (K).

Patient preparation and planning

The cat undergoes general anaesthesia (see Chapter 3) and is placed in sternal recumbency. The rectum is manually evacuated of faeces and a purse-string suture of a synthetic monofilament 2 metric (3/0 USP) material may be placed in the anus (not done in the case illustrated). The tail, tail base and perineal area are fully clipped and prepared aseptically for surgery, and draped.

Both the dorsal and ventral skin incisions are positioned caudal to the proposed level of tail amputation. They are curved so that their convexity is towards the tip of the tail, thus creating a 'clam shell' effect with a dorsal and a ventral flap. The ventral skin flap is designed to be longer than the dorsal skin flap, so that the ventral flap can be folded up over the tail stump and sutured to the dorsal flap, with the suture line separated from the anus, at the end of the procedure.

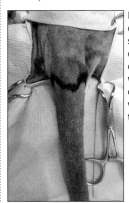

Position of the dorsal skin incision site. The incision is centred on the 3rd caudal vertebra, with a convexity of one caudal vertebral length towards the tail tip.

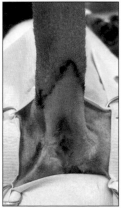

Position of the ventral skin incision site.

Surgical procedure

1 The dorsal incision is made and the flap reflected cranially. The soft tissues are sharply dissected from the caudal vertebrae. Caudal arteries on the dorsolateral and ventrolateral aspects of the vertebrae are ligated or cauterized when they are evident (white arrow).

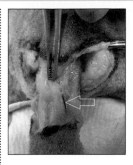

2 The ventral incision is then made in the skin. The tail is then flexed and rotated to determine where the vertebrae articulate; this allows determination of where to incise the ventral muscles of the tail over the appropriate intervertebral disc space with a scalpel.

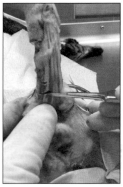

Incising the ventral muscles over the appropriate disc space. The small incision in the more distal tail muscle occurred during incision of the overlying skin.

3 The scalpel blade is inserted into the intervertebral disc space to separate the vertebrae, again from the ventral aspect.

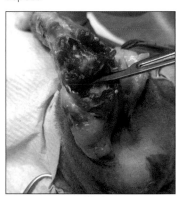

4 The tail is angled first to one side and then to the other, to facilitate using the scalpel to disarticulate the bilateral dorsal articular facets (arrowed) located dorsal to the cranial edge of the intervertebral disc.

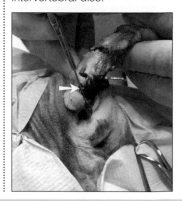

▶

QRG 17.1 *continued*

5 Residual bleeding points are identified, clamped and either ligated or cauterized.

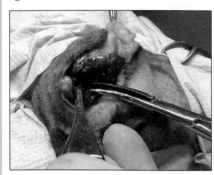

6 The surgical site is then lavaged thoroughly with saline, as the vertebral canal is now open and the nerve roots exposed, placing the cat at increased risk of ascending infection.

7 The ventral flap has been drawn dorsally, moving the suture line away from the anus. The wound is closed in two layers with a continuous subcutaneous layer of monofilament absorbable suture, and either subcuticular or skin sutures depending on the surgeon's preference.

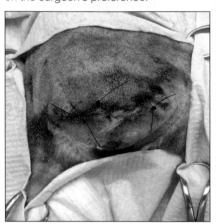

Postoperative care and prognosis

A broad-spectrum antibiotic such as amoxicillin/clavulanate should be administered for 3 days following surgery to reduce the risk of meningeal infection through contamination of the open spinal canal. Appropriate analgesia should also be administered, such as an opioid or an NSAID (see Chapter 3).

Owners should be warned that neurological abnormalities such as incontinence, hindlimb paresis and abnormal perineal sensation may only resolve slowly over weeks to months following surgery, and that neurological function may never return to normal. However, many cats live happily following this injury.

Management of behavioural disorders

Vicky Halls

'Problem' behaviour in cats brought to the attention of veterinary surgeons is based on the individual owner's subjective assessment and perception of what constitutes a problem. Many of the behaviours highlighted by owners will be normal for the species but are misinterpreted by the owner as being 'bad'.

Common behavioural problems in cats

The most common feline behavioural problems seen in veterinary practice are:

- House soiling (inappropriate urination or defecation; see also Chapters 5.20 and 5.21)
- Urine spraying
- Aggression toward other cats
- Aggression toward people
- Anxiety/fear
- Excessive scratching of furniture
- Behavioural problems associated with old age
- Overgrooming (see Chapter 5.26)
- Pica (see Chapter 5.27).

Taking the history

All information needs to be established from the client regarding the cat, the owners, the environment (inside and outside), and the cat's diet and lifestyle, together with the history of the problem. A general behaviour questionnaire is used for this purpose, an example of which is reproduced in the *BSAVA Manual of Feline and Canine Behavioural Medicine, 2nd edition* and is available to BSAVA members at www.bsava.com.

The medical records of all cats in the household should be scrutinized, as these may be helpful in establishing the chronology of the problem and jogging the owner's memory of past events. Some possible indicators of the presence of potential stressors may be evident, e.g. a history of cat bite abscesses, cystitis, allergies/hypersensitivities or recurrent viral infections.

During routine veterinary examinations clients rarely mention behavioural problems, so it is important to incorporate questions about behaviour as part of history-taking during any physical examination, including during visits for routine preventive care (see

Chapter 2). The prevention of behavioural problems, including good early socialization of kittens and continuing education of the pet-owning public (see Chapters 1 and 2), is as significant as any other aspect of total wellness care.

House soiling

Considerations regarding house soiling that are specific to elderly cats are considered later in the chapter.

Inappropriate urination

Urine is normally voided on horizontal surfaces. Quantities of urine passed range from small spots to large volumes.

When urine is passed against vertical surfaces from a standing posture it is more normally associated with urine spray marking (urine spraying; see below).

Periuria is defined as urination in inappropriate places. Behavioural motivation for this includes stress associated with environmental or social issues, lack of early litter training, aversion to the litter tray or substrate in it, lack of indoor litter facilities, bullying from cats outside, and tension in a multi-cat household. There are also a number of medical reasons for periuria, including:

- Cystitis, feline urinary tract disease (FLUTD), feline idiopathic cystitis (FIC; Figure 18.1)

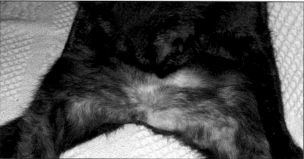

18.1 Overgrooming of the ventrocaudal abdomen and medial thighs associated with the discomfort of FIC in a cat that was presented for inappropriate urination. What appears to be behavioural periuria has often started as a result of FIC, so a careful history and thorough evaluation for FIC is essential.

- Chronic kidney disease, diabetes or other diseases causing polyuria
- Urinary incontinence
- Arthritis (pain or mobility problems)
- Cognitive dysfunction syndrome (see Chapter 17).

Addressing or managing underlying medical issues (see Chapters 13, 14 and 16) may be sufficient to resolve the periuria.

General advice for tackling periuria
This includes:

- Identify and address potential underlying medical issues
- Identify specific stressors and remove or manage them (as for urine spraying; see below)
- Maintain appropriate litter facilities indoors (see also Chapter 2):
  - Provide one litter tray per cat plus one extra, located in separate discrete areas
  - Locate the trays away from busy thoroughfares, sleeping areas, food and water bowls, full-length glass windows and entry and exit points such as cat flaps or doors
  - Use litter substrate that the cat favours (fine, sand-like clumping material with no deodorizers or scent additive is generally preferred)
  - Offer a choice of litter tray type: covered and open. Open trays are generally preferred by cats
  - Use large litter trays (one and a half times the length of the cat from nose to base of tail would be ideal)
  - Ensure the depth of substrate is adequate; 3–4 cm is generally preferred
  - Maintain a regular litter tray cleaning regime
- Do not punish the cat for soiling in the house, as this will further reinforce any underlying anxiety
- When introducing a litter tray, do not place the cat in it (may be considered aversive) nor give a reward for using it
- Any areas where the cat has been soiling should be cleaned thoroughly (as described below for urine spraying).

Inappropriate defecation
Inappropriate defecation can occur in isolation or together with periuria. In either case the general advice given above for tackling periuria would apply. It may also be helpful to deny the cat's access to the preferred location(s) where soiling is taking place. If this is impractical, changing the layout of the area by moving furniture, for example, may help to break the habit.

Urine spraying

Urine spraying is a behaviour seen with both male and female cats (intact and neutered), although the frequency is higher in intact toms. It is a form of territorial marking in which small amounts (<2 ml) of urine are usually deposited on a vertical surface. However, urine spraying has adapted to fulfil other functions in the domestic neutered pet cat, reflecting the emotional state of the animal during socially stressful situations. Caution should be taken in presuming all urine spraying has a primary behavioural motivation, as diseases causing localized pain or discomfort (e.g. FIC involving urethral inflammation, osteoarthritis) may result in a cat adopting a spraying posture to eliminate.

Specific stress triggers for urine spraying
Internal stressors include:

- Inter-cat conflict within a household; this should be differentiated from affiliative behaviour (Figure 18.2)
- Introduction of a new cat into the household
- Environmental upheaval, e.g. building work, new furniture, new baby
- Owner absence/change of work schedule
- Inappropriate punishment
- Attention-seeking in over-attached cats.

Inter-cat conflict
<ul><li>Avoid each other</li><li>Prefer to be facing away from each other when in close proximity</li><li>Fixed staring</li><li>Block access to resources from another cat (e.g. standing in front of a cat flap, litter tray or food bowl to prevent another cat from accessing them)</li><li>Block access to an area by standing in doorways/corridors</li><li>Hissing/growling</li><li>Aggression</li></ul>

Affiliative behaviour
<ul><li>Eat together, often out of the same bowl</li><li>Sleep together, with physical contact</li><li>Groom each other</li><li>Rub against one another</li><li>Nose-to-nose greetings</li><li>Play together</li></ul>

18.2 Inter-cat conflict *versus* affiliative behaviour. Affiliative behaviour suggests sociability in a multi-cat group, i.e. cats belonging to the same social group. Owners are often unaware of the subtle signs of inter-cat conflict and may report that there is no evidence of this unless they are questioned carefully about the signs noted here.

External stressors include:

- Invasion of the home by a strange cat (e.g. a neighbour's cat coming into the house)
- Indirect threat from strange cats (e.g. scent on clothing)
- Presence of a cat flap (giving a sense of vulnerability).

General advice for tackling urine spraying
Any advice given should take into consideration any stress triggers identified. In multi-cat households, presence of inter-cat conflict should be identified (see Figure 18.2) and the cat's core area (see below) recognized, ensuring that this area can be readily accessed by the cat and contains all the essential resources.

> - A cat's **core area** is the location where it feels safe enough to eat, rest, sleep and play without fear of threat. In situations of high conflict this can be as small as the corner of a bedroom (e.g. the cat may choose to spend most of its time underneath a bed or on top of a wardrobe); where there is little or no conflict, the core area may incorporate the majority of the owner's home. ▶

> ■ **Essential resources** to include within the core area include a bed, food, water, litter tray, high perch, hiding place, scratching post and toys. All should be positioned a reasonable distance apart; in particular the litter tray, food and water should all be separated as much as possible.

In addition:

■ Sprayed areas should be cleaned with 10% biological (enzymatic) cleansing solution (rather than an ammonia-based product), rinsed thoroughly, dried and then sprayed with surgical spirit
■ New feeding stations should be placed at cleaned sprayed sites
■ Safe indoor litter trays should be provided, with increased resources
■ Empty litter trays should be propped up against primary spraying sites to provide a controlled environment for spraying
■ Use a feline facial pheromone diffuser or spray (see below).

Some of the following advice may also be applicable, depending on whether the primary stressor is external or internal.

Help with external stressors:

■ Remove full-length curtains or pin them up temporarily to avoid repeated spraying on them
■ Block lower glass panels of full-length windows with opaque adhesive film
■ Commercially available deterrents (e.g. pellets soaked in essence of lion dung) or motion sensor sprinklers, may be useful to keep other cats out of the garden, etc.
■ Install an exclusive-entry cat flap
■ Remove or block external vantage points for any cats outside, e.g. shed roof.

Help with internal stressors:

■ Provide high vantage points indoors and alternative opportunities to mark (e.g. scratching posts) in locations of conflict
■ Install a second cat flap or entry/exit point such as a window or door
■ Maintain litter facilities (see above)
■ Where inter-cat conflict is present (see Figure 18.2), see advice below.

Prognosis

Urine spraying is difficult to resolve but the problem may be reduced or contained to the satisfaction of the owner. Guidance should be offered regarding the long-term welfare of the individual cat if spraying is not resolved; referral to a cat behaviourist may be necessary, as these cases can be complex and multifactorial.

Aggression toward other cats

Cat members of the same household may compete over territory; once cats reach social maturity separate factions (groups) can develop within the same household, with each faction working as a group in its own right. In these circumstances, cats will communicate via scent to avoid contact with each other and resolve disputes using passive aggression and intimidation whenever possible. Signs of passive aggression include staring and blocking thoroughfares and access to resources, such as indoor litter facilities. Active aggression (fighting) will occur if escape and avoidance opportunities are limited or absent.

Causes of (and motivation for) inter-cat aggression
These include:

■ Incompatibility of cats in the same household (Figure 18.3)
■ Redirected aggression, from one cat to another, triggered by acute sense of threat from an external source or novel stimulus
■ Invasion of the core area by a strange cat
■ Defence of the home range in response to a strange cat
■ Illness of a cat within the household (disruption due to potential scent and behaviour changes)
■ Death of a member of a cat group (potentially diminishing the perception of cohesion among the remaining cats)
■ Return from the veterinary clinic or after an absence from the household (failure to be recognized due to scent change)
■ Maternal aggression (queens protecting offspring)
■ Introduction of a new cat
■ Pressures from outside in a densely cat populated area
■ Genetic, acquired predisposition to highly motivated territoriality
■ Misdirected predatory or play behaviour.

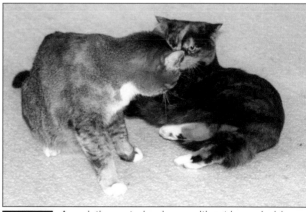

18.3 Agonistic posturing in a multi-cat household. Note the crouched body positions, the ears flattened and facing backwards, and there may be hissing and/or growling between these cats. The intention with this posturing is to prevent fighting. However, such incompatibility may lead to inter-cat aggression.

General advice for tackling inter-cat aggression
This includes:

■ Provide dry food for 'grazing' throughout the day, or divide wet food into several smaller meals to avoid competition at set meal times. Designate several areas within the home as feeding stations to avoid bullying

- Place water bowls throughout the home, located away from food
- Provide high resting places, beds and private areas in sufficient number (one per cat plus one extra)
- Provide scratching posts located near entrances, beds and feeding stations to ensure an appropriate surface is available for marking in areas of potential competition
- Provide indoor litter facilities (one litter tray per cat plus one extra) even if the cats have access to outside
- Provide two separate entry/exit points to the property, i.e. cat flaps, doors or windows, to avoid the risk of guarding or blocking
- If separate social groups have been identified and space is limited, then providing 'one resource per *social group* plus one extra' may be sufficient. Ideally, the cat's core areas should be recognized and each cat's core area should contain all the essential resources (see above).

Aggression toward people

Aggression is a serious problem that can result in significant injury, and sometimes subsequent infection, particularly in the elderly or immunosuppressed, so medical attention is advised for any bites or severe scratches to people. There are numerous causes and motivations; it is misleading and inaccurate to presume that all aggression toward humans is the manifestation of an 'aggressive cat'; the display is an indication of the cat's emotional state *at the time* rather than an innate characteristic of its personality.

There are many ways to categorize aggression, including:

- Fear-related aggression – caused by lack of early socialization
- Play aggression – seen initially in young kittens but can continue into adulthood
- Misdirected predatory behaviour
- Learned aggression – commonly used to deter unwanted attention from humans
- Frustration-related aggression
- Redirected aggression – triggered by acute sense of threat from an external source or novel stimulus
- Maternal aggression
- Idiopathic aggression – referring to those acute outbursts where the trigger or motivation is unknown
- Aggression related to illness/pain – e.g. osteoarthritis, hyperthyroidism, FLUTD, neurological disease.

Aggression toward people is usually the consequence of a variety of complex emotional states, and the assessment of this is beyond the scope of this Manual. Advice or referral to a behaviourist will usually need to be sought, and the reader is encouraged to do this as soon as possible.

General advice for tackling aggression toward people

As there is a serious risk of injury it is unwise to give specific advice without the case being assessed appropriately in the home. However, the safety of all

concerned is paramount and any advice given in response to contact from the owner should focus on limiting the risk of injury, such as the following:

- Arrange for a veterinary evaluation as soon as possible
- Avoid approaching the cat or making eye contact or communicating verbally prior to referral to a behaviour specialist
- Suitable clothing or footwear may be necessary to protect legs and arms
- Shut the cat out of the bedroom at night or, if the aggressive behaviour is ongoing, confine it to a room with all necessary resources while awaiting guidance
- Seek advice or referral from a behaviourist as a matter of urgency if no medical reason for aggressive behaviour is identified.

If the veterinary surgeon finds nothing in the medical examination that may have caused aggressive behaviour, a behaviourist should be involved as a matter of urgency.

Anxiety/fear

Anxiety and/or fear (Figure 18.4; see also Chapter 1) may be caused by:

- Genetic predisposition to timidity
- Inadequate or absent socialization and habituation as a kitten
- A one-off traumatic event
- Age-related insecurity in old cats.

Signs of anxiety
- Tense body
- Lip licking
- Deep swallowing
- Mydriasis
- Hypersensitivity to noise/movement/touch
- Urine retention
- Urine spraying
- Inappropriate urination
- Overgrooming
- Change in normal routine/patterns of behaviour

Signs of fear
- Mydriasis
- Tachypnoea
- Tachycardia
- Tense or rigid body
- Low crouched body posture
- Piloerection (raised fur on the back and tail)
- Sweaty paws
- Trembling
- Aggression
- Escape
- Hiding/freezing/avoiding
- Involuntary elimination

18.4   Signs suggestive of anxiety or fear in cats.

General advice for tackling anxiety
This includes:

- Avoid watching the cat or making physical contact (e.g. stroking); even talking to a cat may cause anxiety
- Do not reassure anxious behaviour, as this can

reinforce the emotional state. Avoid physical punishment
- Give the cat opportunities to escape/hide from challenging situations (Figure 18.5)
- Promote self-confidence by providing stimulation in the environment, access to outdoors and opportunities to express natural behaviour such as hunting behaviour, scratching, climbing and foraging
- Use a feline facial pheromone diffuser in the cat's core area to reinforce security (see below)
- Allow the cat to initiate social interaction with humans
- Confident behaviour can be encouraged by rewarding it with food and play.

See Chapter 1 for ways of minimizing anxiety in the veterinary practice.

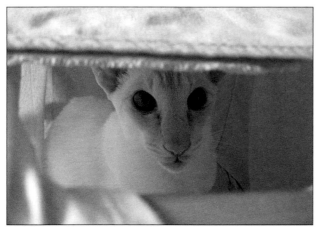

18.5 Hiding may be a sign of stress or anxiety. It is important to provide cats with a place to hide, and to allow them to hide when they choose, as this will reduce their anxiety. It is important that cats are left undisturbed if they have chosen to hide, and are not removed from their hiding place.

Excessive scratching of furniture

Scratching helps maintain healthy claws, exercises the muscles of the forelimbs, and deposits a visual and olfactory signal as a territorial mark. Excessive scratching can occur if there is tension in a multi-cat household. Owners may also look for guidance to protect furniture, wallpaper and carpets, even if the scratching is performed at a 'normal' level.

General advice for tackling scratching
This includes:

- If general scratch damage is occurring, cover the affected area with double-sided (easily removable) adhesive tape or clear perspex sheets
- Provide a variety of rigid vertical and horizontal scratching posts/areas that are suitable for the cat to use at full stretch, placing them near the furniture, wallpaper or carpet that is being damaged
- Rub scratching posts with catnip
- Use a feline facial pheromone spray to deter cats from scratching inappropriate surfaces (see below)
- Seek behavioural advice if scratching is taking place excessively in one or two areas.

Behavioural problems associated with old age

Problem behaviours seen most commonly in elderly cats include:

- House soiling
- Night-time vocalization.

Abnormal or unusual behaviour is often associated with disease and this is particularly relevant in older cats. It is therefore absolutely vital that older cats with behavioural changes are evaluated for medical causes. For example, chronic kidney disease may lead to polyuria with periuria; hypertension may cause behavioural signs such as vocalization.

House soiling
One of the most common problems seen in elderly cats is a breakdown of normal acceptable toilet habits. There are many factors to take into consideration, for example:

- The increased urine production associated with diseases such as chronic kidney disease and diabetes mellitus often results in the litter trays becoming heavily soiled, requiring more frequent maintenance. If litter tray hygiene is not maintained this can result in toileting outside of the litter tray. An increased need to urinate combined with reduced mobility can also contribute to urination occurring outside the litter tray
- Hyperthyroidism may result in urine marking indoors if the cat feels under threat from cats outside, even if it has no previous history of marking
- Cats with painful osteoarthritis and associated mobility problems may have difficulty gaining access to a litter tray
- A breakdown of normal elimination habits is often associated with a decline in cognitive function
- Elderly cats can easily become insecure about defending their territory and be reluctant to eliminate in a previously used site outdoors
- Older cats tend to be more sensitive to changes in the household as their ability to adapt declines with age.

General advice for tackling house soiling in the elderly
All elderly cats, even if they have access outdoors, benefit from the provision of an indoor litter tray. Recommendations for owners include all those given earlier in the chapter on litter trays, plus specific considerations relevant to the elderly, for example:

- Ensure litter trays are on the ground floor or the level where the elderly cat spends most time
- If the cat is senior or geriatric and showing signs of cognitive dysfunction it would be advisable to provide litter tray, food, water, bed and all other important resources in a single room to avoid problems in orientation. A low-sided litter tray enables a cat to enter and exit without the need to negotiate a high step. A fine sand-like substrate is often the most popular; or any material that the cat has always used, would be preferable to frequent changes in the type of litter

- If the cat is passing large volumes of urine (e.g. polydipsic/polyuric cats) then the depth of litter used in the tray needs to be increased. It may be useful to provide a high-sided tray to accommodate the deeper litter *and* place a ramp or steps up to the front and sides for ease of access
- Avoid the use of polythene litter liners as these can get caught in a cat's claws and cause a loss of balance. Highly perfumed litter and litter deodorizers should also be avoided.

Night-time vocalization

It is relatively common for elderly cats to become vocal, particularly at night. The most common causes of night-time vocalization have been found to be:

- Cognitive dysfunction (see Chapter 17)
- Hyperthyroidism (anecdotally seen by the author, pre-clinical signs)
- Hypertension associated with chronic kidney disease, hyperthyroidism, etc.
- Age-related insecurity.

Addressing any medical condition often leads to a complete resolution; in the absence of a clinical cause it would be useful to refer to a pet behaviourist to manage any age-related insecurity or attention-seeking component that may be present.

Feline facial pheromones

Two functional fractions of cat facial secretions have been synthesized artificially and are used to help reduce stress in the cat: F3 and F4. The F3 fraction (e.g. Feliway) is used to promote safety and security during transportation, environmental or social upheaval and moving house. It is also a useful adjunct when treating urine spraying, excessive vertical scratching and inter-cat conflict in multi-cat households. Sprays should be used in corners of rooms, corners of furniture, in the cat's core areas, and in any areas where spraying or vertical scratching is occurring. The F4 fraction (e.g. Felifriend) assists in the development of an atmosphere of confidence between cats and unknown individuals. If applied to the environment or the handler it is reported to encourage cats to approach unfamiliar people. It is important that these products are used according to the manufacturer's instructions to get the best results.

Psychotropic medication

Medication to treat behaviour problems should only be used as part of a behaviour modification programme of treatment, and therefore advice from a behaviourist should be obtained before embarking on such treatments. Psychotropic drugs are metabolized through renal and hepatic pathways, so any contra-indications should be established prior to medication; if it is appropriate to treat, the patient should have regular follow-up biochemical testing to ensure that there are no adverse effects.

Most cats require drug treatment for an extended period of time (4–6 months), so changes may only be evident after several weeks of administration. Although some effects of certain selective serotonin reuptake inhibitors (SSRIs), such as fluoxetine, can be detected within the first week in cats, the full effects usually take 4–6 weeks to become apparent. Similarly, the initial anti-anxiety effects of tricyclic anti-depressants, such as amitriptyline or clomipramine, are seen after 5–7 days, yet more profound changes are seen with additional time. It is normally recommended that drug therapy continues for 1–2 months after the 'problem' behaviour is no longer evident and the dose is then gradually reduced before it is stopped completely. Advice from a veterinary behaviourist should be sought.

Alpha-casozepine is a peptide derived from cow's milk that is marketed as a nutraceutical (Zylkene) for the management of various conditions associated with stress. The peptide binds to benzodiazepine receptors and is therefore considered to have benzodiazepine-like effects, but without any side effects such as sedation. This may be a useful adjunctive treatment for conditions associated with stress; however, as with other medications, it should not replace identification of the underlying triggers causing stress and appropriate management with a behavioural modification programme.

When to refer

As with all specialties, it is the veterinary surgeon's responsibility to refer if expertise is needed beyond what is reasonable in general practice. All reputable pet behaviour counsellors or certified clinical animal behaviourists work only on referral from veterinary surgeons and have the appropriate professional indemnity insurance. It is important to work with someone with particular interest and experience with feline patients.

Most cat behaviour counsellors will make house visits but others may be based at a university, college or veterinary referral centre and offer an in-house clinic where clients will be expected to take their cats. However, it is often possible and more desirable to work with the client alone using video footage, photographs and a floor plan of the home. (A list of certified clinical animal behaviourists can be found on www.asab.nottingham.ac.uk and pet behaviour counsellors on www.apbc.org.uk.)

In some circumstances it may not be possible to reduce the level of stress experienced by the cat displaying the problem behaviour and a decision may be made to re-house the individual to an environment more compatible with its specific requirements.

References and further reading

Bowen J and Heath A (2005) *Behaviour Problems in Small Animals: Practical Advice for the Veterinary Team.* Elsevier Saunders, Philadelphia
Horwitz D and Mills D (2009) *BSAVA Manual of Canine and Feline Behavioural Medicine, 2nd edn.* BSAVA Publications, Gloucester

Infectious diseases

Vanessa Barrs and Julia Beatty

This chapter will focus on some of the more common causes of feline infectious diseases encountered in first-opinion practice, notably cat 'flu, chronic rhinosinusitis, feline infectious peritonitis, retroviral infections and toxoplasmosis. Other infectious agents are covered in chapters on disorders of body systems, including respiratory mycoplasmas (Chapter 10), haemoplasmas (Chapter 20), gastrointestinal parasites and feline parvovirus (Chapter 11) and ectoparasites (Chapter 6).

Feline infectious upper respiratory tract disease (cat 'flu)

Aetiology
Feline infectious upper respiratory tract (URT) disease (cat 'flu) is associated with several different infectious agents, which can cause similar signs. Feline herpesvirus-1 (DNA α-herpesvirus, limited strain variation) (FHV) and feline calicivirus (RNA virus, multiple strains) (FCV) are most commonly involved. Other

agents include *Chlamydophila felis, Mycoplasma* spp. and *Bordetella bronchiseptica*. Co-infections and secondary bacterial infections are common.

Clinical features
FHV/FCV infection
Acute infectious URT disease is most severe in kittens and immunosuppressed adults. Signs include lethargy, anorexia, fever, oculonasal discharge, sneezing, conjunctivitis, oral ulceration and ptyalism.

Oculonasal signs (Figure 19.1a) tend to be more severe in FHV than in FCV infection but dendritic keratitis (see Chapter 8) is the only finding that is pathognomonic for FHV infection. FHV can occasionally cause ulcerative facial and nasal dermatitis (Figure 19.1b).

Oral, especially lingual, ulcers (Figure 19.2a) are typical of acute FCV infection and are less common with FHV. Less common consequences of FCV infection include ulceration of the nasal planum (Figure 19.2b), lips or distant cutaneous sites, polyarthropathy and laryngeal swelling.

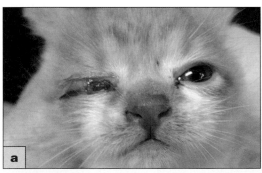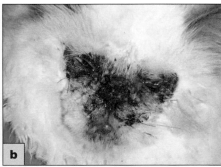

19.1 FHV infection. **(a)** Severe conjunctivitis with associated symblepharon of the right eye and nasal discharge in a kitten. **(b)** Severe ulcerative facial and nasal dermatitis in an adult cat. Skin biopsy samples have been taken, necessitating the suturing shown.

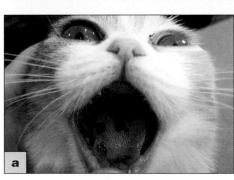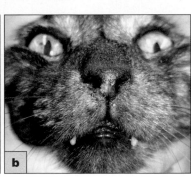

19.2 FCV infection. **(a)** Lingual ulcers in a kitten. **(b)** Ulceration of the nasal planum in an adult cat.

Viral pneumonia can occur with FHV or FCV infection, especially in kittens, but is rare. Outbreaks of 'virulent systemic FCV', characterized by generalized vasculitis, multi-organ failure (cutaneous oedema, ulceration of the head and limbs, respiratory distress, petechiae/ecchymoses, melaena and jaundice) and resulting in high mortality (including adults), have been described. Signs of chronic viral URT disease include rhinosinusitis and ocular manifestations (FHV), or chronic gingivostomatitis (FCV; see Chapter 7).

Bacterial infection

In addition to oculonasal signs and fever, *Bordetella bronchiseptica* infection can cause lymphadenopathy. Kittens <10 weeks old may develop pneumonia.

Chlamydophila felis is the most common infectious cause of conjunctivitis (see Chapter 8). Cats <1 year of age are at greatest risk. Acute infections, characterized by ocular discharge, conjunctival hyperaemia and chemosis, may be accompanied by nasal discharge and sneezing.

Although *Mycoplasma* spp. are commensal bacteria of the conjunctiva and oropharynx, their detection in cats with URT signs implies a role as primary or secondary pathogens.

Diagnosis

FHV/FCV-associated disease

For individual affected cats, identification of the aetiological agent is often not pursued, since a clinical diagnosis is made on the basis of history and presenting signs. Dendritic corneal ulceration identified by fluorescein staining (see Figure 8.2) is pathognomonic for FHV infection. Where there is an outbreak or an ongoing problem in a multi-cat environment, identification of the causal agent can assist in management.

Virus isolation (VI) and PCR on nasal, oropharyngeal or conjunctival swab samples assist in the diagnosis of FHV or FCV infection. PCR is more widely available than VI. Carrier states, viral latency and vaccination influence the interpretation of test results, which must be interpreted with caution (Figure 19.3). Quantification of copy number using qPCR increases the diagnostic sensitivity for detection of clinical illness due to FHV or FCV. High viral loads in clinical specimens suggest active viral replication and involvement in the disease process. Serological tests are not useful, since they do not distinguish between vaccination, active infection and exposure.

Bacterial disease

B. bronchiseptica can be detected by PCR or culture (on selective media to reduce overgrowth by commensal bacteria) of oropharyngeal swabs (or bronchoalveolar lavage fluid where pneumonia is suspected).

C. felis can be detected by PCR of conjunctival swabs, which has very high sensitivity. False negative results can occur if there are insufficient cells but many PCR laboratories now run qPCR for feline internal control genes on submitted swab samples, to ensure that faulty or inadequate sampling does not result in a false negative PCR result. Other diagnostic tests include culture, serology and immunofluorescent antibody testing (IFAT).

Mycoplasma spp. can be detected by PCR or culture; PCR has higher sensitivity.

Possible interpretations	Comments
Positive result	
Clinical illness is due to FCV or FHV	High viral loads detected by qPCR suggest active viral replication and involvement in the disease process
Carrier cat shedding virus (FCV)	Most cats shed virus 30–75 days after clinical recovery, then stop. A minority shed virus continuously for years
Reactivated infection (FHV)	Latency is established in the trigeminal ganglia after primary infection in most cats. Reactivation of viral shedding occurs during periods of stress (e.g. parturition) but may not be associated with clinical illness (recrudescence)
Vaccinated cat shedding virus	Cats recently vaccinated using modified live virus vaccinations may shed vaccine virus. Reactivation and shedding of latent vaccine virus is possible (FHV)
False positive result	Contamination of the sample or in the laboratory but this should be minimized with good laboratory practice
Negative result	
Clinical illness is *not* due to FCV or FHV	A negative qPCR result is not consistent with active viral replication and involvement in the disease process
False negative result	Insufficient DNA/virions on swab [a] Virus inactivation by fluorescein stain or topical anaesthetics during collection or transport (FHV, VI only) Immune clearance of FHV DNA from tissues PCR may not detect all strains of FCV because of sequence variability VI: presence of neutralizing antibodies in clinical samples (FCV)

19.3 Interpreting FCV/FHV reverse transcriptase (RT)-PCR/PCR or virus isolation (VI) results.
[a] Many PCR laboratories now run quantification (q) PCRs for feline internal control genes on submitted swab samples to ensure that faulty or inadequate sampling does not result in a false negative PCR result.

Management

Sick cats

Fluid and electrolyte/acid–base balance should be restored using intravenous fluids.

To ensure nutritional needs are met, patients should be offered palatable, blended, warmed food. A naso-oesophageal (NO) feeding tube (see QRG 5.5.2) should be considered if anorexia persists. Initially, the NO tube may be placed intermittently for each feed in cases where leaving it *in situ* is not well tolerated due to illness. Alternatively, an oesophagostomy tube (see QRG 5.5.3) may be appropriate for these patients, or for patients that are likely to require assisted feeding for a longer period of time.

Nursing management of sick cats should involve cleaning oculonasal discharge with saline, and grooming and wiping the coat with a warm damp cloth once or twice daily. Saline nebulization is useful for maintaining airway hydration. Portable nebulizers can be used for outpatient therapy. Owners can also perform steam therapy in a room with running hot water.

A number of drugs can be used in the treatment of feline infectious URT disease, including antivirals (for FHV), broad-spectrum antibiotics (for secondary bacterial infections), NSAIDs, appetite stimulants and mucolytic drugs (Figure 19.4). Antibiotics for treatment of *B. bronchiseptica* infection should be selected on the basis of susceptibility testing results where available, although empirical treatment with doxycycline can be used if this is not possible.

Control and prevention in multi-cat environments

FHV is inactivated by most disinfectants, antiseptics and detergents. FCV is more environmentally persistent; effective disinfectants include 5% bleach (1:32 dilution), chlorine dioxide and veterinary disinfectants approved for FCV inactivation (e.g. F10SC, Health and Hygiene Pty Ltd).

Shelters: New arrivals should be quarantined separately (unless from the same household) for 14 days.

New kittens introduced into the shelter should be vaccinated on arrival, using modified live vaccine (MLV) from 4–8 weeks of age, every 2 weeks until 16 weeks of age. Very young kittens (<4 weeks) should be quarantined until 7 days after vaccination is started at 4 weeks of age. New adult cats should be vaccinated on admission, and again in 2–4 weeks (Day *et al.*, 2010).

Ongoing effective strategies should be carried out to limit viral transmission, e.g. staff movements and hygiene, cleaning and disinfection protocols, housing design and ventilation.

Breeding catteries:

> **WARNING**
>
> Live vaccines are contraindicated during pregnancy.

Modified live vaccine (MLV) should be given to queens *before* mating. Queens should give birth in isolation and their kittens should be kept isolated until fully vaccinated. Early vaccination should be considered for kittens from queens with a history of viral URT disease in previous litters.

Where all other measures fail, isolation should be considered, with early weaning from 4 weeks of age. Behavioural consequences of early weaning must be borne in mind and socialization must be maximized within the confines of isolation.

Chronic rhinosinusitis

Aetiology

Chronic rhinosinusitis (CR) is idiopathic in most cases. It can occur after severe FHV-induced mucosal damage and turbinate lysis, especially in brachycephalic cats. The initial insult induces an inflammatory response that causes damage to the nasal mucosa and turbinates. This damage affects the structure of the nasal cavity and mucociliary clearance, predisposing the cat to the development of secondary bacterial infections. Ongoing signs result from the immune response to FHV and recurrent, secondary bacterial infection.

Clinical features

CR affects cats of all ages. Typically, cats present with a chronic history (>1 month) of sneezing and nasal discharge. An acute episode of URT signs may also feature in the history. Discharge is more often bilateral than unilateral, and can vary from serous to mucoid or mucopurulent. Epistaxis is present only occasionally and is more commonly associated with nasal neoplasia or fungal infection. In some cases there may also be stertor and dysphonia if inflammation extends into the nasopharynx and/or larynx. On physical examination auscultation of the URT usually reveals harsh inspiratory noises. Submandibular lymph nodes may be mildly enlarged.

Drug	Dose	Indication and comments
Doxycycline	10 mg/kg orally q24h	Treatment of secondary bacterial infections. Treatment of *C. felis* (4–6 weeks to eliminate carrier status, treat in-contact cats), *Mycoplasma* spp and empiric treatment of *B. bronchiseptica*. Ensure complete swallowing of doxycycline with water or food as some formulations are associated with oesophagitis
Amoxicillin/ clavulanate	16.5–20 mg/kg orally q12h	Treatment of secondary bacterial infections. Alternative to doxycycline for *C. felis* in young kittens
Bromhexine	1 mg/kg orally q24h	Mucolytic drug for relief of nasal congestion
Cyproheptadine	0.2–0.5 mg/kg orally q12h	Appetite stimulants (see also Chapter 5.5). Mirtazapine acts more quickly (often within 1–2 hours of dosing) than cyproheptadine
Mirtazapine	1.88–3.75 mg/cat orally q1–3d	
Meloxicam	0.05 mg/kg orally q24h *WITH FOOD*	Analgesia (oral ulceration FCV); antipyretic. Ensure cat is not dehydrated when giving NSAIDs
Famciclovir	30–40 mg/kg orally q12h for 21 days	FHV infection. Demonstrated to improve outcomes for systemic, ophthalmic, clinicopathological, virological and histological variables in cats experimentally infected. Wide dose ranges reported but recent pharmacological study suggested efficacy with lower doses than previously used
Cidofovir (0.5% ophthalmic drops)	1–2 drops into the conjunctival sac q12h for 10 days	FHV keratitis. (Formulate ophthalmic drops by diluting 0.2 ml of the commercially available 75 mg/ml i.v. preparation of cidofovir in 2.8 ml of 1% carboxymethylcellulose, and refrigerate at 4°C). Efficacy in reducing clinical signs and viral shedding demonstrated in experimental infections; efficacy in naturally occurring or recrudescent FHV infections not known
Lysine	500 mg bolus orally q12h	FHV infection, adjunctive therapy. Demonstrated to limit FHV viral replication *in vitro* and *in vivo* but variable efficacy in field studies. Paradoxically may increase shedding
Feline interferon omega	1 million IU/kg s.c. q24–48h *OR* 50,000–100,000 IU orally q24h	Authorized for use in cats with FHV infection. Used with L-lysine in chronic infections. Inhibits FCV replication *in vitro* but efficacy *in vivo* not determined

19.4 Drugs used in the treatment of feline infectious URT disease.

Diagnosis

Most cats are not actively shedding FHV at the time of diagnosis of CR, and thus VI and PCR tests are usually negative. Diagnosis is by exclusion of other differential diagnoses such as neoplasia, fungal infection, foreign body (see Chapter 5.34) or periodontal abscessation.

Bacterial culture of nasal flush samples or nasal mucosal biopsy specimens to detect secondary infections may assist if a single bacterial species is detected, but culture results may represent normal flora. Histological changes vary in nasal mucosal biopsy samples: inflammatory infiltrates can be neutrophilic, lymphoplasmacytic or mixed, and may be accompanied by epithelial erosions, turbinate lysis/remodelling, fibrosis, necrosis and/or glandular hyperplasia.

Management

Treatment is palliative and recurrences are common. Owners should be aware that the condition may be lifelong, with the potential for acute exacerbations. Antiviral drugs (see Figure 19.4) provide benefit in some cases. Supportive care includes treatment of secondary bacterial infection and nasal congestion (Figure 19.5).

Antibiotics should be selected using susceptibility results from culture of nasal wash or biopsy samples, where these are available. Empirical antimicrobial therapy can be given for 6–8 weeks using clindamycin, doxycycline, amoxicillin/clavulanate or azithromycin. Clindamycin and doxycycline penetrate well into the nasal turbinates. If compliance is an issue when longer-term treatment is required, the use of palatable preparations of antimicrobials should be considered.

Steam inhalation or nebulization (10–15 minutes twice daily) is useful to help loosen secretions and encourage sneezing. Antihistamines may alleviate signs in cats with allergy-associated disease (see Figure 19.5). Anti-inflammatory doses of oral corticosteroids or inhaled glucocorticoids can be prescribed for cats that do not respond to other therapies, especially those with lymphocytic–plasmacytic infiltrates.

Corticosteroids should only be used after antibiotic therapy and are best avoided in cats infected with FHV.

Inappetence can be a consequence of CR; feeding small warmed portions of strong-smelling foods may help, and occasionally appetite stimulants (e.g. mirtazapine) may be needed (see Chapter 5.5).

For severely affected cases, intermittent anaesthesia for thorough saline lavage of the nasal cavity can alleviate signs temporarily by reducing accumulated inspissated discharge. This involves intubating the cat and packing the nasopharynx thoroughly to prevent aspiration, before flushing large volumes of warmed sterile saline through each side of the nose, e.g. 50 ml each side. Referral for surgical ablation of the frontal sinuses is a palliative treatment of last resort in severely affected cats.

Feline infectious peritonitis

Aetiology

Feline coronavirus (FCoV) infection is common, especially among cats housed in groups, but most FCoV-infected cats show no clinical signs. FIP is an immune-mediated disease that develops in a small proportion of FCoV-infected cats when mutant viruses capable of replicating within macrophages are thought to emerge, in the face of an inappropriate immune response. Two major lesions can result: immune-mediated vasculitis, associated with leakage of a high-protein effusion into body cavities; and widespread pyogranulomatous inflammation.

Clinical features

FIP can occur in any cat infected with FCoV but most cases occur in young cats (70% <1 year) from a multi-cat environment, such as a breeding cattery or a shelter. Cats <3 or >10 years old are most commonly affected. A stressor, such as rehoming and/or neutering, often precedes the onset of clinical signs. Fluctuating anorexia, lethargy, pyrexia, failure to grow/weight loss, and pale and/or jaundiced mucous membranes are common.

Drug	Dose	Indication
Clindamycin	5.5–11 mg/kg orally q12h	Treatment of secondary bacterial infections/turbinate osteomyelitis
Azithromycin	5–10 mg/kg orally q24h for 5–7 days, then q48–72h for 6–8 weeks	Treatment of secondary bacterial infections
Diphenhydramine	2–4 mg/kg orally q8h	Decongestant
Pseudoephedrine	1 mg/kg orally q8h	Decongestant
0.05% Xylometazoline (Otrivin Paediatric)	1 drop into each nostril q24h for 3 days	Decongestant
Chlorphenamine	1–2 mg/cat orally q12–24h	Antihistamine; may have a sedative effect
Cetirizine	2.5–5 mg/cat orally q12–24h	Non-sedative antihistamine
Clemastine	0.68 mg/cat orally q12h	Non-sedative antihistamine
Fexofenadine	10 mg/cat orally q12–24h	Non-sedative antihistamine
Hydroxyzine	5–10 mg/cat orally q8–12h	Non-sedative antihistamine
Loratadine	5 mg/cat orally q24h	Non-sedative antihistamine
Prednisolone	1–2 mg/kg orally q24h for 1 week, then q48h thereafter	Risk of FHV recrudescence. **Do not use in cats with a history of FHV ocular disease**
Fluticasone	50–250 µg inhalations q12–24h	Requires metered dose inhaler and spacer/mask device

19.5 Additional therapies for treatment of chronic rhinosinusitis (see also Figure 19.4).

Where vasculitis predominates, effusion is a major feature (effusive or wet FIP). Solitary peritoneal effusion is typical (65%; Figure 19.6), but pleural (10%) and bicavitary (25%) effusions are also seen, and so dyspnoea may be a presenting sign. Atypical presentations of effusive FIP include pericardial effusion, ventral oedema (Figure 19.7), scrotal enlargement and polyarthropathy.

Signs associated with non-effusive FIP are more diverse, depending on which organ systems are affected. Ocular changes, including uveitis, keratic precipitates and chorioretinitis (Figure 19.8), and CNS signs (Figure 19.9) are most common (60%), followed by signs referable to abdominal involvement, including renal (Figure 19.10), lymph node and hepatic enlargement or nodular lesions. Atypical presentations of non-effusive disease include cutaneous manifestations and solitary ileocaecocolic, colonic or mesenteric lymph node mass lesions.

FIP is fatal, although signs may wax and wane for weeks or months and periods of apparent remission may occasionally occur.

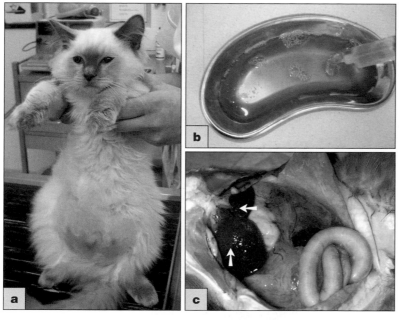

19.6 Effusive FIP. Distended abdomen **(a)** caused by a large volume of peritoneal effusion, comprised of viscous straw-coloured proteinaceous fluid **(b)**. Abdominal effusion and lesions typical of effusive FIP were present in the visceral peritoneum **(c)**, including whitish fibrinous deposits on the spleen and liver (white arrows), intestinal granulomas (yellow arrow) and a thickened omentum.

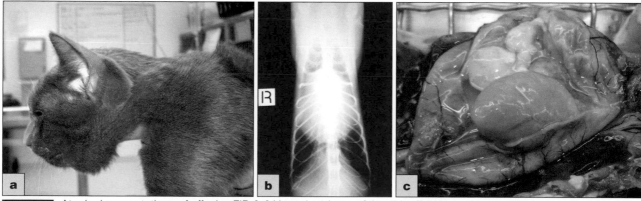

19.7 Atypical presentations of effusive FIP. **(a)** Ventral oedema of the chin. **(b)** Ventrodorsal radiograph with enlarged globoid cardiac silhouette due to a large volume of fibrinous pericardial effusion. **(c)** Pericardial sac of a cat with a pericardial effusion due to FIP, opened on post-mortem examination following euthanasia. The large size of the sac surrounding the heart can be seen; the pericardial fluid was extensive and white fibrinous deposits can be seen within the sac at the top of the image.

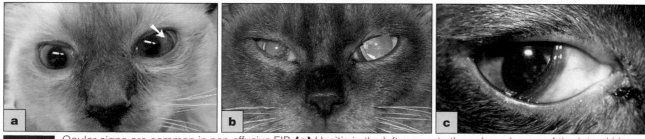

19.8 Ocular signs are common in non-effusive FIP. **(a)** Uveitis in the left eye; note the colour change of the lateral iris from blue to brown (arrowed). **(b,c)** Keratic precipitates or 'mutton-fat deposits' on the inner surface of the cornea of the right eye formed from fibrin and inflammatory cells. The left pupil in (b) is dilated due to chorioretinitis. (Courtesy of Dr Mark Billson, SASH, Sydney, Australia)

- Abnormal mental state and behaviour
- Cerebellar–vestibular signs, e.g. spontaneous nystagmus (especially vertical), head tilt, oculocephalic reflex abnormalities, vestibular ataxia, postural reaction deficits and intention tremor
- Hindlimb ataxia and paresis, progressing to generalized ataxia
- Seizures – generalized motor or partial facial
- Hyperaesthesia to touch and sound
- Cranial nerve deficits

19.9 Common neurological signs in FIP. Neurological signs are referable to multifocal lesion(s) or diffuse disease.

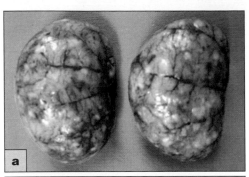
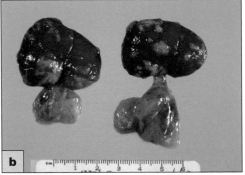
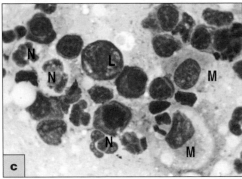

19.10 **(a,b)** Multiple renal nodules with renomegaly in non-effusive FIP. **(c)** Cytology of an ultrasound-guided aspirate from a renal cortical nodule, demonstrating pyogranulomatous inflammation. L = lymphocyte; M = macrophage; N = neutrophil. (Diff-Quik; original magnification X1000 with oil immersion.)

Diagnosis

Diagnosis of FIP is frequently challenging. The gold standard is the demonstration, by immunostaining, of FCoV antigen within macrophages in effusion or tissues, in association with histopathological changes consistent with FIP. In effusive FIP, where immunocytochemistry or immunofluorescence (Figure 19.11) is available and the result is positive, a definitive diagnosis can be made non-invasively. Unfortunately, however, negative immunostaining does not rule out FIP (Figure 19.12).

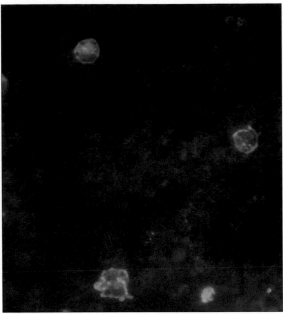

19.11 Light microscopy immunofluorescence preparation of peritoneal effusion from a cat with effusive FIP. Macrophages containing intracytoplasmic FCoV antigen fluoresce bright green. (Courtesy of A/Prof Jacqui Norris, University of Sydney)

Test	Consistent with FIP [a]	Comment
Tests on effusion		
Gross appearance	Viscous, fibrinous, clear to yellow (Figure 19.6b), froths on shaking	Different gross features do not rule out FIP
Total protein	>35 g/l	Corresponds to a *HIGH* protein fluid
Nucleated cell count	<5000 per ml (<5 x10^9/l)	Corresponds to a fluid of *POOR* cellularity
Cytology	Macrophages and neutrophils	
Albumin:globulin ratio	<0.4	>0.8, FIP unlikely
Alpha-1 acid glycoprotein	>1.5 g/l	An acute phase protein. High levels consistent with FIP but specificity not fully evaluated
Immunostaining for FCoV antigen in macrophages	Positive = *DIAGNOSTIC*	PPV 100%; NPV 57%. Negative immunostaining does not rule out FIP if macrophage numbers are low
Rivalta's test	Positive	NPV 96%; PPV 86 %. This test confirms the presence of an exudate and is most useful to *RULE OUT FIP*

19.12 Diagnostic testing in cases of suspected FIP. NPV = negative predictive value; PPV = positive predictive value. [a] Changes listed are commonly but not consistently present. Other aetiologies for effusive disease should be considered, including toxoplasmosis, atypical bacterial infections (e.g. mycoplasmal), neoplasia, right-sided heart failure, post-sinusoidal ascites, and inflammatory liver disease (particularly lymphocytic cholangitis). (continues) ▶

Test	Consistent with FIP [a]	Comment
Tests on other samples		
Complete blood count (EDTA blood)	Non-regenerative anaemia (most common). Stress leucogram esp. lymphopenia (most common). Immune-mediated haemolytic anaemia. Left-shift neutrophilic leucocytosis	CBC changes are common but variable and non-specific
Biochemistry (serum or heparinized plasma)	Hyperglobulinaemia	70% of non-effusive FIP cases. 30–50% effusive cases. Typically a polyclonal gammopathy
	Albumin:globulin ratio <0.4	>0.8, FIP unlikely
	Hyperbilirubinaemia in the absence of identifiable pre/intra/post-hepatic cause. **NB** ALT, ALP and GGT concentrations often normal or only mildly elevated despite hyperbilirubinaemia: this can help increase suspicion of FIP	Impaired transport in the face of high TNF-α levels postulated as mechanism
	Alpha-1 acid glycoprotein >1.5 g/l	An acute phase protein. High levels consistent with FIP but specificity not fully evaluated
CSF analysis (if CNS signs); referral possible	Elevated protein (50–350 mg/dl) and mixed pleocytosis (100–10,000 nucleated cells per ml)	May be difficult to obtain CSF ('dry tap'). Normal CSF does not rule out FIP
Cytology of renal cortical aspirates, or of nodular lesions in other abdominal organs identified on ultrasound examination	Pyogranulomatous inflammation (see Figure 19.10c)	Obtained under sedation with ultrasound guidance. Minimally invasive

19.12 (continued) Diagnostic testing in cases of suspected FIP. NPV = negative predictive value; PPV = positive predictive value. [a] Changes listed are commonly but not consistently present. Other aetiologies for effusive disease should be considered, including toxoplasmosis, atypical bacterial infections (e.g. mycoplasmal), neoplasia, right-sided heart failure, post-sinusoidal ascites, and inflammatory liver disease (particularly lymphocytic cholangitis).

Consistent signalment, history and physical examination findings, including ocular examination, will raise suspicion for FIP. Where an effusion is identified, analysis of the effusion is likely to yield the most diagnostically useful information. If effusion is not apparent on physical examination then ultrasound screening of peritoneal and pleural cavities is indicated.

- Where effusion is available for testing, total protein (TP) and total nucleated cell count (TNCC) should be measured and cytology performed.
- If findings are consistent with FIP (see Figure 19.12) and/or another diagnosis has not been made,

immunostaining is indicated. If immunostaining is positive, a diagnosis of FIP can be made.
- Rivalta's test (Figure 19.13) has a high negative predictive value, so a negative result is useful and shows that the cat is unlikely to have FIP. A positive Rivalta's test is less useful because of the poor specificity of the test (it merely tests for an exudate), although in selected populations (cats <1 year of age where lymphoma and bacterial peritonitis have been ruled out) the positive predictive value is improved. The test can be performed in house.

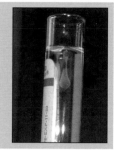

1. Mix one drop of acetic acid with 8 ml of distilled water in a clear tube.
2. Carefully layer one drop of effusion on the surface.

- Negative result: effusion dissipates.
- Positive result: effusion hangs down from the surface but remains as a drop – this confirms the presence of an exudate but does not confirm a diagnosis of FIP.

19.13 Rivalta's test. The image shows a positive test on peritoneal fluid from a cat with effusive FIP. (Courtesy of Dr Dianne Addie)

Other useful tests are listed in Figure 19.12. Serology for FCoV detects exposure to the virus but is not diagnostic for FIP. While high titres of anti-FCoV antibodies may be seen with FIP, they are also seen in FCoV-infected cats without FIP. Additionally, up to 10% of FIP cases have a negative antibody result (likely due to complexing of antibody).

Several FCoV RT-PCR tests are marketed for use in cats, and FCoV levels in tissues and samples from cats with FIP certainly tend to be higher than in those without FIP. Some have suggested that RT-PCRs that detect replicating FCoV are useful in the diagnosis of FIP but conflicting evidence has been published. The usefulness of RT-PCR as a specific diagnostic test for FIP awaits the identification of a consistent mutation(s) associated with FCoV virulence, although progress may have recently been made in identifying a mutation of potential future diagnostic use.

Where intracranial signs are present, MRI findings (Figure 19.14) and CSF analysis (see Figure 19.12) can support an ante-mortem diagnosis of FIP. Referral may be required for these tests.

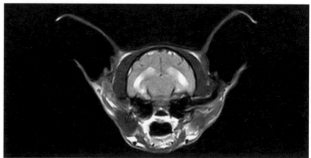

19.14 Referral for MRI may be indicated in cases suspected of having neurological manifestations of FIP. This MRI transaxial post-contrast FLAIR image shows hyperintensity (white) associated with the lateral ventricles, consistent with inflammation. Such periventricular hyperintensity has been described in cats with FIP. Differential diagnoses include viral or bacterial ependymitis, choroiditis and periventricular encephalitis or leucomalacia.

While definitive diagnosis will best guide management decisions, this is not always achievable. Owners must be counselled regarding the weight of circumstantial evidence *versus* the pursuit of definitive diagnosis; surgical biopsy in a debilitated animal will enable immunohistochemistry but this may still not be definitive.

Management

Cats with FIP

The prognosis for FIP is grave. Once the diagnosis is obtained, euthanasia on humane grounds should be considered. There are currently no effective treatments for FIP. Supportive care may be initiated in the short term while owners come to terms with this devastating disease, but prolonged use of supportive care is questionable where quality of life is affected.

In-contact cats

Cats in contact with cases of confirmed FIP will almost certainly be infected with FCoV. However, in general terms their risk of developing FIP is not increased. Where a cat from a single-cat household is euthanased because of FIP, the best way to avoid FIP in the future is to carry out routine disinfection, wait 3 months and then introduce an adult cat that tests seronegative for FCoV (although such FCoV-negative cats may be hard to find).

Feline leukaemia virus infection

FeLV, a gamma-retrovirus, is a significant cause of disease in domestic cats. It is transmitted vertically and horizontally, particularly by close contact but also by aggressive behaviours. The viral RNA is reverse-transcribed into a DNA provirus, which integrates into the host genome. Most exposed cats remain persistently infected but the clinical consequences vary according to how well the infection is contained. There are two major outcomes:

- Progressive infection: Characterized by a high FeLV proviral load. These cats test persistently positive for circulating viral antigen (p27), are at risk from FeLV-associated diseases, and are a source of infection to naïve cats
- Regressive infection: Characterized by a strong immune response that suppresses proviral load, resulting in transient or absent p27 antigenaemia. Risk of FeLV-associated disease is minimal. Regressively infected cats have persistent FeLV proviral loads in the blood, like persistently infected cats, although levels are much lower than in progressively infected cats later in the course of infection. Regressively infected cats are *probably* at little risk of developing FeLV-associated diseases; however, there are reports of reactivation of infection and ensuing viral replication in some cats, so a risk is present.

Abortive infections (characterized by negative test results throughout for antigen and proviral DNA after FeLV exposure) and focal infections (when FeLV infection is restricted to certain tissues, e.g. spleen, lymph nodes, small intestine, or mammary glands) are also described, but seem to be rare.

Clinical features

FeLV-associated disease can occur in cats of any age but is most common in young cats and those housed with other infected cats or allowed to roam. The prognosis for progressively infected cats is poor, with most succumbing to disease within a few years. FeLV causes disease by indirect as well as direct viral effects. Non-specific signs resulting from bone marrow disorders and immunosuppression predominate. Anaemia is a common finding (Figure 19.15) and multiple mechanisms, often presenting concurrently, may be involved (see Chapter 5.4).

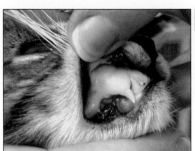

19.15 Severe anaemia manifesting as white gums in a kitten with progressive FeLV infection.

Around 25% of antigenaemic cats develop lymphoid neoplasia, which is typically high grade and of T cell phenotype. The prevalence of FeLV-negative lymphoma has increased significantly in the last 25 years as the worldwide prevalence of FeLV has fallen. FeLV infection is also associated with secondary and opportunistic infections, enteritis, marrow aplasia, reproductive problems and other haemopoietic neoplasms.

Diagnosis

Screening tests

Serological tests that detect circulating p27 antigen are used as screening tests (Figure 19.16). These cage-side enzyme-linked immunosorbent assays (ELISAs) (or similar rapid immunomigration-based tests) require plasma, serum or whole blood, and generally perform well when manufacturers' instructions are followed. Negative p27 antigen test results are generally reliable, whereas positive p27 antigen tests must be confirmed and/or repeated.

Possible interpretations	Comment	Recommendation
Positive p27 antigen test		
The cat is persistently antigenaemic	Cats with progressive infection are at risk from FeLV-related diseases and are a source of infection for naïve cats	Confirm all positive results using IFA, VI or qPCR (DNA). Alternatively, isolate the cat and repeat p27 antigen testing after 60 days but be aware of false positive results if only p27 antigen has been tested for
The cat is transiently antigenaemic	Cats with regressive infection are unlikely to transmit virus under natural conditions. Their risk of FeLV-related disease is low but is incompletely understood currently	
False positive result	Significant when sampling populations with a low prevalence of FeLV, e.g. when healthy cats are tested	

19.16 Interpreting FeLV p27 serology results. (continues) ▶

Possible interpretations	Comment	Recommendation
Negative p27 antigen test		
The cat is uninfected or has regressive infection	This is most likely	If recent exposure cannot be ruled out, repeat p27 antigen testing after 30 days
The cat has early infection	Circulating p27 antigen is not detectable immediately following exposure	
False negative result	Rare – the diagnostic sensitivity of most tests is high	

19.16 (continued) Interpreting FeLV p27 serology results.

Confirmatory testing

Commercial availability of confirmatory tests varies between geographical regions. The laboratory should be contacted for sample requirements. Confirmatory tests include:

- Immunofluorescence (IF): Detects intracellular p27 antigen in leucocytes and platelets on a smear prepared from fresh whole blood or bone marrow aspirates
- Virus isolation (VI): Can be performed on plasma but availability of this test is limited
- qPCR: Detects proviral DNA in exposed cats.

A positive screening test for circulating p27 antigen *and* a positive IF *or* VI result are consistent with progressive infection and a guarded prognosis.

Because any cat exposed to FeLV can test positive for provirus by PCR, this test can only be used to indicate disease risk for an individual cat if a quantitative result is available. A *low* CT value (cycle threshold) correlates with a *high* proviral load and progressive infection.

Repeat p27 antigen testing

Where confirmatory tests are not readily available, p27 antigen testing can be repeated on a second sample taken 60 days after the first. A second positive antigen test is consistent with progressive infection in a cat with appropriate clinical signs; it is important to be aware of the possibility of false positive results, however, which may require that confirmatory testing is performed (see above).

Management

Asymptomatic progressively infected cats

Consultation every 6 months to review the history and to perform physical examination, complete blood count, biochemistry and urinalysis will assist in identifying health problems at the earliest opportunity. Prophylaxis and nutrition can be reviewed at this appointment. The frequency of booster vaccinations for FCV, FHV-1 and FPV should be tailored to the individual's disease risk. Inactivated products are preferred over modified live vaccines in potentially immunocompromised animals (see Chapter 2). Opportunities to hunt should be limited. Management to control spread of FeLV is also required (see below).

Symptomatic progressively infected cats

Sick cats with progressive FeLV infection have a guarded prognosis. The diagnostic investigation is guided by the presenting signs. Specific treatment will depend on the diagnosis and supportive treatment of the clinical signs. Where antibiotics are indicated, bactericidal agents, selected based on susceptibility testing, are preferred. Prolonged courses of treatment may be necessary. Although cats with FeLV-associated lymphoma may respond well to multi-agent chemotherapy (Figure 19.17), this is often not pursued because of the poor overall prognosis associated with FeLV infection.

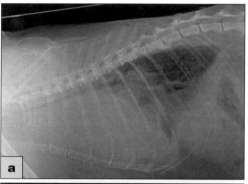
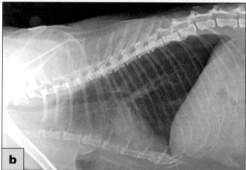

19.17 **(a)** Lateral thoracic radiograph of a 15-year-old male neutered cat with cranial mediastinal lymphoma. The cat tested persistently positive for FeLV p27 antigen and had high levels of provirus on PCR. Note the dorsal tracheal elevation, caudal displacement of the carina and diffuse opacity in the cranial thorax. **(b)** Repeat radiographs in the same cat taken after 9 days of chemotherapy (crisantaspase (L-asparginase), vincristine, cyclophosphamide and prednisolone), showing remission of the lymphoma and normal chest radiography.

Antiviral drug options are limited. Feline interferon omega (10^6 IU/kg s.c. q24h for 5 days) conferred a survival advantage in one study, although the mechanism of action was not determined (de Mari *et al.*, 2004). Euthanasia is indicated where quality of life cannot be maintained.

Strategies for preventing the spread of FeLV

Retroviruses (FeLV and FIV) do not survive for long outside the host, and routine management and disinfection procedures are adequate to prevent spread in the hospital environment. Because of this, hospitalized retrovirus-infected cats do not need to be kept in the isolation ward on the basis of their retrovirus status alone; indeed, this practice may place a potentially immunocompromised cat at greater risk from other infections.

In the home/shelter/cattery setting, the identification and isolation of persistently antigenaemic cats prevents the spread of FeLV. This strategy, coupled with vaccination, has successfully reduced the global prevalence of FeLV. Because of the infectious potential of provirus by inoculation, cats used as blood donors should be negative for p27 antigen and (by PCR) for provirus.

Feline immunodeficiency virus infection

FIV is a retrovirus spread predominantly through biting. Infected cats develop antibodies against the virus but do not clear the infection. It is important to distinguish FIV infection from FIV-associated disease. The prognosis is variable; most FIV-infected cats remain asymptomatic for years. Some infected cats develop FIV-associated diseases, many of which result from immune dysfunction.

Clinical features

Infection is most common in adult, entire, sick, outbred, free-roaming and male cats. There are no pathogno-monic signs of infection. Common clinical problems include gingivostomatitis (Figure 19.18a), haematological abnormalities (particularly cytopenias), muscle wasting, lymphadenomegaly, immune-mediated diseases (Figure 19.18b), and secondary and opportunistic infections (Figure 19.19). Chronic, recurrent and refractory problems are typical (Figure 19.20). FIV infection confers a small increased risk of lymphoma (high-grade, B cell, atypical location) (Figure 19.21). The term 'feline AIDS' can be misleading since this diagnosis is not possible with currently available tests.

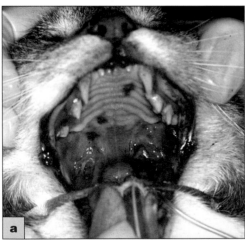

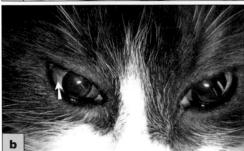

19.18 FIV infection. **(a)** Severe gingivostomatitis and faucitis. **(b)** Anisocoria due to chronic uveitis (right eye); note the relatively increased iris pigmentation (arrowed).

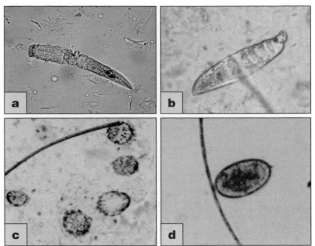

19.19 FIV-infected cats with advanced infection are susceptible to ectoparasitism. **(a)** *Demodex cati.* **(b)** *D. gatoi.* **(c,d)** *Sarcoptes scabiei* mites and egg. (Skin scrapings in paraffin oil, X40 objective lens.)

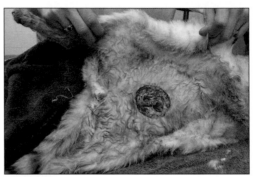

19.20 Non-healing wound in an FeLV-positive cat; the definitive cause was not identified. The haircoat on the ventral abdomen is stained by exudates. Cats with non-healing wounds should be tested for FIV and FeLV infection. Other differentials for non-healing wounds include atypical bacterial infections (e.g. *Mycobacterium* spp.), fungal infections, neoplasia, foreign bodies and corticosteroid therapy.

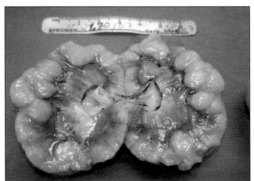

19.21 Longitudinal section through a kidney removed from an FIV-infected cat with high-grade B cell renal lymphoma.

Diagnosis

Screening tests

Serological tests that detect antibodies against FIV are used initially (Figure 19.22). Cage-side ELISA or rapid immunomigration-based tests use plasma, serum or whole blood, are quick and simple to use, and generally perform well when used as instructed. Negative results are usually reliable, whereas positive serological tests may need to be repeated or confirmed.

Possible interpretations	Comment	Recommendation
Anti-FIV antibody-positive		
The cat is infected	If the cat is from a high-risk group, this is the most likely explanation	Confirmatory testing
Maternal antibody is present	Kittens born to infected queens may test positive using serology up to 6 months of age	Repeat serology after 6 months of age *OR* carry out PCR testing (no interval required; useful to check that queen is positive on PCR assay used before testing kittens)
Vaccine-induced antibody is present	Cats vaccinated with Fel-O-Vax FIV (Boehringer Ingelheim), test positive on serology	If the cat is vaccinated or its vaccination status is unknown, PCR testing is indicated
False positive result	Uncommon. Most tests show high diagnostic specificity, but the risk of false positives can be significant in low-risk groups	Where infection risk is low (e.g. in young/purebred/indoor cats) confirmatory testing is indicated
Anti-FIV antibody-negative		
The cat is not infected	This is the most likely explanation. Seronegative but VI-positive cases are extremely rare	Confirmatory testing
Early infection	Seroconversion following exposure may take several weeks	If recent exposure cannot be ruled out, repeat serology after 60 days *or* PCR testing earlier, where available
False negative result	Uncommon. Most tests show high diagnostic sensitivity	If suspicion for FIV infection is high, use alternative antibody test or PCR

19.22   Interpreting FIV serology results.

Confirmatory tests

Anti-FIV antibodies can be detected using immunofluorescence and Western blots. PCR testing detects FIV proviral DNA. This assists the interpretation of positive serology, particularly where vaccination-induced or maternally derived antibody may be present. PCR is usually less sensitive than serology due to the existence of different FIV subtypes; PCR design is therefore difficult due to FIV sequence variation. This is a particular problem in areas where multiple FIV subtypes exist. The laboratory should therefore be consulted for sensitivity and specificity data regarding the FIV subtypes present in the practice's local area, and for sample requirements. It should also be borne in mind that the performance of PCR tests varies between laboratories.

Repeat serology

Where confirmatory tests are not available, serology can be repeated on a second sample, preferably using a different kit. It is not necessary to leave an interval between samples when FIV serology is being repeated to confirm a positive result.

Management

Healthy FIV-infected cats

This is similar to the management of asymptomatic progressively FeLV-infected cats (see above). See also 'Strategies for preventing the spread of FIV', below.

Sick FIV-infected cats

Early and thorough diagnostic investigation is crucial to the management of sick FIV-infected cats; they may, or may not, be showing signs of FIV infection and many will have treatable diseases. Where antibacterials are indicated, bactericidal agents, selected based on susceptibility testing, are preferred. Prolonged courses of treatment may be necessary. FIV-infected cats with lymphoma can respond well to multi-agent chemotherapy, although they should be monitored closely for neutropenia. Options for antiviral treatments are currently limited by evidence of efficacy, side effects and authorization (Levy *et al.*, 2008).

Zidovudine (AZT) (5–10 mg/kg orally or s.c. q12h), feline interferon omega (see Figure 19.4) and human interferon alpha (50 IU sublingually q24h for 7 days on alternating weeks for 6 months, repeat after 2 months) have been used. Where good quality of life cannot be maintained despite specific and/or supportive treatments, or where these options are not available, euthanasia on humane grounds should be considered.

Strategies for preventing the spread of FIV

FIV-infected cats should be neutered and housed indoors. Spread of infection between cats in a stable household is uncommon but can occur. A commercial vaccine (Fel-O-Vax FIV, Boehringer Ingelheim) is available in the USA, Australia and New Zealand. The protection it affords against different FIV isolates/subtypes is variable and its use is controversial.

Toxoplasmosis

Aetiology

Toxoplasmosis is caused by *Toxoplasma gondii,* an intracellular coccidian for which cats are the definitive host. Cats are most commonly infected after ingestion of bradyzoite cysts in meat (typically through eating vertebrate intermediate hosts).

Clinical features

Infection is clinically silent in the majority of cats. In the gut epithelial phase of primary infection, transient small bowel diarrhoea occurs occasionally. Systemic signs can occur during tachyzoite replication in extraintestinal tissues and reflect organ involvement. Risk factors for clinical disease include concurrent infection with FIV or FeLV, having FIP and/or administration of immunosuppressive drugs (e.g. ciclosporin). Hepatic, pulmonary, CNS and pancreatic involvement are common. Clinical signs in acute disseminated infection may include lethargy, anorexia, pyrexia or hypothermia, dyspnoea (due to pulmonary, pleural space or cardiac involvement), jaundice, abdominal distension (peritoneal effusion) and diffuse or multi-focal CNS signs. Acute infections are often fatal, especially in kittens born to queens undergoing primary infections during pregnancy. Focal infections (e.g. uveitis or chorioretinitis) and chronic infections also occur.

Diagnosis

Clinicopathological findings

Clinical examination should include ocular fundoscopy for evidence of chorioretinitis.

Haematological findings are non-specific but may include non-regenerative anaemia, neutrophilic leucocytosis, lymphocytosis, monocytosis and eosinophilia. In severe acute infections there may be neutropenia with a degenerative left shift, lymphopenia and monocytopenia. Abnormalities in serum biochemistry and urinalysis are variable depending on type and severity of organ involvement (e.g. pancreatitis, hepatitis/cholangitis, myositis). Common abnormalities include proteinuria, bilirubinuria, azotaemia, hyperbilirubinaemia and elevations in serum protein, liver enzymes and creatine kinase. In acute illness, serum protein may be decreased.

Thoracic radiographic findings may include a diffuse bronchointerstitial pattern, patchy alveolar infiltrates (Figure 19.23) and pleural effusion. Advanced imaging (ultrasonography, CT, MRI) may assist in detection of effusion and specific organ involvement.

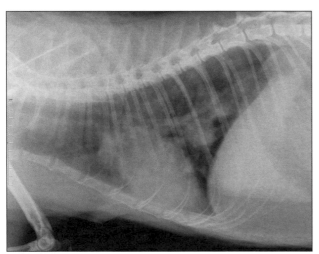

19.23 Lateral thoracic radiograph showing multiple foci of increased opacity (alveolar infiltrates) in a cat with severe toxoplasmosis. (Courtesy of Dr Katherine Briscoe, University of Sydney)

Serology

Serology for the detection of IgG and IgM anti-*T. gondii* antibodies is a useful aid to diagnosis (Figure 19.24) but must be interpreted together with clinical findings. Serological tests that detect some or all classes of antibody include indirect fluorescent antibody (IFA), ELISA, western blot immunoassay and agglutination tests. Using ELISA-based tests, positive IgM titres develop in 80% of cats 1–4 weeks after infection and are usually negative by 16 weeks after infection. Positive IgG titres develop 3–4 weeks after infection and peak 2–4 weeks after initial detection. IgG can be detected in CSF and aqueous humour of both normal and clinically ill cats, but IgM has only been detected in sick cats.

Test result	Interpretation
IgG	
A ≥4-fold increase in titre in paired serum samples taken 2–4 weeks apart	Recent or active infection (true positive)
A <4-fold increase in titre in paired serum samples taken 2–4 weeks apart	No recent or active infection (true negative) Maximal IgG titre occurred before sampling period, or rising titre did not occur, e.g. recrudescent infection (false negative)
A single high positive result (e.g. 1:1000)	Reflects only the presence of *T. gondii* within tissues High titres can persist for many years due to latent infection (bradyzoite tissue cysts)
IgM	
Titre ≥1:64	Recent or active infection (true positive) Persistent high titre beyond the period of active or recent infection (false positive), e.g. some healthy cats, FIV-infected cats, glucocorticoid treatment
Titre <1:64	No recent or active infection (true negative) Did not mount an IgM response (false negative), e.g. 20% healthy cats, recrudescent infection

19.24 Interpreting *Toxoplasma gondii* ELISA serology IgG and IgM results.

Definitive diagnosis

Definitive diagnosis of toxoplasmosis requires cytological, histological or immunohistological detection of *T. gondii* tachyzoites in body cavity effusions, broncho-alveolar lavage fluid, CSF, aqueous humour, tissue aspirates (e.g. from lungs or lymph nodes) or biopsy specimens (Figure 19.25a). Sensitivity is low but specificity is high. Use of immunofluorescent and immuno-histological (Figure 19.25b) methods increases the sensitivity of detection.

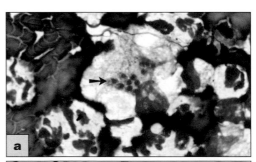

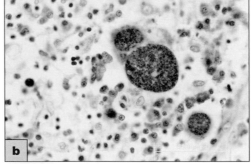

19.25 **(a)** Multiple *Toxoplasma gondii* tachyzoites (arrowed) in a smear of abdominal fluid from a cat with FIP and toxoplasmosis. (Diff-Quik; original magnification X330.) (Courtesy of Dr Amy Lingard, University of Sydney) **(b)** Immunohistochemical staining of a spinal cord sample from a cat with toxoplasmosis. There is positive (brown) staining of multiple, variably sized thin-walled cysts and of free tachyzoites within the neuropil.

Since *T. gondii* DNA can be amplified by PCR in blood, aqueous humour and CSF samples from healthy cats, PCR assays are only useful for confirming the identity of tachyzoites or tissue cysts in clinical specimens.

Oocyst shedding in cats can be detected by centrifugal faecal flotation using Sheather's sugar solution or zinc sulphate. Alternatively, *T. gondii* DNA can be detected in faeces by PCR.

Management

Antibiotic therapy

Options for antibiotic therapy include clindamycin (10–12.5 mg/kg orally or i.v. q12h; note this is higher than standard clindamycin dose), trimethoprim/sulphonamide (15 mg/kg orally q12h) or azithromycin (10 mg/kg orally q24h for a minimum of 4 weeks). Pyrimethamine (0.25–0.5 mg/kg orally q12h) is synergistic when combined with sulphonamides.

Supportive treatments

Intravenous fluid therapy: This should comprise 0.9% NaCl or Hartmann's solution, with appropriate potassium chloride supplementation (see QRG 4.1.3).

Intranasal oxygen therapy: For hospitalized dyspnoeic patients, humidified intranasal oxygen should be administered at 100 ml/kg/min (see QRG 4.2.2).

Assisted feeding: If the cat is inappetent, placement of a naso-oesophageal or oesophagostomy feeding tube should be considered for short-term assisted feeding (see QRGs 5.5.2 and 5.5.3).

Monitoring: Cats with acute toxoplasmosis should be monitored for the development of body cavity effusions, pneumonia, hepatic failure, pancreatitis, encephalomyelitis or myocarditis. In cats that are being treated with sulphonamides or pyrimethamine, haematological monitoring should be performed every 2 weeks for detection of myelosuppression and an alternative antimicrobial used if myelosuppression occurs.

Additional treatments

Depending on the body systems affected, additional supportive therapy may be required, e.g. anticonvulsants in fitting patients, diuretics, ACE inhibitors for congestive heart failure, analgesia for pancreatitis.

Public health concerns

In humans, *T. gondii* can cause severe disease in developing fetuses (if infection is acquired during pregnancy) and in young, old or immunosuppressed people. Most human infection is acquired through ingestion of tissue cysts in infected meat that has not been thoroughly cooked or of oocysts from the environment (e.g. eating contaminated vegetables or eating after gardening without gloves, through contact with soil that contains sporulated oocysts). Infection from contact with a cat is very unlikely since oocysts are passed in feline faeces for a short period (usually ~14 days in the cat's lifetime) and, once passed, take days to sporulate and become infective. If litter trays are cleaned and disinfected daily, any risks from cleaning them should also be minimized.

References and further reading

Chang HW, Egberink HF, Halpin R *et al.* (2012) Spike protein fusion peptide and feline coronavirus virulence. *Emerging Infectious Diseases* **18**, 1089–1095

Day MJ, Horzinek MC and Shultz RD (2010) WSAVA guidelines for the vaccination of dogs and cats. *Journal of Small Animal Practice* **51 (6)**, 338–356

de Mari K, Maynard L, Sanquer A *et al.* (2004). Therapeutic effects of recombinant feline interferon-omega on feline leukemia virus (FeLV)-infected and FeLV/feline immunodeficiency virus (FIV)-coinfected symptomatic cats. *Journal of Veterinary Internal Medicine* **18**, 477–482

Lappin M (2010) Update on the diagnosis and management of *Toxoplasma gondii* infection in cats. *Topics in Companion Animal Medicine* **25**, 136–141

Levy J, Crawford C, Hartmann K *et al.* (2008) 2008 American Association of Feline Practitioners' feline retrovirus management guidelines. *Journal of Feline Medicine and Surgery* **10**, 300–316

Pedersen N (2009) A review of feline infectious peritonitis virus infection: 1963–2008. *Journal of Feline Medicine and Surgery* **11**, 225–258

Useful websites

AAFP, WSAVA and European Advisory Board on Cat Diseases (ABCD) guidelines on feline infectious diseases:

http://catvets.com/professionals/guidelines/publications/?Id=176
http://www.wsava.org/VGG1.htm
http://abcd-vets.org/Pages/guidelines.aspx

Cat group policy statements on a range of infectious diseases:
www.thecatgroup.org.uk

Management of haematological disorders

Séverine Tasker

This chapter deals primarily with the management of anaemia, which is the most common feline haematological abnormality found and managed in practice. Practical QRGs on blood typing and transfusion are also included. Other chapters deal with some other causes of anaemia (e.g. rodenticide toxicity in Chapter 4.9), and advice on the management of collapse in association with anaemia is found in Chapter 4.1. Chapter 5.4 covers the diagnostic approach to anaemia, including making and examining blood smears (see QRG 5.4.1). Further aspects of haematological assessment and an overview of other feline haematological abnormalities and their most frequently recognized causes can be found in QRG 5.4.2; information on the management of some of these disorders can be found in relevant chapters (e.g. flea allergy-associated eosinophilia is dealt with via treatment of the flea allergy; see Chapter 6). The *BSAVA Manual of Canine and Feline Haematology and Transfusion Medicine* should be consulted for further information on less common haematological disorders such as polycythaemia, leukaemias and immune-mediated neutropenia.

Anaemia

Cats tend to tolerate anaemia particularly well, especially if it has developed chronically. This is due to the adaptive mechanisms (physiological – e.g. heart rate increase, haemoglobin structure adaptations; lifestyle – e.g. reduced activity) that come into play when anaemia develops. The need for specific treatment of the anaemia (e.g. by blood transfusion) is partly led by the clinical signs that the cat is showing, which are often more related to the chronicity of the anaemia rather than to its severity. For example, a cat with a PCV of 14% that has developed chronically but is not showing severe clinical signs of anaemia is unlikely to need an immediate blood transfusion.

General treatment for anaemic cats

Supportive care

Any dehydration should be corrected via intravenous fluid therapy (see QRG 4.1.3); haemoconcentration due to dehydration can mask the degree of anaemia, so haematological parameters should be reassessed after rehydration. Encouraging food intake and nutritional support are important if the patient is inappetent (see Chapter 5.5).

WARNING

Any cat with (chronic) severe anaemia may be prone to volume overload, due to increased intravascular volume occurring as a result of the haemodynamic compensatory responses that occur in (chronic) severe anaemia. This makes them susceptible to congestive heart failure if intravenous fluid or Oxyglobin is given too rapidly, so great care must be taken to avoid administering fluids and/or colloids too rapidly or in too great a volume to these cats.

Blood transfusion

If the anaemia is severe (PCV <12%) and/or has developed acutely, **and** significant related clinical signs are present, a blood transfusion (see QRG 20.2) may be required. This should only be done after careful consideration: for example, if the cat's anaemia is regenerative (see Chapter 5.4) it may be that supportive treatment without transfusion is adequate in the short term while the patient replaces its own red blood cells; if the cat has a terminal illness (e.g. neoplasia, FeLV-associated disease) the potential benefit of a blood transfusion to the recipient may not outweigh the risk to the donor for blood collection. Blood transfusion should only be performed after blood typing both the donor and recipient (see QRG 20.1).

Oxygen-carrying haemoglobin

Treatment with oxygen-carrying haemoglobin can be life-saving if blood donors or blood products are not available, or for short-term treatment, especially if circulatory support is also required. Oxyglobin (not authorized in the UK for use in cats) can be used if available (5–10 ml/kg i.v. at a rate of 0.5–1 ml/kg/h; occasionally dose rates up to 2 ml/kg/h may be administered if hypovolaemia is also present). Oxyglobin is a potent colloid, so great care is needed when treating cats prone to circulatory overload (e.g. cats with cardiac disease (including occult hypertrophic cardiomyopathy), renal or respiratory disease, or cats with (chronic) severe anaemia (see warning box)), as pulmonary oedema can result. Haemoglobin values rather than PCV should be used to monitor treatment efficacy.

Treatment for specific causes

Beyond the general treatment of anaemic cats, specific treatment will depend on the underlying disease.

Immune-mediated haemolytic anaemia

If an underlying cause of immune-mediated haemolytic anaemia (IMHA) is apparent (see Chapter 5.4), this should be addressed: for example, if IMHA is suspected to be secondary to drug administration the drug should be stopped; if haemoplasmosis is diagnosed, it should be treated (see below).

Increasing numbers of feline IMHA cases appear to be primary, however, without any underlying cause apparent. These are treated with prednisolone (2–4 mg/kg (start at the lower dose) orally q24h for at least 4 weeks; thereafter tapering the dose gradually (e.g. reduce by 25% every 2–4 weeks)); haematology is monitored prior to each dose reduction to look for evidence of relapse which would preclude the dose reduction. Bilirubin measurements may also help to indicate significant ongoing haemolysis, as hyperbilirubinaemia may be evident. Concurrent use of gastroprotectants (e.g. ranitidine, cimetidine, famotidine, sucralfate) should be considered if high doses of corticosteroids are being used but gut compromise is suspected (e.g. if hypotension is also present).

Some cases of IMHA may fail to respond adequately to corticosteroids alone, and alternative immunosuppressive agents may be required, such as ciclosporin or chlorambucil. Advice can be sought from a specialist if such therapy is required.

Prognosis for feline primary IMHA is generally good with appropriate treatment.

Haemoplasmosis

Mycoplasma haemofelis is the most pathogenic haemoplasma species; infection can be confirmed using a PCR test as cytology is unreliable. Disease may be more severe in cases concurrently infected with retroviruses. Treatment with doxycycline (10 mg/kg orally q24h) for 3–6 weeks is usually appropriate (though see Chapter 3 for details of adverse effects). Fluoroquinolones (e.g. marbofloxacin or pradofloxacin) are an alternative or can be added in if the response to doxycycline alone is inadequate. Response to treatment is monitored via haematology (improvement in parameters occurs with effective treatment) and quantitative PCR tests (a reduction in the amount of haemoplasma DNA should occur with effective treatment). Longer courses of treatment may be required to try and clear infection, although clearance is hard to prove (three negative PCR tests, each a month apart, may be suggestive of clearance) and may be difficult to achieve. Fleas are implicated in transmission, so flea control should be instigated (see Chapter 6). Prognosis is generally good.

Treatment of infection with 'Candidatus Mycoplasma haemominutum' and 'Candidatus Mycoplasma turicensis' is more problematical; indeed, some question the need for treatment of infections with these less pathogenic species. Very few studies have evaluated the response of these species to antibiotics. If anaemia is present, anti-haemoplasma treatment should be instigated, but variable responses to doxycycline and fluoroquinolones occur.

Blood loss

Control of external haemorrhage is indicated, using local pressure, bandages, tourniquets and topical adhesives/tissue glue. Gastroprotectants, as above, are indicated for gastrointestinal bleeding.

For anticoagulant rodenticide toxicity, vitamin K1 should be given (see Chapter 4.9). Vitamin K1 is also often helpful in liver-associated coagulopathies in order to correct clotting times: for example 1.0 mg/kg s.c. q12h two or three times prior to surgical liver biopsy, and every 7–21 days thereafter until the liver disease is controlled.

Autotransfusion

- Transfusion of a cat's own blood can be performed in emergency situations when cavity bleeding has occurred. This should be reserved for haemorrhage only; if sepsis, bile or urine is present alongside blood (e.g. after abdominal trauma) autotransfusion should not be performed.
- Blood should be collected from the cavity using standard techniques as described for thoracocentesis and abdominocentesis (see QRGs 4.2.4 and 5.1.1) but collected into CPDA anticoagulant (1 ml in a 10 ml syringe) and then administered via a filtered giving set.

Systemic causes

Anaemia of inflammatory disease (AID) is usually only mild or moderate, although it can in some cases become quite severe. Generally the underlying disease associated with AID needs to be addressed. Anaemic cats with chronic kidney disease (CKD) should be managed for their renal disease (see Chapter 13), since anaemia is not often a major cause of clinical signs. The use of gastroprotectants should be considered if gastrointestinal ulceration and resulting blood loss is thought to be contributing to the anaemia. Erythropoietin (EPO) drugs can be given if the anaemia is severe and/or symptomatic, although therapy is expensive and can be associated with side effects such as anti-EPO antibody formation, hypertension and seizures. Iron supplementation is usually required alongside EPO treatment. Anti-EPO antibody formation can actually worsen the anaemia, although a newly available EPO analogue called darbepoetin is said to be less associated with anti-EPO antibody formation. Further advice from a specialist should be sought before using EPO.

Primary bone marrow diseases

Primary bone marrow disease can affect one (e.g. anaemia or neutropenia alone) or multiple cell lines (panctyopenia if all three cell lines are affected – anaemia, leucopenia and thrombocytopenia). Most primary bone marrow diseases (e.g. maturation defect myelodysplasia, aplastic anaemia, myeloproliferative diseases) have a poor prognosis, although non-FeLV-associated pure red cell aplasia (PRCA) can respond to immunosuppressive treatment (see below).

If bone marrow disease is found, consideration should be given to stopping the administration of any drugs that could be associated with bone marrow hypoplasia (e.g. griseofulvin (particularly in FIV-infected cats), methimazole, chloramphenicol, some chemotherapeutic agents). Contact with a specialist is advised to discuss possible treatment options for primary bone marrow diseases such as myelodysplasia and myeloproliferative diseases.

Non-FeLV-associated PRCA may respond to immunosuppressive treatment with prednisolone (2–4 mg/kg orally q24h), so empirical treatment for this may be indicated if infectious causes have been ruled out. Other immunosuppressive therapies can be considered if prednisolone alone is not adequate (see IMHA, above).

References and further reading

Chalhoub S, Langston C and Eatroff A (2011) Anaemia of renal disease: what it is, what to do and what's new. *Journal of Feline Medicine and Surgery* **13**, 629–640

Day MJ and Kohn B (2012) *BSAVA Manual of Canine and Feline Haematology and Transfusion Medicine, 2nd edn.* BSAVA Publications, Gloucester

Kohn B, Weingart C, Eckmann V, Ottenjann M and Leibold W (2006) Primary immune-mediated hemolytic anemia in 19 cats: diagnosis, therapy, and outcome (1998-2004). *Journal of Veterinary Internal Medicine* **20**, 159–166

Ottenjann M, Weingart C, Arndt G and Kohn B (2006) Characterization of the anemia of inflammatory disease in cats with abscesses, pyothorax, or fat necrosis. *Journal of Veterinary Internal Medicine* **20**, 1143–1150

Tasker S (2010) Haemotropic mycoplasmas: what's their real significance in cats? *Journal of Feline Medicine and Surgery* **12**, 369–381

Viviano KR and Webb JL (2011) Clinical use of cyclosporine as an adjunctive therapy in the management of feline idiopathic pure red cell aplasia. *Journal of Feline Medicine and Surgery* **13**, 885–895

Wilson HE, Jasani S, Wagner TB *et al.* (2010) Signs of left heart volume overload in severely anaemic cats. *Journal of Feline Medicine and Surgery* **12**, 904–909

QRG 20.1 Feline blood types and blood typing methods
by Suzanne Rudd

Feline blood types

Blood types arise due to the presence of genetically determined antigenic markers on the surface of erythrocytes.

Blood-type incompatibilities are responsible for potentially fatal feline blood transfusion reactions in cats and for neonatal isoerythrolysis (see Chapter 5.4), a major cause of neonatal death.

One blood group system (the AB system) has been extensively defined in cats.

- Blood type A is common
- Blood type B is less common, although prevalent in some pedigree breeds (e.g. British Shorthair, Ragdoll, Birman, Rex)
- Blood type AB is rare.

Recent evidence suggests that other, non-AB blood group systems also exist in cats because blood transfusion reactions have occurred in cats given AB-matched blood transfusions, but these are rare.

Blood typing

- Blood typing can be performed by submitting anticoagulated blood to a commercial laboratory.
- A genetic test for cat blood types is also available in some laboratories; this test, based on PCR and subsequent sequencing, identifies a cat as being *either* blood type A or AB, *or* blood type B, but does not distinguish between types A and AB.
- Two different commercial kits are available for in-house feline blood

typing: Rapid Vet-H (DMS Laboratories) and the Quick Test A+B (Alvedia).

Rapid Vet-H test

The test card has two test 'wells':

- Type A: contains an anti-type A reagent
- Type B: contains an anti-type B reagent.

Interpretation is based on looking for an agglutination reaction in either or both test wells.

The autoagglutination saline screen well contains *no* anti-A or anti-B reagents, and is a control well to ensure that the cat's blood is not already agglutinating spontaneously, as this would give a false AB result. Agglutination in the control well invalidates the test and the Quick Test A+B should then be used, or samples sent to a commercial laboratory.

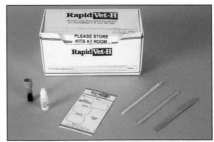

The Rapid Vet-H kit contains a bottle of diluent, plastic pipette, wooden mixing sticks and test card (shown removed from its wrapper). Only EDTA-anticoagulated blood should be used, and 0.5 ml is adequate.

1 Label the card with the cat's details (not shown here for reasons of confidentiality).

2 Apply one drop of diluent on to the control (autoagglutination saline screen), Type A and Type B wells.

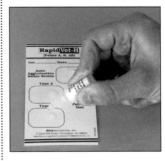

3 Take the EDTA tube and ensure that the blood is thoroughly mixed by inverting the tube three or four times. Apply one drop of blood on to each well using the plastic pipette, taking care not to touch the pipette on to the card.

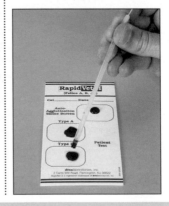

▶

QRG 20.1 *continued*

4 With a mixing stick, mix the blood and diluent around the surface of the control well for 10–20 seconds using a circular motion. Whilst doing this, look to see whether any agglutination becomes visible; this would show up as distinct speckling of the blood (rather than a normal homogeneous appearance) due to clumping of erythrocytes in the well (see later). Autoagglutination (agglutination in the control well) invalidates the test.

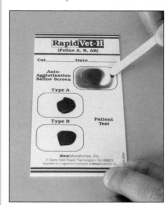

5 If no agglutination is seen in the control well, using the same mixing stick mix the blood and diluent in the Type A well for 10–20 seconds. A moderate amount of pressure when mixing should be used, to ensure that the lyophilized antisera impregnated on the test card mixes well with the blood.

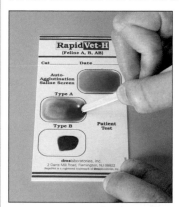

6 Take a *fresh* mixing stick and mix the diluent and blood in the Type B well for 10–20 seconds, pressing firmly to ensure thorough mixing.

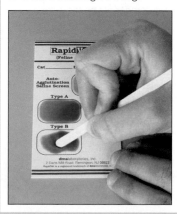

7 Add a further drop of diluent *into the Type A well only.* Lift the card and gently roll it around to allow the diluent to disperse into the blood in the well.

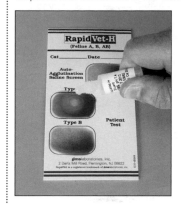

8 Read the results within 2 minutes. Non-significant agglutination can appear in wells after this time, as the test dries, so it must be read within the specified timeframe.

If the test has worked correctly, agglutination should be visible in the Type A, Type B, or both wells.

- If there is agglutination in the Type A well alone, and there is no agglutination in the control well, the cat is blood type A.
- If the agglutination is in the Type B well alone, and there is no agglutination in the control well, the cat is blood type B.
- If agglutination occurs in both the Type A and Type B wells, and there is no agglutination in the control well, the cat is blood type AB.

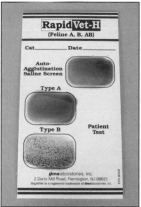

Agglutination is visible in the Type B well only; this cat is blood type B.

Quick Test A+B

A recent study (Seth *et al.*, 2011) found that the Quick Test A+B performed slightly better than the Rapid Vet-H card test. Additionally, the Quick Test A+B method may be more reliable in cats with autoagglutination.

This migration paper strip cartridge test uses monoclonal antibodies to differentiate blood types. It is interpreted by seeing where the red line indicator across the test strip lines up: i.e. adjacent to A, B or both on the slide cover. A control test is also run and is shown to be successfully completed by a red line being visible on the test strip adjacent to C.

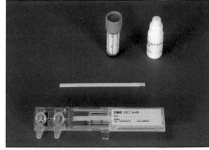

The kit contains the diluent, dipstick, mixing well and test card attached to the test strip (shown here inserted into the mixing well plastic sheath).

For this test you can use blood that has been collected into EDTA, citrate phosphate dextrose, acid citrate dextrose or heparin, or even umbilical cord blood. If the sample to be blood typed is from a cat with severe anaemia (PCV <14%), consideration should be given to spinning and resuspending the blood in a smaller volume of plasma (see below).

1 Label the card with the cat's details before beginning the test (not shown for reasons of confidentiality).

2 Take the bottle of diluent and apply 3 drops into the mixing well.

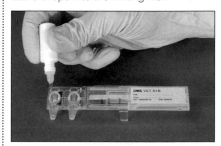

3 Take the dipstick and insert the filter papered end (shown by arrows on the dipstick) into the blood, allowing the blood to be absorbed into the filter paper up to the red and white arrowed indicator.

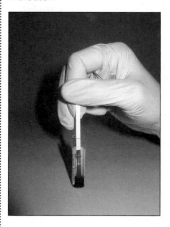

4 Take the dipstick out of the blood, and place it into the mixing well containing the diluent; agitate it for approximately 7 seconds. Discard the dipstick appropriately.

▶

QRG 20.1 *continued*

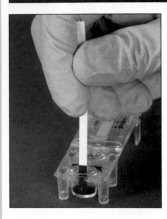

5 Slide the test card and attached test strip out from the plastic sheath.

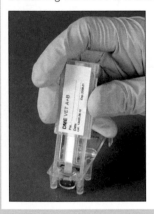

6 Place the test strip attached to the test card into the mixing well containing the blood and diluent.

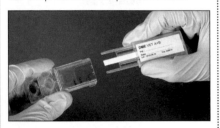

7 Allow the diluted blood to travel up the test strip until it reaches the top of the strip next to the identification label on the test card (arrowed). This should take approximately 2 minutes.

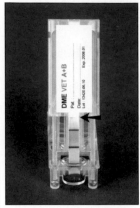

PRACTICAL TIP

If insufficient red blood cells reach the top of the strip, due to the low number present in an anaemic sample, it may be helpful to spin down the blood for 2–3 minutes, remove some of the plasma supernatant and resuspend the remaining red blood cells to provide a higher concentration in the sample. If this is not performed before starting blood typing, a fresh kit will be required.

8 Slide the test card back into the plastic sheath.

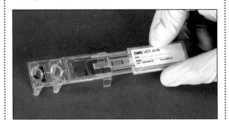

9 Read the test immediately – within 2 minutes. Delays in reading the test will make it invalid.

The control line adjacent to the letter C should always be visible to validate the test. If a line does not appear here, or if no red lines appear at all, the test is invalid.

- A red line adjacent to letters A and C indicates that the cat is blood type A.
- A red line adjacent to letters B and C indicates that the cat is blood type B.
- A red line adjacent to letters A, B and C indicates that the cat is blood type AB.

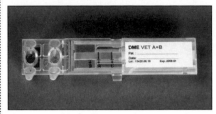

There is a red line adjacent to letters A and C. This cat is blood type A.

Further reading

Day MJ (2012) Feline blood groups and blood typing. In: *BSAVA Manual of Canine and Feline Haematology and Transfusion Medicine, 2nd edn*, ed. MJ Day and B Kohn, pp. 284–288. BSAVA Publications, Gloucester

Seth M, Jackson KV and Giger U (2011) Comparison of five blood-typing methods for the feline AB blood group system. *American Journal of Veterinary Research* **72**, 203–209

QRG 20.2 Blood transfusion

by Suzanne Rudd

Indications

- **Severe anaemia with associated clinical signs,** especially if anaemia has developed acutely with little time for compensatory mechanisms to kick in. If the cat is normovolaemic (e.g. anaemia due to haemolysis), packed red blood cells are most appropriate but if they are unavailable whole blood is usually given.
- **Haemorrhage.** The need for a transfusion may be apparent before anaemia has developed, as the concurrent hypovolaemia (due to loss of plasma from the intravascular compartment) means that the cat's PCV will not fall initially. A transfusion of whole blood is most appropriate.
- **Clotting factor requirement.** Some cats (e.g. cats with severe liver disease, inherited coagulopathies or rodenticide toxicity) are transfused before an invasive

procedure, to provide them with clotting factors contained within fresh plasma. Consideration can be given to separating the red cells and plasma for an individual patient, but this facility may not be available. NB Clotting factors degrade relatively quickly (some within hours) even if blood or plasma is refrigerated.

- **Preparation for anticipated blood loss** during elective surgery in which haemorrhage is very likely to occur.

Blood transfusions are NOT a good source of:

- Platelets for thrombocytopenic patients
- Protein for hypoproteinaemic patients (plasma proteins do not remain in the intravascular compartment for long).

▶

QRG 20.2 *continued*

It is important to be certain that a blood transfusion is definitely the most appropriate treatment (see main text); not every anaemic cat needs a blood transfusion and every treatment option should be considered.

Considerations for the donor cat

It is advantageous for practices to compile a list of potential donors, such as staff pets and also client pets that fulfil the donor suitability criteria. If such a list is not available, the owner of the cat needing a transfusion may have another cat suitable for donating, or may have a relative or friend with a suitable donor cat. There are potential risks to the donor cat, associated with sedation and subsequent blood collection that must be carefully weighed against the potential gain for the recipient cat. It is essential that the client has these risks explained to them and that written consent is obtained before a cat is used for donation.

Requirements for a donor cat include:

- Adequate bodyweight (ideally >5 kg). Weigh the donor cat before donation to ensure that it is large enough to donate the required volume of blood, and to calculate a sedation dose accurately
- Age 1–8 years (ideally 1–5 years)
- Adequate PCV (≥35%). It is essential to check the donor's PCV (done in-house; the sample is best taken from the cephalic vein to ensure minimal trauma to the jugular veins needed for blood collection) *just before donation* to ensure that the donor cat will not become anaemic through donating blood
- A complete normal health check within 6 months prior to donating blood:
  - Complete clinical history, physical examination, routine haematology and biochemistry unremarkable
  - Infectious disease testing (although the environment of the donor can be taken into account; e.g. an indoor-only single-cat household donor may require less screening):
    - FeLV (PCR analysis is best but antigen testing can be done if a rapid result is required)
    - FIV (antibody testing)
    - Haemoplasma PCR screening if time allows
    - *Bartonella* screening if possible (PCR and serology)
    - Cytauxzoonosis, ehrlichiosis, anaplasmosis and neorickettsiosis if important in the country where the donor resides (not appropriate for UK)
- Normal systolic blood pressure (120–149 mmHg) at the time of donation. Low blood pressure may reflect problems, e.g. occult heart disease, that would be exacerbated by sedation. Echocardiography should ideally be performed in all cats prior to donation, to assess for occult heart disease
- Fasted for the last 6 hours, to minimize the risk of regurgitation or vomiting under sedation
- A calm temperament facilitates the process although sedation (see below) of the donor cat is usually required for blood collection as this takes 15–20 minutes
- Correct blood type. It is vital that the recipient and donor cat are of the same blood type (see QRG 20.1), due to the existence of naturally occurring alloantibodies in cats
  - If the recipient has had a transfusion before (>4 days previously; the time taken for antibodies to form against blood-type antigens) it must also undergo cross-matching before receiving any more blood.

Calculations

Donated blood volume

The total blood volume in cats is approximately 66 ml/kg, so a 5 kg cat has around 330 ml of blood. Collection of up to 20% of blood volume (66 ml for a 5 kg cat) is usually safe, but intravenous crystalloid fluids are required to prevent hypovolaemia. Collection of <10% of blood volume from a donor does not usually require intravenous fluid therapy. Usually 50 ml is collected from the donor. ▶

Recipient blood required

Although 50 ml of blood is usually transfused, the amount of blood the recipient needs can be calculated accurately using the following formula:

Volume to be transfused =

$$\frac{66 \times \text{weight of patient (kg)} \times (\text{desired PCV*} - \text{patient PCV})}{\text{PCV of donor}}$$

* The desired PCV is set at ~20%

Alternatively it can be estimated that 2 ml/kg of whole blood increases a patient's PCV by 1%.

However the response to transfusion should be assessed by measurement of PCV after transfusion and by evaluation of improvement in clinical signs.

Equipment and personnel

- **To give the donor intravenous fluids after blood donation ± any additional sedation via a cephalic catheter:** a 22 G intravenous catheter; tape (e.g. Duropore, 3M); T-connector and bung; 5 ml of heparinized saline; swab with surgical spirit; dressing material (e.g. Soffban, Vetwrap); 100 ml of Hartmann's solution; infusion pump, syringe driver or burette.

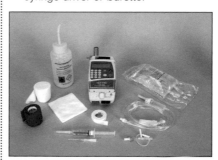

- **To collect blood from the donor and administer it to the recipient:** swab with surgical scrub; swab with surgical spirit; CPDA anticoagulant (from a human blood collection bag); 6 x 10 ml syringes, 15 x 21 G ⁵/₈-inch needles (and if possible 5 x 19 G 1.5-inch needles, not shown); T-connector; 3-way tap; plain 150 ml blood collection bag and blood giving set with filter (for administration of blood – if not available, the blood can be administered in a syringe on a syringe driver, using a syringe filter); artery forceps. Equipment for intravenous cephalic catheter placement in the recipient is also required if not already placed (not shown).

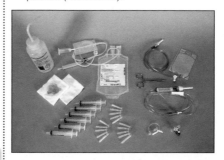

- A phlebotomist, a handler and ideally 2 assistants are required for blood collection.

Preparation

- Draw 1 ml of CPDA anticoagulant (either port can be used; they are identical) into each of the six 10 ml syringes. Ensure that a needle is covering each syringe to keep the CPDA as sterile as possible. Usually 50 ml of blood (five ▶

QRG 20.2 *continued*

syringes full) is collected from the donor, but it is useful to prepare six syringes in case problems occur (e.g. a clot in the syringe necessitating discarding that syringe).

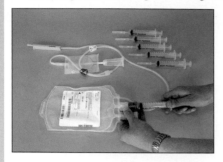

- The T-connector has a needle attached to one end and the 3-way tap attached to the other. CPDA is flushed through these. Attach the first of the CPDA-anticoagulated 10 ml syringes to the open end of the 3-way tap, ready to collect the first 10 ml of blood from the donor.

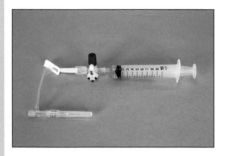

- Tie off the long extension tubing of the small plain blood collection bag (arrow) and clamp it with artery forceps. This will stop the collected blood running down this tube when it is injected into the bag.

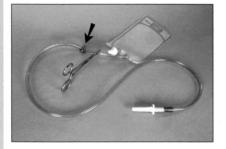

- If not already in place, the recipient should have an intravenous cephalic catheter placed ready for blood administration.

Sedation of the donor

Intramuscular ketamine (5 mg/kg) and midazolam (0.25 mg/kg), given together in the same syringe, is usually used, and gives around 20–30 minutes of sedation. Two separate doses of this sedative combination are prepared in advance; the second dose can be given as a 'top-up' intravenously (in 0.05–0.1 ml increments) in cases where the donor is not sedated for long enough using the intramuscular dose alone.

WARNING

Other sedation combinations can be used but avoid sedatives that lower blood pressure (e.g. alpha-2 agonists) as these would make phlebotomy more difficult.

Blood collection

1 Either before sedation, or immediately once the donor cat is sedated, a catheter is placed into the cephalic vein, with the T-connector and bung, and flushed with 1 ml of heparinized saline.

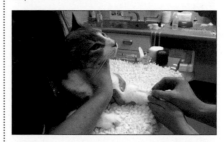

2 The sedated donor cat is placed on its back on a soft bed, blanket or thick towel, with the neck extended for optimal visualization of the jugular vein. Either side of the neck can be used; the area is clipped and prepared aseptically (surgical scrub then spirit) to minimize the risk of contamination of the blood.

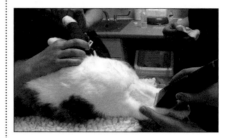

3 The handler then raises the jugular vein at the base of the neck whilst the phlebotomist holds the cat's head in one hand (see QRG 1.2) and has the pre-prepared needle attached to the T-connector, 3-way tap and syringe in the other hand. The 1st assistant should hold the attached syringe ready for blood withdrawal.

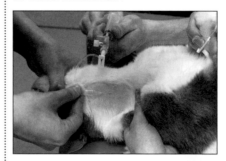

4 The phlebotomist inserts the needle into the jugular vein to its hub and holds the needle steady in position. The 1st assistant begins to withdraw the blood slowly by applying suction on the syringe; this may be done in one continuous motion or by making small suction pulses so as not to collapse the vein.

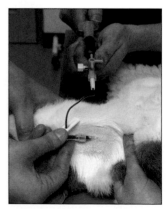

5 When the syringe is full (this can take a few minutes), the 1st assistant should carefully close the 3-way tap to the donor cat. The 1st assistant should have the next prepared syringe to hand (or passed by the 2nd assistant) ready to attach to the 3-way tap (following removal of the needle) to continue collection of blood. ▶

QRG 20.2 *continued*

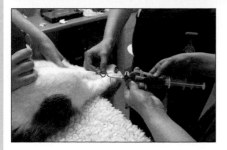

The full syringe is then disconnected from the 3-way tap and handed to the 2nd assistant, who immediately places a capped needle on its end. The 2nd assistant should gently roll the blood-filled syringe for approximately 5 minutes to ensure that the CPDA is mixed thoroughly with the blood.

6 The 3-way tap is turned so that it is open between the patient and syringe, and blood is then withdrawn into the second syringe.

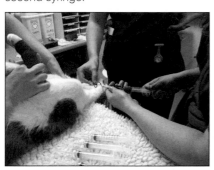

7 Steps 5 and 6 are repeated until five syringes are filled – if the aim is to collect a total volume of 50 ml of blood (the sixth syringe is a spare in case of problems).

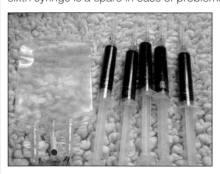

Blood administration

1 All the collected blood is now injected *slowly* (to avoid haemolysis) into the plain blood collection bag through the injection port (indicated by a red spot in the picture above) using the 19 G needles (or 21 G if 19 G are not available), and gently mixed by rotating the bag gently. If any sporadic clots are found whilst injecting the blood (resistance felt to injection), the syringe containing the clot should be discarded.

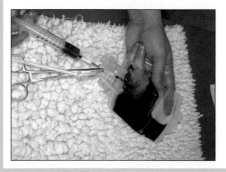

2 The blood giving set with filter is then inserted into the small blood collection bag and the blood run through the giving set, taking care not to make air bubbles or waste any blood.

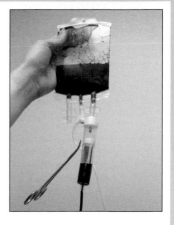

3 The giving set is then attached to the recipient's intravenous cephalic catheter and the transfusion started.

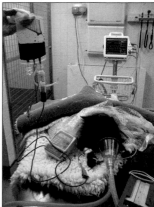

This recipient cat had very severe chronic anaemia due to bone marrow disease; he was given supplementary oxygen by facemask as additional support, as well as warming using blankets and 'hot hands' (not visible).

WARNING

- Blood should not be given through a catheter that contains, or has contained without flushing, calcium-containing fluids (e.g. Hartmann's (lactated Ringer's) solution, Ringer's solution, some colloids).
- The catheter should be flushed with 5 ml of saline before blood administration.

Rate of blood administration

- Transfusion should be started at a rate of 0.25 ml/kg/h for the first 30 minutes.
- If no problems are encountered then the rate can be increased to 0.5 ml/kg/h for a further 30 minutes and then continued at whatever rate is required.
  - If the recipient cat is hypovolaemic, blood can be administered relatively quickly.
  - If the recipient cat is normovolaemic, care should be taken not to administer the transfusion too rapidly.
  - Extra caution is required in cats with cardiac disease or chronic severe anaemia, due to risk of volume overload.
- In all cases transfusion should be completed within 4 hours of collection to minimize risk of bacteraemia.

Monitoring the recipient

Continuous monitoring during the transfusion is required for signs of a transfusion reaction (e.g. weakness, depression, tremors, vocalization, dyspnoea, bradycardia/tachycardia, arrhythmias, weak pulses, salivation, vomiting, diarrhoea, pyrexia or urticaria). Temperature, pulse rate and quality, mucous membrane colour, capillary refill time, and respiratory rate and pattern should be recorded every 5 minutes for the first 30 minutes of the transfusion, reducing to every 10 minutes for the following 30 minutes and then every 15 minutes for the remainder of the transfusion.

If a transfusion reaction is suspected:

- Stop the transfusion immediately
- Consider treatment with: glucocorticoids (e.g. hydrocortisone 2–4 mg/kg i.v. or i.m.); antihistamines ▶

QRG 20.2 *continued*

(e.g. diphenhydramine 1 mg/kg i.v. or i.m.); and/or adrenaline (20 µg/kg of a 1:10,000 solution (100 µg (0.1 mg) per ml) i.v.)

■ Antipyretics (e.g. meloxicam) may be required in some cases
■ If volume overload has resulted in pulmonary oedema, diuretic treatment and oxygen support may be required.

Following transfusion, monitoring of PCV (daily or more frequently if a problem is suspected) for transfusion efficacy and/or development of a haemolytic transfusion reaction is required. Ongoing monitoring of temperature, pulse rate and quality, and respiratory rate and pattern is advised to monitor for other transfusion complications such as volume overload.

Care of the donor after blood collection

■ During or immediately after blood collection, 100 ml of intravenous Hartmann's solution is given to the donor via the cephalic catheter over 1–2 hours.
■ The donor is kept warm, closely monitored (pulse, respiration and mucous membranes every 2–4 hours), and fed as soon as it has recovered from sedation (usually 2–3 hours after sedation).
■ The donor can usually be discharged after 8–12 hours; ensure that the details of the donation (e.g. date, sedation, donated amount and recovery quality) are entered into the cat's records for future reference.

Further reading

Barfield D and Adamantos S (2011) Feline blood transfusions: a pinker shade of pale. *Journal of Feline Medicine and Surgery* **13**, 11–23

Kohn B and Weingart C (2012) Feline transfusion medicine. In: *BSAVA Manual of Canine and Feline Haematology and Transfusion Medicine, 2nd edn*, ed. MJ Day and B Kohn, pp. 308–318. BSAVA Publications, Gloucester

Guidelines for owners of potential blood donors can be found at www.fabcats.org/owners/blood_groups/transfusions_owner.pdf

Practical guidelines for feline blood transfusions are available for both veterinary surgoens and veterinary nurses at www.isfm.net/toolbox/info_sheets/index.html

Videos illustrating blood transfusion procedures can be found at www.felineupdate.co.uk

Management of commonly encountered feline cancers

Mark Goodfellow

This chapter will focus on the management of the most important forms of neoplasia encountered in feline practice: lymphoma; squamous cell carcinoma; cutaneous and visceral mast cell tumours; and injection site sarcomas. Practical guides to removing a lymph node, administering chemotherapy and performing pinnectomy are presented at the end of the chapter. More information on related topics can be found throughout the Manual: approach to an abdominal mass (Chapter 5.2); anorexia (Chapter 5.5); and skin masses, including fine-needle aspiration (Chapter 5.33). Management of gastrointestinal lymphoma, the most common form of this disease, is discussed specifically in Chapter 11, which also includes a practical QRG on biopsy of the gastrointestinal tract and mesenteric lymph node. Practical QRGs on biopsy of various organs can also be found throughout the book, as noted below.

Lymphoma

Lymphoma is the most common tumour of cats and has myriad anatomical presentations. Various systems for classifying feline lymphoma have been suggested, but the most common system categorizes disease into mediastinal, nodal (confined to the peripheral lymph nodes) and extranodal (those involving other organ systems, such as renal or nasal forms). Success of treatment is influenced by anatomical distribution and early identification of disease.

Aetiology

Lymphoma can be induced following FeLV infection. Prior to the introduction of FeLV vaccination and other preventive regimes in the 1980s, cranial mediastinal or multicentric lymphoma were typically seen in young FeLV-positive cats. Disease in young cats is now seen less commonly but lymphoma at all anatomical sites is increasing in prevalence, particularly alimentary and extranodal disease, in older (median age 11 years) FeLV ELISA-negative cats.

While not having a direct oncogenic role, FIV infection also increases the likelihood that an individual will develop lymphoma. Co-infection with FeLV and FIV further increases this risk.

Clinical features

Lymphoma in cats is classified on the basis of anatomical presentation and cases will present with clinical signs dependent on the body system affected (Figures 21.1 and 21.2). At present, alimentary lymphoma is one of the most frequently encountered forms (see Chapter 11). Cats with lymphoma may show non-specific signs of disease (e.g. malaise), regardless of site. This may result from bone marrow

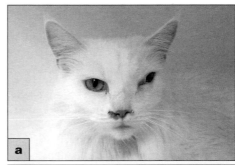

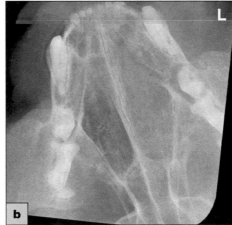

21.1 **(a)** A 4-year-old female unneutered Maine Coon that presented with facial distortion and epistaxis 12 weeks after kittening. **(b)** Intraoral dorsoventral radiographs revealed a soft tissue or fluid opacity throughout the left nasal chamber. On endoscopy, a choanal mass was evident. Assessment of impression smears from biopsy samples revealed a monomorphic population of lymphoblasts, and a diagnosis of nasal lymphoma was made. Radiotherapy was declined by the owner. Treatment with COP chemotherapy resulted in complete remission for 8 months before recurrence of sneezing.

Anatomical site	Presenting signs and features	Main differential diagnoses
Alimentary	See Chapter 11	
Renal	Usually bilateral renomegaly; may be associated with signs of renal insufficiency	Polycystic kidney disease, perinephric pseudocyst, feline infectious peritonitis, bilateral ureteric obstruction
Nasal	Unilateral or bilateral nasal discharge, facial deformity, dyspnoea, and epistaxis	Adenocarcinoma, chronic rhinitis, nasal foreign body, fungal rhinitis (*Cryptococcus*)
Ocular	See Chapter 8	
Mediastinal [a]	Dyspnoea, tachypnoea, non-compressible cranial thorax. Pleural effusion is common, in which neoplastic cells can often be identified. NB Increased incidence in young FeLV-negative Siamese/Orientals, which respond very well to treatment	Thymoma
Nodal or multicentric [a]	Enlargement of one or more peripheral lymph nodes (although true multicentric disease is rare). A distinct form of profound lymphadenopathy of one or more lymph nodes of the head and neck called 'Hodgkin's-like lymphoma' is recognized histopathologically	Reactive lymphadenopathy (peripheral lymphadenopathy without organomegaly is more likely to be reactive than neoplastic in the cat) due to regional inflammation or infection, idiopathic peripheral lymphadenopathy, peripheral lymph node hyperplasia of young cats, bartonellosis, toxoplasmosis, FeLV infection, mycobacterial infections
CNS (intracranial and spinal)	Spinal disease typically affects the thoracolumbar regions, resulting in weakness, ataxia, incontinence and tail flaccidity. Clinical signs are usually non-specific with intracranial disease but may include altered consciousness, ataxia and behavioural change	Intervertebral type 2 disc disease, spinal empyema (e.g. following a cat bite), infectious or inflammatory myelopathies (e.g. FIP), other spinal neoplasia

21.2 Common anatomical forms of feline lymphoma. An individual may present with disease in multiple sites. [a] Forms typically associated with FeLV infection in young cats.

infiltration causing a moderate non-regenerative anaemia and/or a leukaemic profile. Hypercalcaemia and associated clinical signs of polyuria and polydipsia are uncommon in cats (unlike dogs) with lymphoma.

Diagnosis

History and clinical examination will give important clues, but further diagnostic evaluation is always required to exclude other differentials. Haematology and serum biochemistry may suggest occult bone marrow, hepatic or renal involvement or comorbidities. FeLV and FIV testing (see Chapter 19) are appropriate for both diagnosis and predicting prognosis. In the case of nodal forms, cytological examination of a lymph node fine-needle aspirate is not sufficient for diagnosis due to the variety of non-neoplastic lymph node 'syndromes' (e.g. idiopathic peripheral lymphadenopathy, peripheral lymph node hyperplasia of young cats). Biopsy is always required. Ultrasonography allows evaluation of internal lymph nodes, abdominal organs, the cranial mediastinum and pleural space, and facilitates collection of directed fine-needle aspirates. In individuals with extranodal disease, a monomorphic population of lymphoid cells identified on cytology at an ectopic site is sufficient for diagnosis. If there is any doubt, however, Trucut or incisional biopsy or excision of an affected peripheral lymph node (see QRG 21.1) should be performed. Further diagnostics are dependent on anatomical location. For example: in cases of CNS lymphoma, advanced imaging and cytology of cerebrospinal fluid (CSF) may be required, whereas in nasal lymphoma, nasopharyngeal examination (see QRG 5.34.1) and nasal biopsy (see QRG 5.43.2) are most useful.

Management

Definitive treatment

For solitary lymphoma (e.g. ocular or non-Hodgkin's lymphoma) complete surgical excision may be curative, but these represent a minority of cases.

Solitary nasal lymphoma typically responds well to radiotherapy.

Chemotherapy: Systemic chemotherapy (see QRG 21.2) should be considered in all other forms of lymphoma; however, decisions on whether to treat, which protocol to employ and the level of supportive care required are patient-dependent. The patient will need to tolerate frequent visits to the practice for blood sampling and intravenous catheterization for drug administration; if the practicalities of the protocol cause undue distress to the patient, this may be incompatible with a good quality of life. The owner must also be able to devote the necessary time.

Assessing response to an initial short course of chemotherapy can help owners decide whether they wish to pursue protracted treatment. Similarly, the initial choice of treatment should be reviewed, altered or stopped altogether, depending on response and the incidence of adverse effects.

Typically, cats tolerate chemotherapy very well; however, the potential adverse effects of chemotherapy and management strategies must be discussed with the owner. Possible adverse effects include myelosuppression, loss of whiskers, poor hair growth, inappetence, nausea, vomiting and diarrhoea.

- Myelosuppression (and subsequent sepsis) is the most severe risk to the patient, and checking neutrophil count prior to each dose of a myelosuppressive drug is mandatory.
- Inappetence is the commonest adverse effect seen in cats. Every effort should be made to prevent and treat nausea and inappetence aggressively (see Chapter 5.5), as neither is compatible with a good quality of life.
- While the precise extent of the probably small risk to owners is unknown, it is prudent to advise that pregnant women and young children do not handle the patient or its litter tray during the course of the treatment.

Choosing a chemotherapy protocol: There is no single protocol that will be suitable for all patients: anatomical site, type of lymphoma, severity of clinical signs, comorbidities and patient demeanour will all influence the treatment choice. For example, a protocol involving repeated visits to the veterinary practice might be unsuitable for a fractious patient. **Note:** The following protocols are not appropriate for lymphocytic small cell intestinal lymphoma, treatment of which is discussed in Chapter 11.

First-choice chemotherapy protocols typically include cyclophosphamide, vincristine and prednisolone (COP protocol; Figure 21.3), sometimes with addition of doxorubicin (CHOP protocol; Figure 21.3). However, the additional benefit of including doxorubicin is unclear, and therefore COP is an appropriate first-choice protocol for most cases treated in practice. The LMP (chlorambucil + methotrexate + prednisolone; Figure 21.3) or other lower intensity protocols are suitable for cats that have achieved remission with COP or CHOP but where an alternative protocol is required, for example to reduce veterinary visits or adverse effects. In general, 50–70% of cats can be expected to achieve remission on treatment but disease recurrence is expected and the average survival time is approximately 6 months, although a significant proportion of cats in complete remission (~25%) will survive over a year. Initial response to treatment is the strongest prognostic indicator and can occur very quickly, for example within days of starting treatment. Trial therapy can therefore be recommended in all patients. Overall, nasal lymphoma, and mediastinal lymphoma in young FeLV-negative Siamese cats, typically respond well. In contrast, renal lymphoma, and mediastinal lymphoma in young FeLV-positive cats, respond poorly. The immunophenotype is of no prognostic significance in cats.

COP protocol

- **C**yclophosphamide 300 mg/m² i.v./orally, every 21 days [a]
- **V**incristine (**O**) 0.75 mg/m² i.v., every 7 days for 4 weeks then every third week
- **P**rednisolone 2 mg/kg, orally, q24h for 1 week; then 5 mg orally, q48h until relapse or adverse steroid effects, in which case taper dose and discontinue

CHOP protocol

- **C**yclophosphamide 200 mg/m² i.v./orally, weeks 2, 7, 13, 21 [a]
- **D**oxorubicin (**H**) 25 mg/m² i.v., weeks 4, 9, 17, 23
- **V**incristine (**O**) 0.7 mg/m² i.v., weeks 1, 3, 6, 8, 11, 15, 19, 23
- **P**rednisolone 2 mg/kg orally q24h for 28 days; then 1 mg/kg orally, q48h until relapse or adverse steroid effects, in which case taper dose and discontinue

LMP protocol (maintenance only)

- **C**hlorambucil (**L**) 20 mg/m² orally, every 14 days
- **M**ethotrexate 2.5 mg/m² 2–3 times per week [a]
- **P**rednisolone 20 mg/m² orally q48h

21.3 Suggested protocols for treatment of feline lymphoma. For each case, the protocol is modified based on patient response and adverse effects. If adverse effects occur then the drug's dose should be reduced, delayed or omitted; alternatively, if response is suboptimal, an alternate protocol should be considered. More comprehensive oncology texts or the advice of a veterinary oncologist should be consulted before embarking on an unfamiliar treatment course. [a] Consider reformulation of tablets to more suitable sizes for accurate dosing.

Supportive care

The decision of whether, and how, to treat lymphoma is a complex one for both owners and vets. Both parties should agree that the sole aim is maximizing the patient's quality of life, irrespective of the treatment path chosen. Given that response to chemotherapy is one of the strongest prognostic indicators, treatment should be offered and encouraged in all cases. Owners should be counselled that further treatment will depend on the patient's response and tolerance of the chosen protocol. Should a patient not respond or treatment be associated with unacceptable adverse effects, then it is usually in the patient's best interests to alter or cease therapy. Whenever adverse effects occur they should be treated rapidly and aggressively as they diminish quality of life. Assisted feeding, appetite stimulants, analgesia and anti-emetics may all be indicated (see Chapters 3 and 5.5).

Cutaneous squamous cell carcinoma

Aetiology

Cutaneous squamous cell carcinoma (SCC) occurs principally as a result of damage to lightly pigmented or unpigmented areas of skin by ultraviolet (UV) radiation. White cats have a 13-fold increased risk of developing SCC. Multiple cutaneous SCC at other body sites (Bowen's disease – also known as multicentric SCC *in situ*) is of unknown aetiology.

Clinical features

SCC occurs most commonly on the nasal planum (Figure 21.4), eyelid and pinnae of older cats following chronic sunlight exposure. Purebred cats are less likely to develop SCC than DSH or Domestic Longhaired (DLH) cats but whether this is as a result of skin colour, a predominantly indoor lifestyle or genetic make-up is unclear. A third of affected cats have multiple lesions. Lesions may have been present for many months prior to presentation and are slowly progressive. Initially lesions may be minor (an actinic

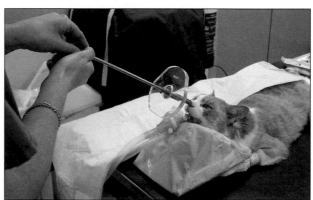

21.4 A 6-year-old male neutered DSH cat receiving strontium[90] plesiotherapy for a superficial SCC of the nasal planum, diagnosed by incisional biopsy. Strontium plesiotherapy was chosen as the lesion was superficial (graded T1 histologically) and because it produces an excellent cosmetic result. Five treatments were administered on an every other day basis. Following treatment, while the treated area remained hairless, the cat was free of disease.

keratosis or carcinoma that has not invaded through the basement membrane (carcinoma *in situ*)), have an easily removed crust, and are often mistaken by owners for cat-scratch wounds. As the lesions progress, they become more erosive and locally infiltrative, presenting as a shallow erosion or crusting. In advanced cases, severe invasion and destruction of underlying tissue occurs, particularly loss of the nasal planum.

Diagnosis
Diagnosis can be achieved by either cytological or histological examination, although only the latter allows assessment of the degree of local infiltration. A small punch biopsy sample (see QRG 5.3.3) from the edge of a lesion is usually sufficient. These tumours rarely metastasize but, given the older population and treatment choices, thoracic radiography, assessment of the draining lymph node, haematology and serum biochemistry are appropriate where possible.

Management
Low-grade lesions, with minimal invasion, respond well to a variety of treatment modalities. In most cases cure or long-term control can be achieved with one or more cycles of the selected treatment. Selection of treatment depends on availability, comorbidities of the patient, expense and the owner's acceptance of the likely cosmetic result. Superficial lesions can be treated with local surgery, strontium[90] plesiotherapy or photodynamic therapy. The last two treatments are particularly suitable for multiple superficial lesions and have good cosmetic results. More invasive lesions require surgical excision (nasal planectomy; pinnectomy (see QRG 21.3)), cryosurgery, external beam radiation or intralesional chemotherapy. All treatments are most successful when lesions are small; control is difficult to achieve after extensive local infiltration (particularly of the nasal planum) has occurred. Single isolated lesions can be successfully managed in practice with surgery, but multiple lesions or lesions that cannot be easily excised, such as those of the eyelid or nasal planum, should be referred for specialist treatment.

Prevention
Limiting sun exposure is the most sensible approach, as topical sunscreens are rapidly groomed off. Local tattooing is ineffective at preventing SCC.

Cutaneous mast cell tumours

Clinical features
Mast cell tumours (MCTs) usually present as solitary, round, hairless, firm cutaneous lesions, often on the head (particularly around the pinnae) and neck. In a minority of cases, multiple lesions may be present or the mass may be diffuse, subcutaneous or plaque-like. Mast cells possess granules containing a variety of vasoactive and inflammatory mediators. Release of these substances following manipulation or trauma either by the patient or by the veterinary surgeon may cause Darier's sign (wheal and flare), pruritus, bleeding or apparent fluctuations in the size of the mass. Two distinct forms (mastocytic and histiocytic; see later) are recognized on the basis of histopathology and, while these may also differ in presentation, they cannot be readily distinguished without sampling.

Diagnosis
Cytology following fine-needle aspiration (FNA) should be performed to exclude other differential diagnoses and because it is diagnostic in most cases of cutaneous MCT. Histologically, feline cutaneous MCT is recognized in two distinct forms:

- Mastocytic – more common form, typically seen in older cats. This is histologically differentiated into the *compact* form, which is behaviourally benign (up to 90% of cases), and the *diffuse* form, which is infiltrative and metastatic
- Histiocytic – less common form, often presenting as multiple lesions in young cats, particularly Siamese. These do not spread and typically regress spontaneously.

Mastocytic MCTs are readily recognized on cytology, but a distinction between diffuse and compact forms cannot be made cytologically. Histiocytic MCTs can be more difficult to diagnose definitively using cytology due to the histiocytic cellular phenotype, vague cytoplasmic granularity and presence of lymphoid cells. Mast cells are common in other inflammatory cutaneous lesions, such as eosinophilic granuloma (see Chapter 6), and this may result in misdiagnosis of MCT. If diagnosis is not achieved with cytology, incisional biopsy is preferred. Biopsy should be planned and performed so that the biopsy site can be subsequently removed completely during definitive excisional surgery.

Management
Surgery
Surgical excision is the preferred modality to treat all forms of cutaneous MCT. Although histiocytic MCTs may regress spontaneously, this should not be relied upon as a mode of therapy. Local resection is sufficient for solitary compact lesions of mastocytic MCT, which make up the majority of cases, while the diffuse form requires more aggressive surgical margins and staging for systemic spread (see below). However, as the distinction between the compact and diffuse forms cannot be made cytologically, the author suggests the following pragmatic approach for all skin masses suspected to be MCTs.

1. Local resection with 0.5–1 cm margins of any MCT diagnosed on cytology (the majority of which will be compact mastocytic or histiocytic MCT). For those rare patients affected by diffuse mastocytic MCT, more aggressive therapy can then be undertaken under the guidance of a veterinary oncologist.
2. Incisional biopsy for those cases in which a firm diagnosis has not been achieved cytologically or that are in a site that would require a more complicated surgical reconstruction should the tumour prove to be of the diffuse mastocytic type (e.g. around the face). In the case of mastocytic MCTs, appropriate surgery and therapy can be planned based on whether a diffuse or compact tumour has been identified.

In all cases, excised material should be submitted for histopathology, the surgical margins assessed and the type of MCT ascertained. A compact mastocytic

MCT requires no further intervention as long as the tumour has been completely excised – the patient should be cured.

Recurrence: Incidence of recurrence is low, even following incomplete excision; when recurrence does occur, it is typically within 6 months. In the case of histiocytic MCTs, a 'watch and wait' policy can be adopted, even following marginal excision, as the majority will regress spontaneously. Patients with a diffuse type of mastocytic MCT should undergo full staging (including cytological assessment of the draining lymph node, two-view thoracic radiography and abdominal ultrasonography) and, if necessary, further surgery or adjuvant therapy following diagnosis. This is best performed under the guidance of a veterinary oncologist and prognosis is likely to be poor.

Other therapies
Antihistamines and cyproheptidine may be of benefit in reducing pruritus of non-resectable lesions caused by histamine and serotonin, respectively. Similarly, antihistamines should be administered prior to surgical manipulation of masses. Cutaneous MCTs are amenable to radiation therapy when unresectable surgically. In contrast to dogs, chemotherapy, including corticosteroids, has no role in the treatment of cutaneous MCT in the cat. The efficacy and role of receptor tyrosine kinase inhibitors (TKIs) is yet to be established. As the majority of feline MCTs are benign, in patients for whom surgery is not possible, treatment is aimed at palliation. Quality of life will tend to be dictated by the local consequences of disease.

Visceral mast cell tumours

Clinical features
Visceral MCTs can occur either primarily in the parenchymal organs (particularly the spleen but also the liver and mesenteric and mediastinal lymph nodes) or in the small intestines, and are typically seen in older cats. Splenic MCT is the most common form (>85%) and the remainder of the discussion will focus on splenic and intestinal forms of the disease.

Cats present with signs of systemic illness, including depression, weight loss, vomiting and (in the intestinal form) diarrhoea, which may contain blood. Typically, the disease course is protracted. Abdominal palpation may reveal splenomegaly, often very marked, an intestinal mass and/or a peritoneal effusion. Systemic spread of visceral MCT may result in cutaneous lesions. Conversely, only rarely does a cutaneous MCT, of the diffuse mastocytic type, precede visceral disease.

Diagnosis

History and clinical examination
The history and clinical examination provide valuable information (see Chapter 5.2). Investigation of cases in which a visceral MCT is suspected should include haematology, biochemistry and Buffy coat cytology (Figure 21.5). A third of cats with intestinal MCTs are anaemic and over half of cases with splenic MCTs will have a circulating mastocytosis, which is specific for MCTs in the cat. The presence of cytopenias alerts to the possibility of bone marrow infiltration, and bone

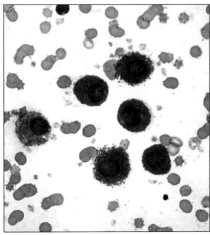

21.5 Multiple mast cells (round cells with round nuclei and cytoplasm that is filled with purple granules) in a Buffy coat smear prepared from a cat with splenic MCT. To prepare a Buffy coat smear: centrifuge EDTA-anticoagulated blood and, with a fine-tipped pipette, gently aspirate the Buffy coat layer with minimal contamination of erythrocytes or plasma; a drop of this aspirate can then be smeared and stained in a similar fashion to whole blood. Alternatively, a microhaematocrit tube containing centrifuged whole blood can be scored and cut at the level of the Buffy coat, and a smear made from a drop of the Buffy coat that is tapped out on to the slide. (Modified Wright's stain; original magnification X1000.) (Courtesy of Roger Powell)

marrow aspiration (see QRG 5.4.3) is advisable in these cases, prior to considering surgery.

Imaging
Abdominal ultrasonography may reveal the presence of splenomegaly or an intestinal mass and can be used to evaluate for metastases to the mesenteric lymph nodes and liver. A splenic MCT may result in either diffuse changes in echogenicity of the splenic parenchyma or, less commonly, can cause multiple nodules throughout the organ. Peritoneal fluid may also be visible. Thoracic radiographs (two orthogonal views) are required for identification of pulmonary metastasis, cranial mediastinal disease and pleural effusion.

Cytology
Fine-needle aspiration of the spleen or intestinal mass can be diagnostic and can help to differentiate MCTs from other causes of splenomegaly (lymphoma, myeloproliferative disease, haemangiosarcoma, splenitis, regenerative anaemias) and intestinal mass (lymphoma, adenocarcinoma). Similarly, cytology of a pleural or peritoneal effusion may reveal a significant population of mast cells and eosinophils.

Management

Surgery
A complete and thorough staging is important prior to considering surgery.

Surgical therapy is appropriate in cases where there is no evidence of gross metastatic disease, even if a circulating mastocytosis is present. Preoperative administration of antihistamines (both H1 and H2 receptor antagonists such as chlorphenamine and cimetidine) is advised to lessen the risk of degranulation of mast cells which could cause hypotension, local coagulation anomalies and gastrointestinal ulceration. During anaesthesia, pulse quality and ideally arterial blood pressure should be monitored closely.

Splenic MCTs: In the case of splenic MCTs, splenectomy, even in the face of mastocytosis, is associated with a prolonged period of good quality of life (12–19 months). Peripheral mastocytosis does not resolve but may lessen, and a subsequent rise can warn of disease progression.

Intestinal MCTs: Intestinal MCTs are associated with a poor prognosis and the majority of cases have diffuse involvement and metastasis at the time of diagnosis. Only in those cases where the disease is localized should resection, with very wide (5–10 cm) surgical margins, be attempted. Survival time is shorter than for those cases with splenic disease but can be many months, and may be extended with systemic chemotherapy.

Other therapies

Adjuvant chemotherapy, using prednisolone, lomustine or vinblastine, may be of some benefit following surgical resection or in non-surgical candidates, including cranial mediastinal disease, or those with widespread metastases. The role of TKIs is as yet unclear. The guidance of a veterinary oncologist should be sought to discuss management options.

Supportive care

Irrespective of treatment modality, the patient's quality of life should be maximized. H1 and H2 antagonists may reduce the risk of gastrointestinal ulceration, gastric hyperacidity and nausea. Supportive care, including encouragement to eat, use of appetite stimulants and when necessary anti-emetics and analgesic drugs, should always be considered.

Feline injection site sarcoma

Feline injection site sarcoma (FISS) describes a group of aggressive, highly locally infiltrative sarcomas, usually with a relatively low metastatic rate (up to about 25% cases metastasize), typically found in the interscapular region, at a site of previous injection (Figure 21.6).

Aetiology

Previously known as feline vaccination-associated sarcoma (VASA) or vaccine-associated fibrosarcoma (VAFS), it is now recognized that these tumours can be caused by a variety of foreign agents in the subcutis, including vaccines, microchips, long-acting antibiotics and lufenuron. However, prior use of adjuvanted vaccines for rabies or FeLV is most commonly implicated. The number of previous vaccinations at the same site also plays a role. In the predisposed cat an inflammatory response is elicited, which ultimately undergoes neoplastic transformation.

Clinical features

FISS manifests as a mass at an injection site months or years following an injection. FISS can occur at any age but is more common in middle-aged cats. Once detected, tumour growth is usually rapid. The mass

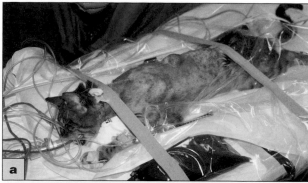
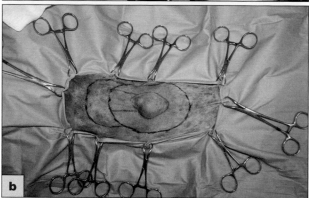
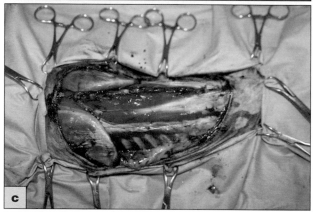

21.6 **(a)** A 4-year-old male neutered Bengal presented with a firm plum-sized dorsal mass, noted 2 months after routine vaccination. Incisional biopsy confirmed FISS. Neo-adjuvant epirubicin resulted in a halving of the size of the mass and it was noticeably softer on palpation. Despite its discrete appearance, contrast CT revealed cranial extension. **(b)** Surgical margins of 3 cm were inked around the mass, with a further 3 cm margin rostrally, given the occult extension of disease detected on CT. **(c)** To achieve a deep margin of excision, the trapezius and rhomboideus muscles, with portions of the latissimus dorsi and the tips of the dorsal vertebral spinous processes, were removed. Closure of the large deficit required careful deadspace management and a layered anatomical closure. Following surgical excision, a further course of adjuvant chemotherapy was administered. The patient was in excellent health, without evidence of recurrence, 24 months after the final dose of chemotherapy.

may be: relatively mobile and apparently confined to the subcutaneous tissue; or deeply attached to the underlying musculature. Irrespective of the external appearance, wide infiltration of the surrounding structures is likely. These sarcomas are typically of low metastatic potential and are associated with few systemic clinical signs, but are rapidly growing and locally aggressive. Very large masses may become traumatized or may ulcerate.

Diagnosis

An aggressive investigative approach is required for the rapid identification of FISS, in order to achieve optimal management. The main differential diagnosis is an injection site abscess, and the Vaccine Associated Feline Sarcoma Task Force (VAFSTF) proposed a rule of 3-2-1 to assist in determining timing of intervention (Figure 21.7).

- Perform biopsy on any mass that is still present THREE months after vaccination/injection.
- Perform biopsy on any mass at an injection site that is greater than TWO centimetres in diameter.
- Perform biopsy on any mass that is increasing in size within ONE month after vaccination/injection.

21.7 The 3-2-1 approach to injection site masses. (Guidelines proposed by the VAFSTF; for complete document see www.avma.org.)

Cytology of tumour aspirates is unreliable and histopathology is required for definitive diagnosis. An incisional wedge biopsy should be planned, if necessary with advice from a specialist oncological surgeon, and performed so that subsequent definitive surgical removal will include the entire biopsy site. Tru-cut needle biopsy may result in misdiagnosis due to the small sample size and heterogenous nature of the tumour. Excisional biopsy should not be attempted for diagnosis, as this invariably results in incomplete excision, reducing the effectiveness of subsequent surgeries.

Management

There is no sole effective treatment for FISS; instead a multimodal approach including radical surgery and adjunctive/neo-adjuvant chemotherapy and/or radiotherapy is associated with the best outcome. Referral to a special centre is therefore always preferable where possible. If definitive specialist treatment is not possible or available, management should be directed toward palliation. Surgical resection by non-specialist surgeons has been associated with rapid tumour recurrence, typically within a couple of months, and so is likely to be of little benefit to the patient.

Staging

Metastasis occurs in up to 25% of cases and is typically to the lungs. At least two fully inflated orthogonal thoracic radiographs are required in order to assess for metastatic disease prior to performing surgery. Aggressive surgery is not warranted in the face of metastatic disease. Thoracic CT has a higher sensitivity for evaluation of the thorax for metastases than does radiography, and also aids surgical planning as the tumour volume may be twice that estimated by palpation.

Surgery

Time to recurrence is substantially increased if surgery is performed by a specialist when the tumour is small. Aggressive surgical margins of at least 2 cm (but ideally 3–5 cm) lateral and deep to the tumour mass, crossing at least one facial plane are required. This may include the dorsal spinous processes of vertebrae and the dorsal border of the scapula. Intensive supportive care (including assisted feeding and analgesia) is required postoperatively.

Tumour recurrence occurs in a significant proportion of cases with apparently tumour-free margins in the 2 years following surgery. This recurrence rate, even in the face of aggressive surgery, confirms that curative-intent surgical resection should not be attempted except by a specialist surgeon as part of a multimodal treatment regime.

Chemotherapy and radiotherapy

These are employed either to reduce tumour size prior to excision (i.e. neo-adjunctive), or following surgery (i.e. adjunctive) to reduce residual disease. There is consensus that a multimodal approach increases time to recurrence and overall survival, but the most effective protocol has yet to be determined. Typically, anthracyclines such as epirubicin are the cytotoxic agents employed. Further details on treatment protocols can be found in the *BSAVA Manual of Canine and Feline Oncology*.

Outcome

With multimodal therapy, survival times vary depending on the protocol but are typically several years.

Prevention

As this tumour is iatrogenic, it is vital for veterinary surgeons to minimize the risk of tumour formation by an approach to vaccination appropriate to an individual patient's risk (see Chapter 2). Veterinary surgeons should vaccinate as infrequently as possible, while ensuring adequate immunity. Where possible, vaccines and other injections should be administered at sites that would be more amenable to more aggressive surgical resection (e.g. distal limb).

References and further reading

Dobson J and Lascelles BDX (2011) *BSAVA Manual of Canine and Feline Oncology, 3rd edn*. BSAVA Publications, Gloucester

Martano M, Morello E and Buracco P (2011) Feline injection-site sarcoma: past, present and future perspectives. *Veterinary Journal* **188**, 136–141

Moore A and Ogilvie GK (2000) *Feline Oncology: A Comprehensive Guide to Compassionate Care*. Wiley Blackwell, Oxford

Morrison WB, Starr RM and the Vaccine-Associated Feline Sarcoma Task Force (2001) Vaccine-associated feline sarcomas. *Journal of the American Veterinary Medical Association* **218**, 697–702

Watson P and Lindley S (2010) *BSAVA Manual of Canine and Feline Rehabilitation, Supportive and Palliative Care*. BSAVA Publications, Gloucester

Withrow SJ and MacEwen EG (2001) *Small Animal Clinical Oncology, 4th edn*. WB Saunders, Philadelphia

QRG 21.1 Lymph node excision
by Geraldine Hunt

- Lymph nodes are usually removed for the purpose of obtaining a definitive diagnosis for lymphadenomegaly (differential diagnoses include lymphoma, inflammatory conditions such as *Mycobacterium avium* infection, and lymph node hyperplasia), staging a neoplastic process, or as part of oncological surgery itself.
- The most accessible lymph nodes are the mandibular and popliteal; however, it is sometimes necessary to remove the superficial cervical (prescapular), inguinal, axillary, retropharyngeal, medial iliac (sublumbar), tracheobronchial or sternal nodes. The superficial cervical, mandibular and popliteal nodes are palpable even when normal. The axillary and inguinal nodes are rarely palpable when normal.
- The abdominal nodes (hepatic, cranial mesenteric, pancreatic, ileocolic) are often not removed *in toto*, due to their close proximity to the intestinal vasculature, and wedge or suture amputation biopsy samples are taken instead (see QRG 11.1 for biopsy of mesenteric lymph node).
- Removal of the intrathoracic or medial iliac lymph nodes is rarely undertaken in general practice.

Equipment

- Right-angled dissecting forceps or mosquito forceps
- Brown–Adson forceps
- Metzenbaum scissors
- 2 or 1.5 metric (3/0 or 4/0 USP) monofilament absorbable suture material

Surgical procedure for removal of a popliteal lymph node

1 Before starting surgery, palpate the lymph node through the skin and clip and prepare the site.

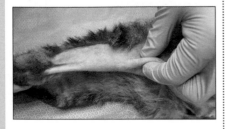

2 Make a skin incision directly over the node.

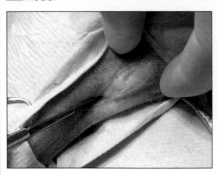

3 Expose the lymph node and the attachments between its capsule and the surrounding tissues using blunt dissection with mosquito or right-angled forceps.

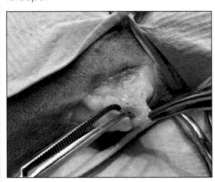

PRACTICAL TIP

In general, lymph nodes reside at the junction between two body parts, between flexor surfaces of joints, or where visceral structures divide. They are usually surrounded by fatty tissue, which can make localization and identification difficult if they are not enlarged. Lymph nodes possess a capsule, and are usually tan-coloured or grey. A single blood vessel enters on the medial aspect, and sometimes the lymph node can be found by first identifying a blood vessel within a fat pad and then tracking it to the node. Small lymph nodes in the inguinal and popliteal fat pads can be notoriously hard to find, and surgeons should concentrate on identifying anatomical structures that the lymph node should be associated with (such as the inguinal canal in the case of the inguinal lymph node, or the arterial supply to the popliteal lymph node, which can be found travelling caudally from the flexor surface of the stifle).

4 A small blood vessel (white arrow) will often indicate where the node (encircled) is located within the fat pad. Once the node has been identified it can be grasped gently, using Brown–Adson forceps, and traction applied. This helps to clarify which structures are actually attached to it, and which are simply in close proximity. Gentle traction also helps to stabilize the tissues being dissected, as the node may otherwise have a tendency to slide away from the dissecting instruments, making the procedure longer and more frustrating.

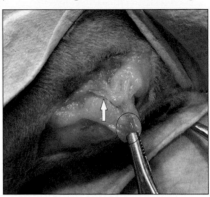

WARNING

- Care should be taken not to perforate the capsule or damage the lymph node architecture.
- Dissection should proceed close to the capsule, directly over the node, rather than into the surrounding tissues, as nodes are often associated with larger blood vessels and nerves.

5 The vascular supply to the lymph node should be divided using electrocautery, a battery-operated cautery pen or the absorbable suture material.

6 Connective tissue attachments remaining after the blood vessel has been ligated can be divided with sharp or blunt dissection.

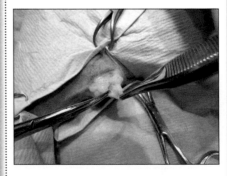

7 The dissection site should be lavaged with saline and inspected for ongoing bleeding. The loose connective tissue is then closed, avoiding deep bites into tissue that may contain nerves or blood vessels, and the skin is closed according to the surgeon's preference. ▶

QRG 21.1 *continued*

WARNING

For adherent lymph nodes with neovascularization from surrounding structures, a combination of blunt dissection using a fine surgical suction tip, and monopolar or bipolar cautery, with use of surgical clips for larger vessels, is necessary. Removal of large, adherent lymph nodes should only be attempted if this equipment is available.

Other lymph nodes

Mandibular

The proximity between the mandibular lymph node, mandibular salivary gland and retropharyngeal lymph nodes can create confusion. The mandibular lymph node is most superficial, sitting cranioventral to the salivary gland. It is sometimes removed accidentally by novice surgeons trying to remove the salivary gland. The mandibular lymph node is a lentil-shaped structure. The salivary gland is identifiable because of its larger size, its dome-shaped appearance when the superficial tissues are dissected and its distinct capsule that separates from the glandular structure underneath when perforated.

Retropharyngeal

The retropharyngeal lymph nodes sit just below the wings of the atlas vertebra and can be accessed by first approaching the mandibular salivary gland, then continuing the dissection dorsal to the salivary gland into the deeper tissues. As soon as the retropharyngeal lymph node is identified, it should be grasped with Babcock forceps and firmly exteriorized while the soft tissue dissection is completed. Exteriorizing the lymph node as much as possible helps avoid problems with damage to the vagosympathetic trunk, glossopharyngeal nerve, hypoglossal nerve and internal carotid artery, all of which travel close to it.

Mesenteric or ileocolic

Following exploratory laparotomy, biopsy of the mesenteric lymph node (see QRG 11.1) or ileocolic lymph node can be performed.

Complications

Complications that can occur after lymph node excision include haematoma and seroma, and neurovascular damage (especially with the retropharyngeal lymph nodes).

QRG 21.2 Chemotherapy for lymphoma
by Mark Goodfellow

BEFORE intravenous cytotoxic drug therapy

Calculate the cat's body surface area based on its *current* (not a previous) bodyweight *using a table specific to cats* (BSA for bodyweight is different in dogs). Then calculate the dose of drug required. Ideally, two people should perform these calculations independently, to ensure accuracy. Doses should be **rounded down** to the closest tablet size or measurable volume.

Bodyweight (kg)	Body surface area (m²)
2.0	0.159
2.5	0.184
3.0	0.208
3.5	0.231
4.0	0.252
4.5	0.273
5.0	0.292
5.5	0.311
6.0	0.330
6.5	0.348
7.0	0.366
7.5	0.383
8.0	0.400

Within 2 days prior to *every* administration, check a haematology sample to ensure that the patient has sufficient neutrophils (>3 x10⁹/l) and platelets (automated or manual count of >120 x10⁹/l). Assessment of a total granulocyte or leucocyte count is not sufficient, but many in-practice machines are able to quantify neutrophils specifically. If there is any doubt, assessment by an external laboratory is advisable. *If the neutrophil count is insufficient, delay treatment and recheck haematology after 48 hours.*

Prior to use of any drug, consult reference texts for specific treatment strategies in the event of extravasation, so that appropriate measures can be taken immediately.

Preparing the drug

WARNING

Cytotoxic drugs are mutagenic and carcinogenic to humans, and personnel cannot be too cautious when handling these agents. Appropriate PPE should be worn.

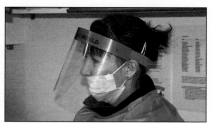

Aerosolization and contamination of clothing represent the greatest risks for staff carrying out chemotherapy. Whenever possible a facemask and visor, an impervious gown (specifically manufactured for use when administering chemotherapy) with elasticated cuffs, and nitrile gloves should be worn to minimize exposure.

Collect all required materials prior to starting and line the working area with an absorbent plastic-backed material (e.g. incontinence sheets). Pre-label the syringe to contain the cytotoxic agent carefully and clearly.

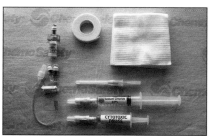

Appropriate equipment for the safe administration of cytotoxic drugs, on an absorbent mat. A Smart-Site vented vial access device allows withdrawal of cytotoxic drug into a syringe capped with a Texium needle-free injection device in a closed manner, preventing aerosolization and self-injection. A Smart-Site needle-free T connector is attached to the patient's intravenous cannula to allow drug administration in a similarly closed manner. Prior to drug administration, the intravenous cannula is flushed copiously with normal saline.

WARNING

Because aerosolization of drugs represents the greatest hazard to personnel, the following should ideally be performed in a biological safety cabinet or using a needleless system with Luer-lok syringes (numerous affordable needle-free systems exist for use in practice). ▶

QRG 21.2 *continued*

WARNING

- When withdrawing liquids from vials, do not inject air first as this increases the risk of leakage.
- When withdrawing needles from vials, wrap the vial in an alcohol-soaked swab to catch any droplets.
- Do not recap syringes or, if absolutely essential, do so with great care.

Preparation of the patient

Place the cat in a quiet well ventilated area, ensuring that it is comfortable.

- Ideally, the patient should be on an absorbent plastic-backed material (e.g. incontinence sheet) in case of cytotoxic spills.
- Ensure that sufficient aid is available to restrain the cat appropriately.
- Ensure that other personnel do not enter the room during drug administration (e.g. place a sign on the door saying 'Chemotherapy in progress. Do not enter').

Place a 22 G intravenous cannula into the chosen peripheral vein (e.g. cephalic vein; see QRG 4.1.1). When possible use a different limb for venous access on subsequent occasions. NB Should the first attempt fail, an alternative vein should be used for a second attempt.

- Some cytotoxic drugs are vesicants and any escape of drug perivascularly will cause severe tissue necrosis. Do not use butterfly catheters or give cytotoxic drugs 'off the needle'.
- Flush the cannula to ensure correct placement using normal (0.9%) saline. NB Heparinized saline precipitates some chemotherapy drugs (e.g. doxorubicin) and should therefore be avoided.
- Use of a pre-flushed T connector or similar extension set will allow subsequent administration without the need to hold the patient's paw.

Administering the drug

1 Remove any dressings that were applied to the cannula site, in order that the catheterized vein can be observed and palpated throughout the chemotherapy procedure.

2 Slowly inject the drug.

PRACTICAL TIP

If an extension set has not been used, hold the patient's limb and the syringe in the same hand, to prevent accidental disconnection if the cat moves.

WARNING

Should leakage or extravasation of drug be suspected during the infusion, or if the patient appears to resent infusion, administration should cease immediately.

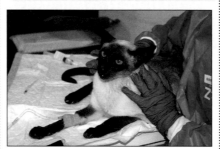

Administration of vincristine to an 11-year-old Siamese with lymphoblastic alimentary lymphoma. Note that the operator's gloves are pulled over the elasticated cuffs. All dressings have been removed from the cannula site and the cat's leg has been extended. Use of a Y connector allows freedom for the cat to move slightly. A bolus of intravenous fluids is being administered concurrently.

3 Flush copiously with 5 ml of normal (0.9%) saline after drug administration.

4 Cover the injection site with a swab (to prevent flicking droplets of potentially contaminated blood into the environment) and remove the intravenous cannula. Securely bandage the swab in place.

WARNING

Place all potentially contaminated materials into a separate bag for disposal in accordance with local regulations. All contaminated syringes and needles should be disposed of *en bloc* in a designated Hazardous Waste 'sharps' bin.

Aftercare

- Record the route (including which limb) and dose of chemotherapy administered accurately.
- Remind the owner that litter tray waste should be handled with caution (wearing gloves) and separately bagged for disposal, as cytotoxic drugs or their metabolites may be excreted for at least 48 hours.
- Prescribe appropriate anti-emetics for the owner to administer if they are concerned that the cat is nauseous and/or inappetent. For example, maropitant (1 mg/kg orally for up to 5 consecutive days; unauthorized) or metoclopromide (0.2–0.5 mg/kg orally q8h).
- Whenever a patient is unwell following chemotherapy, consider whether myelosuppression may have resulted in sepsis, even in the absence of pyrexia. In such cases, perform a complete haematological assessment and, if necessary, prescribe broad-spectrum antibiotics (amoxicillin/clavulanate 12.5 mg/kg orally q12h and metronidazole 10 mg/kg orally q12h).
- If the cat experiences adverse effects such as vomiting, diarrhoea or inappetence, consider a dose reduction of 20% for subsequent doses of the cytotoxic drug. Also consider a dose reduction if neutropenia results in a treatment delay.

QRG 21.3 Pinnectomy
by Geraldine Hunt

- Pinnectomy is usually performed for the treatment of squamous cell carcinoma (SCC) or advanced actinic (solar) dermatitis.
- Years of solar damage to the skin can lead to the need for pinnectomy, and it should be noted that any skin

remaining on the pinna is at risk of developing the same lesions in the future. Complete pinnectomy (as described here) is therefore usually preferable over trimming of the affected portion only.

- SCC lesions should be removed with

a margin of at least 1 cm of normal-appearing pinna. Ideally, biopsy should be performed to confirm the disease process prior to pinnectomy, but in geographical regions with a high incidence of SCC (e.g. Australia), presumptive diagnosis is often ▶

QRG 21.3 continued

made on the basis of clinical appearance and behaviour in order to save the owner from additional expense and the cat from additional surgical procedures.
- Pinnectomy is often performed bilaterally, due to the bilateral nature of lesions, and symmetry between the two sides will improve the cosmetic result.

Equipment

- No. 10 scalpel blade and handle
- Curved non-crushing clamps, e.g. Cooley or Satinsky non-crushing vascular forceps

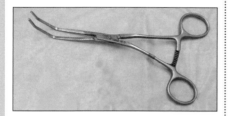

- Brown–Adson thumb forceps
- 1.5 metric (4/0 USP) synthetic monofilament absorbable suture material

Patient preparation

Anaesthetize the patient (see Chapter 3) and place them in sternal recumbency with the head elevated on a small sandbag or rolled towel. Clip the ear (or both ears if bilateral pinnectomy is required), including the skin at the base of the ear. Flush the ear canal and clean it of debris, and pack the ear canal with cotton wool. Aseptically prepare the ear pinna.

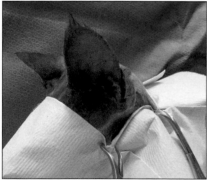

The pinnae have both been clipped and draped in preparation for bilateral surgery.

Procedure

1 Stretch the skin of the dorsal surface of the pinna towards the tip of the ear and place a non-crushing curved clamp across the base of the pinna; this provides a guide for incision, holds the skin in place and provides haemostasis. A Cooley (shown) or Satinsky vascular clamp is ideal if available. Otherwise, a Doyen bowel clamp or some other non-crushing clamp may be used, but will result in a different cosmetic appearance due to the wider radius of its curvature.

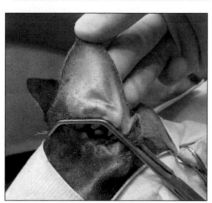

2 The pinna is then amputated: preserving at least 2–3 mm of loose skin distal to the clamp on the dorsal part of the ear to allow suturing over the exposed cartilage. Once the clamp has been positioned close to the base of the ear, providing a curved 'stub' to the base of the ear, divide the pinna sharply, directly alongside the upper edge of the clamp, using a scalpel or curved scissors. The clamp is then left in place for a few minutes for haemostasis before it is removed prior to suturing the wound. The amputated pinna can be submitted for histopathology if required and/or used as a template for pinnectomy for the contralateral side (see later).

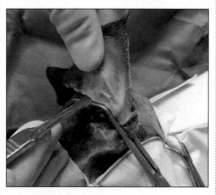

3 After a few minutes, the clamp is removed and suturing commences, taking care to pull the thicker, haired loose skin of the dorsal (outside) pinna over the cut edge of the exposed auricular cartilage to suture it to the thinner skin of the inner pinna. This inner skin is more closely attached to the underlying cartilage and sutures should take a small bite of cartilage as well, to anchor the skin securely.

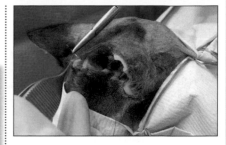

4 A continuous suture of the absorbable suture material can be used for closure, as shown here. Alternatively, the surgeon may prefer to place non-absorbable sutures in any pattern that achieves adequate skin closure with coverage of the cut edge of the cartilage.

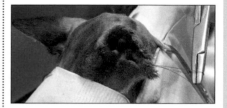

5 The amputated pinna from the first ear is used as a template for the second side; it is laid back-to-back on the outside of the second ear as shown, guiding placement of the atraumatic clamp. Amputation of the second pinna proceeds in an identical way to the first.

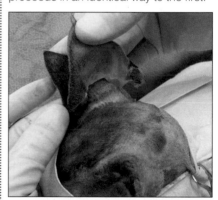

6 An Elizabethan collar should be placed postoperatively to avoid premature suture removal or excessive bleeding due to self-trauma. The cat may need to be sedated or anaesthetized for suture removal. The cosmetic appearance of bilateral pinnectomy is usually very acceptable.

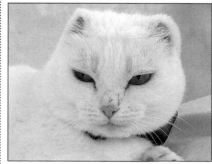

Appearance of a different cat several weeks after bilateral pinnectomy. (Courtesy of Dr S Kuan)

Appendix

Suture patterns

Geraldine Hunt

In the images shown, red lines indicate the line of the surgical incision, and yellow lines indicate where the needle and suture material pass through the tissue.

Single interrupted suture

Placement of a single interrupted suture

A single interrupted suture is placed as shown, before being tied with a square knot (see below).

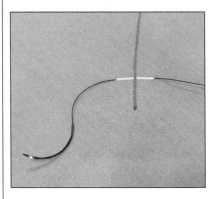

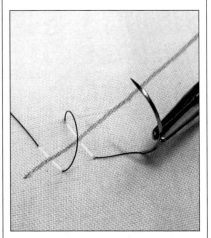

Tying off a suture using a square knot

1 The long end of the suture is wrapped twice around the needle-holders, before grasping the short end.

2 The short end is pulled to the opposite side.

3 The long end is wrapped once around the needle-holders before grasping the short end.

4 The short end is pulled to the opposite side to complete the first square knot. The knot is then tightened. At least two square knots are required to secure a single interrupted suture.

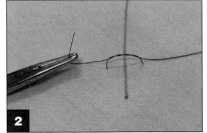

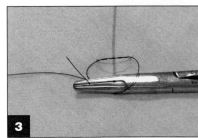

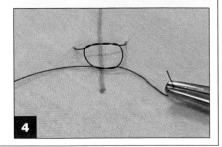

Cruciate suture

The needle is passed through the tissues as indicated by the yellow lines. The two sides of the suture should be spaced evenly.

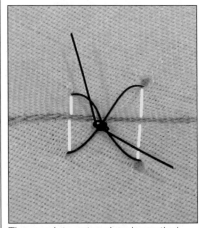

The cruciate suture has been tied using two square knots, as described above.

Simple continuous suture

Placement of a simple continuous suture

The continuous suture is started with a single interrupted suture and square knot, but the arm of the suture attached to the needle is left intact (i.e. not cut).

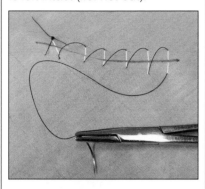

Tying off a simple continuous suture

After the last pass from one side of the wound to the other, the needle is returned through the near side to create a loop in the suture material (star). The long end (arrow) is then tied to the loop using two square knots, as described above.

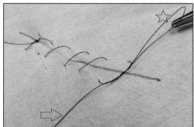

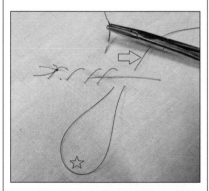

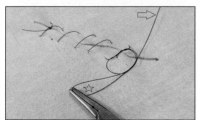

Completing the first square knot.

Cushing suture

A Cushing suture is a continuous suture where the tissue bites are taken parallel to the wound edge (yellow lines), rather than across it (as seen earlier with the simple continuous suture). The Cushing suture is started and completed in a similar manner as the simple continuous suture.

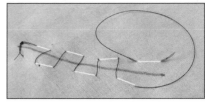

Horizontal mattress suture

A horizontal mattress suture is placed as shown and tied with a square knot (see above).

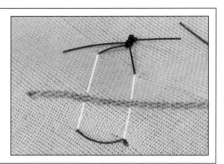

Subcuticular suture

The subcuticular suture is commenced using a buried knot; the suture material is passed from deep to superficial, leaving the free end in the deep tissues (A). The suture then crosses the wound and is passed from superficial to deep, so that the needle end (B) is coming out from the deep tissues. A and B are tied using a square knot to create the buried knot. A continuous suture pattern is then performed, as described above.

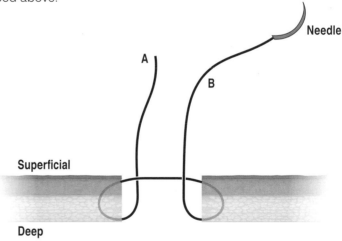

The subcuticular suture is completed using another buried knot. The suture is passed from superficial to deep, then turned on itself and passed from deep to superficial to form a deep loop (A). The suture is then passed to the other side of the incision and passes from superficial to deep, so that the needle end is now coming from deep within the wound (B). A and B are tied using a square knot so that the knot is buried.

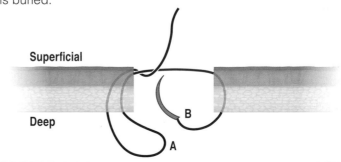

Index